# ANEMIA

Edited by **Donald S. Silverberg**

**Anemia**
Edited by Donald S. Silverberg

**Published by InTech**
Janeza Trdine 9, 51000 Rijeka, Croatia



**Publishing Process Manager** Silvia Vlase

**Technical Editor** Teodora Smiljanic

**Cover Designer** InTech Design Team

Additional hard copies can be obtained from orders@intechopen.com

Anemia, Edited by Donald S. Silverberg
p. cm.
ISBN 978-953-51-0138-3

# Meet the editor

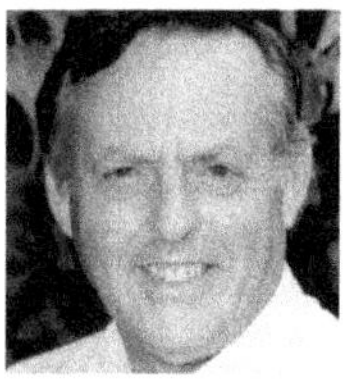

Dr. Donald S. Silverberg graduated from the Medical School University of Manitoba in 1962, and has completed his residency training in internal medicine and nephrology at the Mayo Clinic Rochester, Minnesota (1962-1966) and at the University of Lund, Sweden (1966-1967). He has been living in Israel and practicing nephrology since 1976, and currently works at the Tel Aviv Medical Center. During his scientific career, Dr. Silverberg has authored over 160 articles in peer-reviewed journals and has been on the editorial board of the Journal of Human Hypertension. At present he is on the editorial board of the Journal of Nephrology. Dr. Silverberg's research interests include: IV iron and Erythropoietin in the anemia of hemodialysis, peritoneal dialysis, chronic renal failure, congestive heart failure and COPD, sleep apnea and hypertension.

# Contents

# Preface

This book provides an update on a variety of aspects of anemia. It begins with a review of the impact of anemia on morbidity and mortality (1). It then examines the various mechanisms involved in the production of anemia including the role of programmed cell death (2), membrane shedding from RBCs as a mechanism of membrane modulation and damage control (3) the role of oxidative stress (4) and the various other mechanisms involved in the production of anemia in chronic disease including inflammation, nitric oxide, and iron deficiency (5). A recent example of the anemia of chronic disease is the anemia associated with Chronic Obstructive Lung Disease and this is then reviewed (6 ).

The next major subject is a discussion of the diagnostic evaluation of anemia including the differential diagnosis (7). The extremely common and important subject of the role of nutrition in anemia is then discussed which begins with an overview of the role of nutrition in production of anemia (8) and then examines in more detail the role of nutritional anemia in developing countries (9-13) including risk factors in children (11), prevention and control (9-13). Two examples are given about attempts to control iron deficiency anemia in developing countries (12,13). The role of nutrition in the anemia of cancer patients is then reviewed (14). The next subject is a review of all aspects of the anemia of pregnancy (15). This is followed by a review of the clinical management of haemolytic disease of the fetus and newborn (16).

Two common causes of anemia due to infection are then discussed – trypanosomiasis (17,18), and malaria (19,20). This is followed by an update of the mechanisms and treatment of two genetic diseases, sickle cell anemia (21) and thalassemia (22). The anemia of Paroxysmal Nocturnal Hemoglobinuria is then discussed (23). This is followed by a review of Fanconi anemia and leukemia (24). Finally the role of toxin-induced anemia is examined in one paper examining aluminium toxicity (25) and another the hemolysis and anemia induced by dapsone hydroxylamine (26).

This book thus provides a wealth of up to date and useful information for all those interested in various aspects of anemia.

**Dr. Donald S. Silverberg**
Tel-Aviv Medical Center
Israel

# 1

# Morbidity and Mortality in Anemia

Fawzia Ahmed Habib, Intessar Sultan and Shaista Salman
*Taibah University-College of Medicine-Al Madinah Al Munawara*
*Kingdom of Saudi Arabia*

## 1. Introduction

A growing body of research suggests that anemia is independently associated with morbidity and mortality in the general population as well as in patients with chronic diseases where the prevalence of anemia is high (1-4). Anemia prognosis depends on the underlying cause of the anemia. However, the severity of the anemia, its etiology, and the rapidity with which it develops can each play a significant role in the prognosis. Similarly, the age of the patient and the existence of other co-morbid conditions influence outcome. Higher mortality rates are almost always observed in patients with anemia. Many studies (5-11) identified anemia as an independent factor impacting mortality and provided the evidence that management of anemia, independent of other risk factors, improves mortality rates. In one study (3), independent of the underlying disease, anemia was associated with increased mortality in chronic kidney disease, congestive heart failure and acute myocardial infarction patients; increased morbidity in chronic kidney disease, congestive heart failure and cancer radiotherapy patients; and decreased quality of life in chronic kidney disease and cancer patients. In addition to its impact upon mortality, anemia also significantly influences morbidity. Multiple studies support this assertion especially in patients with chronic kidney disease and heart failure (12-17).

## 2. Morbidity and mortality among patients with certain types of anemia

### 2.1 Aplastic anemia

In the early 1930s aplastic anemia was considered almost inevitably fatal. However, the morbidity and mortality of this disease have decreased dramatically since the introduction of bone marrow transplantation and immunosuppressive therapy. Survival figures in aplastic anemia from several studies have shown biphasic curves, with the highest mortality rates within the first 6 months after diagnosis. Five-year survival rates have been described to range from 70% to 90% and to be similar among patients treated with either bone marrow transplantation or immunosuppression (18). Patients who undergo bone marrow transplantation have additional issues related to toxicity from the conditioning regimen and graft versus host disease (19). With immunosuppression, approximately one third of patients does not respond. For the responders, relapse and late-onset clonal disease, such as paroxysmal nocturnal hemoglobinuria, myelodysplastic syndrome, and leukemia, are risks (20). In one retrospective institutional analysis, predictors for response to immmunosuppresion at 6 months were younger age, higher baseline absolute reticulocyte, lymphocyte, and neutrophil counts with the five-year survivals ranging from 92 in the responders to 53% in the non responders (21). Two factors determines the clinical outcome in aplastic anemia, the severity of the pancytopenia and patient age. In a retrospective review from the European Group for Blood and Marrow Transplantation (EBMT), the relative risk for a poor outcome following immunosuppressive treatment was 3.4 for patients with very severe anemia and 1.5 in those with severe anemia compared with less severe cases. In the EBMT, the 5-year survival rate varied inversely and significantly with age. Also, at any degree of severity, the outcome was worse in older patients. The increase in mortality in the older patients was mainly due to infection or bleeding. Most infections were acquired from endogenous microbial flora of the skin and gastrointestinal tract (22).

### 2.2 Vitamin B12 deficiency anemia

Pernicious anemia is associated with a two- to threefold excess risk of intestinal-type gastric cancer but, the actual degree of risk varies with the duration of disease and geographic location. Pernicious anemia is also associated with an increased risk of gastric carcinoid tumors, presumably due to prolonged achlorhydria with compensatory hypergastrinemia, and argyrophilic cell hyperplasia. There is also a suggested excess of oesophageal cancer among these patients (23). In the analysis of the Oxford Vegetarian Study (24), low vitamin B12 intake could explain the increased death rate (2.2 times) from mental and neurological diseases among vegetarians compared to non-vegetarians. Specific neurologic problems associated with vitamin B12 deficiency consist of subacute combined degeneration of the dorsal (posterior) and lateral spinal columns, axonal degeneration of peripheral nerves and central nervous system symptoms including memory loss, irritability, and dementia (25).

In some cases, B12-deficient dementia may be misdiagnosed as Alzheimer's disease (26). The cognitive decline in older subjects associated with subclinical vitamin B12 deficiency is difficult to explain but a role for increased homocysteine level is possible. People with Alzheimer's disease were found to have elevated homocysteine, reduced B12, or reduced folate levels (27). On the other hand studies found elevated homocysteine to be associated with risk of Alzheimer's disease (26). Selhub et al. (27) analyzed data from 8,083 people, including whites, blacks, and Hispanics. They found that elevated homocysteine levels (> 11.4 µmol/l for men, > 10.4 µmol/l for women) were associated with B12 levels less than 338 pg/ml. A level of 430 pg/ml provides a safety factor for homocysteine and other potential problems. Elevated homocysteine is associated with increased mortality, with an increased risk of 33% per 5 µmol/l increase in homocysteine (28,29) with increased risk for coronary artery, cerebrovascular, and peripheral vascular diseases and venous thrombosis (30). A 2008 meta-analysis of vitamin supplementation and cognitive function found little benefit to people already diagnosed with dementia, but did improve cognition in elderly people with elevated homocysteine but who were not diagnosed with dementia (31). Another 2008 study found that vitamin supplementation did not slow cognitive decline in people with mild to moderate Alzheimer's disease (32).

Vitamin B12 deficiency appears to be associated with an increased risk of osteoporosis (33,34), and hip and spine fractures (35), possibly due to suppression of osteoblast activity (36,37). Even subtle degrees of B12 deficiency may be associated with bone loss (38), although this has not been shown in all studies (39). Supplementation with vitamin B12 and folate has been shown to reduce hip fractures in a group of elderly Japanese patients with residual hemiplegia after an ischemic stroke. However, there is insufficient data to recommend this therapeutic approach in other populations at high risk for fracture.

### 2.3 Folic acid deficiency anemia

Studies found that both maternal plasma folate and vitamin B12 are independent risk factors for neural tube defects (40). In a literature review, Ray et al examined 8 studies that demonstrated that folate deficiency was a risk factor for placental abruption/infarction (41). Several observational and controlled trials have shown that neural tube defects can be reduced by 80% or more when folic acid supplementation is started before conception (42). In countries like the United States and Canada, the policy of widespread fortification of flour with folic acid has proved effective in reducing the number of neural tube defects (43). Although the exact mechanism is not understood, a relative folate shortage may exacerbate an underlying genetic predisposition to neural tube defects. Diminished folate status is associated with enhanced carcinogenesis. A number of epidemiologic and case-control studies have shown that folic acid intake is inversely related to colon cancer risk (44). With regard to the underlying mechanism, Blount et al showed that folate deficiency can cause a massive incorporation of uracil into human DNA leading to chromosome breaks (45). Another study by Kim et al suggested that folate deficiency induces DNA strand breaks and hypomethylation within the *p53* gene (46). Low folate and high homocysteine levels are a risk factor for cognitive decline in high-functioning older adults (47) and high homocysteine level is an independent predictor of cognitive impairment among long-term stay geriatric patients (48). Despite the association of high homocysteine level and poor cognitive function, homocysteine-lowering therapy using supplementation with vitamins B-12 and B-6 was not associated with improved cognitive performance after two years in a double-blind, randomized trial in healthy older adults with elevated homocysteine levels (49).

### 2.4 Thalassemia

Iron excess in patients with thalassemia is associated with early death if untreated. Several publications provide evidence that the heart is unquestionably the most critical organ affected by iron jeopardizing survival of thalassemia patients. In a study of 97 thalassemia patients (50), 36% of patients between the ages of 15 and 18 showed detectable cardiac iron, the risk of cardiac disease increases as patient's age increases. For the full cohort, the estimated survival without cardiac disease was 80% after 5 years of chelation therapy, 65% after 10 years and only 55% after 15 years. At the New York Academy of Sciences, Seventh Symposium on Thalassemia (51), the causes of death reported in 240 thalassemia major patients in Italy born between 1960-1984 were cardiac disease (71%), infections (12%), liver (6%) and other causes (11%). Another review of information available to the Cooley's Anemia Foundation shows that 11% of its 724 registered patients (77 total) died over the time period January 1999 - July 31, 2008. The data demonstrate that heart disease in these young patients remains the leading cause by far.

Since 1999, there has been a marked improvement in survival in thalassaemia major in the UK (52), similar change with improved survival has been reported from Italy (53,54) and Cyprus (55). This improvement has been mainly driven by a reduction in deaths due to cardiac iron overload. The most likely causes for this include the introduction of T2* cardiac magnetic resonance imaging technique to quantify myocardial iron overload and appropriate intensification of iron chelation treatment, alongside other improvements in clinical care. With a reduction in deaths from iron overload, infection may become a leading cause of death in thalassaemia in the future. Splenectomy increases risk of infection with Pneumococcus and Haemophilus influenzae and deferoxamine therapy increases risk of infection with Yersinia enterocolitica, and there have been at least 3 deaths from these infections. However, the most frequently isolated organism was Klebsiella. An increased risk of Klebsiella infection in thalassaemia has previously been reported from South East Asia (56,57), and some forms of Klebsiella can use deferoxamine as an iron source (58), but it remains to be clarified whether Klebsiella infection is related to iron chelation therapy. Hepatocarcinoma is also a growing problem for hepatitis C positive patients, and improved antiviral treatments are needed. Fortunately, transmission of hepatitis C by blood transfusion is now very rare, so this risk may be limited to older patients (52).

### 2.5 Sickle cell anemia

The greatest burden of sickle cell anemia (SCA) is in sub-Saharan Africa (SSA), and estimates suggest that 50–80% of these patients will die before adulthood (59). Identification of risk factors has led to improved survival through targeted interventions. In the West, reported risk factors for death include infections, low hemoglobin and fetal hemoglobin (HbF), high white blood cell count and hemolysis (60-62). Comprehensive care includes prompt treatment of acute events and prophylaxis against infections, mainly with oral penicillin and vaccination against *Streptococcus pneumoniae.* Countries that have introduced these interventions have achieved significant reductions in mortality; with up to 94% surviving to 18 years in the USA (63) and 99% to 20 years in the UK (64). In most African countries, the lack of an evidence-base has led to inertia in terms of implementation of these interventions, such as penicillin prophylaxis. In Africa, available mortality data are sporadic and incomplete. Many children are not diagnosed, especially in rural areas, and death is often attributed to malaria or other comorbid conditions (65). The mortality rates in SCA amongst a hospital-based cohort in Tanzania (66) was 1.9 per 100 PYO which is similar to 3 per 100 PYO reported from the USA before use of penicillin prophylaxis (67), with the highest incidence of death was in the first 5 years of life. Evidence from previous research suggests that infection is the most likely cause of death in this period, with the proportion of deaths from infection reported to be 50% in the USA (60, 68), 28% in Jamaica (69) and 20% in Dallas (63). The prevention of pneumococcal infection with penicillin and the introduction of pneumococcal conjugate vaccine has been shown to be effective in reducing mortality (70) with improved survival rates of 84% in Jamaica (69), 86% by 18 years in Dallas (64) and 99% in London (65). One review reported 42% reduction in mortality in SCA in USA, 0 to 3 years old, between two eras, 1995–1998 and 1999–2002 (71). There is compelling justification for implementation of these interventions in Africa to prevent deaths due to infections (65,66).

Sudden death is not uncommon among SCA patients. A retrospective/prospective review of 21 autopsy cases from sickle cell patients who died suddenly between 1990 and 2004 demonstrated higher-than-expected percentages of acute and chronic sickle cell-related lung injury such as fat embolism (33.3%) and pulmonary hypertension (33.3%), with right ventricular hypertrophy (33.3%) (72). In Sickle cell trait (SCT) under unusual circumstances serious morbidity or mortality can result from complications related to polymerization of deoxy-hemoglobin S. Although rare, sudden death is the most serious complication of sickle cell trait. SCT has a substantially increased age-dependent risk of exercise-related sudden death as in military basic training and civilian organized sports. A retrospective review of all soldiers in basic training found that those with SCT had a 40-fold increased risk of sudden exertional death (73). Sudden death may occur in susceptible persons when poor physical conditioning, dehydration, heat stresses or hypoxic states precipitate sickling of the abnormal erythrocytes. Most of the death mechanisms are related to the biological consequences of diffuse microvascular occlusion due to sickling, although a significant number of such sudden deaths remain unexplained after thorough autopsy. Rare mechanisms encountered include acute splenic sequestration (74). Other problems may also be encountered in SCT patients including increased urinary tract infection in women, gross hematuria, complications of hyphema, splenic infarction with altitude hypoxia or exercise and life-threatening complications of exertional heat illness (exertional rhabdomyolysis, heat stroke, or renal failure). In addition, some disease associations have been noted with sickle cell trait which might not result from polymerization of hemoglobin S but from linkage to a different gene mutation. There is an association with renal medullary carcinoma, early end stage renal failure in autosomal dominant polycystic kidney disease, and surrogate end points for pulmonary embolism (75).

### 2.6 Paroxysmal nocturnal hemoglobinuria

Most patients with paroxysmal nocturnal hemoglobinuria (PNH) die from venous thrombotic events. Stroke is a common cause of morbidity and mortality in PNH and it is almost exclusively a result of cerebral venous thrombosis. Case reports of ischemic stroke complicating PNH have implicated a similar propensity for arterial events caused by the disease. PNH is a rare cause of arterial stroke with reported 9 cases but it should be considered in young stroke patients with abnormal blood findings (76).

## 3. Morbidity and mortality of anemia in high risk groups

### 3.1 Effect of anemia on maternal mortality and morbidity

Maternal anemia is a ubiquitous pregnancy complication, and has been associated with an array of adverse perinatal and reproductive outcomes. It is estimated that 20% of maternal deaths in Africa can be attributed to anemia. In combination with obstetric hemorrhage, anemia is estimated to be responsible for 17-46% of cases of maternal death (77). A review of symptoms associated with maternal deaths in Bangladesh led researchers to conclude that anemia had played a secondary role in nearly all cases (78). Estimates of maternal mortality resulting from anemia range from 34/100,000 live births in Nigeria to as high as 194/100,000 in Pakistan (79). The risk of death is greatly increased with severe anemia. There is little evidence of increased risk associated with mild or moderate anemia. Viteri (80) reported that anemic pregnant women are at greater risk of death during the perinatal period and that anemia is the major contributory or sole cause of death in 20-40% of the 500 000 maternal deaths/year. A study from Indonesia illustrated the much higher risk of maternal death in anemic women from rural areas than from urban areas, possibly as a result of problems with timely access to obstetric care (81). On the basis of the evidence available, it seems reasonable to assume that the risk of maternal mortality is greatly increased with severe anemia. The data available only confirm an associative—not a causal—relationship. Nevertheless, the strength of this relationship makes it appropriate to presume that it is causal. It must also be noted that there are currently no agreed international standards or sets of criteria for attributing death to anemia (82). Except in South Asia and Papua New Guinea, the reported rates of severe anemia do not appear to exceed 10% of pregnant women (79). In a large Indonesian study, the maternal mortality rate for women with a

hemoglobin concentration <100 g/L was 70.0/10000 deliveries compared with 19.7/10000 deliveries for non-anemic women (81). However, the authors believed that the relation of maternal mortality with anemia reflected a greater extent of hemorrhage and late arrival at admission rather than the effect of a prenatal anemic condition. In another study, approximately one-third of the anemic women had megaloblastic anemia due to folic acid deficiency and two-thirds had hookworm. The cutoff for anemia was extremely low (<65 g hemoglobin/L), and the authors stated that although anemia may have contributed to mortality, it was not the sole cause of death in many of the women (83). It has been suggested that maternal deaths in the puerperium may be related to a poor ability to withstand the adverse effects of excessive blood loss, an increased risk of infection, and maternal fatigue; however, these potential causes of mortality have not been evaluated systematically (84).
Maternal morbidity resulting from anemia includes diminished work capacity and physical performance have been reported as a result mostly of iron deficiency anemia. Anemia leads to abnormalities in host defense and neurological dysfunction. Increased risks of premature labor and low birth weight have also been reported in association with anemia in pregnancy (80).

### 3.2 Effect of anemia on infant mortality and morbidity

There is substantial evidence that maternal iron deficiency anemia increases the risk of preterm delivery and subsequent low birth weight, and accumulating information suggests an association between maternal iron status in pregnancy and the iron status of infants postpartum. Preterm infants are likely to have more perinatal complications, to be growth-stunted, and to have low stores of iron and other nutrients. Lower birth weights in anemic women have been reported in several studies (85-87). In one study, the odds for low birth weight were increased across the range of anemia, increasing with lower hemoglobin in an approximately dose-related manner (88). Welsh women who were first diagnosed with anemia (hemoglobin <104 g/L) at 13–24 wk of gestation had a 1.18–1.75-fold higher relative risk of preterm birth, low birth weight, and prenatal mortality (89). After controlling for many other variables in a large Californian study, Klebanoff et al., (90) showed a doubled risk of preterm delivery with anemia during the second trimester but not during the third trimester. In Alabama, low hematocrit concentrations in the first half of pregnancy but higher hematocrit concentrations in the third trimester were associated with a significantly increased risk of preterm delivery (91). When numerous potentially confounding factors were taken into consideration, analysis of data from low-income, predominantly young black women in the United States showed a risk of premature delivery (<37 wk) and subsequently of having a low-birth-weight infant that was 3 times higher in mothers with iron deficiency anemia on entry to care (92). Similar relations were observed in women from rural Nepal, in whom anemia with iron deficiency in the first or second trimester was associated with a 1.87-fold higher risk of preterm birth, but anemia alone was not (88). In an analysis of 3728 deliveries in Singapore, 571 women who were anemic at the time of delivery had a higher incidence of preterm delivery than did those who were not anemic (93). An association between maternal anemia and lower infant Apgar scores was reported in some studies. In 102 Indian women in the first stage of labor, higher maternal hemoglobin concentrations were correlated with better Apgar scores and with a lower risk of birth asphyxia (94). In the Jamaican Perinatal Mortality Survey of >10000 infants in 1986, there was an ≈50% greater chance of mortality in the first year of life for those infants whose mothers had not been given iron supplements during pregnancy (95). Trials that included large numbers of iron-deficient women showed that iron supplementation improved birth weight (86,96) and Apgar scores (97). In rural populations in China antenatal supplementation with iron-folic acid was associated with longer gestation and a reduction in early neonatal mortality compared with folic acid. Multiple micronutrients were associated with modestly increased birth weight compared with folic acid, but, despite this weight gain, there was no significant reduction in early neonatal mortality (98).

### 3.3 Effect of anemia on children and adolescents mortality and morbidity

Apart from previously mentioned morbidity and mortality from hereditary anemia among children, by far the most common cause of anemia in this age group is chronic iron deficiency anemia (IDA). There is reasonably good evidence that mental and motor developmental test scores are lower among infants with IDA. Although some aspects of cognitive function seem to change with iron therapy, lower developmental IQ and achievement test scores have still been noted after treatment. A variety of non-cognitive alterations during infant developmental testing has also been observed, including failure to respond to test stimuli, short attention span, unhappiness, increased fearfulness, withdrawal from the examiner, and increased body tension. Exploratory analyses suggest that such behavioral abnormalities may account for poor developmental test performance in infants with IDA. There has been a steady accumulation of evidence that IDA limits maximal physical performance, sub-maximal endurance, and spontaneous activity in the adult, resulting in diminished work productivity with attendant economic losses. However, it is important to consider that studies that attempt to separate indicators of malnutrition, such as iron deficiency, from other types of environmental deprivation may be inappropriately separating factors that occur together naturally and that therefore cannot be differentiated (99). The behavioral effects of IDA may be due to changes in neurotransmission. In a recent review that focuses on human studies, short- and long-term alterations associated with iron deficiency in infancy can be related to major dopamine pathways (100). It is widely accepted that long-term consequences of iron deficiency are often irreversible. Several studies have found that reversal of the anemia did not improve standardized test scores (101,102). One study (103) examined a group of Costa Rican children at five years of age. Children who had moderately severe IDA (hemoglobin less than 10 g per dL [100 g per L]) in infancy scored significantly lower on standardized tests at five years of age, despite a return to normal hematologic status and growth.

However, there is accumulating evidence for the potential benefits of preventing iron deficiency in infancy and treating it before it becomes chronic or severe. A recent study (104) of the preschool-aged Chinese children found that children who had chronic IDA in infancy displayed less positive social and emotional development. In contrast, the behavior and affect of children whose anemia was corrected before the age of 24 months were comparable to those of children who were non-anemic throughout infancy. The persistence of poorer cognitive, motor, affective, and sensory system functioning during childhood highlights the need to prevent iron deficiency in infancy and to find interventions that lessen the long-term effects of this widespread nutrient disorder.

Iron deficiency is also implicated in such neurologic sequelae as irritability, lethargy, headaches, and infrequently papilledema, pseudotumor cerebri, and cranial nerve abnormalities. Although only a few cases (30 cases) in the literature support the association between IDA and increased intracranial tension, it may be more common than previously thought. The underlying mechanisms remain unknown, but cerebral venous thrombosis should be carefully excluded (105). Rarely has iron deficiency been recognized as a significant cause of stroke in the adult or pediatric populations (106,107). One case series reported 6 children, 6 to 18 months of age, who presented with an ischemic stroke or venous thrombosis after a viral prodrome. All patients had iron deficiency as a consistent finding among the group, and other known etiologies of childhood stroke were excluded (108)

### 3.4 Effect of anemia on mortality and morbidity in elderly people

In the past decade, anemia has been associated with a number of negative outcomes in elderly people. In a report from the Netherlands, community-dwelling subjects older than 85 years with anemia had higher 5-year mortality rates than subjects with normal hemoglobin levels (109,110). In a cohort of older women with mild-to-moderate physical disability, Chaves et al noted an increase in mortality associated with hemoglobin levels less than 110 g/L (111). In a study of 1744 community-dwelling persons aged 71 years or older, anemia is independently associated with increased mortality over 8 years for both races and sex. Anemia also is a risk factor for functional and cognitive decrease (1).

In an analysis of 5888 community-dwelling older adults enrolled in the Cardiovascular Health Study (2), anemia was associated with increased risk for hospitalization and mortality in older adults. In another community-based study of more than 17 000 older adults more than 66 years (4), anemia was significantly associated with risk for all-cause hospitalization, hospitalization secondary to cardiovascular disease, and all-cause mortality. In both studies, the association between hemoglobin and mortality was not linear; with the risk for death increased at both extremes of hemoglobin. As this risk occurs at hemoglobin levels that are currently considered normal, consideration should be given to refining the current definition of anemia in older adults to reflect this continuum of risk (2, 4).

Not only anemia in elderly is a strong predictor of death, it has also been associated with various conditions such as decreased physical performance, disability in daily living, mobility disabilities, cognitive impairment, depression, falls and fractures, frailty, admission to hospital and diminished quality of life (112-114). However in the presence of common comorbidities among elderly, anemia could be considered as a risk marker rather than a risk factor. In the Leiden 85-plus Study (115), a population-based prospective follow-up study of 562 people aged 85 years, anemia in very elderly people was found to be associated with an increased risk of death, independent of comorbidity. However, the associated functional decline appears to be attributed mainly to comorbidity.

### 3.5 Effect of anemia on mortality and morbidity in patients with cancer

Anemia is common in cancer patients, although the prevalence is influenced both by the type of malignancy and the choice of treatment. Individual studies have compared the survival of patients with and without anemia and have shown reduced survival times in patients with various malignancies associated with anemia including carcinoma of the lung, cervix, head and neck, prostate, lymphoma, and multiple myeloma. A systemic, quantitative review in 2001 (116) estimated the overall increase in risk of death with anemia to 65% (CI: 54-77%). In addition, an intriguing association has also been observed between anemia and disease progression among patients undergoing radiotherapy, particularly in those with cervical carcinoma or with squamous cell carcinoma of the head and neck. Harrison et al found that two thirds of women with cervical carcinoma are anemic at baseline, and 82% are anemic during radiotherapy (117). Correlations between anemia, tumor tissue oxygenation, local recurrence, and survival have been demonstrated in other studies (118,119). In one study including cases of head and neck cancer, 75% of patients undergoing combined chemotherapy and radiotherapy become anemic (120) and anemia has been associated with worse local regional control and survival rates (121). However, there is presently little evidence that anemia treatment per se impacts the tumor response to chemotherapy alone.

### 3.6 Effect of anemia on mortality and morbidity in patients with cardiac diseases

Substantial evidence suggests that anemia is an independent risk factor for worse outcomes in patients with heart failure (CHF) and ischemia heart disease including myocardial infarction. Anemia is a common comorbidity in CHF. Compared with nonanemic patients the presence of anemia also is associated with worse cardiac clinical status, more severe systolic and diastolic dysfunction, a higher beta natriuretic peptide level, increased extracellular and plasma volume, a more rapid deterioration of renal function, a lower quality of life, and increased medical costs (122-129).

In a systematic review and meta-analysis published in 2008, after a minimal follow-up of 6 months, 46.8% of anemic patients died compared with 29.5% of non-anemic patients irrespective to the cause of CHF. In studies that analyzed hemoglobin as a continuous variable, a 1-g/dL decrease in hemoglobin was independently associated with significantly increased mortality risk (130).

The associations between hemoglobin and outcomes was studied in 2653 patients randomized in the CHARM Program in the United States and Canada. Anemia was common in heart failure, regardless of left ventricular ejection fraction (LVEF). Lower hemoglobin was associated with higher LVEF yet was an independent predictor of adverse mortality and morbidity outcomes (131). On the contrary, a large nationally representative study of older patients in the United States hospitalized with HF demonstrated no graded relationship between lower hematocrit values and increased mortality and suggest that although anemia is an independent predictor of hospital readmission, its relationship with increased mortality in HF patients is largely explained by the severity of comorbid illness. The authors suggest that anemia may be predominantly a marker rather than a mediator of increased mortality risk in older patients with HF (132).

In heart failure, the causes of anemia and the associations between anemia and outcomes are probably multiple and complex. The anemia in CHF mainly is caused by a combination of renal failure and CHF-induced increased cytokine production, and these can both lead to reduced production of erythropoietin (EPO), resistance of the bone marrow to EPO stimulation, and to cytokine-induced iron-deficiency anemia caused by reduced intestinal absorption of iron and reduced release of iron from iron stores. The use of angiotensin-converting enzyme inhibitor and angiotensin receptor blockers also may inhibit the bone marrow response to EPO. Hemodilution caused by CHF also may cause a low hemoglobin level (129). The potential mechanisms linking anemia to increased mortality risk in CHF have not been characterized but may be related to changes in ventricular loading conditions and cardiac structure, altered neurohormonal activation, or reduced free radical scavenging capacity. It is also possible that anemia is a marker of more severe underlying myocardial disease (133).

In several controlled and uncontrolled studies, correction of the anemia with subcutaneous erythropoietin (EPO) or darbepoetin in conjunction with oral and intravenous iron has been associated with an improvement in clinical status, number of hospitalizations, cardiac and renal function, and quality of life. However, larger, randomized, double-blind, controlled studies still are needed to verify these initial observations. The effect of EPO may be related partly to its nonhematologic functions including neovascularization; prevention of apoptosis of endothelial, myocardial, cerebral, and renal cells; increase in endothelial progenitor cells; and anti-inflammatory and antioxidant effects (129).

In ischemic heart disease, both advanced age and the presence of flow-limiting coronary stenosis markedly impaired cardiac compensatory response to anemia, even without concomitant acute myocardial injury. These conditions, among other limits to the patients' physiologic reserve, may explain why levels of hemoglobin tolerated by younger individuals would not be tolerated by the elderly. They may also explain why elderly patients with acute myocardial infarction represent a group at extremely high risk for death, despite infarct sizes similar to those of younger patients (3).

The clinical utility of blood transfusion in anemic cardiovascular disease populations is controversial. According to the guidelines from the American College of Physicians and the American Society of Anesthesiology, the "transfusion threshold" for patients without known risk factors for cardiac disease is a hemoglobin level in the range of 6 to 8 g/dL. In one study, patients hospitalized with acute myocardial infarction, blood transfusion was associated with a significantly lower 30-day mortality rate among patients with a hematocrit <30% on admission (134). But in 838 critically ill patients (26% with cardiovascular disease), maintaining hemoglobin at 10 to 12 g/dL did not provide additional benefits on 30-day mortality compared with maintaining hemoglobin at 7 to 9 g/dL (135). Blood transfusion may be associated with other adverse effects including immunosuppression with increased risk of infection, sensitization to HLA antigens, and iron overload. Given this profile of risks and benefits, transfusion may be considered as an acute treatment for severe anemia on an individualized basis but does not appear to be a viable therapeutic strategy for the long-term management of chronic anemia in CHF (135,136).

Pilot studies have found that in a large number of HF patients it's safe to raise hemoglobin with erythropoietin-stimulating therapies and there is a suggestion that raising hemoglobin in anemic HF patients may lead to improved outcomes (136). A prospective, randomized trial studied the treatment of anemia in patients with moderate-to-severe CHF (NYHA class III to IV) whose left ventricular ejection fraction was less than 40% of normal. Patients who received treatment had a 42.1% improvement in NYHA class, compared with the control cohort who had a decrease of 11.4%. Number of hospital days, need for diuretic therapy, and renal function impairment were all significantly greater in the control group than in the treated group (137).

The Study of Anemia in Heart Failure Trial (STAMINA-HeFT) is a large multicenter, randomized, double-blind, placebo-controlled trial. In this study treatment of anemia with erythropoiesis-stimulating agents (ESAs) (darbepoetin alfa) was not associated with significant clinical benefits. But in the post hoc analysis of outcomes among the treated group, an increase of 1.0 g/dL or more in hemoglobin is required to achieve benefit in reduction of all-cause mortality or heart failure-related hospitalization (138). However, further observational and experimental studies are needed to help identify optimal treatment algorithms for both ESAs and iron that maximize clinical benefit while minimizing adverse outcomes. A pragmatic approach to the care of patients with HF needs definitive anemia treatment goals that are dynamic and disease specific, rather than those that adopt a more simplistic hemoglobin-specific approach.

### 3.7 Effect of anemia on mortality and morbidity in patients with end stage renal diseases

Anemia is associated with higher mortality rates and possibly heart disease in patients with kidney disease. However, the available evidence is limited as concluded in a systematic literature review published in 2006 (139). In a retrospective review (140) of nearly 20 000 of patients undergoing maintenance hemodialysis, hemoglobin levels of 8.0 g/dL or less were associated with a 2-fold increase in odds of death when compared with hemoglobin levels ranging between 10.0 and 11.0 g/dL. A similar study (141) of nearly 100 000 hemodialysis patients confirmed that a hematocrit higher than 30% was associated with a lower mortality. Compared with patients with a hematocrit higher than 30%, the overall relative risk of death was between 33% and 51% higher for the group with a hematocrit less than 27%, and between 12% and 20% higher for the group with a hematocrit of 27% to 30%, with and without adjustments for severity of disease. Subsequent analyses have determined that hematocrit levels maintained between 33% and 36% were associated with the lowest risk of death (142). Another study showed that in patients undergoing maintenance hemodialysis, the risk of hospitalization declines with hematocrit improvement, with a 16% to 22% lower hospitalization rate for patients with hematocrit values between 36% and 39% compared with patients with hematocrits between 33% and 36% (12). Also, prospective clinical trials of patients with end-stage renal disease have demonstrated a relationship among hematocrit, left ventricular dilatation, and left ventricular hypertrophy (LVH) (13-17,143).

The optimal management of anemia in patients with end-stage renal disease is controversial. Appropriate use of ESAs and intravenous iron can effectively manage the anemia of chronic kidney disease and end-stage renal disease (ESRD) (144-146), several randomized trials have reported an increased risk of mortality and cardiovascular events in patients treated to achieve higher hematocrit levels (145-147). A large cohort of incident US hemodialysis patients found that dialysis units that treated severe anemia more aggressively with ESAs and intravenous iron had a one-year mortality rate that was 5 percent lower than in units that treated more conservatively. But the same aggressive treatment for milder anemia brought a 10 percent increase in the rate of mortality (147).

### 3.8 Effect of anemia on mortality and morbidity in patients with end stage renal diseases and heart failure

Anemia also may play a role in increasing cardiovascular morbidity in chronic kidney insufficiency, diabetes, renal transplantation, asymptomatic left ventricular dysfunction, left ventricular hypertrophy, acute coronary syndromes including myocardial infarction and chronic coronary heart disease, and in cardiac surgery. Renal failure, cardiac failure, and anemia therefore all interact to cause or worsen each other--the so-called cardio-renal-anemia syndrome (129). The reciprocal relationships among these 3 components of cardiorenal anemia have been the subject of a number of trials with inconsistent and sometimes paradoxic results (148). Cardiovascular disease (CVD) is a significant complication in chronic kidney disease (CKD) and a major cause of death in dialysis patients. Clinical studies have shown that anemia is associated with reduced survival in patients with renal disease, heart failure or both. Low haemoglobin (Hb) has been identified as an independent risk factor for LV growth in CKD patients, suggesting that there is a direct link between anemia and adverse cardiac outcomes. This suggests that correction of anemia may improve prognosis. In patients with chronic kidney disease and CHF, treatment of anemia improves many of the abnormalities seen in CHF: it reduces LVH (149-151);

prevents left ventricular dilatation (152); and increases left ventricular ejection fraction, (153-154), stroke volume, and cardiac output (153).

The evidence for an association between anemia and an increased risk of adverse cardiovascular outcomes in patients with CKD is strong. The relationship between anemia and adverse outcomes is complex. While it is likely to be indirect to some extent, evidence also suggests that there may be a causal link between low hemoglobin levels and the development of CVD. Treatment of anemia with epoetin has been shown to improve cardiac function and to produce regression of LVH in CKD patients, whether or not they are receiving dialysis. Furthermore, consistent treatment with epoetin before the initiation of dialysis is associated with a reduced risk of developing cardiac disease in patients with CKD. Normalizing Hb levels in patients with advanced CVD has a limited effect on changes in LV geometry, however, and - at least under certain circumstances -may increase their risk of death. The degree of CVD could affect other factors, such as vascular reactivity, which may determine whether partial or full correction of anemia is appropriate for a particular individual (154).

## 4. References


[1] Denny SD, Kuchibhatla MN, Cohen HJ. Impact of anemia on mortality, cognition, and function in community-dwelling elderly. Am J Med.2006;119(4):327-334.

[2] Zakai NA, Katz R, Hirsch C, et al. A prospective study of anemia status, hemoglobin concentration, and mortality in an elderly cohort: the Cardiovascular Health Study. Arch Intern Med. 2005;165(19):2214-2220.

[3] Nissenson AR, Goodnough LT, Dubois RW. Anemia: not just an innocent bystander? Arch Intern Med. 2003;163(12):1400-1404.

[4] Culleton BF, Manns BJ, Zhang J, et al. Impact of anemia on hospitalization and mortality in older adults. Blood 2006;107(10): 3841-3846 .

[5] Ma J, Ebben J, Xia H, et al. Hematocrit levels and associated mortality in hemodialysis patients. J Am Soc Nephrol. 1999;10:610-619.

[6] Collins A, Xia H, Ebben J, et al. Change in hematocrit and risk of mortality. J Am Soc Nephrol. 1998;9(suppl A):204A.

[7] Collins AJ, Li S, St Peter W, et al. Death, hospitalization, and economic associations among incident hemodialysis patients with hematocrit values of 36 to 39%. J Am Soc Nephrol.2001;12: 2465-2473.

[8] Maeda K, Tanaka Y, Tsukano Y, et al. Multivariate analysis using a linear discriminate function for predicting the prognosis of congestive heart failure. Jpn Circ J. 1982;46:137-142.

[9] Carson JL, Duff A, Poses RM, et al. Effect of anemia and cardiovascular disease on surgical mortality and morbidity. Lancet. 1996;348:1055-1060.

[10] Hebert PC, Wells G, Sweeddale M, et al. Does transfusion practice affect mortality in critically ill patients? Am J Respir Crit Care Med. 1997;155:1618-1623.

[11] McClellan WM, Flanders WD, Langston RD, et al. Anemia and renal insufficiency are independent risk factors for death among patients with congestive heart failure admitted to community hospitals: a population-based study. J Am Soc Nephrol. 2002;13:1920-1936.

[12] Besarab A, Bolton WK, Browne JK, et al. The effects of normal as compared with low hematocrit values in patients with cardiac disease who are receiving hemodialysis and epoetin.N Engl J Med. 1998;339:584-590.

[13] Foley RN, Parfrey PS, Harnett JD, Kent GM, Murray DC, Barre PE. The impact of anemia on cardiomyopathy, morbidity, and mortality in end stage renal disease. Am J Kidney Dis.1996;28:53-61.
[14] Levin A, Thompson CR, Ethier J, et al. Left ventricular mass index increase in early renal disease: impact of decline in hemoglobin. Am J Kidney Dis. 1999;34:125-134.
[15] Levin A, Singer J, Thompson CR, Ross H, Lewis M. Prevalent left ventricular hypertrophy in the predialysis population: identifying opportunities for intervention. Am J Kidney Dis.1996;27:347-354.
[16] Silverberg JS, Rahal DP, Patton R, Sniderman AD. Role of anemia in the pathogenesis of left ventricular hypertrophy in end-stage renal disease. Am J Cardiol. 1989;64:222-224.
[17] Canella G, LaCanna G, Sandrini M, et al. Reversal of left ventricular hypertrophy following recombinant human erythropoietin treatment of anaemic dialysed uraemic patients. Nephrol Dial Transplant. 1991;6:31-37.
[18] Young, NS. Aplastic anaemia. Lancet 1995; 346:228.
[19] Kojima S, Matsuyama T, Kato S, Kigasawa H, Kobayashi R, Kikuta A, et al. Outcome of 154 patients with severe aplastic anemia who received transplants from unrelated donors: the Japan Marrow Donor Program. Blood. Aug 1 2002;100(3):799-803.
[20] Orazi A, Czader MB. Myelodysplastic syndromes. Am J Clin Pathol. Aug 2009;132(2):290-305.
[21] Scheinberg, P, Wu, CO, Nunez, O, Young, NS. Predicting response to immunosuppressive therapy and survival in severe aplastic anaemia. Br J Haematol 2009; 144:206.
[22] Tichelli, A, Socie, G, Henry-Amar, M, et al. Effectiveness of immunosuppressive therapy in older patients with aplastic anemia: A report from the European Blood and Marrow Transplant (EBMT) Severe Aplastic Anaemia Working Group. Ann Intern Med 1999; 130:193. NS.
[23] Ye W and Nyrén O. Risk of cancers of the oesophagus and stomach by histology or subsite in patients hospitalised for pernicious anaemia. Gut. 2003 July;52(7): 938–941.
[24] Appleby PN, Key TJ, Thorogood M, Burr ML, Mann J. Mortality in British vegetarians. Public Health Nutr. 2002 Feb;5(1):29-36.
[25] Green, R, Kinsella, LJ. Editorial: Current concepts in the diagnosis of cobalamin deficiency. Neurology 1995; 45:1435.
[26] Van Dam F, Van Gool WA. Hyperhomocysteinemia and Alzheimer's disease: A systematic review. Arch Gerontol Geriatr. 2009 May-Jun;48(3):425-30. Epub 2008 May 13. Review.
[27] Selhub J, Bagley LC, Miller J, Rosenberg IH. B vitamins, homocysteine, and neurocognitive function in the elderly. Am J Clin Nutr. 2000 Feb;71(2):614S-620S.
[28] Hoogeveen EK, Kostense PJ, Jakobs C, Dekker JM, Nijpels G, Heine RJ, Bouter LM, Stehouwer CD. Hyperhomocysteinemia increases risk of death, especially in type 2 diabetes: 5-year follow-up of the Hoorn Study. Circulation. 2000 Apr 4;101(13):1506-11.
[29] Vollset SE, Refsum H, Tverdal A, Nygard O, Nordrehaug JE, Tell GS, Ueland PM. Plasma total homocysteine and cardiovascular and non cardiovascular mortality: the Hordaland Homocysteine Study. Am J Clin Nutr. 2001 Jul;74(1):130-6.
[30] Humphrey LL, Fu R, Rogers K, Freeman M, Helfand M. Homocysteine level and coronary heart disease incidence: a systematic review and meta-analysis. Mayo Clin Proc. 2008 Nov;83(11):1203-12

[31] Malouf R, Grimley Evans J. Folic acid with or without vitamin B12 for the prevention and treatment of healthy elderly and demented people. Cochrane Database Syst Rev. 2008 Oct 8;(4):CD004514.
[32] Aisen PS, Schneider LS, Sano M, Diaz-Arrastia R, van Dyck CH, Weiner MF, Bottiglieri T, Jin S, Stokes KT, Thomas RG, Thal LJ; Alzheimer Disease Cooperative Study. High-dose B vitamin supplementation and cognitive decline in Alzheimer disease: a randomized controlled . JAMA. 2008 Oct 15;300(15):1774-83.
[33] Dhonukshe-Rutten, RA, Lips, M, de Jong, N, et al. Vitamin B-12 status is associated with bone mineral content and bone mineral density in frail elderly women but not in men. J Nutr 2003; 133:801.
[34] Tucker, KL, Hannan, MT, Qiao, N, et al. Low plasma vitamin B12 is associated with lower BMD: the Framingham Osteoporosis Study. J Bone Miner Res 2005; 20:152.
[35] Goerss, JB, Kim, CH, Atkinson, EJ, et al. Risk of fractures in patients with pernicious anemia. J Bone Miner Res 1992; 7:573.
[36] Carmel, R, Lau, KH, Baylink, DJ, et al. Cobalamin and osteoblast-specific proteins. N Engl J Med 1988; 319:70.
[37] Kim, GS, Kim, CH, Park, JY, et al. Effects of vitamin B12 on cell proliferation and cellular alkaline phosphatase activity in human bone marrow stromal osteoprogenitor cells and UMR106 osteoblastic cells. Metabolism 1996; 45:1443.
[38] Stone, KL, Bauer, DC, Sellmeyer, D, Cummings, SR. Low serum vitamin B-12 levels are associated with increased hip bone loss in older women: a prospective study. J Clin Endocrinol Metab 2004; 89:1217.
[39] Cagnacci, A, Baldassari, F, Rivolta, G, et al. Relation of homocysteine, folate, and vitamin B12 to bone mineral density of postmenopausal women. Bone 2003; 33:956. Kumar, N. Copper deficiency myelopathy (human swayback). Mayo Clin Proc 2006; 81:1371.
[40] Afman LA, Van Der Put NM, Thomas CM, Trijbels JM, Blom HJ. Reduced vitamin B12 binding by transcobalamin II increases the risk of neural tube defects. QJM. 2001 Mar;94(3):159-66.
[41] Ray JG, Laskin CA. Folic acid and homocyst(e)ine metabolic defects and the risk of placental abruption, pre-eclampsia and spontaneous pregnancy loss: A systematic review. Placenta. Sep 1999;20(7):519-29.
[42] Wolff T, Witkop CT, Miller T, Syed SB. Folic acid supplementation for the prevention of neural tube defects: an update of the evidence for the U.S. Preventive Services Task Force. Ann Intern Med. May 5 2009;150(9):632-9.
[43] Honein MA, Paulozzi LJ, Mathews TJ, et al. Impact of folic acid fortification of the US food supply on the occurrence of neural tube defects. JAMA. Jun 20 2001;285(23):2981-6
[44] Gatof D, Ahnen D. Primary prevention of colorectal cancer: diet and drugs. Gastroenterol Clin North Am. Jun 2002;31(2):587-623, xi..
[45] Blount BC, Mack MM, Wehr CM, et al. Folate deficiency causes uracil misincorporation into human DNA and chromosome breakage: implications for cancer and neuronal damage. Proc Natl Acad Sci U S A. Apr 1 1997;94(7):3290-5..
[46] Kim YI, Pogribny IP, Basnakian AG, et al. Folate deficiency in rats induces DNA strand breaks and hypomethylation within the p53 tumor suppressor gene. Am J Clin Nutr. Jan 1997;65(1):46-52..
[47] Kado DM, Karlamangla AS, Huang MH, Troen A, Rowe JW, Selhub J. Homocysteine versus the vitamins folate, B6, and B12 as predictors of cognitive function and

decline in older high-functioning adults: MacArthur Studies of Successful Aging. Am J Med. Feb 2005;118(2):161-7.
[48] Adunsky A, Arinzon Z, Fidelman Z, Krasniansky I, Arad M, Gepstein R. Plasma homocysteine levels and cognitive status in long-term stay geriatric patients: a cross-sectional study. Arch Gerontol Geriatr. Mar-Apr 2005;40(2):129-38. x
[49] McMahon JA, Green TJ, Skeaff CM, Knight RG, Mann JI, Williams SM. A controlled trial of homocysteine lowering and cognitive performance. N Engl J Med. Jun 29 2006;354(26):2764-72.
[50] Borgna-Pignatti C, Rugolotto S, DeStefano P, Zhao H, Cappellini MD, Del Vecchio GC, et al. Survival and complications in patients with thalassemia major treated with transfusion and deferoxamine. Haematologica 2004;89:1187-93.
[51] Borgna-Pignatti C, Rugolotto S, Piga, A, DiGregorio F, Gamberi M.R., Sabato V, Melevendi C, Cappellini MD, Verlato G; Survival and Disease Complications in Thalassemia Major. Annuals of the New York Academy of Sciences, Volume 850, 1998
[52] Modell B , Khan M, Darlison M, Westwood MA, Ingram D and Pennell DJ. Improved survival of thalassaemia major in the UK and relation to T2* cardiovascular magnetic resonance. Journal of Cardiovascular Magnetic Resonance 2008, 10:42
[53] Piga A, Gaglioti C, Fogliacco E, Tricta F: Comparative effects of deferiprone and deferoxamine on survival and cardiac disease in patients with thalassemia major: a retrospective analysis. Haematologica 2003, 88:489-96.
[54] Borgna-Pignatti C, Cappellini MD, De Stefano P, Del Vecchio GC, Forni GL, Gamberini MR, Ghilardi R, Piga A, Romeo MA, Zhao H, Cnaan A: Cardiac morbidity and mortality in deferoxamine- or deferiprone-treated patients with thalassemia major. Blood 2006, 107:3733-7.
[55] Telfer P, Coen PG, Christou S, Hadjigavriel M, Kolnakou A, Pangalou E, Pavlides N, Psiloines M, Simamonian K, Skordos G, Sitarou M, Angastiniotis M: Survival of medically treated thalassemia patients in Cyprus. Trends and risk factors over the period 1980-2004. Haematologica 2006, 91:1187-92.
[56] Chung BH, Ha SY, Chan GC, Chiang A, Lee TL, Ho HK, Lee CY, Luk CW, Lau YL: Klebsiella infection in patients with thalassemia. Clin Infect Dis 2003, 36:575-9.
[57] Wang SC, Lin KH, Chern JP, Lu MY, Jou ST, Lin DT, Lin KS: Severe bacterial infection in transfusion-dependent patients with thalassemia major. Clin Infect Dis 2003, 37:984-8.
[58] Khimji PL, Miles AA: Microbial iron-chelators and their action on Klebsiella infections in the skin of guinea-pigs. Br J Exp Pathol 1978, 59:137-47.
[59] Weatherall D, Akinyanju O, Fucharoen S, Olivieri N, Musgrove P (2006) Inherited Disorders of Hemoglobin. In: Jamison D, editor. Disease Control Priorities in Developing Countries 2nd ed. New York: Oxford University Press. pp. 663–80.
[60] Leikin SL, Gallagher D, Kinney TR, Sloane D, Klug P, et al. (1989) Mortality in children and adolescents with sickle cell disease. Cooperative Study of Sickle Cell Disease. Pediatrics: 84(3): 500–8.
[61] Platt OS, Brambilla DJ, Rosse WF, Milner PF, Castro O, et al. (1994) Mortality in sickle cell disease. Life expectancy and risk factors for early death. N Engl J Med: 330(23): 1639–44.
[62] Kato GJ, McGowan V, Machado RF, Little JA, Taylor Jt, et al. (2006) Lactate dehydrogenase as a biomarker of hemolysis-associated nitric oxide resistance,

priapism, leg ulceration, pulmonary hypertension, and death in patients with sickle cell disease. Blood: 107(6): 2279–85.

[63] Quinn CT, Rogers ZR, Buchanan GR (2004) Survival of children with sickle cell disease. Blood: 103(11): 4023–7.

[64] Telfer P, Coen P, Chakravorty S, Wilkey O, Evans J, et al. (2007) Clinical outcomes in children with sickle cell disease living in England: a neonatal cohort in East London. Haematologica: 92(7): 905–12.

[65] Obaro S (2009) Pneumococcal Disease in Sickle Cell Disease in Africa: Does Absence of Evidence Imply Evidence of Absence? Arch Dis Child.

[66] Makani J, Cox SE, Soka D, Komba AN, Oruo J, et al. (2011) Mortality in Sickle Cell Anemia in Africa: A Prospective Cohort Study in Tanzania. PLoS ONE 6(2): e14699

[67] Powars D, Chan LS, Schroeder WA (1990) The variable expression of sickle cell disease is genetically determined. Semin Hematol: 27(4): 360–76

[68] http://www.plosone.org/article/info%3Adoi%2F10.1371%2Fjournal.pone.0014699 - pone.0014699-Leikin1

[69] Lee A, Thomas P, Cupidore L, Serjeant B, Serjeant G (1995) Improved survival in homozygous sickle cell disease: lessons from a cohort study. BMJ: 311(7020): 1600–590

[70] Vichinsky EP (1991) Comprehensive care in sickle cell disease: its impact on morbidity and mortality. Semin Hematol: 28(3): 220–6

[71] Yanni E, Grosse SD, Yang Q, Olney RS (2009) Trends in pediatric sickle cell disease-related mortality in the United States, 1983-2002. J Pediatr: 154(4): 541–5.

[72] Graham JK, Mosunjac M, Hanzlick RL, Mosunjac M. Sickle cell lung disease and sudden death: a retrospective/prospective study of 21 autopsy cases and literature review. Am J Forensic Med Pathol. 2007 Jun;28(2):168-72.

[73] Murray MJ, Evans P. Sudden exertional death in a soldier with sickle cell trait. Mil Med. 1996 May;161(5):303-5.

[74] Mitchell BL. Sickle cell trait and sudden death--bringing it home. J Natl Med Assoc. 2007 Mar;99(3):300-5.

[75] John N. A Review of Clinical Profile in Sickle Cell Traits. OMJ. 25, 3-8 (2010)

[76] Audebert H; Planck J; Eisenburg M; Schrezenmeier H; Haberl RL. Cerebral Ischemic Infarction in Paroxysmal Nocturnal Hemoglobinuria: Report of 2 Cases and Updated Review of 7 Previously Published Patients. Journal Of Neurology 2005, 252(11),1379-1386.

[77] World Bank, WHO, UNFPA. Preventing the tragedy of maternal deaths. A report on the International Safe Motherhood Conference Nairobi, Kenya, 1987. Geneva: WHO.

[78] Alauddin M. Maternal mortality in rural Bangladesh. The Tangail District. Stud Fam Plann 1986; 17: 13–21.

[79] World Health Organization. Prevention and Management of Severe Anaemia in Pregnancy. Geneva: WHO; 1993.

[80] Viteri FE, Torun B. Anemia and physical work capacity. In: Garby L (ed) Clinics in Haematology, vol. 3, WB Saunders, 1974; 609–26

[81] Chi I, Agoestina T, Harbin J. Maternal mortality at twelve teaching hospitals in Indonesia: an epidemiologic analysis. Int J Gynaecol Obstet 1992; 39: 87–92

[82] Llewellyn-Jones D. Severe Anemia in pregnancy (as seen in Kuala-Lumpur, Malaysia). Aust N Z J. Obstet Gynaecol 1965;5:191-7.

[83] Rush D. Nutrition and maternal mortality in the developing world. Am J Clin Nutr 2000; 72 (Suppl.): 212–40.

[84] Broek NV. Anaemia and micronutrient deficiencies. Reducing maternal death and disability during pregnancy Br Med Bull (2003) 67 (1): 149-160.
[85] Hemminki E, Rimpela U. Iron supplementation, maternal packed cell volume, and fetal growth. Arch Dis Child 1991;66:422-5.
[86] Agarwal KN, Agarwal DK, Mishra KP. Impact of Anemia prophylaxis in pregnancy on maternal hemoglobin, serum ferritin and birth weight. Indian J Med Res 1991;94:277-80.
[87] Singla PN, Tyagi M, Kumar A, Dash D, Shankar R. Fetal growth in maternal anemia. J Trop Pediatr 1997;43:89-92.
[88] Dreyfuss M. Anemia and iron deficiency during pregnancy: etiologies and effects on birth outcomes in Nepal. PhD dissertation. Johns Hopkins University, Baltimore, 1998.
[89] Murphy JF, O'Riordan J, Newcombe RJ, Coles EC, Pearson JF. Relation of hemoglobin levels in first and second trimesters to outcome of pregnancy. Lancet 1986;1:992-5.
[90] Klebanoff MA, Shiono PH, Selby JV, Trachtenberg AI, Graubard BI. Anemia and spontaneous preterm birth. Am J Obstet Gynecol 1991;164:59-63.
[91] Lu ZM, Goldenberg RL, Cliver SP, Cutter G, Blankson M. The relationship between maternal hematocrit and pregnancy outcome. Obstet Gynecol 1991;77:190-4.
[92] Scholl TO, Hediger ML, Fischer RL, Shearer JW. Anemia vs iron deficiency: increased risk of preterm delivery in a prospective study. Am J Clin Nutr 1992;55:985-8.
[93] Singh K, Fong YF, Arulkumaran S. Anemia in pregnancy—a cross-sectional study in Singapore. Eur J Clin Nutr 1998;52:65-70
[94] Rusia U, Madan N, Agarwal N, Sikka M, Sood S. Effect of maternal iron deficiency Anemia on foetal outcome. Indian J Pathol Microbiol 1995;38:273-9.
[95] Greenwood R, Golding J, McCaw-Binns A, Keeling J, Ashley D. The epidemiology of perinatal death in Jamaica. Paediatr Perinat Epidemiol 1994;8:143-57.
[96] Hemminki E, Starfield B. Routine administration of iron and vitamins during pregnancy: review of controlled clinical trials. Br J Obstet Gynaecol 1978;85:404-10.
[97] Preziosi P, Prual A, Galan P, Daouda H, Boureima H, Hercberg S. Effect of iron supplementation on the iron status of pregnant women: consequences for newborns. Am J Clin Nutr 1997;66:1178-82.
[98] Zeng L, Dibley MJ, Cheng Y, Dang S, Chang S, Kong L, Yan H. Impact of micronutrient supplementation during pregnancy on birth weight, duration of gestation, and perinatal mortality in rural western China: double blind cluster randomised controlled trial. BMJ. 2008;337:a2001.
[99] Lozof B. Iron and learning potential in childhood. Bull N Y Acad Med. 1989;65(10):1050-1088
[100] Lozoff B. Early Iron Deficiency Has Brain and Behavior Effects Consistent with Dopaminergic Dysfunction. J. Nutr. 2011; 141:4 740S-746S
[101] Mackler B, Person F, Miller LR. Iron-deficiency in the rat: biochemical studies of brain metabolism. Pediatr Res 1978;12:217-20.
[102] Voorhess ML, Stuart MJ, Stockman JA, et al. Iron-deficiency and increased urinary norepinephrine excretion. J Pediatr 1975;86: 542-7.
[103] Oski FA, Honig AS. The effects of therapy on the developmental score of iron-deficient infants. J Pediatr 1978;92:21-4.
[104] Chang S, Wang L, Wang Y, Brouwer ID, Kok FJ, Lozoff B, Chen C. Iron-Deficiency Anemia in Infancy and Social Emotional Development in Preschool-Aged Chinese Children. PEDIATRICS Vol. 127 No. 4 April 1, 2011

[105] Biousse V, Rucker JC, Vignal C, Crassard I, Katz BJ, Newman NJ. Anemia and papilledema. American Journal of Ophthalmology 135(4),437-446, 2003
[106] Habis A, Hobson WL, Greenberg R. Cerebral sinovenous thrombosis in a toddler with iron deficiency anemia. Pediatr Emerg Care. 2010 Nov;26(11):848-51).
[107] Maguire JL, deVeber G, Parkin PC. Association between iron-deficiency anemia and stroke in young children. Pediatrics. 2007 Nov;120(5):1053-7.
[108] Hartfield DS, Lowry NJ, Keene DL, Yager JY. Iron deficiency: a cause of stroke in infants and children. Pediatr Neurol. 1997 Jan;16(1):50-3).
[109] http://bloodjournal.hematologylibrary.org/content/107/10/3841.
[110] Izaks GJ, Westendorp RG, Knook DL. The definition of anemia in older persons. JAMA 1999;281:1714–7.
[111] Chaves PH, Xue QL, Guralnik JM, et al. What constitutes normal hemoglobin concentration in community-dwelling disabled older women?J Am Geriatr Soc 2004; 52:1811–6.
[112] Beghé C, Wilson A, Ershler WB. Prevalence and outcomes of anemia in geriatrics: a systematic review of the literature. Am J Med 2004;116 (Suppl 7A):3S–10S.
[113] Eisenstaedt R, Penninx BW, Woodman RC. Anemia in the elderly: current understanding and emerging concepts. Blood Rev 2006;20:213–26.
[114] Lipschitz D. Medical and functional consequences of anemia in the elderly. J Am Geriatr Soc 2003;51(Suppl 3):S10–3.
[115] Paltiel O, Clarfield AM "Anemia in elderly people: Risk marker or risk factor?" CMAJ 2009
[116] Caro JJ, Salas M, Ward A, et al: 2001; Anemia as an independent prognostic factor for survival in patients with cancer: A systemic, quantitative review. Cancer 91:2214-2221,
[117] Harrison LB, Shasha D, White C, Ramdeen B. Radiotherapy-associated anemia: the scope of the problem. Oncologist. 2000;5(suppl 2):1-7.
[118] Bush RS. The significance of anemia in clinical radiation therapy. Int J Radiat Oncol Biol Phys. 1986;12:2047-2050.
[119] Grogan M, Thomas GM, Melamed I, et al. The importance of hemoglobin levels during radiotherapy for carcinoma of the cervix. Cancer. 1999;86:1528-1536.
[120] Lee JS, Scott C, Komaki R, et al. Concurrent chemoradiation therapy with oral etoposide for locally advanced inoperable non-small-cell lung cancer: radiation therapy oncology group protocol 91-06. J Clin Oncol. 1996;14:1055-1064.
[121] Fein DA, Lee WR, Hanlon L, et al. Pretreatment hemoglobin level influences local control and survival of T1-T2 squamous cell carcinomas of the glottic larynx. J Clin Oncol.1995;13:2077-2083.
[122] Kalra PR, Bolger AP, Francis DP, Genth-Zotz S, Sharma R, Ponikowski PP, Poole-Wilson PA, Coats AJ, Anker SD. Effect of anemia on exercise tolerance in chronic heart failure in men. Am J Cardiol 2003;91:888-891.
[123] Ezekowitz JA, McALister FA, Armstrong PW. Anemia is common in heart failure and is associated with poor outcomes. Insights form a cohort of 12 065 patients with new-onset heart failure. Circulation 2003;107:294-299.
[124] Anand IS, Kuskowski MA, Rector TS, Florea VG, Glazer RD, Hester A, Chiang YT, Aknay N, Maggioni AP, Opasich C, Latini R, Cohn JN. Anemia and change in hemoglobin over time related to mortality and morbidity in patients with chronic heart failure: results from Val HeFT. Circulation 2005;112:1121-1127.

[125] Sharma R, Francis DP, Pitt B, Poole-Wilson PA, Coats AJ, Anker SD. Haemoglobin predicts survival in patients with chronic heart failure: a substudy of the ELITE II trial.Eur Heart J 2004;25:1021-1028.
[126] Horwich TB, Fonarow GC, Hamilton MA, Maclellan WR, Borenstein J. Anemia is associated with worse symptoms, greater impairment in functional capacity and a significant increase in mortality in patients with advance heart failure. J Am Coll Cardiol 2002;39:1780-1786.
[127] Mozaffarian D, Nye R, Levy WC. Anemia predicts mortality in severe heart failure. The prospective randomized amlodipine survival evaluation (PRAISE). J Am Coll Cardiol 2003;41:1933-1939.
[128] Anand I, McMurray JV, Whitmore J, Warren M, Pham A, McCamish MA, Burton PBJ. Anemia and its relationship to clinical outcome in heart failure. Circulation2004;110:149-154.
[129] Silverberg DS, Wexler D, Iaina A, Schwartz D. The interaction between heart failure and other heart diseases, renal failure, and anemia. Semin Nephrol. 2006 Jul;26(4):296-306.
[130] Groenveld HF, Januzzi JL, Damman K, Wijngaarden J, Hillege HL, van Veldhuisen DJ, and Meer PV, Anemia and Mortality in Heart Failure Patients. A Systematic Review and Meta-Analysis. J Am Coll Cardiol, 2008; 52:818-827
[131] Swedberg K, Pfeffer M, Granger C, Held P, McMurray J, Ohlin G, Olofsson B, Ostergren J, Yusuf S. Candesartan in heart failure--assessment of reduction in mortality and morbidity (CHARM): rationale and design. Charm-Programme Investigators. J Card Fail. 1999 Sep;5(3):276-82.
[132] Kosiborod M, Curtis JP, Wang Y, Smith GL, Masoudi FA; Foody; Havranek EP; Krumholz HM. Anemia and Outcomes in Patients With Heart Failure. A Study From the National Heart Care Project. Arch Intern Med. 2005;165:2237-224.
[133] Mitka M. Researchers probe anemia-heart failure link. JAMA. 2003;290:1835–1838.
[134] Wu WC, Rathore SS, Wang Y, Radford MJ, Krumholz HM. Blood transfusion in elderly patients with acute myocardial infarction. N Engl J Med. 2001;345:1230 –1236.
[135] Hebert PC, Wells G, Blajchman MA, Marshall J, Martin C, Pagliarello G, Tweeddale M, Schweitzer I, Yetisir E. A multicenter, randomized, controlled clinical trial of transfusion requirements in critical care: Transfusion Requirements in Critical Care Investigators, Canadian Critical Care Trials Group. N Engl J Med. 1999;340:409–417.
[136] Tang Y and Katz SD. Anemia in Chronic Heart Failure: Prevalence, Etiology, Clinical Correlates, and Treatment Options. Circulation 2006, 113:2454-2461.
[137] Silverberg OS, Wexler D, Sheps D, et al. The effect of correction of mild anemia in severe, resistant congestive heart failure using subcutaneous erythropoietin and intravenous iron: a randomized controlled study. J Am Coll Cardiol. 2001;37:1775-1780
[138] Ghali JK, Anand I, Abraham WT, et al. Randomized, double-blind, placebo-controlled trial to assess the impact of darbepoetin alfa treatment on exercise tolerance in anemic patients with symptomatic heart failure: results from STAMINA-HeFT. European Society of Cardiology Heart Failure 2006 Congress; June 17-20, 2006; Helsinki, Finland. Abstract 549
[139] Volkova N, Arab L. Evidence-based systematic literature review of hemoglobin/hematocrit and all-cause mortality in dialysis patients. Am J Kidney Dis. 2006 Jan;47(1):24-36.

[140] Ma J, Ebben J, Xia H, et al. Hematocrit levels and associated mortality in hemodialysis patients. J Am Soc Nephrol. 1999;10:610-619.
[141] Collins A, Xia H, Ebben J, et al. Change in hematocrit and risk of mortality. J Am Soc Nephrol. 1998;9(suppl A):204A.
[142] Collins AJ, Li S, St Peter W, et al. Death, hospitalization, and economic associations among incident hemodialysis patients with hematocrit values of 36 to 39%. J Am Soc Nephrol.2001;12: 2465-2473.
[143] Collins A, Ma JZ, Ebben J, et al. Impact of hematocrit on morbidity and mortality. Semin Nephrol. 2000;20:345-349.
[144] Eschbach JW, Abdulhadi MH, Browne JK, et al. Recombinant human erythropoietin in anemic patients with end-stage renal disease: results of a phase III multicenter clinical trial. Ann Intern Med. 1989;111(12):992-1000.
[145] Singh AK, Szczech L, Tang KL, et al; CHOIR Investigators. Correction of anemia with epoetin alfa in chronic kidney disease. N Engl J Med. 2006;355(20):2085-2098.
[146] Pfeffer MA, Burdmann EA, Chen CY, et al; TREAT Investigators. A trial of darbepoetin alfa in type 2 diabetes and chronic kidney disease. N Engl J Med. 2009; 361(21):2019-2032.
[147] Brookhart MA, Schneeweiss S, Avorn J, Bradbury BD, Liu J; Winkelmayer WC. Comparative Mortality Risk of Anemia Management Practices in Incident Hemodialysis Patients. JAMA. 2010;303:857-864
[148] Kazory A and Ross EA, Anemia: The Point of Convergence or Divergence for Kidney Disease and Heart Failure? J Am Coll Cardiol, 2009; 53:639-647.
[149] Low I, Grutzmacher P, Bergmann M, Schoeppe W. Echocardiographic findings in patients on maintenance hemodialysis substituted with recombinant human erythropoietin. Clin Nephrol. 1989;31:26-30.
[150] Low-Friedrich I, Grutzmacher P, Marz W, Bergmann M, Schoeppe W. Therapy with recombinant human erythropoietin reduces cardiac size and improves heart function in chronic hemodialysis patients. Am J Nephrol. 1991;11:54-60.
[151] Goldberg N, Lundin AP, Delano B, Friedman EA, Stein RA. Changes in left ventricular size, wall thickness, and function in anemic patients treated with recombinant human erythropoietin. Am Heart J. 1992;124:424-427.
[152] Foley RN, Parfrey PS, Morgan J, et al. A randomized controlled trial of complete vs partial correction of anemia in hemodialysis patients with asymptomatic concentric LV hypertrophy or LV dilatation. J Am Soc Nephrol. 1998;9:208.
[153] Linde T, Wikstrom B, Andersson LG, Danielson BG. Renal Anemia treatment with recombinant human erythropoietin increases cardiac output in patients with ischemic heart disease. Scand J Urol Nephrol. 1996;30:115-120.
[154] Eckardt KU. Managing a fateful alliance: Anemia and cardiovascular outcomes. Nephrol Dial Transplant. 2005 Jun;20 Suppl 6:vi16-20.

# 2

# Erythrocyte: Programmed Cell Death

Daniela Vittori, Daiana Vota and Alcira Nesse
*Department of Biological Chemistry, School of Sciences, University of Buenos Aires, and IQUIBICEN - National Council of Scientific and Technical Investigation*
*Argentina*

## 1. Introduction

Erythrocytes are produced by a complex and finely regulated process of erythropoiesis. It starts with a pluripotential stem cell that, in addition of its self replication capacity, can give rise to separate cell lineages. Erythropoiesis passes from the stem cell through the multipotent progenitor CFU-GEMM (colony-forming unit granulocyte erythroid monocyte and megakaryocyte), and then BFU-E (burst-forming unit erythroid) and CFU-E (colony-forming unit eryhtroid), to the first recognizable erythrocyte precursor in the bone marrow, the pronormoblast. This cell gives rise to a series of progressively smaller normoblasts with increasing content of hemoglobin. The nucleus is finally extruded from the late normoblast leading to mature red blood cell through the reticulocyte stage. Erythropoiesis ends with the mature circulating red cell, which is a non-nucleated biconcave disc, performing its function of oxygen delivery. In this process, the glycoprotein hormone erythropoietin has been known as the major humoral regulator of red cell production. It is now well established that erythropoietin stimulates erythropoiesis, at least in part, by protecting erythroblasts from apoptosis.

Human mature erythrocytes are terminally differentiated cells that are devoid of mitochondria, as well as of nucleus and other organelles. In circulation, the red cell is constantly tested for its capacity to undergo marked cellular deformation. This ability to change its shape is essential for optimal cell function, since the resting diameter of the human red cell far exceeds that of the capillaries and splenic endothelial slits through which it must pass (Mohandas & Groner, 1989). A two dimensional network of proteins interacting between transmembrane location and cytoplasmic surface of the plasma membrane gives the red blood cell its properties of elasticity and flexibility that allows the success of this journey.

The mature erythrocyte is unable to self-repair and has no capacity to synthesize proteins. Therefore, its lifespan is finite and is shortened further when the cell's environment becomes hostile or when the erythrocyte's ability to cope with damaging extracellular influences becomes impaired. The erythrocyte limited lifespan implies that, as in other cells, life and death are well regulated for erythrocytes, in spite of their lack of capacity for protein synthesis (Bosman et al., 2005).

In the present review, we aim to show updated information concerning erythrocyte death in order to contribute to the understanding of the physiopathological relationship of this process with the development of anemia.

## 2. Anemia

The term anemia is derived from ancient Greek for "bloodlessness". It is a condition involving abnormal reduction of hemoglobin content. In healthy adults, there is steady-state equilibrium between the rate of release of new red cells from the bone marrow into the circulation and the rate of removal of senescent red cells from the circulation by reticuloendothelial system. Balance disruption appears by decreased cell production, increased destruction or both, leading then to anemia. Different mechanisms which may lead to anemia are blood loss, decreased red cell lifespan, acquired or congenital defects, ineffective erythropoiesis, and impairment of red cell formation.
In this chapter we focus on anemia resulting from accelerated clearance of red blood cells from circulating blood before hemolysis.

## 3. Erythrocyte death

Apoptosis is a regulated process of self-destruction characterized by a series of changes affecting the nucleus, cytoplasm and plasma membrane of the cell, and leading to the rapid capture and ingestion of the dying cell by macrophages. Programmed death allows the elimination of cells without release of intracellular proteins which would otherwise cause inflammation.
It is well known that eukaryotic cells use a similar death program. Moreover, erythrocyte precursors, which are true organelle-containing cells, are susceptible to apoptosis induction. Instead, human mature erythrocytes have been considered as unable to undergo programmed cell death due to their lack of mitochondria, nucleus, and other organelles. Increasing evidence is now available to demonstrate that mature erythrocytes can undergo a rapid self-destruction process sharing several features with apoptosis, including cell shrinkage, plasma membrane microvesiculation, shape changes, cytoskeleton alterations associated with protein degradation, and loss of plasma membrane phospholipid asymmetry leading to the externalization of phosphatidylserine. As described, erythrocyte death is characterized by some features that are shared by apoptosis. To distinguish the death of erythrocytes from apoptosis of nucleated cells, some authors suggest the term "eryptosis" (Lang KS et al., 2005).
Erythrocyte lifespan is limited to approximately 120 days and is ended by a process of senescence during which aging erythrocytes suffer changes that display molecules that are recognized by macrophages leading to their clearance from peripheral blood by reticuloendothelial system (Bratosin et al., 1998). Programmed erythrocyte death prevents intravascular hemolysis and allows the elimination of cells without inflammation. Even though this is one of the processes that regulate effective erythropoiesis, a disturbance of the fine equilibrium between erythrocyte production and cell destruction may be caused by the presence of factors that create a harmful environment.
The knowledge of the mechanism of the erythrocyte death is of the highest importance since, apart from its association with anemia, it could lead to improvements of the storage conditions in blood banks by increasing the time of viability of stored red blood cells (Bratosin et al., 2002).

## 4. Mechanism of suicidal erythrocyte death

As mentioned above, mature erythrocytes can undergo a rapid self-destruction process leading to increased intracellular calcium content, modifications of the erythrocyte

morphology, metabolic disruption, membrane protein modifications, and externalization of phosphatidylserine, thereby activating a clearance mechanism involving heterophagic removal in the reticuloendothelial system.
Data describing cell changes and mechanism involved in erythrocyte premature death are stated below.

### 4.1 Intracellular calcium content

It is well established that two properties of red blood cells, deformability and elasticity, are dramatically affected by calcium ions. Thus, a rise in internal $Ca^{2+}$ leads to changes in cell shape and volume, increased cellular rigidity and hemolysis (Weed et al., 1969; Palek et al., 1974; Kirkpatrick et al., 1975). Such alterations seem to arise from $Ca^{2+}$ interactions with various molecular targets. These include both low-affinity associations with membrane phospholipids (Chandra et al., 1987) and high-affinity ones with specific membrane proteins, especially the Ca-dependent K channel (Romero, 1976) as well as with some cytoskeletal proteins (Wallis et al., 1993). It was observed that the presence of the bivalent-cation ionophore A23187 did not induce erythrocyte death in the absence of extracellular $Ca^{2+}$, nor in the presence of both $Ca^{2+}$ and the $Ca^{2+}$ chelator EDTA, thus characterizing erythrocyte death as an active process requiring $Ca^{2+}$ entry into the cells (Bratosin et al., 2001).
Since internal $Ca^{2+}$ is subjected to metabolic control via an ATP-dependent extrusion mechanism (Ca pump) (Schatzmann, 1983), it is expected that the decreased ATP content attained during red cell aging should lead to raised cellular $Ca^{2+}$. The homeostasis of $Ca^{2+}$ in these cells is carried out by the concerted action of just two mechanisms: the active extrusion already mentioned and the entry through defined $Ca^{2+}$ channels (Romero & Romero, 1999).
Different factors that may cause cellular stress, such as hyperosmotic shock, oxidative stress, or energy depletion, are capable of $Ca^{2+}$ channel activation in the erythrocyte, including the nonselective cation channel TRPC, with subsequent increased entry of $Ca^{2+}$ (Föller el al., 2008). It has been reported that free $Ca^{2+}$ concentration, cell-shrinkage, and phospholipid scrambling were significantly lower in $Cl^-$-depleted TRPC6 -/- erythrocytes than in wildtype mouse erythrocytes, which let the authors conclude that human and mouse erythrocytes express TRPC6 cation channels which participate in cation leak and $Ca^{2+}$-induced suicidal death (Föller el al., 2008).
The increase in erythrocyte cytosolic $Ca^{2+}$ concentration further stimulates $Ca^{2+}$-sensitive $K^+$ channel (Gardos channel). The subsequent efflux of $K^+$ hyperpolarises the cell membrane, which drives $Cl^-$ exit in parallel to $K^+$. The cellular loss of KCl with osmotically obliged water leads to cell shrinkage. It has been reported that cell shrinkage leads to formation of ceramide. This compound can also contribute to the triggering of cell membrane scrambling (Lang et al., 2004), one of the typical features of suicidal erythrocyte death.
Another important effect caused by a raise in intracellular $Ca^{2+}$ concerns the activation of different enzymes, including calpain. This endogenous protease primarily cleaves the Ca pump, then band 3 protein and finally some cytoskeletal proteins.

### 4.2 Enzyme activity

#### 4.2.1 Enzymes of the glycolytic pathways

Band 3, the anion-exchange protein, also binds various cytoskeletal proteins as well as hemoglobin and cytoplasmic glycolytic enzymes. It has been shown that mild oxidants, such as potassium ferricyanade, diamide, and hydrogen peroxide stimulate red blood cell glycolysis in proportion to the elevation of band 3 tyrosine phophorylation. Band 3 sequences surrounding tyrosine residues have been associated with intracellular binding of several cytosolic proteins, including hemoglobin and the glycolytic enzymes aldolase, phosphofructokinase, and glyceraldehyde-3-phosphate dehydrogenase. *In vitro*, the tyrosine phosphorylation of band 3 prevented the binding of these glycolytic enzymes. Since these enzymes are inhibited in their bound state, the functional consequence of N-terminal band 3 tyrosine phosphorylation would be an enhanced rate of glycolysis in the intact cells (Harrison et al., 1991; Mallozi et al., 1995). This mechanism of erythrocyte metabolic regulation can stimulate or reduce energy production in times of special needs, such as during a free radical attack.

### 4.2.2 Enzymes involved in thiol metabolism and protection against oxidative damage

Activities of some cytoplasmic enzymes decline during erythrocyte aging or when they are induced to programmed cell death. Oxidative stress as well as antioxidant depletion cause decreased activity of erythrocyte catalase (CAT), superoxide dismutase (SOD), and glutathione peroxidase (GPX). However, the enzyme behavior seems to depend on the biological model as well as the oxidant agent, since there are some reports showing activation of CAT, SOD, and GPX which has been associated with the metabolic response to cell injure.

### 4.2.3 Proteases

Members of the caspase family contain a cystein residue in their active center and exist as zymogens that need to be activated by proteolytic cleavage adjacent to aspartates. During apoptosis, caspases function either as initiators (e.g. caspase-8 and -9) in response to proapoptotic signals or as effectors (e.g. caspase-3) (Berg et al., 2001). Mature erythrocytes contain considerable amounts of caspase-3 and caspase-8 whereas other essential components of the mitochondrial apoptotic cascade such as caspase-9, Apaf-1 and cytochrome c are absent. Strikingly, although caspase-3 and -8 were functionally active *in vitro*, they did not become activated by various proapoptotic stimuli. Cysteine protease inhibitors prevented programmed erythrocyte death induced by $Ca^{2+}$ influx, and allowed erythrocyte survival *in vitro* and *in vivo*. However, the cysteine proteases involved seem not to be caspases, since caspase-3, while present in erythrocytes, was not activated during cell death, and cytochrome c, a critical component of the apoptosome, was lacking. Therefore, $Ca^{2+}$-induced erythrocyte death appeared to proceed in the absence of caspase activation (Bratosin et al., 2001). In opposition, pretreatment of red cells with the caspase-8 or the caspase-3 specific inhibitors blocked the oxidative stress-induced inhibition of aminophospholipid translocase activity, leading to the conclusion that caspase-8 dependent caspase-3 activation could play a role in the phosphatidylserine externalization (Mandal et al., 2005). Other authors observed that treatment of erythrocytes with peroxynitrite under conditions in which the oxidant diffuses to the intracellular compartment led to phosphatidylserine translocation in parallel with activation of caspases (Pietraforte et al., 2007). Taking together, the abovementioned results suggest that the role of caspases in the mature human erythrocytes needs to be clarified.

The major $Ca^{2+}$-activated cysteine protease found to be involved in the process of cell death is calpain. Following an increase of cytosolic calcium, calpain translocates from the cytosol to the membrane where it undergoes autoproteolytic activation. Although caspases were found inactive in senescent erythrocytes or cells treated with calcium ionophores, activation of the cysteine protease calpain was readily induced in response to elevated calcium levels (Berg et al., 2001). Red blood cells exposed to the oxidative agent peroxynitrite also showed an increase of the active form of μ-calpain (Matarrese et al., 2005). In contrast, calpain inhibitors did not affect phosphatidylserine exposure suggesting that it is presumably a protease-independent event in erythrocytes. A possible explanation may be that increased intracellular calcium is sufficient to disrupt phospholipid asymmetry by activating an aminophospholipid scramblase and inactivating aminophospholipid translocase.

The activation of calpain in normal human erythrocytes incubated in the presence of $Ca^{2+}$ and ionophore A23187 led to the decline of the $Ca^{2+}$-dependent ATPase activity of the cells, which was prevented by preloading of the erythrocyte with an anticalpain antibody. The decline of the pump activity corresponded to the degradation of the pump protein and was inversely correlated to the amount of the natural inhibitor of calpain, calpastatin, present in the cells. Results suggested that the Ca pump and band 3 were the most sensitive proteins to calpain-induced degradation (Salamino et al., 1994).

Calpain was also responsible for phosphotyrosine phosphatase 1B (PTP1B) cleavage in platelets (Frangioni et al., 1993) and in cell lines with erythroid differentiation ability (Callero et al., 2011), which was accompanied by stimulation of its enzymatic activity. Reversible oxidation of PTP1B *in vitro* strongly facilitated the association with calpain and led to greatly increased calpain-dependent cleavage (Trümpler et al., 2009). Both oxidative environment and increased intracellular $Ca^{2+}$ may account for the altered tyrosyl phosphorylation that may have important implications in the programmed erythrocyte death.

### 4.3 Phosphatydilserine externalization

Alterations in the transbilayer distribution of phospholipids in erythrocyte membrane have significant physiologic consequences. Phospholipids in the plasma membrane of mammalian cells are not randomly distributed between the two leaflets of the membrane bilayer. Choline-containing phospholipids phosphatidylcholine and sphingomyelin dominate the outer leaflet, while the aminophospholipids phosphatidylethanolamine and phosphatidylserine are major components of the inner leaflet (Williamson & Schlegel, 2002). Of these phospholipids, only phosphatidylserine demonstrates an absolute distribution, and the appearance of this lipid on the external surface has significant consequences for the red blood cell (Daleke, 2008). Several functional roles for asymmetric phospholipid distribution in plasma membranes have been suggested. For instance, several regulatory and structural proteins including protein kinase C (Palfrey & Waseem, 1985), annexin (Meers & Mealy, 1994), and membrane skeletal proteins, such as spectrin (O'Toole et al., 1999), appear to localize to the cytoplasmic face of the membrane through their interaction with phosphatidylserine (Manno et al., 2002).

Although asymmetric lipid synthesis and chemical modification make some contribution, ATP-dependent directional lipid transport is the primary mechanism for generation and maintenance of lipid asymmetry. The latter transport is catalyzed by an enzyme called the aminophospholipid translocase, a P-type ATPase that specifically and rapidly transports the aminophospholipids, phosphatidylethanolamine and phosphatidylserine, from the outer to the inner leaflet of the plasma membrane (Tang et al., 1996). At least one membrane protein is required to facilitate a rapid loss of lipid asymmetry. Although no protein mediating this function has been identified they are called "phospholipid scramblases". The bivalent cation $Ca^{2+}$ plays an important role in the regulation of lipid scrambling. In erythrocyte, once activated by $Ca^{2+}$, the scrambling pathway remains active for at least 2 h (Williamson et al., 1992). Scramblase creates a proteinaceous aqueous pore that facilitates migration of the polar headgroup of the lipids across the hydrophobic core of the bilayer, while keeping the acyl chain moieties in the core of the bilayer (Bevers & Williamson, 2010).

Whether triggered by injury, disease or cell activation, the movement of phosphatidylserine to the surface of the cell alters rheologic and hemostatic properties of the membrane. Erythrocytes with surface-exposed phosphatidylserine adhere to one another and to vascular endothelial cells (Daleke, 2008). Thus, the regulation and control of the distribution of phospholipid asymmetry are essential for maintenance erythrocyte mechanical stability and proper cell function. Furthermore, asymmetric distribution of aminophospholipids has significant effects on cell shape and on membrane mechanical stability. Ghosts that maintained their asymmetric lipid distribution had normal discoid morphology whereas ghosts in which asymmetric lipid distribution was lost exhibited echinocytic morphology (Manno et al., 2002). Understanding the cause of perturbations of transbilayer distribution of phospholipids and the molecular mechanism by which they are regulated is essential for ameliorating some of the consequences of erythrocyte membrane abnormalities.

In summary, phosphatidylserine translocation, now generally accepted as a hallmark of cells in apoptosis, results from the inhibition of aminophospholipid translocase activity and activation of scramblase. Surface exposure of phosphatidylserine on apoptotic cells presents a recognition and engulfment signal for removal by phagocytosis competent cells even before the development of morphological changes usually associated with death (Schlegel & Williamson, 2001).

### 4.4 Erythrocyte morphology

The volume of red cells decreases with cell aging and substantial amount of hemoglobin is lost from circulating erythrocytes during total lifespan. This is probably due to loss of potassium and to loss of membrane via microvesiculation, resulting in cellular dehydration, membrane protein removal, and increased density.

Vesicle formation appears to be accompanied by the breakdown of band 3 protein. It has been postulated that removal of senescent erythrocytes by macrophages is mediated by senescent cell-specific autoantigens originated on band 3, the anion exchanger and the major membrane protein of the erythrocyte (Kay, 2005). In accordance, Willekens et al. (2008) confirmed that vesiculation is not only associated with the removal of membrane-bound hemoglobin, but is associated with generation of senescent cell antigen, a neoantigen that originates from band 3 after its breakdown in senescent red blood cells. Based on results from immunological analysis of vesicles and taken into consideration the existence of an efficient body mechanism to remove these vesicles, the authors concluded that vesiculation constitutes a mechanism for the removal of erythrocyte membrane patches containing removal molecules, thereby postponing the elimination of otherwise healthy erythrocytes.

Allan and Thomas (1981) found the importance of a raised intracellular $Ca^{2+}$ concentration in the microvesiculation process. Plasma membrane microvesiculation, induced *in vitro* by $Ca^{2+}$, was found identical to that expressed by the very small subpopulation of *in vivo* senescent erythrocytes purified from peripheral blood of healthy donors (Bratosin et al., 2001). Recent comparative proteomic analysis of erythrocytes and their vesicles provide new clues to the mechanisms involved in erythrocyte death (Bosman et al., 2010).

The structure and molecular interaction of proteins within the complex assembly of the erythrocyte cytoskeleton explain the particular shape and shape transformations of these cells. Spectrin, band 3, actin, ankyrin, and other cytoskeletal proteins play an important role for membrane integrity, typical discocyte form, and elasticity of red blood cells. Conversely, protein damage has been implicated in altered erythrocyte morphology.

The shape of $Ca^{2+}$-loaded erythrocytes changed from normal discocytes to echinocytes or spheroechinocytes with plasma membrane microvesiculation (Bratosin et al., 2001; Vota et al., 2010) (Figure 1). Morphological changes induced by A23187 in the presence of $Ca^{2+}$ were associated with cell shrinkage, one of the characteristic features of apoptosis that distinguishes this active and regulated self-destruction process from the passive and chaotic event of necrosis induced by plasma membrane damage (Bratosin et al., 2001).

On the other hand, stomatocytes were the main morphological cell transformation associated to *in vitro* (Vota et al., 2010) and *in vivo* (Richards et al., 2007; Antonelou et al., 2011) oxidative stress (Figure 1).

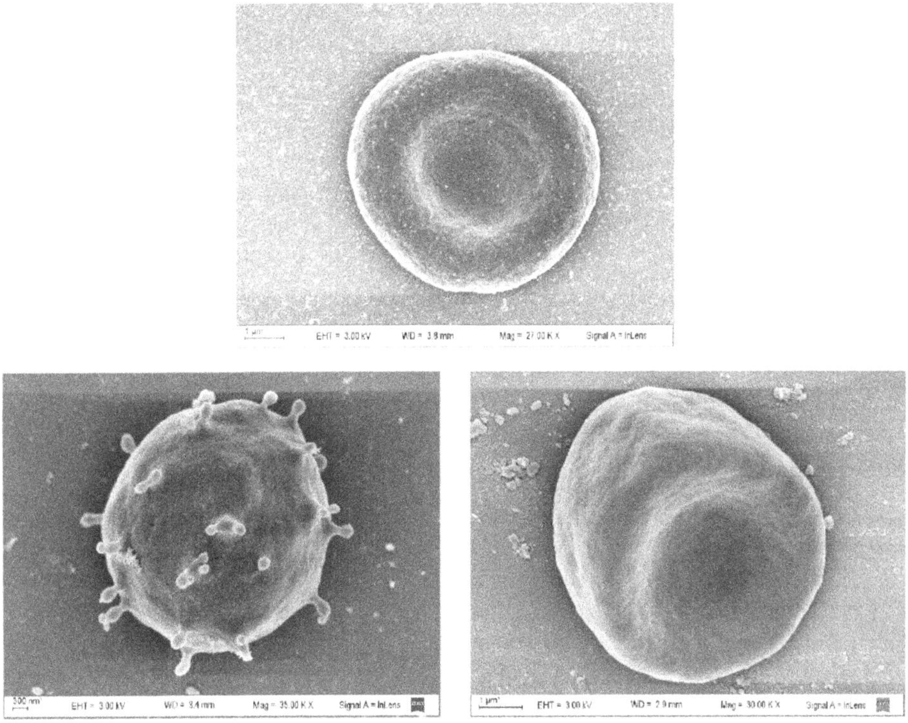

Fig. 1. Altered shapes of erythrocytes subjected to proeryptotic agents. The normal discoid biconcave shape (top) turned to spherocyte with microvesiculation due to increased intracellular calcium concentration (left bottom) or to stomatocyte induced by oxidative stress (right bottom). Results obtained in our laboratory.

### 4.5 Protein modifications

Erythrocyte membrane proteins are susceptible to covalent modification by the lipid peroxidation products generated by an oxygen radical attack. *In vitro* and *in vivo* assays in which erythrocyte metabolic alterations were associated to oxidant environments induced increased lipoperoxidation (Quintanar-Escorza et al., 2010; Calderón-Salinas et al., 2011).

The cytoplasmic domain of band 3 serves as a center of erythrocyte membrane organization and constitutes the major substrate of erythrocyte tyrosine kinases. Tyrosine phosphorylation of band 3 is induced by several stimuli, including malaria parasite invasion, cell shrinkage, normal cell aging, and oxidative stress (Harrison et al., 1991).
Erythrocytes contain protein tyrosine kinase activity, with band 3 protein being the major substrate for the kinases (Brunati et al., 1996). Besides, phosphotyrosine phosphatase was found associated to band 3 protein. This phosphatase is normally highly active and prevents the accumulation of band 3 phosphotyrosine. However, in A23187-treated erythrocytes increased intracellular $Ca^{2+}$ was found to promote band 3 tyrosine phosphorylation via dissociation of phosphotyrosine phosphatase from band 3 (Zipser et al., 2002).
Tyrosine phosphorylation of band 3 markedly reduced its affinity for ankyrin, leading to release of band 3 from the spectrin/actin membrane skeleton, enhancement of the lateral mobility of band 3 in the bilayer, and progressive vesiculation. Because release of band 3 from its ankyrin and adducin linkages to the cytoskeleton can facilitate changes in multiple membrane properties, the authors suggested that tyrosine phosphorylation of band 3 may produce changes in erythrocyte biology that allow the cell to respond to initial stress (Ferru et al., 2011).
Another marker of red blood cell apoptosis is band 3 clustering, which generates a cell surface epitope identified by autologous IgG antibodies and may act as a signal for the removal of erythrocytes from circulation (Kay et al., 1989).
The nitration of tyrosine residues in proteins occurs through the action of reactive oxygen and nitrogen species such as peroxynitrite, the product of the reaction between nitric oxide and superoxide anion. The nitrated peptides were able to activate *lyn*, an erythrocyte *src* tyrosine kinase. It suggested a mechanism of peroxynitrite-mediated signaling that may be correlated with upregulation of tyrosine phosphorylation (Mallozi et al., 2001).

## 5. Processes that induce premature erythrocyte death

Eryptosis can be triggered by different injuries such as energy depletion, osmotic shock or oxidative stress.

### 5.1 Energy depletion

As mentioned in Section 4.1, the reduced calcium-ATPase activity due to energy depletion leads to decreased calcium efflux and this in turn accelerates the transmembrane movement of potassium and chloride, resulting in cell dehydration.
Energy stress also impairs the replenishment of glutathione and thus weakens the antioxidative defense of erythrocytes (Bilmen et al., 2001). Accordingly, this condition similarly activates cation channels affecting calcium flux (Duranton et al., 2002). On the other hand, phosphatidylserine and phosphatidylethanolamine are maintained in the cell inner leaflet by an ATP-dependent transporter known as flippase (Williamson & Schlegel, 2002). Membrane-bound $Mg^{2+}$-ATPases seem to play a key role in the maintenance of the membrane lipid organization. This subfamily of ATPases has been reported to actively translocate aminophospholipids across membranes. Decreased ATP-dependent transport may be very well one of the consequences of phosphatidylserine exposure (Soupene & Kuypers, 2006). Besides, energy depletion involves activation of PKC and PKC-dependent phosphorylation of membrane proteins with subsequent stimulation of eryptosis (Föller et al., 2008).

### 5.2 Osmotic shock

Osmotic shock is found among the well-known inducers of apoptotic cell death. The cellular mechanisms involved in the triggering of apoptosis following cell exposure to hypertonic extracellular fluid have been deeply studied in nucleated cells. Erythrocytes have similarly been shown to bind annexin following osmotic shock.

Erythrocytes incubated in a hyperosmotic environment released prostaglandin E2 (PGE2), which in turn activated nonselective cation channels (Kaestner & Bernhardt, 2002; Lang PA et al., 2005), and increased the cytosolic $Ca^{2+}$ concentration. Activation of the cell volume- and redox potential-sensitive cation channel and subsequent $Ca^{2+}$ entry contributed to the development of erythrocyte cell membrane scrambling. Osmotic cell shrinkage was involved in the stimulation of sphingomyelinase which caused sphingomyelin degradation with subsequent release of ceramide in erythrocytes (Lang et al., 2004). Ceramide then activated scramblase leading to breakdown of phosphatidylserine asymmetry of the cell membrane. The ability of ceramide to induce this kind of erythrocyte death was somewhat surprising, as erythrocytes lack mitochondria, crucial elements in the ceramide-triggered signaling cascade in nucleated cells (Lang et al., 2004). Thus, at least in erythrocytes, ceramide must trigger annexin binding through a pathway distinct from that described in nucleated cells.

### 5.3 Oxidative stress

Increasing intracellular oxidants by altering ambient oxygen concentrations or lowering antioxidant levels accelerates the onset of erythrocyte senescence whereas lowering ambient oxygen or increasing reactive oxygen species (ROS) scavenging appears to delay senescence. In general, conditions that induce senescence often appear to be accompanied by a rise in intracellular ROS levels. Polyunsaturated fatty acids within the membrane, an oxygen rich environment, and iron-rich hemoglobin make red cells susceptible to peroxidative damage. The product of membrane lipid peroxidation can affect the anion transport function and activity of enzymes of the glycolytic pathway associated to band 3 (Dumaswala et al., 1999).

By virtue of its potent oxidant and nitrating ability, peroxynitrite has been proposed as an important mediator of inflammation-induced tissue injury and dysfunction, and it is considered the most efficient nitrating species of biological relevance (Szabó et al., 2007). The red blood cells are, in fact, the major scavengers of peroxynitrite in blood and it has been calculated that at 45% hematocrit about 40–45% of peroxynitrite crosses the cell membrane and quickly reacts with hemoglobin, while the remainder reacts extracellularly with carbon dioxide (Romero & Radi, 2005). In an *in vitro* experimental system mimicking the oxidative imbalance detectable *in vivo*, peroxynitrite acted both extra- and intracellularly as a function of cell density and carbon dioxide concentration, inducing the appearance of distinct cellular biomarkers as well as modulation of metabolism (Pietraforte et al., 2007). Intracellular oxidations, due mostly to direct reactions of peroxynitrite with glutathione and hemoglobin (methemoglobin), lead to decreased ATP and the appearance of apoptotic signs, such as clustering of band 3, externalization of phosphatidylserine, and activation of caspases. Surface/membrane oxidations were principally due to indirect radical reactions causing oxidation of surface thiols, formation of membrane-associated 3-nitrotyrosine, and downregulation of glycophorins A, the latter being considered a senescence biomarker (Matarrese et al., 2005; Pietraforte et al., 2007; Metere et al., 2009).

## 6. *In vivo* erythrocyte death and possible prevention

Oxidative stress is a term used to describe the body's prolonged exposure to oxidative factors that cause more free radicals than the body can neutralize. Under this condition, free radical formation may play a role in the pathophysiology of several diseases. There is evidence that erythrocytes undergo oxidative changes in conditions where free radical formation is known to be high such as rheumatoid arthritis (Richards et al., 2007), diabetes (Manuel y Keenoy et al., 2001; Calderón-Salinas et al., 2011), and hemodialysis treatment (Zachee et al., 1988). Oxidative damage was also considered the cause of decreased deformability and altered rheology of erythrocytes found in individuals with chronic fatigue syndrome, a condition that may be triggered by certain infectious diseases, multiple nutrient deficiencies, food intolerance, or extreme physical or mental stress (Richards et al., 2007). Erythrocyte alterations would have the physiological effect of reducing oxygen delivery to the tissues. In several models, 2,3-diphosphoglycerate (2,3-DPG) levels were increased and this effect may be explained as a compensation since 2,3-DPG have the effect of decreasing oxygen affinity. Therefore, this would allow more oxygen to be delivered to the tissues.

Any erythrocyte disorder facilitating erythrocyte shrinkage, could, to the extent as it leads to activation of the cell volume regulatory cation channels, trigger premature apoptosis and thus accelerate erythrocyte death. Red blood cells from patients with sepsis (Kempe et al., 2007), sickle cell disease (Wood et al., 1996), thalassemia (Kuypers et al., 1998), glucose-6-phosphate dehydrogenase deficiency (Lang et al., 2002), and phosphate depletion (Birka et al., 2004) are more sensitive to apoptotic stimuli, a property correlating with the shortened erythrocyte lifespan in these disorders. Membrane lipid disorders play an important role in the pathology of hemoglobinopathies, leading to premature removal (anemia) and imbalance in hemostasis (e.g. lipid breakdown products of phosphatidylserine-exposed cells result in vascular dysfunction) (Neidlinger et al., 2006).

Altered phosphorylation of erythrocyte cytoskeletal proteins and increased ROS production result in disruption of cytoskeleton stability in healthy and sickle cell erythrocytes (George et al., 2010).

Significant modifications in red blood cell structure and membrane proteome in end stage renal disease patients were observed in the context of increased ROS accumulation. The intrinsic oxidative stimuli related to the uremic state were closely associated with membrane cytoskeleton instability, loss of surface area through vesiculation, and transformation of normal discocytes. The observed alterations might contribute to premature erythrocyte death and to the progression of anemia (Antonelou et al., 2011).

Under normal conditions, red blood cells are continuously exposed to ROS from both internal and external sources. In healthy erythrocytes, significant oxidative damage is prevented by a very efficient antioxidant system, consisting of enzymatic and nonenzymatic pathways. Enzymes for preventing oxidative denaturation in erythrocytes include superoxide dismutase, catalase, glutathione peroxidase and glutathione reductase which sustain glutathione regeneration, and NADH-methemoglobin reductase. In addition to primary antioxidant defense systems that prevent the generation of free radicals or radical chain reactions, secondary systems have been proposed. These include proteases that preferentially degrade proteins damaged by oxidation. Endogenous non-enzymatic antioxidants also provide defense against oxidative damage: they are lipophylic (vitamin E, carotenoids, melatonin) and water soluble compounds (vitamin C, gluthatione, ceruloplasmin, uric acid) (Burak Çimen, 2008).

Free radicals are produced as intermediate products of normal metabolic functions. Thus, antioxidants function as modulators of cellular homeostasis including detoxification of radicals and metals as well as potent free radical scavengers.

Erythropoietin, the hormone that is the principal regulator of red blood cell production, prevents apoptosis of erythroid progenitors, supporting their survival. It is well known that the target cells for erythropoietin are the progenitors of erythrocytes found in the hematopoietic organs. However, early works have shown prolonged red blood cell survival during treatment with recombinant human erythropoietin (Schwartz et al., 1992; Polenakovic & Sikole, 1996), suggesting a contribution to the maintenance of corrected hematocrit values. Later, other works were performed to elucidate mechanisms of action of erythropoietin upon mature erythrocytes. Myssina et al. (2003) reported that erythropoietin inhibited cell death through a direct effect via erythropoietin receptor on mature erythrocytes. Unlike the general knowledge of the absence of erythropoietin receptors in reticulocytes, the authors detected the expression of about six erythropoietin binding sites per mature red blood cell. In this work, they postulated that erythropoietin bound to erythrocytes inhibited the volume-sensitive cation channel responsible for calcium entry, and thus blocked phosphatidylserine translocation. More investigation is needed to elucidate the erythropoietin effects upon erythrocytes, since it is well known that erythropoietin induces increased intracellular $Ca^{2+}$ concentration in human erythroid progenitors when they are activated via binding of the hormone with its specific receptor.

On the other hand, a direct effect of erythropoietin on mature erythrocytes might be possible, since erythropoietin similar to other proteins would protect red cell membranes from lipid peroxidation by scavenging hydroxyl radicals generated by oxidative stress. Chattopadhyay et al. (2000) reported that the oxidative damage brought about by copper (II) ascorbate upon red blood cells was due to generation of hydroxyl radical and that erythropoietin was able to protect the membrane from oxidative damage.

In a preliminary study, mature erythrocytes from patients with chronic renal insufficiency exhibited higher annexin binding when compared with red blood cells from healthy individuals. Moreover, the number of cells expressing phosphatidylserine externalization decreased after dialysis only when patients received erythropoietin immediately before dialysis (Myssina et al., 2003). Irrespective the erythropoietin mechanism it seems that the hormone does not only inhibit apoptosis of erythroid progenitor cells, but blunts the suicidal death of mature erythrocytes. This protective antieryptotic mechanism may ameliorate erythrocyte death *in vivo*, resulting in increased lifespan of circulating cells.

## 7. Conclusion

The human red blood cell, by lacking nucleus or any other subcellular organelle, represents the final differentiation stage of the erythroid series. After a limited period in circulation, aged cells become sequestered and removed by macrophages from the reticuloendothelial system. This fate implies that erythrocyte life and death should be well regulated.

Senescence of red blood cells occurs along their lifespan in the vascular system. During aging, erythrocytes display molecules that lead to recognition and removal of old damaged cells by the immune system. Current evidence indicates that neoantigens on altered band 3 and phosphatidylserine exposed at the outside of erythrocytes are the main signals for cell removal and phagocytosis. Vesicles, generated as an integral part of the aging process probably to remove damaged membrane patches, disappear rapidly from circulation. The formation of vesicles as well as changes in electrolyte movements lead to decreased cell volume. Disruption of cell metabolism, hemoglobin denaturalization, changes in cytoskeletal protein interaction, protein phosphorylation/dephosphorylation disbalance, and membrane protein modifications are among the factors responsible for the appearance of morphological alterations.

Considering that senescence represents the time-dependent induction of erythrocyte self-destruction process, premature cell death due to proeryptotic factors could greatly contribute to the development of anemia.
Energy depletion, oxidative stress, and osmotic shock are the most common events that can produce erythrocyte damage, leading to premature eryptosis (Fig. 2). The common feature is the increased intracellular calcium concentration due to either calcium channel activation or depressed calcium pump. Calcium accumulation in turn activates the potassium channel favoring this cation efflux, followed by chloride and water exit, which in conjunction generate cell shrinkage. Calpain, activated by calcium, affects cytoskeletal proteins inducing membrane destabilization and blebbling, and is involved in scramblase activation, thus facilitating phosphatydilserine translocation.

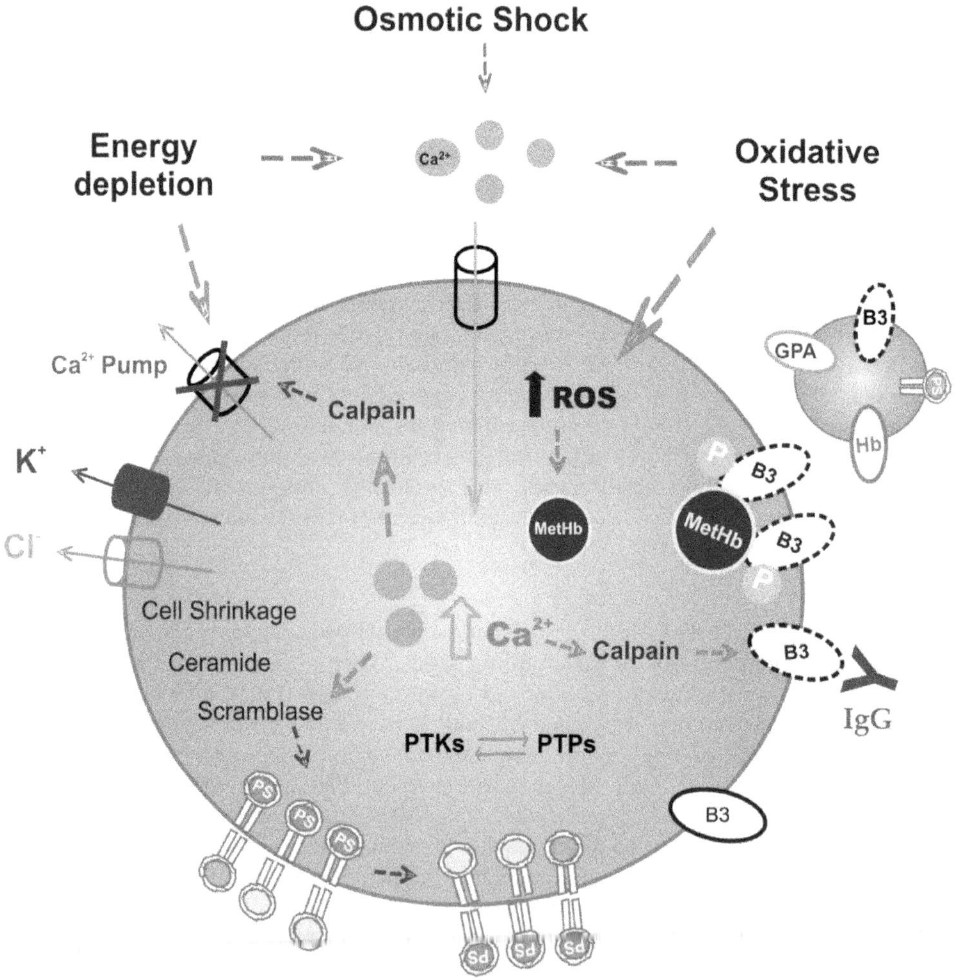


Fig. 2. Mechanisms involved in programmed erythrocyte death. B3: band 3; ROS: reactive oxygen species; Hb: hemoglobin; MetHb: methemoglobin; GPA: glycophorin A; PTKs: phosphotyrosine kinases; PTPs: phosphotyrosine phosphateses; PS: phosphatidylserine.

Additional increase in intracellular oxidants by altering ambient oxygen concentrations or lowering antioxidant levels also accelerates the onset of senescence. Concurrent effects mediated by oxidized hemoglobin and by protein phosphorylation due to disbalance in the kinase/phosphatase ratio are directed towards erythrocyte damage, and consequently to eryptosis.

It is evident that elucidation of mechanisms that regulate eryptosis is a complex issue because of technical problems in obtaining purified cell fractions of a well-defined cell age or in the correct manipulation of erythrocytes *in vitro*, and especially due to the low probability to test hypothesis of programmed erythrocyte death *in vivo*. However, to get an insight into this mechanism is essential for understanding the pathological circumstances surrounding anemia associated to many different diseases.

## 8. Acknowledgments

Dr. Daniela Vittori and Dr. Alcira Nesse are research scientists from the CONICET (National Council for Scientific and Technical Research, Argentina), and Lic. Daiana Vota is recipient of a fellowship from CONICET. The three authors are teachers at the Department of Biological Chemistry (School of Sciences, University of Buenos Aires, Argentina).

## 9. References

Allan, D. & Thomas, P. (1981). Ca2+-induced biochemical changes in human erythrocytes and their relation to microvesiculation. *Biochem J* 198, 433-440.

Antonelou, M.H., Kriebardis, A.G., Velentzas, A.D., Kokkalis, A.C., Georgakopoulou, S-C., & Papassideri I.S. (2011). Oxidative stress-associated shape transformation and membrane proteome remodeling in erythrocytes of end stage renal disease patients on hemodialysis. *J Proteom* doi:10.1016/j.jprot.2011.04.009.

Berg, C.P., Engels, I.H., Rothbart, A., Lauber, K., Renz, A., Schlosser, S.F., Schulze-Osthoff, K., & Wesselborg. S. (2001). Human mature red blood cells express caspase-3 and caspase-8, but are devoid of mitochondrial regulators of apoptosis. *Cell Death Differ* 8, 1197-1206.

Bevers, E.M. & Williamson, P.L. (2010). Phospholipid scramblase: an update. *FEBS Letters* 584, 2724-2730.

Bilmen, S., Aksu, T.A., Gümüslü, S., Korquin, D.K., & Canatan, D. (2001). Antioxidant capacity of G-6-PD-deficient erythrocytes. *Clin Chim Acta* 303, 83-86.

Birka, C., Lang, P.A., Kempe, D.S., Hoefling, L., Tanneur, V., Duranton, C., Nammi, S., Henke, G., Myssina, S., Krikov, M., Huber, S.M., Wieder, T., & Lang, F. (2004). Enhanced susceptibility to erythrocyte "apoptosis" following phosphate depletion. *Pflugers Arch* 448, 471–477.

Bosman, G.J., Willekens, F.L., & Werre, J.M. (2005). Erythrocyte aging: a more than superficial resemblance to apoptosis? *Cell Physiol Biochem* 16, 1-8.

Bosman, G.J., Lasonder, E., Groenen-Döpp, Y.A., Willekens, F.L., Werre, J.M., & Novotný, V.M. (2010). Comparative proteomics of erythrocyte aging in vivo and in vitro. *J Proteom* 73, 396-402.

Bratosin, D., Mazurier, J., Tissier, J.P., Estaquier, J., Huart, J.J., Ameisen, J.C., Aminoff, D., & Montruil, J. (1998). Cellular and molecular mechanisms of senescent erythrocyte phagocytosis by macrophages. A review. *Biochemie* 80, 173-195.

Bratosin, D., Estaquier, J., Petit, F., Arnoult, D., Quatannens, B., Tissier, J-P., Slomianny, C., Sartiaux, C., Alonso, C., Huart, J-J., Montreuil, J., & Ameisen, J.C. (2001). Programmed cell death in mature erythrocytes: a model for investigating death effector pathways operating in the absence of mitochondria. *Cell Death Differ* 8, 1143-1156.

Bratosin, D., Estaquier, J., Ameisen, J.C., & Montreuil, J. (2002). Molecular and cellular mechanisms of programmed cell death: impact on blood transfusion. *Vox Sang* 83, 307-310.

Brunati, A.M., Bordin, L., Clari, G., & Morel, V. (1996). The Lyn-catalyzed Tyr phosphorylation of the transmembrane band 3 protein of the human erythrocytes. *Eur J Biochem* 240, 394-399.

Burak Çimen, M.Y. (2008). Free radical metabolism in human erythrocytes. *Clin Chim Acta* 390, 1-11.

Calderón-Salinas, J.V., Muñoz-Reyes, E.G., Guerrero-Romero, J.F., Rodríguez-Morán, M., Bracho-Riquelme, R.L., Carrera-Gracia, M.A., & Quintanar-Escorza, M.A. (2011). Eryptosis and oxidative damage in type 2 diabetic mellitus patients with chronic kidney disease. *Mol Cell Biochem* doi: 10.1007/s11010-011-0887-1.

Callero, M.A., Vota, D.M., Chamorro, M.E., Wenker, S.D., Vittori, D.C., & Nesse, A.B. (2011). Calcium as a mediator between erythropoietin and protein tyrosine phosphatase 1B. *Arch Biochem Biophys* 505, 242-249.

Chandra, R., Joshi, P.C., Bajpai, V.K., & Gupta, C.M. (1987). Membrane phopholipid organization in calcium-loaded human erythrocytes. *Biochim Biophys Acta* 902, 253-262.

Chattopadhyay, A., Das Choudhury, T., Bandyopadhyay, D., & Datta A. (2000). Protective effect of erythropoietin on the oxidative damage of erythrocyte membrane by hydroxyl radical. *Biochem Pharmacol* 59, 419-425.

Daleke, D.L. (2008). Regulation of phospholipid asymmetry in the erythrocyte membrane. *Curr Opin Hematol* 15, 191-195.

Dumaswala, U.J., Jacobsen, D.W., Jain, S.K., & Sukalski, K.A. (1999). Protein and lipid oxidation of banked human erythrocytes: role of glutathione. *Free Radic Biol Med* 27, 1041-1049.

Duranton, B., Huber, S.M., & Lang, F. (2002). Oxidation induced a Cl(-)-dependent cation conductance in human red blood cells. *Cell Biol Toxicol* 18, 381-396.

Ferru, E., Giger, K., Pantaleo, A., Campanella, E., Grey, J., Ritchie, K., Vono, R., Turrini, F., & Low, P. (2011). Regulation of membrane-cytoskeletal interactions by tyrosine phosphorylation of erythrocyte band 3. *Blood* 117, 5998-6006.

Föller, M., Kasinathan, R. S., Koka, S., Lang, C., Shumilina, E., Birnbaumer, L., Lang, F., & Huber, S. M. (2008). TRPC6 contributes to the $Ca^{2+}$ leak of human erythrocytes. *Cell Physiol Biochem* 21, 183–192.

Frangioni, J.V., Oda, A., Smith, M., Salzman, E., & Neel, B.G. (1993). Calpain-catalyzed cleavage amd subcellular relocation of protein phosphotyrosine phosphatase 1B (PTP-1B) in human platelets. *EMBO J* 12, 4843-4856.

George, A., Pushkaran, S., Li, L., An, X., Zheng, Y., & Mohandas, N. (2010). Altered phosphorylation of cytoskeleton proteins in sickle red blood cells: The role of protein kinase C, Rac GTPases, and reactive oxygen species. *Blood Cells Mol Dis* 45, 41-45.

Harrison, M.L., Rathinavelu, P., Arese, P., Geahlen, R.L., & Low, P.S. (1991). Role of Band 3 tyrosine phosphorylation in the regulation of erythrocyte glycolysis. *J Biol Chem* 266, 4106-4111.

Kaestner, L. & Bernhardt, I. (2002). Ion channels in the human red blood cell membrane: their further investigation and physiological relevance. *Bioelectrochemistry* 55, 71-74.

Kay, M.M., Flowers, N., Goodman, J., & Bosman, G. (1989). Alteration in membrane protein band 3 associated with accelerated erythrocyte aging. *Proc Natl Acad Sci (USA).* 86, 5834-5838.

Kay, M. (2005). Immunoregulation of cellular life span. *Ann N Y Acad Sci* 1057, 85-111.

Kempe, D.S., Akel, A., Lang, P.A., Hermle, T., Biswas, R., Muresanu, J., Friedrich, B., Dreischer, P., Wolz, C., Schumacher, U., Peschel, A., Götz, F., Döring, G., Wieder, T., Gulbins, E., & Lang, F. (2007). Suicidal erythrocyte death in sepsis. *J Mol Med (Berl)* 85, 273-281.

Kirkpatrick, F.H., Hillman, D.G., & La Celle, P.L. (1975). A23187 and red cells: changes in deformability, $K^+$, $Mg^{2+}$, $Ca^{2+}$ and ATP. *Experientia* 31, 653-654.

Kuypers, F.A., Yuan, J., Lewis, R.A., Snyder, L.M., Kiefer, C.R., Bunyjaratvej, A. Fucharoen, S., Ma, L., Styles, L., de Jong, K., & Schrier, S.L. (1998). Membrane phospholipid asymmetry in human thalassemia. *Blood* 91, 3044-3051.

Lang, K.S., Roll, B., Myssina, S., Schittenhelm, M., Scheel-Walter, H.G., Kanz, L., Fritz, J., Lang, F., Huber, S.M., & Wieder, T. (2002). Enhanced erythrocyte apoptosis in sickle cell anemia, thalassemia, and glucose-6-phosphate dehydrogenase deficiency. *Cell Physiol Biochem* 12, 365-372.

Lang, K.S., Myssina, S., Brand, V., Sandu, C., Lang, P.A., Berchtold, S., Huber, S.M., Lang, F., & Wieder, T. (2004). Involvemnt of ceramide in hyperosmotic shock-induced death of erythrocytes. *Cell Death Differ* 11, 231-243.

Lang, K.S., Lang, P.A., Bauer, C., Duranton, C., Wieder, T., Huber, S., & Lang, F. (2005). Mechanisms of suicidal erythrocyte death. Cell Physiol Biochem 15, 195-202.

Lang, P.A., Kempe, D.S., Myssina, S., Tanneur, V., Birka, C., Laufer, S., Lang, F., Wieder, T., & Huber S.M. (2005). PGE(2) in the regulation of programmed erythrocyte death. *Cell Death Differ* 12, 415-428.

Mallozi, C., Di Stasi, A.M., & Minetti, M. (1995). Free radicals induce reversible membrane-cytoplasm translocation of glyceraldehydes-3-phosphate dehydogenase in human erythrocytes. *Arch Biochem Biophys* 321, 345-352.

Mallozi, C., Di Stasi, A.M., & Minetti, M. (2001). Nitrotyrosine mimics phosphotyrosine binding to the SH2 domain of the *src* family tyrosine kinase *lyn*. *FEBS Letters* 503, 189-195.

Mandal, D., Mazumder, A., Das, P., Kundu, M., & Basu, J. (2005). Fas-, caspase-8, and caspase-3-dependent signaling regulates the activity of the aminophospholipid translocase and phosphatidylserine externalization in human erythrocytes. *J Biol Chem* 280, 39460-39467.

Manno, S., Takakuwa, Y., & Mohandas N. (2002). Identification of a functional role for lipid asymmetry in biological membranes: Phosphatidylserine-skeletal protein interactions modulate membrane stability. *Proc Natl Acad Sci (USA)* 99, 1943-1948.

Manuel y Keenoy, B., Vertommen, J., & De Leeuw, I. (2001). Divergent effects of different oxidants on glutathione homeostasis and protein damage in erythrocytes from diabetic patients: effects of high glucose. *Mol Cell Biochem* 225, 59-73.

Matarrese, P., Straface, E., Pietraforte, D., Gambardella, L., Vona, R., Maccaglia, A., Minetti, M., & Malomi, W. (2005). Peroxynitrite induces senescence and apoptosis of red blood cells through the activation of aspartyl and cysteinyl porteases. *FASEB J* 19, 416-8.

Meers, P. & Mealy, T. (1994). Phospholipid determinants for the annexin V binding sites and the role of tryptophan 187. *Biochemistry* 33, 5829-5837.

Metere, A., Iorio, E., Pietraforte, D., Podo, F., & Minetti, M. (2009). Peroxynitrite signaling in human erythrocytes: Synergistic role of hemoglobin oxidation and band 3 tyrosine phospsorylation. *Arch Biochem Biophys* 484, 173-182.

Mohandas, N., & Groner, W. (1989). Cell membrane and volume changes during red cell development and aging. *Ann N Y Acad Sci* 554,217-224.

Myssina, S., Huber, S.M., Birka, C., Lang, P.A., Lang, K.S., Friedrich, B., Risler, T., Wieder, T, & Lang, F. (2003). Inhibition of erythrocyte cation channels by erythropoietin. *J Am Soc Nephrol* 14, 2750-2757.

Neidlinger, N.A., Larkin, S.K., Bhagat, A., Victorino, G.P., & Kuypers, F.A. (2006). Hydrolysis of phosphatidylserine-exposing red blood cells by secretory phospholipase A2 generates lysophosphatidic acid and results in vascular dysfunction. *J Biol Chem* 28, 775-781.

O'Toole, P.J., Wolfe, C., Ladha, S., & Cherry, R.J. (1999). Rapid diffusion of spectrin bound to a lipid surface. *Biochim Biophys Acta* 1419, 64-70.

Palek, J., Stewart, G., & Lionetti, F.J. (1974). The dependence of shape of human erythrocyte ghosts on calcium, magnesium, and adenosine triphosphate. *Blood* 44, 583-597.

Palfrey, H.C. & Waseem, A. (1985). Protein kinase C in the human erythrocyte. Translocation to the plasma membrane and phosphorylation of bands 4.1 and 4.9 and other membrane proteins. *J Biol Chem* 260, 16021-16029.

Pietraforte, D., Matarrese, P., Straface, E., Gambardella, L., Metere, A., Scorza, G., Leto, T., Malorni, W., & Minetti, M. (2007). Two different pathways are envolved in peroxynitrite-induced senescente and apoptosis of human erythrocytes. *Free Radical Biol Med* 42, 202-214.

Polenakovic, M. & Sikole, A. (1996). Is erythropoietin a survival factor for red blood cells? *J Am Soc Nephrol* 7, 1178-1182.

Quintanar-Escorza, M.A., González-Martínez, M.T., Intriago-Ortega, M.P., & Calderón-Salinas, J.V. (2010). Oxidative damage increases intracellular free calcium $[Ca^{2+}]_i$ concentration in human erythrocytes incubated with lead. *Toxicol In Vitro* 24, 1338-1346.

Richards, R.S., Wang, L., & Jelinek, H. (2007). Erythrocyte Oxidative Damage in Chronic Fatigue Syndrome. *Archiv Med Res* 38, 94-98.

Romero, N. & Radi, R. (2005). Hemoglobin and red blood cells as tools for studying peroxinitrite biochemistry. *Methods Enzymol* 396, 229-245.

Romero, P.J. (1976) The role of membrane-bound Ca in ghost permeability to Na and K. *J Membrane Biol* 29, 329-343.

Romero, P.J. & Romero, E.A. (1999). The role of calcium metabolism in human red blood cell ageing: A Proposal. *Blood Cells Mol Dis* 15, 9-19.

Salamino, F., Sparatore, B., Melloni, E., Michetti, M., Vioti, P.L., Pontremoli, S., & Carafoli, E. (1994). The plasma membrane calcium pump is the preferred calpain substrate within the erythrocyte. *Cell Calcium* 15, 28-35.

Schatzmann, H.J. (1983). The red cell calcium pump. *Annu Rev Physiol* 45, 303-312.

Schlegel, R.A. & Williamson, P. (2001). Phosphatidylserine, a death knell. *Cell Death Differ* 8, 551-563.

Schwartz, A.B., Kahn, S.B., Kelch, B., Kim K.E., & Pequignot, E. (1992). Red blood cell improved survival due to recombinant human erythropoietin explained effectiveness of less frequent, low dose subcutaneous therapy. *Clin Nephrol* 38, 283-289.

Soupene, E. & Kuypers, F.A. (2006). Identification of an erythroid ATP-dependent aminophospholipid transporter. *Brit J Hematol* 133, 436-438.

Szabó, C., Ischiropoulos, H., & Radi, R. (2007). Peroxynitrite: biochemistry, pathophysiology and development of therapeutics. *Nature Rev* 6, 662-680.

Tang, X., Halleck, M.S., Schlegel, R.A., & Williamson, P. (1996). A subfamily of P-type ATPases with aminophospholipid transporting activity. *Science* 272, 1495-1497.

Trümpler, A., Schlott, B., Herrlich, P., Greer, P., & Böhmer, F-D. (2009). Calpain-mediated degradation of reversibly oxidized protein-tyrosine phosphatase 1B. *FEBS J* 276, 5622-5633.

Vota, D., Callero, M., Chamorro, M.E., Crisp, R., Nesse, A., & Vittori, D. (2010). Mechanisms involved in premature self-destruction of red blood cells under different eryptosis stimuli. *Haematologica* 95 (s2), 304.

Wallis, C.J., Babitch, J.A., & Wenegieme, E.F. (1993). Divalent cation binding to erythrocyte spectrin. *Biochemistry* 32, 5045-5050.

Weed, R.I., La Celle, P.L., & Merrill, E.W. (1969). Metabolic dependence of red cell deformability. *J Clin Invest* 48, 795-809.

Willekens, F.L., Werre, J.M., Groenen-Döpp, Y.A., Roerdinkholder-Stoelwinder, B., de Pauw, B., & Bosman, G.J. (2008). Erythrocyte vesiculation: a self-protective mechanism? *Brit J Haematol* 141, 549-556.

Williamson, P, Kulick, A., Zachowski, A., Schlegel, R.A., & Devaux, P.F. (1992). $Ca^{2+}$ induces transbilayer redistribution of all major phospholipids in human erythrocytes. *Biochemistry* 31, 6355-6360.

WIliamson, P. & Schlegel, R.A. (2002). Transbilayer phospholipids movement and the clearance of apoptotic cells. *Biochim Biophys Acta* 1585, 53-63.

Wood, B.L., Gibson, D.F., & Tait, J.F. (1996). Increased phosphatidylserine exposure in sickle cell disease: flow-cytometric measurements and clinical associations. *Blood* 88, 1873-1880.

Zachee, P., Emonds, M., Lins, R., & Boogaerts, M. (1988). Red blood cells, the scavengers for toxic free radicals during haemodialysis. *Nephrol Dial Transplant* 4, 104-105.

Zipser, Y., Piade, A., Barbul, A., Korenstein, R., & Kosower, N.S. (2002). Ca2+ promotes erythrocyte band 3 tyrosine phosphorylation via dissociation of phosphotyrosine phosphatase from band 3. *Biochem J* 368, 137-144.

# 3

# Phosphatidylserine Shedding from RBCs – A Mechanism of Membrane Modulation and Damage Control

Eitan Fibach
*Hematology, Hadassah – Hebrew University Medical Center, Jerusalem Israel*

## 1. Introduction

Normally, phospholipids (PLs) are distributed across the membrane of all cells, including the RBCs, asymmetrically [1]: aminophospholipids such as phosphatidylserine (PS) are mainly localized in the cytoplasmic leaflet of the membrane, whereas lipids with a choline head (e.g., phosphatidylcholine) are mainly localized in the outer leaflet [2]. The PS distribution across the cell membrane is in a dynamic equilibrium; while the enzyme aminophospholipid translocase inserts it inward, the scramblase causes its externalization. Some of this external PS is shed into the extracellular medium either as membrane-bound vesicles [3] or as membrane-free PS [4]. In RBCs, exposed PS is one of the signals of senescence, mediating the removal of old or damaged RBCs from the circulation [5]. Shedding of PS may reduce this signal and thus function to moderate RBC removal [6]. PS externalization and shedding are also associated with development of RBCs in the bone marrow, fulfilling various structural and functional purposes [7]. In the present review I we summarize our studied on changes in PS distribution and shedding during maturation and ageing of erythroid cells.

## 2. Methodologies

For these studies we have employed two analytical methodologies, Nuclear Magnetic Resonance (NMR) spectroscopy [4] and flow cytometry [8]. Using $^{1}$H- and $^{31}$P-NMR procedures, we measured absolute concentrations of metabolites in aqueous and organic extracts of the cells [9-12].

Flow cytometry was employed to measure various parameters of cellular oxidative stress: generation of reactive oxygen species (ROS) and membrane lipid peroxides, the intracellular content of reduced glutathione [13], as well as the contents of the labile iron [14] and calcium (Ca). These measurements are based on changes in the fluorescence intensities of specific probes.

To measure the cellular distribution of PS and its shedding from erythroid cells, we developed a two-step fluorescence inhibition assay [8]. PS is usually estimated by staining cells with annexin V which specifically binds to PS. Fluorochrome-conjugated annexin V is used to determine the percentage of PS-carrying cells by flow cytometry [15, 16]. This method is applicable to populations containing a significant fraction of positive cells, for example, following exposure to an apoptosis-inducing agent. However, in vivo, at a given time, only a small fraction of any cell population is apoptotic, making their determination statistically unreliable. In addition, this procedure does not yield information regarding the inner PS, which is not exposed on the outer surface of the cells, nor on the PS shed into the surrounding medium. Moreover, the method refers usually only to strongly positive cells, giving the impression that the process occurs in an "all or none" fashion, neglecting cells with less than maximal amount of bound annexin V. Most importantly, the procedure provides relative comparison rather than absolute quantitative values.

To overcome these limitations, we developed a novel flow cytometry methodology that provides a quantitative measurement of the external PS as well as the intracellular and shed PS. The procedure entails two steps: In the first step, the outer PS of intact cells or the total PS of cell lysates and supernatants, or human serum is bound to excess amount of fluorescent-annexin V. In the second step, the residual, non-bound fluorescent-annexin V is quantified by binding to PS exposed on apoptotic cells (e.g., 6-day old HL-60 cells) which serve as an indicator reagent. The fluorescence of these indicator cells is reciprocally proportional to the amount of PS on the measured cells in the first step [8].

## 3. PS exposure and shedding during the lifespan of RBCs in the circulation

During their life in the circulation, RBCs are exposed to several stress situations, which are (i) physical, occurring when they squeeze through small capillaries, (ii) hyperosmotic, when they travel through the kidney medulla, and (iii) oxidative, when they pass the oxygenated lung. These stress conditions affect the RBC composition and properties, leading to their senescence and eventually to their elimination from the circulation.

One of the signals of senescence is PS externalization. PS-carrying RBCs undergo phagocytosis (erythrophagocytosis) by macrophages in the reticulo-endothelial system (extravascular hemolysis) [5]. Under normal conditions this occurs in humans after 120 days, but under pathological conditions this process is accelerated, thereby shortening the life-span of RBCs, causing hemolytic anemia. These hemolytic anemias are hereditary, such as the hemoglobinopathies, thalassemia and sickle cell disease, or acquired, such as the myelodysplastic syndromes.

Using the methodologies described above, we studied the externalization and shedding of PS in RBCs during their senescence and compared RBCs derived from the peripheral blood of normal donors and patients with hemolytic anemias. $^{31}$P-NMR analysis indicated that compared to normal RBCs, thalassemic RBCs have lower concentrations of total cellular PS which was associated with increased PS shedding [4]. Flow cytometry measurements, using fluorescent annexin V as a probe, confirmed these results and further demonstrated that despite of the decreased total cellular PS, in thalassemic RBCs, the PS exposed on their outer membrane was significantly increased. This was reflected not only by moderate increase in the percentage of annexin V positive cells as measured by the direct method, but also by a significant increase in exposed PS on the entire population as measured by the indirect method. The increased PS exposure reflected the balance between the decrease in the inner membrane PS and the increase in the shedding of PS into the extracellular milieu. The increased PS shedding by thalassemic RBCs was also reflected in the higher PS concentration in sera of thalassemic patients compared with normal donors. It should be mentioned that while shedding is often described in the context of microparticles, i.e., membrane-bound vesicles [3], we have shown that the majority of the shed PS is membrane-free [8].

PS shedding has a profound effect on the membrane composition and functionality. The PLs and cholesterol are the major lipid membrane components. Using a $^1$H-NMR, we determined their ratio in normal and thalassemic RBC membranes and in supernatants following in vitro incubation [6]. The results indicated a significant decrease in PLs in the membranes and an increase in the supernatants, while cholesterol was only slightly decreased in the membrane and was minimal in the supernatants. These changes resulted in an increased cholesterol/PL ratio in the RBC membranes. Thalassemic RBCs demonstrated a higher basal cholesterol/PL ratio than normal RBCs. These findings suggest that shedding is a selective process involving mainly PLs and leading to relative accumulation of cholesterol in the membrane.

PS shedding and the consequential changes in the membrane composition and properties affect its functionality. It increased its osmotic resistance and the susceptibility of RBCs to undergo erythrophagocytosis. Using cultured macrophages, we have shown that while PS externalization increased phagocytosis, the shed PS prevented it, probably by competitive binding to PS receptors on the macrophages [6].

PS shedding may play a role in the functioning and fate of mature RBCs in the circulation:

a. Shedding of PS-enriched membranes [3, 4] might cause size reduction which characterizes RBC senescence as well as microcytic anemias. Shedding might serve mainly to rejuvenate the plasma membrane of the RBCs by removing its damaged components [17].
b. The cholesterol content of the RBC plasma membrane was reported to affect its mechanical properties (fluidity) [18, 19]. During physiological aging, senescent RBCs showed an increased cholesterol/PL ratio followed by greater membrane strength [20]. We have shown that in RBCs PS shedding and relative accumulation of cholesterol are associated with a greater osmotic resistance [6].
c. PS externalization has been suggested as one of the mechanisms of senescent RBC clearance from the circulation by PS receptor carrying reticuloendothelial system macrophages [5]. We have shown that whereas PS externalization increases phagocytosis, PS shedding decreases it [4]. The latter effect may be attributed to a decrease in the exposed PS, as well as competition by the shed PS for the macrophage PS receptors. Thus, the balance between PS externalization and shedding may play a role in controlling the fate/lifespan of the RBCs in the circulation under both physiological and pathological conditions, e.g., in thalassemia where RBCs were shown to have increased PS shedding [4, 8].
d. Finally, it is worth mentioning that PS has procoagulant properties [21]. Exposed and shed PS could be involved in normal and pathological homeostasis [1]. Thus, thalassemic patients with increased exposed and shed PS are prone to thromboembolic complications [22, 23].

## 4. PS shedding during development of erythroid cells

RBCs are produced in the bone marrow by a well regulated process (erythropoiesis) that involves proliferation and maturation. PS externalization and shedding have important roles in this process [7]. We studied normal human bone marrow cells as well as two in vitro models of erythropoiesis, primary cultures of human erythroid precursors and a murine erythroleukemia cell line. The human erythroid precursors are derived from progenitors present in the peripheral blood of normal donors. They are stimulated by the physiological inducer erythropoietin to proliferate and mature into hemoglobin-containing nucleated orthochromatophilic normoblasts. This system provides a reliable *in vitro* model that recapitulates many aspects of erythroid maturation [24]. The murine cells, derived originally from the spleen of viral induced leukemia, were stimulated to undergo erythroid maturation by hexamethylene bis acetamide [25] [26]. In all these systems, both PS exposure and shedding were found to be high in early precursors, and to be reduced during maturation.

Several suggestions might be raised regarding the role of PS shedding in the maturation of erythroid cells:

a. Size reduction characterizes not only RBC senescence in the circulation, but also erythroid maturation in the bone marrow. During their maturation erythroid precursors undergo a gradual and continuous, but a significant, reduction in size [27, 28]. This is an important functional adaptation generating mature RBCs small enough to pass through narrow capillaries. It also generates a high surface to volume ratio that promotes gas exchange between the RBCs and tissue cells during this passage. Shedding of PS-enriched membranes [3, 4] during maturation might be the cause or the outcome of the size reduction process. We have shown that inhibition of PS externalization/shedding prevented size reduction in differentiating erythroid cells [7], favoring the first possibility.
b. Apoptosis of nuclear cells involves PS externalization [29]. RBC production is regulated by apoptosis of erythroid precursors, which is controlled by erythropoietin, serving as an anti-apoptotic agent [30]. We found that depletion of erythropoietin during maturation of cultured erythroid precursors results in PS externalization, suggesting that this process is involved in the apoptosis of erythroid precursors as part of normal or pathological (ineffective) erythropoiesis (e.g., in the myelodysplastic syndrome or thalassemia), while PS shedding may have an opposite effect.
c. During their early development in the bone marrow, erythroid precursors are found in erythroblast islands, where they surround a central macrophage [31]. A diverse array of adhesion proteins expressed on the erythroblast surface mediate its interaction with both stromal cells and the extracellular matrix [32, 33]. It is possible that the outer PS on these precursors may assist in their attachment to macrophages carrying PS receptors, thus forming the erythroblast islands. Outer PS shedding (in addition to PS internalization) may lessen this adhesion and facilitate the release of erythroid precursors from the island as they mature. This possibility awaits experimental confirmation.
d. During maturation, erythroid precursors expel their cellular organelles, including the nucleus, mitochondria and ribosomes, by exocytosis through membrane-bound vesicles [34, 35]. Recent results indicated that enucleation is caused by the coalescence of vesicles at the nuclear-cytoplasmic junction, whereas, mitochondria are eliminated through selective autophagy [36]. Plasma membrane remodeling by PS redistribution might also be part of this process. Yoshida et al. have shown that "the nuclei are engulfed by macrophages only after they are disconnected from reticulocytes, and that phosphatidylserine, which is often used as an 'eat me' signal for apoptotic cells, is also used for the engulfment of nuclei expelled from erythroblasts" [37].

## 5. Mechanisms involved in PS shedding

We studied several mechanisms in relation to the above described changes in PS distribution: the oxidative status of the cells, changes in Ca-flux and microtubule (MT) polymerization.

## 6. Oxidative stress

The oxidative status of cells depends on the balance between oxidants (such as ROS) and antioxidants. Under pathological conditions, the balance leans towards generation of excess oxidants, which is accompanied by reduced content of antioxidants, resulting in oxidative stress. Although free radicals have important roles in normal physiology, such as in signal transduction, in excess they interact with and damage various components of the cells (e.g., proteins, lipids and nucleic acids). Many diseases are associated with oxidative stress, including hemolytic anemias. Although these anemias vary as to their etiology, in all cases the damage to erythroid cells is mediated by oxidative stress [38]. Using flow cytometry, we have demonstrated oxidative stress in normal mature RBCs treated with various oxidants: increased generation of ROS and membrane lipid peroxides and decreased content of reduced glutathione - the main cellular antioxidant. Similar results were obtained in RBCs derived from patients with thalassemia, sickle cell disease, myelodysplastic syndromes (MDS), paroxysmal nocturnal hemoglobinuria, spherocytosis and other hemolytic anemias. $^{1}$H-NMR analysis demonstrated oxidative stress in such RBCs by a high lactate/pyruvate ratio [4].

Oxidative stress reduces the activity of the enzyme translocase [39], causing the equilibrium that exists between the PS on the inner and the outer membrane leaflets to lean towards externalization. We have found that oxidatively stressed RBCs (old vs. young RBCs, thalassemic vs. normal RBCs, oxidant treated vs. non treated normal RBCs) have less total cellular PS but more exposed and shed PS [6]. Ameliorating the oxidative stress, e.g., by treating thalassemic cells with an antioxidant (e.g., vitamin C or N-acetyl cysteine) resulted in opposite results [8].

As mentioned above, in RBCs, exposed PS is one of the signals of senescence [5] and that it induces erythrophagocytosis. This process is accelerated in hemolytic anemias resulting in short survival of RBCs in the circulation. Although in patients with hemolytic anemia the proliferation of erythroid precursors in the bone marrow is increased (by stimulating the production of erythropoietin in the kidneys), when the condition is chronic the production of mature RBCs is futile due to increased premature death (by apoptosis) and lack of maturation of the erythroid precursors (ineffective erythropoiesis) [40]. The supply of mature, functional, RBCs is thus insufficient.

The main cause of oxidative stress in hemolytic anemias is iron overload due to increased iron absorption and repeated blood transfusions. When the iron content in the serum exceeds the binding capacity of transferrin, the iron-transport protein, surplus iron appears as "non-transferrin bound iron", which is taken up by cells, including RBCs, by mechanisms that are transferrin receptor-independent [41]. The incoming iron accumulates intra-cellularly as "labile iron pool" [42, 43], which is of redox potential due to its participation in chemical (Haber-Weiss and Fenton) reactions that generate ROS.

The oxidative status affects PS externalization/shedding also in developing erythroid cells. It is modulated throughout maturation; from being very high in early erythroid precursors it is reduced considerably as the cells mature. This change is most probably related to the decrease in the metabolic rate. Most of the ROS produced by cells are originated in the mitochondria in the process of oxidative energy production [38]. Erythroid maturation involves a loss of mitochondria and a decrease in energy production which results in lower generation of ROS and consequently, in lower PS externalization and shedding.

## 7. Ca-flux

Increase in the intracellular Ca concentration is a well-known mechanism of PS [44]. We studied the relationship between the oxidative state, changes in Ca-flux and PS shedding [6]. It was found that the oxidatively stressed thalassemic RBCs with their increased PS shedding have high Ca content which could be corrected by treatment with antioxidants. The low Ca content and PS-shedding of normal RBCs could be increased by treatment with oxidants. Modulating the Ca content of normal RBCs by treatment with the Ca ionophore A23187 or by varying the Ca concentration in the medium confirmed that increasing the inward Ca flux induced PS externalization and shedding.

## 8. Microtubule (MT) polymerization

Several lines of evidence suggest an interaction between the plasma membrane PLs and cytoskeleton components [45, 46], including the MTs [47,48] - the key components of the cytoskeleton [49]. MTs are made up of αβ-tubulin heterodimers [49], and they readily polymerize and depolymerize in cells. MTs are involved in a variety of cellular processes such as cell division, maintenance of cell shape, cell signaling and migration, and cellular transport [50] as well as maturation and stress. During erythroid maturation, MTs undergo dramatic changes in distribution to become absent in mature mammalian RBCs [51]. It has been shown that at early stages of maturation of murine erythroid precursors MTs are radially arranged just under the plasma membrane. Addition of the MT depolymerization promoters, colchicine or vinblastine, caused MTs to disappear completely. This, however, did not affect enucleation [51]. Addition of paclitaxel (Taxol), which enhances MT polymerization and stabilization, to these cells caused the resulting pre-mature RBCs (reticulocytes) to contain abnormally high numbers of polymerized MTs [51]. Treatment of patients with Taxol caused PS externalization and short survival of their RBCs [52].

We investigated the effect of MT depolymerization in developing erythroid cells on their membrane PS distribution and shedding using cultured human and murine erythroid precursors. Cells were treated with the MT depolymerization enhancer - colchicine and inhibitor - Taxol. The effect of these modulators was studied on the constitutive shedding as well as shedding induced by the Ca-ionophore A23187 [53]. We found that treatment with colchicine and Taxol markedly increased both the constitutive and the induced PS externalization. PS shedding, however, was increased by colchicine, but was inhibited by Taxol.

As discussed above, PS shedding is one of the mechanisms of membrane remodeling [54], including changes in the membrane cholesterol/PL ratio [4, 8]. Using $^1$H-NMR, we showed that colchicine, by enhancing shedding, increased the cholesterol/PL ratio, whereas Taxol, by inhibiting shedding, decreased this ratio.

Many compounds that alter the polymerization dynamics of MTs block mitosis, and consequently, induce cell death by apoptosis [55]. One of these compounds, Taxol, a promoter of MT polymerization and stabilization, is being used for treatment of patients with various malignancies such as breast cancer [56] or ovarian cancer [57]. A significant side effect of this treatment is severe anemia which was related to the effect of Taxol on PS externalization of mature RBC [52]. In line with the importance of PS shedding in erythroid development, the present finding that Taxol affects PS shedding may suggest that anemia in patients treated with Taxol might be also due to its effect on erythropoiesis in the bone marrow.

## 9. Summary

PS externalization and shedding undergo a bi-phasic modulation in erythroid cells: both are decreased during maturation but increased during aging. This redistribution of PS is the outcome of multiple factors and mechanisms, including changes in the cellular oxidative status, Ca concentration and MT polymerization which affect the inward and outward PS flow and PS shedding. These dynamic processes are ongoing continuously and simultaneously, and may have opposite effects. For example, PS exposure on thalassemic RBCs, induced by their high intracellular oxidative status and Ca concentration, is blunted by increased PS shedding. Only when PS externalization overcomes the ability to remove it by shedding are thalassemic RBCs removed by erythrophagocytosis. Further study on the roles played by PS shedding in the production and clearance of RBCs is crucial for understanding its effect on the pathological consequences of hemolytic anemias and for the planning of novel therapeutic modalities to overcome them.

## 10. References

[1] R.F. Zwaal, P. Comfurius, E.M. Bevers, Surface exposure of phosphatidylserine in pathological cells, Cell Mol Life Sci 62 (2005) 971-988.

[2] J.A. Op den Kamp, Lipid asymmetry in membranes, Annu Rev Biochem 48 (1979) 47-71.

[3] K. Pattanapanyasat, E. Noulsri, S. Fucharoen, S. Lerdwana, P. Lamchiagdhase, N. Siritanaratkul, H.K. Webster, Flow cytometric quantitation of red blood cell vesicles in thalassemia, Cytometry B Clin Cytom 57 (2004) 23-31.

[4] I. Freikman, J. Amer, J.S. Cohen, I. Ringel, E. Fibach, Oxidative stress causes membrane phospholipid rearrangement and shedding from RBC membranes--an NMR study, Biochim Biophys Acta 1778 (2008) 2388-2394.

[5] M. Foller, S.M. Huber, F. Lang, Erythrocyte programmed cell death, IUBMB Life 60 (2008) 661-668.

[6] I. Freikman, I. Ringel, E. Fibach, Oxidative Stress-Induced Membrane Shedding from RBCs is Ca Flux-Mediated and Affects Membrane Lipid Composition, J Membr Biol 240 (2011) 73-82.

[7] I. Freikman, E. Fibach, Distribution and shedding of the membrane phosphatidylserine during maturation and aging of erythroid cells, Biochim Biophys Acta 1808 (2011) 2773-280.

[8] I. Freikman, J. Amer, I. Ringel, E. Fibach, A flow cytometry approach for quantitative analysis of cellular phosphatidylserine distribution and shedding, Anal Biochem 393 (2009) 111-116.

[9] J. Schiller, K. Arnold, Application of high resolution 31P NMR spectroscopy to the characterization of the phospholipid composition of tissues and body fluids - a methodological review, Med Sci Monit 8 (2002) MT205-222.
[10] D.J. Philp, W.A. Bubb, P.W. Kuchel, Chemical shift and magnetic susceptibility contributions to the separation of intracellular and supernatant resonances in variable angle spinning NMR spectra of erythrocyte suspensions, Magn Reson Med 51 (2004) 441-444.
[11] I. Spasojevic, V. Maksimovic, J. Zakrzewska, G. Bacic, Effects of 5-fluorouracil on erythrocytes in relation to its cardiotoxicity: membrane structure and functioning, J Chem Inf Model 45 (2005) 1680-1685.
[12] J.E. Raftos, S. Whillier, B.E. Chapman, P.W. Kuchel, Kinetics of uptake and deacetylation of N-acetylcysteine by human erythrocytes, Int J Biochem Cell Biol 39 (2007) 1698-1706.
[13] J. Amer, E. Fibach, Oxidative status of platelets in normal and thalassemic blood, Thromb Haemost 92 (2004) 1052-1059.
[14] E. Prus, E. Fibach, Flow cytometry measurement of the labile iron pool in human hematopoietic cells, Cytometry A 73 (2008) 22-27.
[15] J. Amer, O. Zelig, E. Fibach, Oxidative status of red blood cells, neutrophils, and platelets in paroxysmal nocturnal hemoglobinuria, Exp Hematol 36 (2008) 369-377.
[16] F.A. Kuypers, R.A. Lewis, M. Hua, M.A. Schott, D. Discher, J.D. Ernst, B.H. Lubin, Detection of altered membrane phospholipid asymmetry in subpopulations of human red blood cells using fluorescently labeled annexin V, Blood 87 (1996) 1179-1187.
[17] F.L. Willekens, J.M. Werre, Y.A. Groenen-Dopp, B. Roerdinkholder-Stoelwinder, B. de Pauw, G.J. Bosman, Erythrocyte vesiculation: a self-protective mechanism?, Br J Haematol 141 (2008) 549-556.
[18] H.A. Wilson-Ashworth, Q. Bahm, J. Erickson, A. Shinkle, M.P. Vu, D. Woodbury, J.D. Bell, Differential detection of phospholipid fluidity, order, and spacing by fluorescence spectroscopy of bis-pyrene, prodan, nystatin, and merocyanine 540, Biophys J 91 (2006) 4091-4101.
[19] L.J. Gonzalez, E. Gibbons, R.W. Bailey, J. Fairbourn, T. Nguyen, S.K. Smith, K.B. Best, J. Nelson, A.M. Judd, J.D. Bell, The influence of membrane physical properties on microvesicle release in human erythrocytes, PMC Biophys 2 (2009) 7.
[20] P. Caprari, A. Scuteri, A.M. Salvati, C. Bauco, A. Cantafora, R. Masella, D. Modesti, A. Tarzia, V. Marigliano, Aging and red blood cell membrane: a study of centenarians, Exp Gerontol 34 (1999) 47-57.
[21] M.S. Tallman, D. Hakimian, H.C. Kwaan, F.R. Rickles, New insights into the pathogenesis of coagulation dysfunction in acute promyelocytic leukemia, Leuk Lymphoma 11 (1993) 27-36.
[22] A. Eldor, E.A. Rachmilewitz, The hypercoagulable state in thalassemia, Blood 99 (2002) 36-43.
[23] A. Ruf, M. Pick, V. Deutsch, H. Patscheke, A. Goldfarb, E.A. Rachmilewitz, M.C. Guillin, A. Eldor, In-vivo platelet activation correlates with red cell anionic phospholipid exposure in patients with beta-thalassaemia major, Br J Haematol 98 (1997) 51-56.

[24] E. Fibach, D. Manor, A. Oppenheim, E.A. Rachmilewitz, Proliferation and maturation of human erythroid progenitors in liquid culture, Blood 73 (1989) 100-103.
[25] R.C. Reuben, R.L. Wife, R. Breslow, R.A. Rifkind, P.A. Marks, A new group of potent inducers of differentiation in murine erythroleukemia cells, Proc Natl Acad Sci U S A 73 (1976) 862-866.
[26] E. Fibach, R.C. Reuben, R.A. Rifkind, P.A. Marks, Effect of hexamethylene bisacetamide on the commitment to differentiation of murine erythroleukemia cells, Cancer Res 37 (1977) 440-444.
[27] A. Cueff, R. Seear, A. Dyrda, G. Bouyer, S. Egee, A. Esposito, J. Skepper, T. Tiffert, V.L. Lew, S.L. Thomas, Effects of elevated intracellular calcium on the osmotic fragility of human red blood cells, Cell Calcium 47 (2010) 29-36.
[28] J. Jandl, Blood - Textbook of Hematology, Little, Brown and Co., Boston, 1996.
[29] P.A. Leventis, S. Grinstein, The distribution and function of phosphatidylserine in cellular membranes, Annu Rev Biophys 39 (2010) 407-427.
[30] U. Testa, Apoptotic mechanisms in the control of erythropoiesis, Leukemia 18 (2004) 1176-1199.
[31] M.C. Bessis, J. Breton-Gorius, Iron metabolism in the bone marrow as seen by electron microscopy: a critical review, Blood 19 (1962) 635-663.
[32] J.A. Chasis, N. Mohandas, Erythroblastic islands: niches for erythropoiesis, Blood 112 (2008) 470-478.
[33] S. Soni, S. Bala, M. Hanspal, Requirement for erythroblast-macrophage protein (Emp) in definitive erythropoiesis, Blood Cells Mol Dis 41 (2008) 141-147.
[34] S.C. Gifford, J. Derganc, S.S. Shevkoplyas, T. Yoshida, M.W. Bitensky, A detailed study of time-dependent changes in human red blood cells: from reticulocyte maturation to erythrocyte senescence, Br J Haematol 135 (2006) 395-404.
[35] J. Liu, X. Guo, N. Mohandas, J.A. Chasis, X. An, Membrane remodeling during reticulocyte maturation, Blood 115 (2010) 2021-2027.
[36] P.A. Ney, Normal and disordered reticulocyte maturation, Curr Opin Hematol 18 (2011) 152-157.
[37] H. Yoshida, K. Kawane, M. Koike, Y. Mori, Y. Uchiyama, S. Nagata, Phosphatidylserine-dependent engulfment by macrophages of nuclei from erythroid precursor cells, Nature 437 (2005) 754-758.
[38] E. Fibach, E. Rachmilewitz, The role of oxidative stress in hemolytic anemia, Curr Mol Med 8 (2008) 609-619.
[39] A. Lopez-Revuelta, J.I. Sanchez-Gallego, A.C. Garcia-Montero, A. Hernandez-Hernandez, J. Sanchez-Yague, M. Llanillo, Membrane cholesterol in the regulation of aminophospholipid asymmetry and phagocytosis in oxidized erythrocytes, Free Radic Biol Med 42 (2007) 1106-1118.
[40] S. Rivella, Ineffective erythropoiesis and thalassemias, Curr Opin Hematol 16 (2009) 187-194.
[41] E. Prus, E. Fibach, Uptake of non-transferrin iron by erythroid cells, Anemia 2011 (2011) 945289.
[42] W. Breuer, M. Shvartsman, Z.I. Cabantchik, Intracellular labile iron, Int J Biochem Cell Biol 40 (2008) 350-354.
[43] E. Prus, E. Fibach, The labile iron pool in human erythroid cells, Br J Haematol 142 (2008) 301-307.

[44] F. Lang, K.S. Lang, P.A. Lang, S.M. Huber, T. Wieder, Mechanisms and significance of eryptosis, Antioxid Redox Signal 8 (2006) 1183-1192.

[45] G.R. Chichili, W. Rodgers, Cytoskeleton-membrane interactions in membrane raft structure, Cell Mol Life Sci 66 (2009) 2319-2328.

[46] K.F. Meiri, Membrane/cytoskeleton communication, Subcell Biochem 37 (2004) 247-282.

[47] E. Reaven, S. Azhar, Effect of various hepatic membrane fractions on microtubule assembly-with special emphasis on the role of membrane phospholipids, J Cell Biol 89 (1981) 300-308.

[48] J.M. Caron, R.D. Berlin, Interaction of microtubule proteins with phospholipid vesicles, J Cell Biol 81 (1979) 665-671.

[49] B. van der Vaart, A. Akhmanova, A. Straube, Regulation of microtubule dynamic instability, Biochem Soc Trans 37 (2009) 1007-1013.

[50] B. Bhattacharyya, D. Panda, S. Gupta, M. Banerjee, Anti-mitotic activity of colchicine and the structural basis for its interaction with tubulin, Med Res Rev 28 (2008) 155-183.

[51] S.T. Koury, M.J. Koury, M.C. Bondurant, Cytoskeletal distribution and function during the maturation and enucleation of mammalian erythroblasts, J Cell Biol 109 (1989) 3005-3013.

[52] P.A. Lang, J. Huober, C. Bachmann, D.S. Kempe, M. Sobiesiak, A. Akel, O.M. Niemoeller, P. Dreischer, K. Eisele, B.A. Klarl, E. Gulbins, F. Lang, T. Wieder, Stimulation of erythrocyte phosphatidylserine exposure by paclitaxel, Cell Physiol Biochem 18 (2006) 151-164.

[53] E.N. Dedkova, A.A. Sigova, V.P. Zinchenko, Mechanism of action of calcium ionophores on intact cells: ionophore-resistant cells, Membr Cell Biol 13 (2000) 357-368.

[54] T.J. Greenwalt, The how and why of exocytic vesicles, Transfusion 46 (2006) 143-152.

[55] M.A. Jordan, Mechanism of action of antitumor drugs that interact with microtubules and tubulin, Curr Med Chem Anticancer Agents 2 (2002) 1-17.

[56] J.C. Chang, E.C. Wooten, A. Tsimelzon, S.G. Hilsenbeck, M.C. Gutierrez, Y.L. Tham, M. Kalidas, R. Elledge, S. Mohsin, C.K. Osborne, G.C. Chamness, D.C. Allred, M.T. Lewis, H. Wong, P. O'Connell, Patterns of resistance and incomplete response to docetaxel by gene expression profiling in breast cancer patients, J Clin Oncol 23 (2005) 1169-1177.

[57] W.P. McGuire, W.J. Hoskins, M.F. Brady, P.R. Kucera, E.E. Partridge, K.Y. Look, D.L. Clarke-Pearson, M. Davidson, Cyclophosphamide and cisplatin compared with paclitaxel and cisplatin in patients with stage III and stage IV ovarian cancer, N Engl J Med 334 (1996) 1-6.

# 4

# Anemia Caused by Oxidative Stress

Yoshihito Iuchi
*Yamaguchi University*
*Japan*

## 1. Introduction

Anemia is considered to be one of the major health problems. According to the World Health Organization, about 30 percent of people throughout the world suffer from anemia. The most common cause of anemia is iron deficiency; however, recent work has shown that reactive oxygen species (ROS) of erythrocytes are one of the principal causative factors of anemia. Elevation of ROS in erythrocytes could occur either by activation of ROS generation or by suppression of antioxidative/redox system. When erythrocytes experience an excessive elevation of ROS, oxidative stress develops. ROS are known to contribute to the pathogenesis of several hereditary disorders of erythrocytes, including sickle cell anemia, thalassemia, and glucose-6-phosphate dehydrogenase (G6PD) deficiency.

Deficiency of antioxidant enzymes such as superoxide dismutase 1 (SOD1) or peroxiredoxin II (Prx II) induces elevation of oxidative stress in erythrocytes and causes anemia, while deficiency of catalase or glutathione peroxidase does not. In addition to the abnormalities of antioxidant enzymes, some transcription factors such as p45NF-E2 or Nrf2 can cause anemia. In this chapter, I provide some evidence of the involvement of oxidative stress in anemia.

## 2. Oxidative stress-mediated destruction of erythrocytes

### 2.1 Cellular oxidative stress and anti-oxidative system

Under normal physiological conditions, there is a balance between the ROS and the defense system of antioxidant enzymes and antioxidants, which prevents or limits oxidative damage. ROS are produced as a result of intracellular metabolic activity. During this process, ROS such as superoxide ($\bullet O_2^-$), hydrogen peroxide ($H_2O_2$), and hydroxyl radical ($\bullet$OH) are produced, even in healthy individuals. Oxidative stress is the result of an imbalance between oxidants and antioxidants. Increased pro-oxidants and/or decreased antioxidants trigger a cascade of oxidative reactions. Oxidative stress can damage specific molecular targets (lipids, proteins, nucleotides, etc.), resulting in cell dysfunction and/or death. Enzymes that participate in ROS production include xanthine oxidase (XO), nicotinamide adenine dinucleotide phosphate (NADPH) oxidase, nitric oxide synthase (NOS), cytochrome P450, cyclo-oxygenase (COX), and lipoxygenase. Major defence mechanisms against ROS include enzymatic (superoxide dismutase (SOD), catalase, glutathione peroxidase (GPx), peroxiredoxin (Prx)) as well as non-enzymatic systems (reduced glutathione (GSH), ubiquinols, uric acid, vitamins C and E, flavonoids, carotenoids).

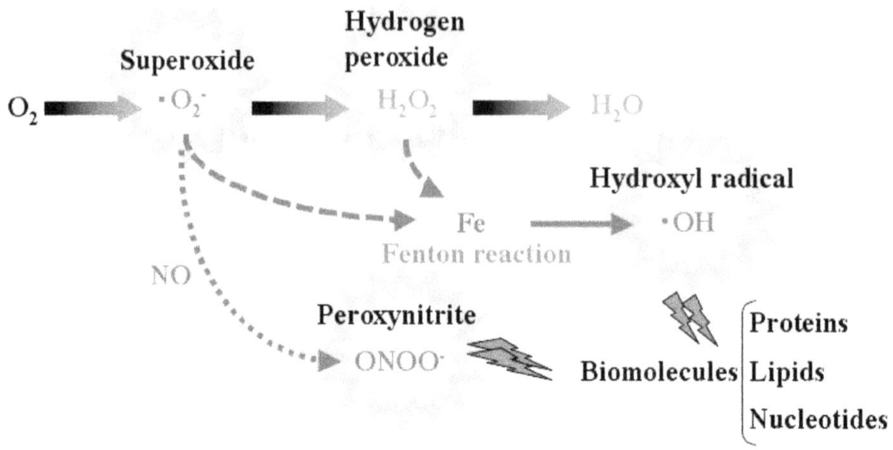


Fig. 1. Reactive oxygen species (ROS) generated in the cell.

### 2.2 Oxidation of erythrocyte membrane caused by ROS

During the binding of oxygen to form oxy-hemoglobin (oxy-Hb), one electron is transferred from iron to the bound oxygen forming a ferric-superoxide anion complex. The shared electron is normally returned to the iron when oxygen is released during deoxygenation. However, the electrons can remain and transform oxygen into superoxide anions. In this process, iron is left in the ferric state and Hb is transformed into methemoglobin (met-Hb). The autoxidation of Hb occurs spontaneously and transforms 0.5–3% of Hb into met-Hb per day. In addition to this physiological process, met-Hb can be produced by endogenous oxidants, such as $H_2O_2$, nitric oxide (NO), and hydroxyl radicals. Since met-Hb cannot bind oxygen, this is the first step in the formation of harmful hemichromes (Rice-Evans & Baysal, 1987). In normal conditions, spontaneous production of met-Hb from autoxidation and conversion of met-Hb back to Hb are in balance. However, in pathological conditions, increased oxidative stress or impaired antioxidant defence will enhance production of met-Hb and generation of ROS. Hemichrome formation depends on the amount of met-Hb formed and is accelerated by ROS such as superoxide or $H_2O_2$. Superoxide produced by one electron reduction of oxygen would reduce ferri-hemichrome to ferro-hemichrome. In the Fenton reaction, ferro-hemichrome catalyzes decomposition of $H_2O_2$ to hydroxyl radical. Hydroxyl radical is an extremely reactive free radical that can react with various biomolecules such as membrane lipids. Peroxidation of membrane lipids, most notably the polyunsaturated fatty acids arachidonic acid and linoleic acid, generates a wide array of molecules, such as lipid hydroperoxides, which are secondary lipid peroxidation products (for example, malondialdehyde and 4-hydroxynonenal, HNE). Lipid peroxidation products can damage membrane structure with the formation of membrane pores, alter water permeability, decrease cell deformability, and enhance IgG binding and complement activation. Finally, disruption of the normal asymmetrical distribution of membrane phospholipids occurs. This may enhance exposure of phosphatidylserine (PS) on the outer cell surface. Erythrocytes that have PS exposed on the outer surface are recognized and engulfed by macrophages with PS-specific receptors, resulting in their degradation (Carrell et al., 1975; Hebbel, 1985; Nur et al., 2011).

At the same time, ROS can be used for killing harmful microorganisms. However, ROS not only participate in pathogen killing but also induce activation of inflammatory mediators and production of adhesion molecules and membrane damage. The increased intra- and extra-erythrocytic oxidative stress induces lipid peroxidation and membrane instability, contributing to accelerated hemolysis. Increased levels of hydroperoxides cause erythrocyte membrane damage and deformity and, ultimately, lead to cell death.

### 2.3 Band 3-mediated erythrocyte removal

Band 3, also termed the anion exchanger, is a major erythrocyte membrane protein, constituting 25% of the total erythrocyte membrane protein. It has two independent domains: the membrane-spanning domain, which catalyzes anion exchange and contains the antigenic determinants recognized by naturally occurring antibodies (NAbs), and the cytoplasmic domain (Pantaleo et al., 2008). A very important feature of hemichrome/free heme/iron damage is its non-random occurrence in space. The highly damaging feature of hemichromes is their tight association with the cytoplasmic domain of band 3, which, following their binding, leads to band 3 oxidation and clusterization. These band 3 clusters show increased affinity for NAbs, which activate complement and finally trigger phagocytosis-mediated erythrocyte removal. This band 3/hemichrome complex was found not only in pathological conditions in which oxidative stress in erythrocytes is thought to be elevated, but also in senescent erythrocytes (Arese et al., 2005).

## 3. Relationship between human hereditary anemia and oxidative stress

### 3.1 Sickle cell disease

Sickle cell disease (SCD) is a hemoglobinopathy clinically characterized by chronic hemolysis. Chronic activation and damage of endothelial cells by sickle erythrocytes, heme, polymorphonuclear neutrophils (PMNs), and inflammatory mediators contribute to progressive microvascular damage in all organs, including the brain, lungs, and kidneys. SCD is an inherited disorder of hemoglobin synthesis. SCD has the same single base pair mutation (GAG to GTG, Glu to Val) in the β globin molecule of sickle cells (HbS).

Chronic oxidative stress constitutes a critical factor in endothelial dysfunction, inflammation, and multiple organ damage in SCD (Nur et al., 2011). There are several causes of oxidative stress in SCD. Major sources of ROS in SCD are thought to be the (i) enhanced rate of HbS auto-oxidation, (ii) increased xanthine oxidase activity in SCD aortic endothelium, and (iii) higher number of leucocytes, which produce twice the fluxes of superoxide in SCD (Wood & Granger, 2007).

Endothelial dysfunction in patients with SCD has been related to inflammation, high levels of production of ROS and reactive nitrogen species, and erythrocyte adhesion to blood vessel walls. There have been several studies showing that patients with SCD have a high level of oxidative damage, assessed through lipid peroxidation. In turn, oxidative stress is associated with chronic hemolysis. Sickle erythrocytes have a high frequency of phosphatidyl serine exposure, which is due to oxidative stress, suggesting that oxidative stress might play a role in intravascular hemolysis. Hypertension in patients with SCD was found to be related to ROS, which can directly deactivate endothelial nitric oxide synthase (eNOS), reducing nitric oxide (NO) levels, an important vasodilator (Rusanova et al., 2010).

### 3.2 Thalassemia

The thalassemia syndrome is one of the most common genetic disorders affecting a single gene or gene cluster. The various thalassemia disorders are caused by insufficient production of one of the two types of globin chains that constitute the hemoglobin tetramer. In α thalassemia , α globin production is reduced or absent, and in β thalassemia, β globin production is impaired. The α and β thalassemias are characterized by the presence of a pool of unpaired hemoglobin chains. While α or β hemoglobin chains are stable when part of the $\alpha_2\beta_2$ hemoglobin tetramer, the unpaired α or β hemoglobin chains are unstable and subject to high rates of auto-oxidation. The auto-oxidation of the unpaired hemoglobin chains leads to the generation of superoxide and $H_2O_2$, and subsequent release of globin-free heme and iron (Bunn, 1967; Shinar & Rachmilewitz, 1990). β thalassemic erythrocytes exhibit a significant decrease in the NADPH/NADP ratio similar to that seen in severe G6PD-deficiency anemia (see next chapter). As a consequence of this decrease, both catalase activity and GSH concentration are decreased (Scot, 2006). Expression of peroxiredoxin (Prx) II, an antioxidant enzyme that detoxifies $H_2O_2$, is increased in β thalassemic mouse erythrocytes (Matte et al., 2010). These findings indicate that this high expression of PrxII has a compensatory effect against elevated oxidative stress in thalassemic erythrocytes (Rund & Rachmilewitz, 2005).

### 3.3 Glucose-6-phosphate dehydrogenase (G6PD) deficiency

Glucose-6-phosphate dehydrogenase (G6PD) deficiency was first discovered in African-American subjects. The fact that it seemed to be limited to one ethnic group suggested that it has a genetic basis. Because it was shown that transmission was generally from mother to son, it became apparent that G6PD deficiency is an X-linked disorder. G6PD deficiency is one of the glycolytic enzymopathies that frequently cause hemolytic anemia. G6PD deficiency is the most common erythrocyte enzyme defect, affecting over 400 million people (Beutler, 2008).

G6PD deficiency is mainly caused by point mutations in the G6PD gene. About 140 mutations have been described: most are single base changes, leading to amino acid substitutions (Cappellini & Fiorelli, 2008). The most frequent clinical manifestations of G6PD deficiency are neonatal jaundice and acute hemolytic anemia, which is usually triggered by an exogenous agent. Some G6PD variants cause chronic hemolysis, leading to congenital non-spherocytic hemolytic anemia. The appearance of Heinz bodies both in vivo and in vitro in G6PD-deficient cells and their inability to protect their GSH against drug challenge suggested that a major component of the hemolytic process is the inability of the erythrocytes to protect sulfhydryl groups against oxidative stress (Fig. 2, Cohen & Hochstein, 1961). However, it has been shown that, in mice, targeted disruption of the gene encoding glutathione peroxidase has little effect on oxidation of hemoglobin of murine cells challenged with peroxides.

G6PD provides erythrocytes with important protection against oxidative stress. G6PD is a key regulatory enzyme of the pentose phosphate pathway (also called hexose monophosphate shunt), which is essential for the supply of reduced NADPH. NADPH enables cells to counterbalance oxidative stress that can be triggered by several oxidant agents, and to preserve the reduced form of glutathione. NADPH is pivotal to the cellular antioxidative defence systems in most organisms. Since erythrocytes do not contain mitochondria, the pentose phosphate pathway is their only source of NADPH; therefore, defence against oxidative damage is dependent on G6PD.

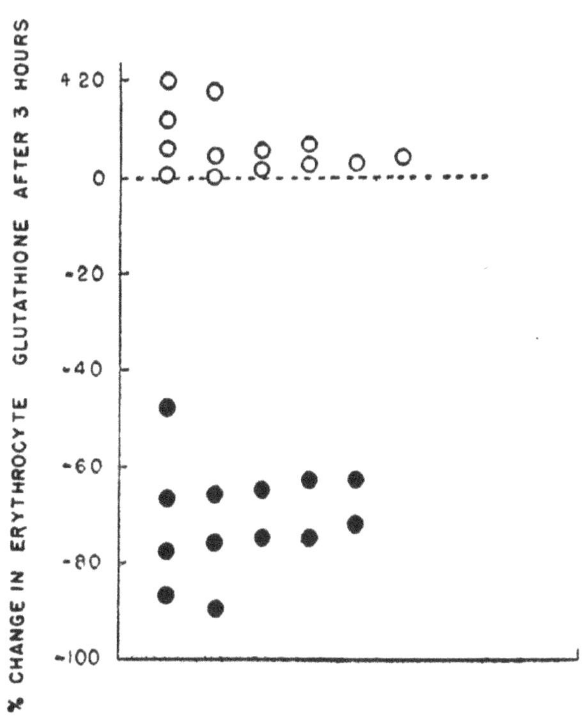


Fig. 2. Percentage change in reduced glutathione (GSH) in erythrocytes of 13 individuals with G6PD deficiency (solid circles) and 13 individuals with normal G6PD activity (open circles) after 3 hours of hydrogen peroxide diffusion (Cohen & Hochstein, 1961).

## 4. Animal model of anemia

### 4.1 Deficiency of antioxidant enzymes

#### 4.1.1 Superoxide dismutase 1 (SOD1) deficiency

Among the known antioxidative proteins, superoxide dismutase (SOD) is thought to play a central role because of its ability to scavenge superoxide anions, the primary ROS generated from molecular oxygen in cells (Fridovich, 1995). SOD1-deficient mice have been generated by several groups. Unexpectedly, SOD1-deficient mice grow normally but develop female infertility (Ho et al., 1998; Matzuk et al., 1998), cochlear hair cell loss (McFadden et al., 1999), and vascular dysfunction (Didion et al., 2002). Adding to these phenotypes, SOD1-deficient mice exhibit severe anemia, even in infant mice (Iuchi et al., 2007; Starzyński et al., 2009). Anemia appears to be caused by shortened lifespan of erythrocytes. Increased ROS due to SOD1 deficiency makes their erythrocytes vulnerable to oxidative stress. In addition to SOD1 deficiency, GPx activity and protein levels of GPx1 were significantly lower in erythrocytes. Since GPx1 protein is prone to oxidative inactivation, oxidized GPx1 would be removed by the protease that degrades oxidized proteins in erythrocytes.

While most mammalian cells possess two intracellular SOD isoforms to protect against ROS, erythrocytes lack mitochondria and, as a result, carry only the SOD1 protein to scavenge superoxide anions. Erythrocytes of SOD1-deficient mice, therefore, face severe oxygen toxicity compared with other tissues. Erythrocytes that are hyperoxic bind oxygen in the lungs (~21%), and release oxygen in peripheral tissues, which are relatively hypoxic (~2%). Thus, erythrocytes undergo cyclic exposure to hyperoxic and hypoxic environments, generating large amounts of superoxide via auto-oxidation of hemoglobin.

The continuous destruction of oxidized erythrocytes in SOD1-deficient mice appears to induce the formation of autoantibodies against certain erythrocyte components, for example, carbonic anhydrase II, and the immune complex is deposited in the kidney glomeruli. Therefore, these mice exhibit autoimmune hemolytic anemia (AIHA)-like symptoms when they reach old age. This pathophysiological symptom is thought as a secondary effect of elevated oxidative stress in SOD1-deficient erythrocytes.

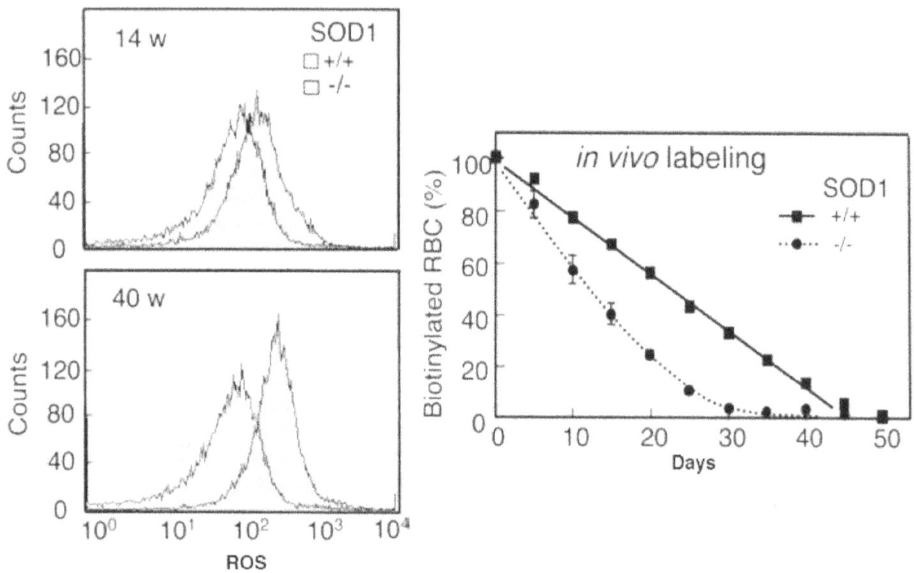


Fig. 3. Elevated ROS (left panels) and shortened lifespan (right panel) of erythrocytes in SOD1-deficient mice (Iuchi et al., 2007).

### 4.1.2 Catalase deficiency

Human erythrocytes contain large amounts of catalase. While the catalase and NADPH/GSH/GPx system is very important for disposal of $H_2O_2$ in human erythrocytes, genetic deficiencies of catalase do not predispose erythrocytes to peroxide-induced destruction (Jacob et al., 1965). Mice lacking the catalase gene develop normally (Ho et al., 2004). A link between catalase deficiency and anemia has not been reported.

### 4.1.3 Glutathione peroxidase-1 (GPx1) deficiency

The role of glutathione peroxidase in erythrocyte anti-oxidant defense was examined using erythrocytes from mice with genetically engineered disruption of the glutathione peroxidase-1 (GPx1) gene. Because GPx1 is the sole glutathione peroxidase in erythrocytes, all erythrocyte GSH peroxidase activity was eliminated. Oxidation of hemoglobin and membrane lipids was determined during oxidant challenge from cumene hydroperoxide and $H_2O_2$. As a result, no difference was detected between wild-type erythrocytes and GPx1-deficient erythrocytes, even at high levels of $H_2O_2$ exposure. Thus, GPx1 appears to play little or no role in the defense of erythrocytes against exposure to peroxide (Johnson et al., 2000).

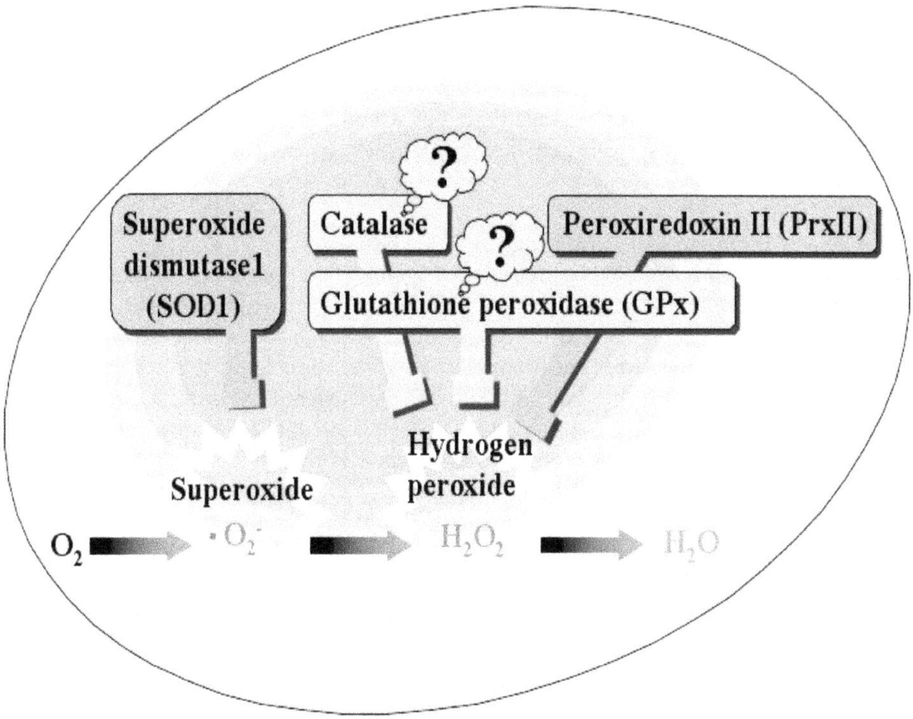


Fig. 4. Do SOD1 and PrxII actually work in erythrocytes?

#### 4.1.4 Peroxiredoxin II (PrxII) deficiency

A number of proteins also protect cells against oxidative stress. SOD, GPx, and catalase are commonly known antioxidant enzymes and have been extensively characterized. Recently, a new family of antioxidative proteins, collectively referred to as Prxs (peroxiredoxins), have been identified. Six distinct gene products are known in the Prx family in mammals (Fujii & Ikeda, 2002). Thioredoxin-dependent peroxidase activity appears to be common to most Prx family members, and in addition, other divergent biological functions have been elucidated for individual Prx members. However, the most well-characterized function of Prx family members is the ability to modulate hydrogen peroxide signaling in response to various stimuli (Rhee et al., 2005).

Mice deficient in Prx II, which is abundantly expressed in all types of cells, were healthy in appearance and fertile. However, they had splenomegaly caused by the congestion of red pulp with hemosiderin accumulation. Erythrocytes from these mice contained markedly higher levels of ROS. The Prx II-deficient mice had significantly decreased hematocrit levels, but increased reticulocyte counts and erythropoietin levels, indicative of a compensatory action to maintain hematologic homeostasis in the mice (Lee et al., 2003).

For a long time, it was considered that catalase and GPx constitute the erythrocyte defense against $H_2O_2$, and there has been continuous debate about which of these is more significant

(Cohen & Hochstein, 1963; Gaetani et al., 1989; Gaetani et al., 1996). Until recently, little attention has been paid to the antioxidant role of Prxs in erythrocytes, even though Prx II is the third most abundant cytoplasmic erythrocyte protein. These mice possess fully functional catalase and GPx. Erythrocytes also possess PrxI and PrxVI, although at lower levels than PrxII. It is reported that PrxII expression and content were markedly increased in erythrocytes from β thalassemic mouse models compared with those in wild-type mice (Matte et al., 2010). This indicates that PrxII has a non-redundant function in protecting healthy erythrocytes against oxidative damage and plays a crucial role even in pathological conditions.

### 4.2 Deficiency of transcription factor

In many cases, transcriptional activation of genes that play an important role in detoxification of xenobiotics and defense against oxidative stress is mediated partly by the antioxidant response element (ARE). For example, AREs have been found in promoter sequences of genes including nicotinamide adenine dinucleotide phosphate–quinone oxidoreductase, heme oxygenase, glutathione-S-transferases, and glutamylcysteine synthetase (Favreau et al., 1995; Inamdar et al., 1996; Jaiswal et al., 1994; Mulcahy et al., 1995; Prestera et al., 1995). The ARE consensus sequence is very similar to the NF-E2–like sequence of the β globin locus control region, which was found to be essential for globin gene expression. Multiple proteins can interact with the NF-E2 consensus sequence. The cap 'n' collar (CNC)–bZIP factor family of proteins was identified from searches for proteins that bind and activate the NF-E2 site of the β-globin locus control region. This multiple-protein family includes p45NF-E2, NF-E2–related factor (Nrf)1, and Nrf2. The similarities among CNC family members are most notable in the basic-DNA binding region and another homology domain (Moi et al., 1994).

#### 4.2.1 p45NF-E2 deficiency

p45NF-E2 is a member of the cap 'n' collar (CNC)-basic leucine zipper family of transcriptional activators that is expressed at high levels in various types of blood cells. It plays a crucial role in megakaryocyte maturation and platelet biogenesis. Mice with disruption of p45NF-E2 have severe platelet deficiency due to defective megakaryocyte maturation. In addition, p45NF-E2 knockout mice exhibit anemia characterized by the presence of hypochromic erythrocytes and reticulocytosis. Erythrocytes from p45NF-E2–deficient mice are sensitive to oxidative stress. Erythrocytes from p45NF-E2–deficient mice accumulated high levels of free radicals when exposed to oxidants, and this correlated with increased formation of met-Hb and loss of membrane deformability. In addition, severe anemia developed in p45NF-E2 deficient mice treated with oxidative-stress–inducing drugs, and mutant erythrocytes had decreased survival.

Because CNC factors may represent an important class of regulators of antioxidant gene expression by means of the ARE, one possibility is that p45NF-E2 is involved in regulating oxidative stress-response genes in erythrocytes. It is possible that a compensated hemolytic state contributes to the erythroid abnormalities observed in p45NF-E2 knockout mice.

#### 4.2.2 Nrf2 deficiency

The NF-E2-related factor 2 (Nrf2) transcription factor regulates genes related to ROS scavenging and detoxification. Although Nrf2 is expressed widely and is important for cellular antioxidant potential, Nrf2 knockout mice develop and grow normally (Chan et al., 1996). Young Nrf2 knockout mice are not anemic, whereas targeted disruption of either NF-E2 or Nrf1 resulted in anemia. In aged mice, however, disruption of Nrf2 causes regenerative immune-mediated hemolytic anemia due to increased sequestration of damaged erythrocytes. Splenomegaly and spleen toxicity in Nrf2-deficient mice raised the possibility of hemolytic anemia and splenic extramedullary hematopoiesis in Nrf2-deficient mice. Nrf2-deficient erythrocytes are highly sensitive to $H_2O_2$-induced hemolysis in vitro, further suggesting that Nrf2-deficient erythrocytes are highly susceptible to stress. In addition, Nrf2-deficient erythrocytes showed increased met-Hb formation after incubation with high concentrations of $H_2O_2$, suggesting that Hb in Nrf2-deficient erythrocytes is more easily oxidized than that in Nrf2 WT erythrocytes (Lee et al., 2004). A unique feature of the Nrf2-ARE pathway (the programmed cell life pathway) (Li et al., 2002) is that it coordinately up-regulates many protective detoxification and antioxidant genes, which can synergistically increase the efficiency of the erythrocyte defense system against oxidative stress.

#### 4.2.3 Nrf1 deficiency

Nrf1 knockout mice have also been reported to develop anemia in early stages of embryo, and they die in utero (Chan et al., 1998). Nrf1 knockout mice have abnormal fetal liver erythropoiesis as a result of a defect in the fetal liver microenvironment specific for erythroid cells. Anemic phenotype of Nrf1-deficient mice is not due to the oxidative stress in erythrocytes, but due to abnormal erythropoiesis.

## 5. Relationship between hereditary sideroblastic anemia and SOD2 deficiency

### 5.1 Hereditary sideroblastic anemia

Iron overload is a feature of human disorders including sideroblastic anemia (SA). Excess iron is toxic because it can catalyze the generation of ROS that damage cellular molecules. Some genetic lesions have been identified as causes of hereditary or acquired SA. As defined genetic lesions, dysfunction in one of the mitochondrial metabolic pathways has been observed: heme synthesis, iron homeostasis and transport, or electron transport. These lesions result in abnormal use of erythroid mitochondrial iron, causing pathologic iron deposition (Napier et al., 2005). Identified lesions affect nuclear-encoded mitochondrial proteins or the mitochondrial genome. The heme biosynthetic pathway was identified as a primary cause of SA. However, other pathways, including mitochondrial oxidative phosphorylation and iron-sulfur cluster biosynthesis, were also identified as primary defects in SAs. They may secondarily affect heme metabolism (Rouault & Tong, 2005; Martin, 2006). Two X-linked sideroblastic anemias (XLSAs) exist, one caused by mutations of an erythroid-specific form of the heme biosynthetic enzyme aminolevulinic acid (ALA)–synthase 2 (ALAS2) (Cotter et al., 1994), and one caused by mutation of a putative mitochondrial iron-transport protein, ATP-binding cassette, member 7 (ABC7) (Allikmets et al., 1999).

### 5.2 SOD2-deficiency anemia

SOD2-deficiency anemia is another example of mitochondrial dysfunction resulting in an erythroid-specific SA-like phenotype. Although genetically deficient mice of SOD1 have a normal lifespan along with exhibiting an anemic phenotype (Iuchi et al., 2007), inactivation of SOD2 results in embryonic or neonatal lethality. Because of its mitochondrial location, SOD2 is the principal defense against the toxicity of superoxide generated by oxidative phosphorylation in mitochondria. The SOD2-deficient phenotype is associated with pathologic evidence of mitochondrial injury and oxidative damage to biomolecules, as well as severe damage to cardiac muscle. Hematopoietic stem cell-specific SOD2-deficient mice were generated by transplantation of SOD2-deficient mouse HSCs, and sideroblastic anemia-like symptom was the major phenotype in the transplanted animals (Friedman et al., 2001). This model suggests that oxidative stress in mitochondria affects the reduced heme biogenesis and accumulation of iron deposits in erythroid cells, and plays an important role in the pathogenesis of sideroblastic anemia.

It is interesting to note that peroxiredoxin II (Prx II), a member of the thioredoxin peroxidase family, was decreased in SOD2-deficient cells, but showed an increase with antioxidant treatment (Friedman et al., 2004). Knockout of Prx II causes hemolytic anemia (Lee et al., 2003) with evidence of increased oxidative damage to mature RBCs. This suggests that Prx II may be an important target of oxidative damage in SOD2-deficient cells. These findings suggest that mitochondrial dysfunction with excessive ROS production and with excess iron accumulation plays a critical role in causing SA.

## 6. Therapeutic supplementation of antioxidant for anemia

### 6.1 N-acetylcysteine (NAC) and its derivatives

N-acetylcysteine (NAC) is one of the precursors of GSH. In vitro and animal studies have demonstrated that treatment of blood cells with NAC increases the intracellular concentration of the reduced form of GSH and decreases oxidative stress (Amer et al., 2006; Nur et al., 2011). Treatment of sickle cell patients with NAC at a dose of 2,400 mg per day increased intracellular GSH and reduced dense cell formation (Pace et al., 2003). NAC is also effective for antioxidant enzyme-deficient mice. Administration of NAC (1.0% in drinking water) to SOD1-deficient mice significantly suppressed ROS in erythrocytes and partly improved the anemia (Iuchi et al., 2007).

Recently, several new derivatives of NAC have been developed. Among these new agents, the amide form of NAC, N-acetylcysteine amide (AD4), in which the carboxylic group is neutralized, is more lipophilic and has better membrane permeability than NAC. AD4 is also effective for its antioxidant effects. In vitro treatment of blood cells from β thalassemic patients with AD4 elevated the reduced glutathione (GSH) content of erythrocytes, platelets, and polymorphonuclear leukocytes, and reduced their ROS. These effects resulted in significantly reduced sensitivity of thalassemic erythrocytes to hemolysis and phagocytosis by macrophages. Intra-peritoneal injection of AD4 to β thalassemic mice reduced the parameters of oxidative stress. The superiority of AD4, compared with NAC, in reducing oxidative stress markers in thalassemic cells both in vitro and in vivo has been demonstrated (Amer, J. et al., 2008).

### 6.2 Vitamin E

Vitamin E, a fat-soluble antioxidant, has been identified as an essential erythropoietic factor for certain species of animals. Treatment with vitamin E increased the number of colony forming units of erythroid precursors, enhanced erythropoiesis, and thus corrected the experimentally induced anemia in an animal model. Results of some of clinical trials suggested that vitamin E might prevent some types of human anemia due to its putative role in promoting erythropoiesis, enhancing the stability of erythrocyte membrane proteins and lipids, and reducing oxidative stress-induced erythrocyte injury. Supplementation of vitamin E was tried for patients with some types of inherited hemolytic anemia. Some of these trials have shown that there was an improvement in hemolysis, as evidenced by longer erythrocyte lifespan, in elevated hemoglobin level, and decreased reticulocyte count (Corash et al., 1980; Hafez et al., 1986). On the other hand, some groups indicated no change in hematologic status after treatment with high doses of vitamin E (Newman et al., 1979; Johnson et al., 1983).

In patients suffering from homozygous β thalassemia, supplementation of vitamin E was effective in reducing plasma levels of lipid peroxidation end products and a significant improvement in the hemoglobin levels (Das et al., 2004). A 4- to 8-week-long supplementation with vitamin E given to children with various types of thalassemia was shown to decrease $H_2O_2$-mediated erythrocyte hemolysis and increase the resistance to oxidative damage. Supplementation with vitamin E in children suffering from sickle cell anemia was shown to reduce the percentage of sickled erythrocytes, increased resistance of erythrocytes to lysis, and enhanced blood hemoglobin concentration (Jilani & Iqbal, 2011).

## 7. Conclusion

In recent years, many studies have implicated oxidative stress in anemia complicated with some infectious diseases. For example, malaria infection results in decreased antioxidant enzymes and substances such as catalase, GPx, SOD, GSH, ascorbate, and plasma tocopherol. The development of new antioxidant drugs with a function based on ROS reduction might constitute a promising tool not only for hereditary anemia but also for the control of the infection-mediated anemia.

## 8. References

Allikmets, R., Raskind, W. H., Hutchinson, A., Schueck, N. D., Dean, M., & Koeller, D. M. (1999) Mutation of a putative mitochondrial iron transporter gene (ABC7) in X-linked sideroblastic anemia and ataxia (XLSA/A). *Hum. Mo.l Gene.t* 8, 743–749.

Amer, J., Atlas, D. & Fibach, E. (2008) N-acetylcysteine amide (AD4) attenuates oxidative stress in beta-thalassemia blood cells. *Biochim. Biophys. Acta* 1780, 249–255.

Amer, J., Ghoti, H., Rachmilewitz, E et al. (2006) Red blood cells, platelets and polymorphonuclear neutrophils of patients with sickle cell disease exhibit oxidative stress that can be ameliorated by antioxidants. *Br. J. Haematol.* 132, 108-113.

Arese, P., Turrini, F. & Schwarzer, E. (2005) Band 3/Complement-mediated recognition and removal of normally senescent and pathological human erythrocytes. *Cell. Physiol. Biochem.* 16, 133-146.

Bunn, H. F. & Jandl, J. H. (1967) Exchange of heme among hemoglobins and between hemoglobin and albumin. *J. Biol. Chem.* 243, 465–475.

Carrell, R.W., Winterbourn, C. C. & Rachmilewitz, E. A. (1975) Activated oxygen and hemolysis. *Br. J. Hematol.* 30, 259-264.

Chan, J. Y., Kwong, M., Lo, M., Emerson, R., Kuypers, F. A. (2001) Reduced oxidative-stress response in red blood cells from p45NFE2-deficient mice. *Blood*, 97, 2151-2158.

Chan, J. Y., Kwong, M., Lu, R., Chang, J., Wang, B., Yen, T. S., Kan, Y. W. (1998) Targeted disruption of the ubiquitous CNC-bZIP transcription factor, Nrf-1, results in anemia and embryonic lethality in mice. *EMBO J*, 17, 1779–1787.

Chan, K., Lu, R., Chang, J. C. & Kan, Y. W. (1996) NRF2, a member of the NFE2 family of transcription factors, is not essential for murine erythropoiesis, growth, and development. *Proc. Natl. Acad. Sci. USA* 93, 13943–13948.

Cohen, G. & Hochstein, P. (1963) Glutathione peroxidase: primary agent for elimination of hydrogen peroxide in erythrocytes. *Biochemistry*. 2, 1420-1428.

Corash, L., Spielberg, S. & Bartsocas, C. (1980) Reducedchronichaemo- lysisduring high-dosevitamin E administration in Mediterranean type glucose-6-phosphate dehydrogenase deficiency. *N. Engl. J. Med.* 303, 416-420.

Cotter, P. D., Rucknagel, D. L. & Bishop, D. F. (1994) X-linked sideroblastic anemia: identification of the mutation in the erythroid- specific delta-aminolevulinate synthase gene (ALAS2) in the original family described by Cooley. *Blood* 84, 3915–3924.

Das, N., Das Chowdhury, T., Chattopadhyay, A . & Datta, A. G. (2004) Attenuation of oxidative stress-induced changes in thalassemic erythrocytes by vitamin E. *Pol. J. Pharmacol.*, 56, 85-96.

Didion, S. P., Ryan, M. J., Didion, L. A., Fegan, P. E., Sigmund, C. D. & Faraci, F. M. (2002) Increased superoxide and vascular dysfunction in CuZnSOD- deficient mice. *Circ. Res.* 91, 938–944.

Favreau, L. V., Pickett, C. B. (1995) The rat quinone reductase antioxidant response element: identification of the nucleotide sequence required for basal andinducible activity and detection of antioxidant response element-binding proteins in hepatoma and non-hepatoma cell lines. *J Biol Chem.* 270, 24468-24474.

Friedman, J. S., Rebel, V. I., Derby, .R, Bell, K., Huang, T. T., Kuypers, F. A., Epstein, C. J. & Burakoff, S. J. (2001) Absence of mitochondrial superoxide dismutase results in a murine hemolytic anemia responsive to therapy with a catalytic antioxidant. *J. Exp. Med.* 193(8), 925-934.

Friedman, J. S., Lopez, M. F., Fleming, M. D., Rivera, A., Martin, F. M., Welsh, M. L., Boyd, A., Doctrow, S. R. & Burakoff, S. J. (2004) SOD2-deficiency anemia: protein oxidation and altered protein expression reveal targets of damage, stress response, and antioxidant responsiveness. *Blood* 104(8), 2565-73.

Fridovich, I. (1995) Superoxide radical and superoxide dismutases. *Annu. Rev. Biochem.* 64, 97–112.

Fujii, J. & Ikeda, Y. (2002) Advances in our understanding of peroxiredoxin, a multifunctional, mammalian redox protein. *Redox Rep.* 7(3), 123-130.

Gaetani, G. F., Ferraris, A. M., Rolfo, M., Mangerini, R., Arena, S. & Kirkman, H. N. (1996) Predominant role of catalase in the disposal of hydrogen peroxide within human erythrocytes. *Blood.* 87, 1595-1599.

Gaetani, G. F., Galiano, S., Canepa, L., Ferraris, A. M. & Kirkman, H. N. (1989) Catalase and glutathione-peroxidase are equally active in detoxification of hydrogen- peroxide in human-erythrocytes. *Blood.* 73, 334-339.

Hafez, M., Amar, E. S., Zedan, M., Hammad, H., Sorour, A. H., el-Desouky, E. S. &Gamil, N. (1986) Improved erythrocyte survival with combined vitamin E and selenium therapy in children with glucose-6-phosphate dehydrogenase deficiency and mild chronic hemolysis. *J. Pediatr.* 108(4), 558-561.

Hebbel, R. P. (1985) Auto-oxidation and a membrane-associated "Fenton reagent": A possible explanation for development of membrane lesions in sickle erythrocytes. *Clinics in Hematol* 14, 129-140.

Ho, Y. S., Gargano, M., Cao, J., Bronson, R. T., Heimler, I. & Hutz, R. J. (1998) Reduced fertility in female mice lacking copper-zinc superoxide dismutase. *J. Biol. Chem.* 273, 7765–7769.

Ho, Y. S., Xiong, Y., Ma, W., Spector, A. & Ho, D. S. (2004) Mice Lacking Catalase Develop Normally but Show Differential Sensitivity to Oxidant Tissue Injury. *J Biol Chem.* 279 (31), 32804–32812.

Inamdar, N. M., Ahn, Y. I., Alam, J. (1996) The heme-responsive element of the mouse heme oxygenase-1 gene is an extended AP-1 binding site that resembles the recognition sequences for MAF and NF-E2 transcription factors. *Biochem Biophys Res Commun.* 221, 570-576.

Iuchi, Y., Okada, F., Onuma, K., Onoda, T., Asao, H., Kobayashi, M. & Fujii, J. (2007) Elevated oxidative stress in erythrocytes due to an SOD1 deficiency causes anemia and triggers autoantibody production. *Biochem. J.* 402: 219-227.

Jacob, H. S., Ingbar, S. H. & Jandl, J. H. (1965) Oxidative hemolysis and erythrocyte metabolism in hereditary acatalasia. *J Clin Invest.* 44, 1187-1199.

Jaiswal, A.K. (1994) Antioxidant response element. *Biochem Pharmacol.* 48, 439-444.

Jilani, T. & Iqbal, M. P. (2011) Does vitamin E have a role in treatment and prevention of anemia's ? *Pak. J. Pharm. Sci.* 24(2), 237-242.

Johnson, G. J., Vatassery, G. R., Finkel, B. & Allen, D. W. (1983) High-dose vitamin E does not decrease the rate of chronic hemolysisin G-6-PD deficiency. *N. Engl. J. Med.* 303, 432-436.

Johnson, R. M., Goyette, G., Ravindranath, Y. & Ho, Y. (2000) Red cells from glutathione peroxidase-1-deficient mice have nearly normal defenses against exogenous peroxides. *Blood.* 96, 1985-1988.

Lee, T. H., Kim, S. U., Yu, S. L., Kim, S. H., Park, S., Moon, H. B., Dho, S. H., Kwon, K. S., Kwon, H. J., Han, Y. H. et al. (2003) Peroxiredoxin II is essential for sustaining life span of erythrocytes in mice. *Blood* 101, 5033–5038.

Lee, J. M., Chan, K., Kan, Y. W., Johnson, J. A. (2004) Targeted disruption of Nrf2 causes regenerative immune-mediated hemolytic anemia. *Proc Natl Acad Sci USA*, 101(26), 9751-9756.

Li, J., Lee, J. M., Johnson, J. A. (2002) Microarray analysis reveals an antioxidant responsive element-driven gene set involved in conferring protection from an oxidative stress-induced apoptosis in IMR-32 cells. *J. Biol. Chem.* 277, 388–394.

Martin, F. M., Bydlon, G. & Friedman, J. S. (2006) SOD2-deficiency sideroblastic anemia and red blood cell oxidative stress. *Antioxid. Redox Signal.* 8(7-8), 1217-1225.

Matte, A., Low, P. S., Turrini, F., Bertoldi, M., Campanella, M. E., Spano, D., Pantaleo, A., Siciliano, A. & De Franceschi L. (2010) Peroxiredoxin-2 expression is increased in beta-thalassemic mouse red cells but is displaced from the membrane as a marker of oxidative stress. *Free Radic Biol Med.* 2010 49(3), 457-466.

Matzuk, M. M., Dionne, L., Guo, Q., Kumar, T. R. & Lebovitz, R. M. (1998) Ovarian function in superoxide dismutase 1 and 2 knockout mice. *Endocrinology* 139, 4008–4011.

McFadden, S. L., Ding, D., Reaume, A. G., Flood, D. G. & Salvi, R. J. (1999) Age-related cochlear hair cell loss is enhanced in mice lacking copper/zinc superoxide dismutase. *Neurobiol. Aging.* 20, 1–8.

Moi, P., Chan, K., Asunis, I., Cao, A., Kan, Y. W. (1994) Isolation of NF-E2- related factor 2 (Nrf2), a NF-E2-like basic leucine zipper transcriptional activator that binds to the tandem NF-E2/AP1 repeat of the beta-globin locus control region.Proc. *Natl. Acad. Sci. USA* 91, 9926–9930.

Mulcahy, R. T., Gipp, J. J. (1995) Identification of a putative antioxidant response element in the 59-flanking region of the human gamma- glutamylcysteine synthetase heavy subunit gene. *Biochem Biophys Res Commun.* 209, 227-233.

Napier, I., Ponka, P. & Richardson, D. R. (2005) Iron trafficking in the mitochondrion: Novel pathways revealed by disease. *Blood* 105, 1867–1874.

Newman, G. J., Newman, T. B., Bowie, L. J. & Mendelsohn, J. (1979) An examinationof the role of vitamin E in G-6-PD deficiency. *Clin. Biochem.* 12, 149-151.

Nur, E., Biemond, B. J., Otten, H. M., Brandjes, D. P & Schnog, J. B. (2011) Oxidative stress in sickle cell disease; pathophysiology and potential implications for disease management. *Am. J. Hematol.* 86, 484–489.

Pace, B. S., Shartava, A., Pack-Mabien, A., Mulekar, M., Ardia, A. & Goodman, S. R. (2003) Effects of N-acetylcysteine on dense cell formation in sickle cell disease. *Am. J. Hematol.* 73(1), 26-32.

Pantaleo, A., Giribaldi, G., Mannu, F., Arese P. & Turrini, F. (2008) Naturally occurring anti-band 3 antibodies and red blood cell removal under physiological and pathological conditions. *Autoimmun. Rev.* 7(6), 457-462.

Prestera, T. & Talalay, P. (1995) Electrophile and antioxidant regulation of enzymes that detoxify carcinogens. *Proc. Nat.l Acad. Sci. USA.* 92, 8965-8969

Rhee, S. G., Kang, S. W., Jeong, W., Chang, T. S., Yang, K. S. & Woo, H. A. (2005) Intracellular messenger function of hydrogen peroxide and its regulation by peroxiredoxins. *Curr. Opin. Cell Biol.* 17, 183–189.

Rice-Evans, C. & Baysal, E. (1987) Iron-mediated oxidative stress in erythrocytes. *Biochem. J.* 244, 191-196.

Rouault, T. A. & Tong, W. H. (2005) Opinion: Iron-sulphur cluster biogenesis and mitochondrial iron homeostasis. *Nat. Rev. Mol. Cell. Biol.* 6, 345–351.

Rund, D., & Rachmilewitz, E. (2005) β-Thalassemia. *N. Engl. J. Med.* 353, 1135-1146.

Rusanova, I., Escames, G., Cossio, G., de Borace, R. G., Moreno, B., Chahboune, M., López, L. C., Díez, T. & Acuña-Castroviejo, D. (2010) Oxidative stress status, clinical outcome, and β-globin gene cluster haplotypes in pediatric patients with sickle cell disease. *Eur J Haematol.* 85(6), 529-537.

Scot, M. D. (2006) H2O2 injury in β thalassemic erythrocytes: Protective role of catalase and the prooxidant effects of GSH. *Free Radic. Biol. & Med.* 40, 1264–1272. Rund, D., & Rachmilewitz, E. (2005) β-Thalassemia. *N. Engl. J. Med.* 353, 1135-1146.

Shinar, E. & Rachmilewitz, E. (1990) Oxidative denaturation of red blood cells in thalassemia. *Semin. Hematol.* 27(1), 70-82.

Starzyński, R. R., Canonne-Hergaux, F., Willemetz, A., Gralak, M. A., Woliński, J., Styś, A., Olszak, J. & Lipiński, P. (2009) Haemolytic anaemia and alterations in hepatic iron metabolism in aged mice lacking Cu,Zn-superoxide dismutase. *Biochem. J.* 420(3), 383-390.

Wood, K. C. & Granger, D. N. (2007) Sickle cell disease: Role of reactive oxygen and nitrogen metabolites. *Clinic Exp Pharmacol Physiol* 34, 926–932.

# 5

# Iron and Nitric Oxide in Anemia of Chronic Disease (ACD)

Oluyomi Stephen Adeyemi[1], Adenike Faoziyat Sulaiman[2] and Musbau Adewumi Akanji[2]
[1]*Redeemer's University, Department of Chemical Sciences, Mowe,*
[2]*University of Ilorin, Department of Biochemistry, Ilorin*
*Nigeria*

## 1. Introduction

Anemia of chronic disease (ACD) may also be referred to as anemia of inflammation and this develops in subjects with diseases involving acute or chronic immune activation. Anemia, which could be described as an immunopathological feature in most established infection, may also be a consequence of host response to invading pathogens. Infections with pathogens normally activate macrophages triggering a strong cytokine production among which are tumor necrosis factor (TNF), γ-interferon (IFN-γ) and nitric oxide (NO). The immune response mounted against such infections is required for parasite clearance but its persistence can cause collateral damage to the host with occurrence of anemia as the major pathology. Inflammation results as a part of this natural immune response. The inflammation triggers the release of chemicals that signal the iron regulation mechanism to adopt a defense mode. Thus this type of anemia is usually characterised by an imbalance between erythrophagocytosis and erythropoiesis, which is linked to, perturbed iron (Fe) homeostasis including altered Fe sequestration and recycling by macrophages and/or sustained and overproduction of NO. The exact mechanism of ACD is not fully understood although studies suggest that the syndrome may partly be due to the influence of hepcidin production on iron metabolism. Moreover complex relationships between Fe and NO has been demonstrated and may be linked to iron deficient anemia during infection.

Both iron and nitric oxide play important roles in the progression and outcome of ACD essentially through the promotion of free radical generation and/or altered homeostasis. Increased iron status may promote free hydroxyl radical generation in cellular systems and thus potentiate cellular damage. Subsequently continuous and sustained production of nitric oxide resulting from persistent infection could contribute to oxidative damage via the formation of peroxynitrite, a very reactive free radical, which may promote lipid peroxidation of key biomolecules and membranes. It should also be noted that production of nitric oxide during infection episodes affects iron metabolism and vice versa. This suggest that a delicate homeostatic balance exist between iron and nitric oxide in living cells such that a disruption or perturbation of this strictly regulated balance would physiologically affect the cellular system. The fact that strong link that has been demonstrated between iron and nitric oxide indicates that the duo play crucial physiological roles in cellular processes.

## 2. Iron metabolism

Iron metabolism may be referred to as the set of biochemical reactions maintaining the homeostasis of iron. Iron is an essential but potentially harmful nutrient. The control of this necessary but potentially toxic substance is an important part of many aspects of human health and disease. Iron contributes to many important physiologic functions in the body essentially because of its unusual flexibility to serve as both an electron donor and acceptor. Iron being critical to a number of synthetic and enzymatic processes by play unique roles in electron transfer and oxygen utilization as heme and non-heme bound proteins. Although most of the body iron is part of hemoglobin molecule where iron serves a key role in oxygen transport, it is also required for proper maintenance of immune functions affecting leukocytes, endothelial cells and cytokine production. Iron also have capacity to promote free radical generation through the Fenton and/or Haber-Weiss reactions, thereby triggering secondary chain reactions in the oxidative modification of lipids, proteins and DNA within cellular systems. Unless appropriately chelated or removed, iron, due to its catalytic action in one-electron redox reactions, plays a key role in the formation of harmful oxygen radicals that may ultimately cause oxidative damage to vital cell structures. To ensure iron availability and to eliminate the toxicity of free iron in addition to its accessibility for invading pathogens, mammals have evolved a strictly regulated system for iron homeostasis. Metabolism of iron is highly regulated within narrow limits. Iron can be recycled and thus conserved by the body. Cellular systems are equipped with exclusive mechanisms that maintain adequate amounts of iron for synthesis of physiologically functional iron-containing molecules and yet keep "free iron" at its lowest possible concentration. Many proteins, hormones and iron itself have been demonstrated to affect iron metabolism by various mechanisms at different regulatory levels. Physiologically, the cellular system acquires iron from plasma glycoprotein, transferrin (Tf). In most cases body iron is sequestered and recycled by the reticuloendothelial system, which breaks down senescent red blood cells (RBCs). Iron metabolism in mammals is a highly regulated phenomenon. This process, which ensures iron availability to meet cellular demand, is necessary in order to eliminate toxicity and free accessibility for invading pathogens.

Iron demands are met obviously through two main sources; acquisition from diet, iron is an absolute requirement for most forms of life, including humans, most microorganisms, plants and animals; therefore it is found in a wide variety of food sources. And also from destruction of heme and non-heme proteins which in most cases are being recycled for reutilization.

### 2.1 Iron acquisition from diet

Dietary iron represents a viable source for acquisition of iron to meet the body demands. The absorption of dietary iron is a variable and dynamic process that ensures the amount of iron absorbed compared to the amount ingested is typically low. The efficiency of iron absorption from diet depends largely on the source and demand for iron. Heme iron (obtainable from animal and plant foods) is best absorbed compared to non-heme iron (iron salts). Dietary iron is absorbed in the duodenum by enterocytes of the mucosal cells. The dietary iron must be part of a protein or be in its ferrous ($Fe^{2+}$) state in order to be absorbed. An enzyme, ferric reductase located on the enterocytes' brush border, Dcytb, reduces ferric $Fe^{3+}$ to $Fe^{2+}$ by lowering the pH. A transport protein called divalent metal transporter-1 (DMT-1 also called Nramp-2) then transport the iron across the enterocyte's cell membrane and into the cell cytosol. The mucosal cells can either store the iron as ferritin which is accomplished by oxidizing $Fe^{2+}$ to $Fe^{3+}$ and subsequent binding to apoferritin to form ferritin (FHC) or translocate the iron through ferroportin-1 (FPN-1) to the portal circulation, which is finally delivered to tissues and the erythroid bone marrow. Hephaestin, a ferroxidase found in the mucosal cells and capable of oxidizing $Fe^{2+}$ to $Fe^{3+}$ may assist ferroportin-1 in transfer of iron. Each of the steps involved in dietary iron acquisition is strictly regulated in response to body need for iron. For instance, cells in response to iron deficiency anemia produce more Dcytb, DMT-1 and ferroportin-1 thus implicating genetic involvement. Several factors including total iron stores, the extent to which bone marrow is producing new red blood cells, the concentration of hemoglobin in the blood, and the oxygen content of the blood all contribute to the rate of iron absorption through the mucosal cells. Infection or inflammation may also affect the rate of iron absorption from diet. Lesser iron is usually absorbed during inflammation and/or infection episodes leading to ACD precipitation. Dcytb is confined to iron transport across the duodenum, while ferroportin-1 is distributed throughout the body on all iron storing cells suggesting that ferroportin-1 is central to cellular iron availability. And indeed, recent discoveries have indicated inflammation leading to hepcidin-induced restriction on iron release from enterocytes via the regulation of ferroportin-1 as responsible for ACD.

## 2.2 Iron bound proteins

Iron is usually bound to hemoglobin, myoglobin, cytochromes, transferrin, lactoferrin and/or ferritin to restrict pathogen access to iron, although most microorganisms or pathogens have developed sophisticated iron-acquiring system that are able to compete successfully with iron-binding proteins of the host. In mammals hemoglobin of red blood cells contain more than 60% of body iron. Much of the remaining is in storage form in ferritin. In physiological conditions, tissue macrophages, in particular liver-associated Kupffer cells recover $Fe^{2+}$ via engulfment of senescent red blood cells (RBCs) from circulation. In addition, these cells internalize the iron-containing hemoglobin; degrade it extracting $Fe^{2+}$ through the action of heme-oxygenase-1 (HO-1) resulting in the release of ferrous iron ($Fe^{2+}$), carbon (II) oxide and bilverdin. Iron is then transported from the phagosome into the cytosol via the DMT-1, the main $Fe^{2+}$ transporter, from where it can be either stored intracellularly via ferritin (FHC) or exported extracellularly via ferroportin-1(FPN-1) depending on the demand for iron. The extracellular $Fe^{2+}$ after conversion to ferric iron ($Fe^{3+}$) through ceruloplasmin (CP), will bind to transferrin (Tf) and transported mainly to the bone marrow to fuel erythropoiesis. Consequently, limitations in iron ($Fe^{3+}$) availability may exert a strong negative impact on erythropoiesis and contribute to ACD. Hence maintaining physiological levels of RBCs relies on a subtle balance between RBC uptake and RBC generation as well as iron homeostasis.

Unique to iron homeostasis are cytosolic iron regulatory proteins (IRP1 and IRP2). These proteins, which are responsive to circulating iron levels, affect iron metabolism by binding to specific nucleotide sequences, termed iron-responsive elements (IREs). Iron-responsive elements (IREs) are usually present in mRNAs for numerous proteins involved in iron metabolism. The binding of IRP1 and IRP2 to IREs affect proteins involved in iron uptake (transferrin receptor-1; TfR1 and DMT-1), utilization (erythroid d-aminolevulinic acid synthase), storage (ferritin) and export (ferroportin-1). IRP1 is a 98-kDa bifunctional protein with mutually exclusive functions of RNA binding and aconitase activity and shares a 30%

identity with mitochondrial aconitase an enzyme of the Krebs cycle. IRP2, a second IRE-binding protein, was initially identified in rat hepatocytes, and had been cloned from a variety of mammalian tissues and cells subsequently. Recent discoveries have shown that IRP2 shares 62% amino acid sequence identity with IRP1 but differs in a unique way by possessing a 73-amino acid insertion in its N-terminal region as well as lacking the [Fe-S] cluster. IRP2 does not have aconitase activity, probably due to the absence of the [Fe-S] cluster. The Fe-S cluster in IRP1 may serve to sense iron level signals. Observations from the several investigations implicated cellular iron as an important factor in the interactions of IRPs with IREs with a consequence affecting the regulation of iron metabolism. When cellular iron becomes depleted, IRP1 and 2 acquire high affinity binding state. The binding of IRPs to the IRE in the 5`- untranslated region (UTR) of ferritin mRNA blocks the translation of ferritin, whereas the association of IRPs with IREs in the 3`- UTR of TfR mRNA stabilizes this transcript. On the other hand, when intracellular iron is abundant, IRP1 acquires aconitase activity and loses IRE binding activity, while IRP2 is degraded, resulting in efficient translation of ferritin mRNA and rapid degradation of TfR mRNA. Also contributing to the regulation of systemic iron homeostasis is the circulating peptide hormone, hepcidin. Hepcidin is usually increased during inflammatory conditions. This ensures cellular iron effluxes are limited by (i) binding to ferroportin-1 and (ii) inducing its internalization.

## 3. Influence of iron and nitric oxide interaction on anemia

RBCs circulate throughout the body engaged in gaseous exchange, oxygen transport, and carbon (iv) oxide removal. Erythropoiesis (Epo) must maintain steady state levels of circulating RBCs and respond to acute challenges. The bone marrow is a highly dynamic organ that produces two to three million red cells every second. These red cells are filled with haemoglobin and are replaced after 75-150 days. This process is controlled by the hypoxia sensing mechanism of the kidney, which responds by modulating the output of Epo, which in turn determines the level of erythropoietic activity. When red cell production fails to match red cell destruction, the result is anaemia.

Iron deficiency anaemia is one of the most common disorders in the world. It however remains an under managed feature of many gastroenterological conditions. About one third of inflammatory bowel disease (IBD) patients suffer from recurrent anaemia. Anaemia has significant impact on the quality of life of affected patients. Chronic fatigue, a frequent IBD symptom itself, is commonly caused by anaemia and may debilitate patients as much as abdominal pain or diarrhoea. Both iron deficiency and anaemia of chronic disease (ACD) contribute mostly to the development of anaemia in IBD. Cobalamin or folate deficiency and various other causes of anaemia such as haemolysis occur infrequently. IBD associated anaemia has been successfully controlled with a combination of iron sucrose and erythropoietin, which then positively affect the misled immune response in IBD.

NO is known to increase the affinity of the intracellular iron-regulatory protein for iron-responsive elements in transferrin receptor and ferritin mRNAs, and a recent study has indicated that NO may affect iron metabolism through disruption of the iron-sulfur complex of iron-regulatory protein 1.

The effects of NO on the regulation of cellular iron metabolism and on the erythropoiesis in anemia of chronic disease has been described extensively; however, there are few studies on the NO production during the various stages of iron deficiency anemia and during iron supplementation. Moreover, data for correlation coefficients between NO production and erythropoiesis in iron deficiency anemia are limited.

### 3.1 Infection influences iron homeostasis leading to anemia

Infections or inflammation conditions in most cases are characterized by anemia (ACD) with profound changes in iron homeostasis usually mediated by cytokines. Following n exposure to a wave of pathogen particles, the host immune system becomes activated leading to the production of cytokines initially by the T-helper cells type-1 (Th-1) and subsequently by T-helper cells type-2 (Th-2). The initial activation of macrophages promotes largely the production of pro-inflammatory cytokines. These cytokines including mainly tumor necrosis factor (TNF), γ-interferon (IFN-γ) and nitric oxide (NO) are key to host defence against the invading pathogens but on the other hand are crucial to promoting inflammatory condition. Inflammation, being a major pathogenic feature during chronic infection may ensue secondary to release of these pro-inflammatory signals by activated macrophages. Also noteworthy is the fact that though the released cytokines are meant to provide an environment necessary for parasite clearance but may also have some physiological effects which include the alteration of iron and subsequently nitric oxide homeostasis with far reaching consequence to the initiation and progression of ACD.

Central to iron homeostasis is the activation of macrophages essentially following exposure to infection. Macrophages are normally responsible for the processing of hemoglobin iron from senescent red blood cells (RBCs) and subsequent supply to the bone marrow for erythropoiesis. As explained earlier, the intracellular iron homeostasis is under the control of cytoplasmic iron regulatory proteins (IRP1 and IRP2), which regulate the expression of several proteins by binding to iron-responsive elements (IREs) on the respective mRNA. Furthermore in addition to its activity being regulated by cellular iron, cytokines also modulate the binding activity of IRP. Cytokines are produced by activated macrophages following contact with infectious agent. The immune cells so activated release cytokines among which is the nitric oxide (NO), tumor necrosis factor-alpha (TNF-α) and interleukin-1 (IL-1) amongst others. The T-helper cells type-1 (Th-1)-derived cytokines have been demonstrated to also affect iron homeostasis by different mechanisms. Interleukin-1 (IL-1) and tumor necrosis factor (TNF) are able to induce hypoferramia by modulating iron metabolism. Pro-inflammatory and anti-inflammatory cytokines produced by T-helper cells type-1 and 2 respectively are major contributors to development of ACD by influencing iron homeostasis. Cytokines do not only affect iron metabolism, but also have inhibitory effects on erythropoiesis by blocking proliferation and differentiation of erythroid progenitor cells limiting their ability to respond to erythropoietin as well as causing deficiency in the production of erythropoietin.

The mononuclear phagocytes acquire iron as a result of erythrophagocytosis during the normal process of removal of senescent blood red cells (RBCs). However the mechanisms involved in the liberation of iron by these cells in order for it to be returned to the circulation is yet to be understood clearly. It is assumed that during inflammatory disease or infection, there is tendency for macrophages to retain more iron in order to restrict pathogen access and this can eventually lead to anemia (ACD).

However, the ability of macrophage-produced nitric oxide (NO) in aiding the release of iron taken up by macrophages through phagocytosis and thereby contributing greatly to the maintenance of iron homeostasis have been demonstrated by several investigators. The role of NO in such scenario involving the reduction of ferritin synthesis and mobilization for intracellular iron seem to oppose the effect of other cytokines such as tumor necrosis factor-alpha (TNF-α) and interleukin-1 (IL-1) which promote iron retention through increased ferritin synthesis. NO production by macrophages is inducible upon introduction of foreign or infectious agent. The implication is that, when an active infection leading to activated macrophages stimulate the production of cytokines in order to get rid of the infectious agent and/or infection, NO acts in opposition to the other cytokines with a resultant effect of maintaining iron homeostasis. Whereas the other cytokines such as tumor necrosis factor-alpha (TNF-α) and interleukin-1 (IL-1) act in a concerted manner to ensure iron sequestration and retention by macrophages so as to minimise the iron level available to invading parasites and by so doing disrupt iron homeostasis, the NO counterbalances these effects by ensuring that iron deficit is minimal essentially through increasing the expression of transferrin receptor (TfR), reduction of ferritin synthesis and activation of IRP1.

## 4. Iron sequestration during infection

Regulating iron balance is necessary especially during infection. Invading pathogens require iron for replication and establishment of infection. Thus it is essential to regulate iron balance such that there is sufficient iron to meet body demands without making too much available to the invading parasites. Although divergent views and conflicting data exist as to the relationship between iron deficiency and infection, recent discoveries have demonstrated that iron depletion protects against and could control infection as well as minimise inflammatory related conditions. Beyond this, the interaction between host and infectious agent is an exciting and complex phenomenon. Yet no theory or experimental model has fully explained it. Several lines of evidence existing illustrate the unique role that iron plays in modulating the battle for survival between mammalian host and the invading pathogens with each organism displaying a unique and competitive mechanism for iron acquisition and maintenance. These mechanisms, which involve enormous genetic investments, are iron responsive and thus able to adapt to the different phases of infection with a variety of tactics on both sides. For instance, in response to poor iron availability in host, pathogens produce siderophores to take the element from host proteins. In response, the mammalian protein lipocalin-2 binds to several kinds of siderophores preventing the pathogen from accessing siderophores-bound iron. However, to evade this strategy, some pathogens produce a glycosylated form of the siderophores preventing its sequestration by lipocalin-2.

## 5. Role of nitric oxide in modulating iron regulatory proteins

In Biological systems, Nitric Oxide (NO), a small free-radical molecule, has been implicated in a vast array of cellular activities, which ranges from acting as a cytotoxic host defence molecule to being an intercellular signal. Two major routes of NO delivery to cells and tissues have being identified; this could be via Nitric oxide donors as: S-nitroso-N-acetyl Penicillamine (SNAP) and sodium nitroprusside (SNP) or via L-arginine in a reaction catalyzed by nitric oxide synthase.

The activity of iron regulatory protein (IRP), is modulated by both NO donors, SNAP and SNP. This may consequently affect iron uptake through transferrin receptor expression. IRP-

1 and IRP-2 are used by cells, to adjust intracellular iron concentration to levels that are adequate for their metabolic needs, but below the toxicity threshold. The proteins therefore, not only sense the status of cytoplasmic iron but also controls Ferritin and transferrin receptor.

The element regulated by the two IRPs, Fe, is essential for all fundamental and vital activities in the cells, so much so that, its deprivation threatens cell survival. While low iron body stores results in iron deficiency, a number of disease states have been pathogenically linked to excess body iron stores. These include acquired or genetic iron overload as well as delocalization of intracellular iron as seen in inflammation and atherosclerosis.

The Two-sided element can be of an advantage or disadvantage to the cell, depending on whether it serves as a micronutrient (advantage) or as a catalyst of free radical reactions (disadvantage). Oxygen radical generation is not the only type of cellular free radical known; the production of nitrogen radicals has also being established. The capacity of readily exchanging electrons makes iron not only essential for fundamental cell functions, but also a potential catalyst for chemical reactions involving free-radical formation and subsequent oxidative stress and cell damage. Cellular iron levels are therefore carefully regulated not only to maintain the body's required concentrations but also to minimize the pool of potentially toxic 'free iron'.

Iron and nitric oxide are intimately associated in various biological processes. Nitric oxide is one of the major pathophysiological stimuli that modulate the activity of IRP-1, a key effector molecule involved in the regulation of intracellular iron metabolism. IRP-1 is a cytoplasmic aconitase (converting citrate into isocitrate) when it contains a [4Fe-4S] cluster, and an RNA-binding protein after complete removal of the metal center. By binding to specific mRNA sequences, the iron responsive elements (IREs), IRP-1 modulates ferritin mRNA translation and transferrin receptor stability.

Contrarily, IRP-2 does not assemble a cluster nor possess aconitase activity, despite structural and functional similarities to IRP-1, it however possess a distinct pattern of tissue expression and is modulated via proteasome-mediated degradation. NO preferentially targets [Fe-S] clusters and the inhibition of aconitase is involved in the cytotoxic effect of NO. Its involvement in a variety of physiological and pathological processes necessitates establishing the role it plays in the IRP-mediated regulation of iron metabolism. The loss of IRP-2 is highly expressed in macrophages even when IRP-1 is activated, this may not be unconnected with the fact that, the improved ferritin synthesis and a decreased transferrin receptor mRNA is accompanied by cytokine-mediated activation of macrophages. While down-regulation of IRP-1 protein levels by NO may have a role to play, IRP-2 has a greater affinity for target IREs.

NO has a number of effects on the key regulators of cellular iron homoeostasis, IRP-1 and IRP-2 in response to fluctuations in the level of the 'labile iron pool', as a result various agents and conditions may affect IRP activity, thereby modulating iron and oxygen radical levels in different patho-biological states. The number of mRNAs regulated through IRE-IRP interactions is on the increase, thereby expanding the role of IRPs from just being iron-regulatory proteins to other roles in essential metabolic pathways.

For instance, the concentration of NO is regulated in the respiratory chain (RC) by a balance between its production and its utilization. This in turn regulates mitochondrial oxygen uptake and energy supply. Cell damage resulting from high concentrations of NO involves

inhibition of a number of cellular processes, such as DNA synthesis and mitochondrial respiration.
While some of these effects may be direct, others arise from the reaction of NO with $O_2$ to form peroxynitrite ($ONOO^-$). NO and $ONOO^-$ can cause damage thereby disrupting cellular functions. To differentiate the sites at which both interact with the respiratory chain from the mechanism of inhibition, NO binds to cytochrome c oxidase, the terminal member of the mitochondrial respiratory chain, and NO, as recently reported, may act as an inhibitor of this enzyme at physiological concentrations in a reversible and competitive reaction with oxygen.
$ONOO^-$ however has little or no effect on cytochrome C oxidase, but inhibits respiratory complexes I–III in an apparently reversible manner. Reaction of NO with molecular oxygen results in oxidation products that can react with low molecular weight and protein-associated thiols, such as cysteine, glutathione, and albumin, to form S-nitrosothiols. It is now established that NO shows antioxidant properties, contrary to the deleterious effects of the reactive nitrogen oxide species formed from NO and oxygen.
Since NO biochemistry is dominated by free-radical reactions, its interaction with other free-radical species could lead to either inhibition or potentiation of oxidative damage effect. Iron–sulfur clusters have long been recognized as molecular targets of NO.
Several reports have shown that NO does increase IRP-1 activity and two possible mechanism or hypothesis of such activation have been suggested for the NO effect: The first is the induction of cytoplasmic aconitase's disassembly and switching to IRP-1 when NO bind to its Fe–S cluster, while the second is NO induction of cellular iron release and reduction of the labile iron pool, effects that would be compensated by spontaneous disassembly of the aconitase cluster or by the synthesis of cluster-free IRP-1. A decrease in aconitase activity may not always be accompanied by a consistent increase in IRP-1 activity, as this is dependent on the iron status of the cell. Iron depleted cells, for instance, may respond to nitrogen reactive species by increasing their IRP-1 activity, a process reflecting disassembly of the aconitase cluster by NO or $ONOO^-$.
IRP-2 is invariably inactivated by NO or $ONOO^-$ or in macrophages committed to the formation of reactive nitrogen species after stimulation with cytokines. This effect is attributed to redox modifications of –SH residues exposed by the cluster-free IRP-2, and to redox modifications followed by proteasome-mediated protein degradation. Thus, IRP-2 degradation may account for the enhanced ferritin synthesis and reduced TfR mRNA content observed in cytokine-stimulated macrophages producing NO and $ONOO^-$. The effect of nitrogen reactive species on IRP may therefore explain the iron sequestration pattern that characterizes macrophages under inflammatory conditions. Current on-going patho-physiological studies across the globe will in the nearest future reveal how to use this mechanism to minimize formation and release of free radicals in diseased tissues.

## 6. Concluding remark

The pathophysiology of ACD may largely be attributed to iron homeostasis, which is affected by several factors. The foregoing discussion has clearly depicted the faces of underlying and intriguing factors that work independently or interdependently to contribute to the initiation and progression of ACD. These factors among which are cytokines produced mainly by activated macrophages in response to prevailing cellular condition at a particular time, more often are responsible for ACD development and also may predict its outcome. In normal physiological state, abundance of iron limits its acquisition from diet and promotes ferritin synthesis while nitric oxide working in concert with iron proteins increases mobilization for intracellular iron. However, all of these processes become perturbed secondary to introduction of other factors. For instance, in the presence of an infection, production of pro-inflammatory cytokines will promotes ACD while an early skewing toward producing anti-inflammatory signals may reverse the situation. In this regard, iron sequestration and retention by macrophages play key role in ACD. In such cases there is abundance of iron stored away in ferritin and not accessible by erythroid cells hence increased erythrophagocytosis without a commensurate erythropoiesis may precipitate anemia. Of crucial importance are the roles played by intracellular iron levels and nitric oxide in affecting iron homeostasis and eventually ACD. In the absence of an infection however, anemia may develop following inadequate iron supply to meet cellular demands.

## 7. References

Adeyemi O.S., Akanji M.A., Johnson T.O., Ekanem J.T. (2011). Iron and nitric oxide balance in African Trypanosomosis: Is there really a link? *Asian J. Biochem.* 6(1): 15 - 28.

Barisani, D., Cairo, G., Ginelli, E., Marozzi A. and Conte D. (2003). Nitric Oxide Reduces Nontransferrin-Bound Iron Transport in HepG2 Cells. *Hepatology*, Volume 29, Issue 2

Beckman, J.S., Beckman, T.W., Chen, J., Marshall, P.A. and Freeman, B.A. (1990). Apparent hydroxyl radical production by peroxynitrite: implications for endothelial injury from nitric oxide and superoxide. *Proc. Natl. Acad. Sci.* USA 87, 1620–1624.

Bolanos, J.P., Heales, S.J.R., Land, J.M. and Clark, J.B. (1995). Effect of peroxynitrite on the mitochondrial respiratory chain: differential susceptibility of neurons and astrocytes in primary culture. *J. Neurochem.* 64, 1965–1972.

Boveris, A., Lores Arnaiz, S., Alvarez, S., Costa, L.E. and Valdez, L. (2000). The mitochondrial production of free radicals. In: Yoshikawa, T., Toyokumi, S., Yamamoto, Y., Naito, Y. (Eds.), *Free Radicals in Chemistry, Biology and Medicine.* OICA International, London, pp. 256–261.

Brown, G.C. and Cooper, C.E. (1994). Non-molar concentrations of nitric oxide reversibly inhibit synaptosomal respiration by competing with oxygen at cytochrome oxidase. *FEBS Lett.* 356, 295–298.

Brudvig, G.W., Stevens, T.H., Morse, R.H. and Chan, S.I. (1980). Reactions of nitric oxide with cytochrome c oxidase. *Biochemistry*:19, 5275–5285.

Cairo G., and Pietrangelo, A. (2000). Iron regulatory proteins in pathobiology. Review Article. *Biochem. J.* 352, 241-250.

Cairo, G. and Pietrangelo, A. (2000). Iron regulatory proteins in pathobiology. *Biochem. J.* 352, 241–250.

Cairo, G., Castrusini, E., Minotti, E. and Bernelli-Zazzera, A. (1996). Superoxide and hydrogen peroxide-dependent inhibition of iron regulatory protein activity: a protective stratagem against oxidative injury. *FASEB J.* 10, 1326–1335.

Cairo, G., Recalcati, S., Pietrangelo, A. and Minotti, G. (2002). The iron regulatory protein: targets and modulators of free radical reactions and oxidative damage. *Free Radic. Biol. Med.* 32, 1237–1243.

Cleeter, M.W.J., Cooper, J.M., Darley-Usmar, V.M., Moncada, S. and Schapira, A.H.V. (1994). Reversible inhibition of cytochrome c oxidase, the terminal enzyme of the mitochondrial respiratory chain by nitric oxide. *FEBS Lett.* 345, 50–54.

Drapier, J. C. and Bouton, C. (1996). Modulation by nitric oxide of metalloprotein regulatory activities. *BioEssays:* 18, 549-556.

Fritsche, G., Larcher, C., Schennach, H. and Weiss, G. (2001). Regulatory interactions between iron and nitric oxide metabolism for immune defense against Plasmodium falciparum infection. *J. Infect. Dis.* 183:1388–1394.

Galleano, M., Aimo, L., Borroni, M.V. and Puntarulo, S. (2001). Nitric oxide and iron overload. Limitations of ESR detection by DETC. *Toxicology.* 167, 199–205.

Galleano, M., Simontacchi, M., and Puntarulo, S. (2004). Nitric oxide and iron: effect of iron overload on nitric oxide production in endotoxemia. Review Article. *Molecular Aspects of Medicine.* 25: 141–154.

Giulivi, C., Poderoso, J.J., Boveris, A., (1998). Production of nitric oxide by mitochondria. *J. Biol. Chem.* 273, 11038–11043.

Gow, A.J. and Stamler, J.S. (1998). Reactions between nitric oxide and haemoglobin under physiological conditions. *Nature:* 391, 169–173.

Hanson, E.S. and Leibold, E.A. (1999). Regulation of the iron regulatory proteins by reactive nitrogen and oxygen species. *Gene. Expr.* 7, 367–376.

Hida, A.I., Kawabata, T., Minamiyama, Y., Mizote, A. and Okada, S. (2003). Saccharated colloidal iron enhances lipopolysaccharide-induced nitric oxide production *in vivo. Free Radic. Biol. Med.* 34, 1426–1434.

Kagan, V.E., Kozlov, A.V., Tyurina, Y.Y., Shvedova, A.A. and Yalowich, J.C. (2001). Antioxidant mechanisms of nitric oxide against iron-catalized oxidative stress in cells. Antiox. *Redox Signal* 3, 189–202.

Kim, S., and Ponka, P. (2000). Effects of interferon-gamma and lipopolysacharide on macrophage iron metabolism are mediated by nitric oxide-induced degradation of iron regulatory protein 2. *J. Biol. Chem.* 275, 6220–6226.

Knowles, R.G. (1997). Nitric oxide, mitochondria and metabolism. *Biochem. Soc. Trans.* 25, 895–901.

Knowles, R.G. and Moncada, S. (1994). Nitric oxide synthases in mammals. *Biochem. J.* 298, 249–258.

Komarov, A.M., Kramer, J.H., Tong Mak, I. and Weglicki, W.B. (1997a). EPR detection of endogenous nitric oxide in postischemic heart using lipid and aqueous-soluble dithiocarbamate-iron complexes. *Mol. Cell. Biochem.* 175, 91–97.

Komarov, A.M., Mattson, D.L., Tong Mak, I. and Weglicki, W.B. (1998). Iron attenuates nitric oxide level and iNOS expression in endotoxin-treated mice. *FEBS Lett.* 424, 253–256.

Komarov, A.M., Tong Mak, I. and Wegliki, W.B. (1997b). Iron potentiates nitric oxide scavenging by dithiocarbamates in tissue of septic shock mice. *Biochim. Biophys. Acta.* 1361, 229–234.

Kubrina, L.N., Mikoyan, V.D., Mordvintcev, P.I. and Vanin, A.F. (1993). Iron potentiates bacterial lipopolisaccharide-induced nitric oxide formation in animal organs *Biochim. Biophys. Acta.* 1176, 240– 244.

Lipinski P., Drapier, J.C., Oliveira L., Retmanska H., Sochanowicz B. and Kruszewski M. (2000). Intracellular iron status as a hallmark of mammalian cell susceptibility to oxidative stress: a study of L5178Y mouse lymphoma cell lines differentially sensitive to $H_2O_2$. *Blood;* 95: 2960–6.

Lizasoain, I., Moro, M.A., Knowles, R.G., Darley-Usmar, V. and Moncada, S. (1996). Nitric oxide and peroxynitrite exert distinct effects on mitochondrial respiration, which are differentially blocked by glutathione or glucose. *Biochem. J.* 314, 887–898.

Mikoyan, V.D., Kubrina, L.N., Serezhenkov, V.A., Stukan, R.A., and Vanin, A.F. (1997). Complexes of $Fe_2$ with diehyldithiocarbamate or N-methyl-D-glucamine dithiocarbamate as traps of nitric oxide in animal tissues: comparative investigations. *Biochim. Biophys. Acta.* 1336, 225–234.

Mikoyan, V.D., Voevodskaya, N.V., Kubrina, L.N., Malenkova, I.V. and Vanin, A.F. (1995). The influence of antioxidants and cicloheximide on the level of nitric oxide in the livers of mice *in vivo. Biochim. Biophys. Acta.* 1269, 19–24.

Moncada, S. and Higgs, E.A. (1995). Molecular mechanisms and therapeutic strategies related to nitric oxide. *FASEB J.* 9, 1319–1330.

Moncada, S., Palmer, R.M.J. and Higgs, E.A. (1991). Nitric oxide: physiology, pathophysiology and pharmacology. *Pharmacol. Rev.* 43, 109–142.

Nathan, C., and Xie, Q.W. (1994). Nitric oxide synthases: roles, tolls, and controls. *Cell:* 78, 915–918.

Obolenskaya, M.Y., Vanin, A.F., Mordvintcev, P.I., Meulsch, A., and Decker, K. (1994). EPR evidence of nitric oxide production by regenerating rat liver. *Biochem. Biophys. Res. Commun.* 202, 571–576.

Pippard, M.J. (1994). Secondary iron overload. In: Powell, L.W. (Ed.), *Iron Metabolism in Health and Disease.* W.B. Saunders, London, pp. 271–309.

Proudfoot, L., Nikolaev, A.V., Feng, G.J., Wei, W.Q., Ferguson, M.A., Brimacombe, J.S., and Liew, F.Y. (1996). Regulation of the expression of nitric oxide synthase and leishmanicidal activity by glycoconjugates of Leishmania lipophosphoglycan in murine macrophages. *Proc. Natl. Acad. Sci.* USA 93, 10984–10989.

Radi, R., Rodriguez, M., Castro, L., and Telleri, R. (1994). Inhibition of mitochondrial electron transport by peroxinitrite. *Arch. Biochem. Biophys.* 308, 89–95.

Recalcati, S., Taramelli, D., Conte, D. and Cairo, G. (1998). Nitric oxide-mediated induction of ferritin synthesis in J774 macrophages by inflammatory cytokines: Role of selective iron regulatory protein-2 down-regulation. *Blood.* 91, 1059–1066

Rubbo, H., Radi, R., Trujillo, M., Telleri, R., Kalyanaraman, B., Barnes, S., Kirk, M., and Freeman, B.A. (1994). Nitric oxide regulation of superoxide and peroxynitrite-dependent lipid peroxidation. Formation of novel nitrogen-containing, oxidized lipid derivatives. *J. Biol. Chem.* 269, 26066–26075.

Starzynski, R.R., Gonçalves, A.S., Muzeau, F., Tyrolczyk, Z., Smuda, E., Drapier, J.C., Beaumont, C., and Lipinski, P. (2006). STAT5 proteins are involved in down-regulation of iron regulatory protein 1 gene expression by nitric oxide. *The Biochemical Journal,* 400(2): 367-75.

Stuehr, D.J., (1999). Mammalian nitric oxide synthases. *Biochim. Biophys. Acta* 1411, 217–230.

Taha, Z., Kiechle, F., and Malinski, T. (1992). Oxidation of nitric oxide by oxygen in biological systems monitored by porphyrinic sensor. *Biochem. Biophys. Res. Commun.* 188, 734–739.

Takenaka, K., Suzuki, S., Sakai, N., Kassel, F., and Yamada, H. (1995). Transferrin induces nitric oxide synthase mRNA in rat cultured aortic smooth muscle cells. *Biochem. Biophys. Res. Commun.* 213, 608–615.

Tiesjema, R.H., and van Gelder, B.F. (1974). Biochemical and biophysical studies on cytochrome c oxidase. XVI. Circular dichroic study of cytochrome c oxidase and its ligand complexes. *Biochim. Biophys. Acta.* 347, 202–214.

Torres, J., Darley-Usmar, V., and Wilson, M.T. (1995). Inhibition of cytochrome c oxidase in turnover by nitric oxide: mechanism and implications for control of respiration. *Biochem. J.* 312, 169–173.

Vanin, A.F. (1999). Iron diethyldithiocarbamate as spin trap for nitric oxide detection. *Meth. Enzymol.* 301, 269–279.

Weinberg, E.D. (2000). Modulation of intramacrophage iron metabolism during microbial cell invasion. *Microbes. Infect.* 2, 85–89.

Weiss, G., Werner-Felmayer, G., Werner, E. R., Grunewald, K., Wachter, H. and Hentze, M. W. (1994). Iron regulates nitric oxide synthase activity by controlling nuclear transcription. *J. Exp. Med.* 180, 969-976

Wink, D.A., Nims, R.W., Darbyshire, J.F., Christodoulou, D., Hanbauer, I., Cox, G.W., Laval, F., Cook, J.A., and Krishna, M.C. (1994). Reaction kinetics for nitrosation of cysteine and glutathione in aerobic nitric oxide solutions at neutral pH. Insights into the fate and physiological effects of intermediates generated in the $NO/O_2$ reaction. *Chem. Res. Toxicol.* 7, 519–525.

# 6

# Diagnostic Evaluation of Anaemia

Vikrant Kale and Abdur Rahmaan Aftab
*Gastroenterology Department,*
*St.Luke's Hospital, Kilkenny*
*Ireland*

## 1. Introduction

Anaemia is one of the major signs of disease. It is never normal and its cause(s) should always be sought.
The history, physical examination, and simple laboratory testing are all useful in evaluating the anaemic patient.
The workup should be directed towards answering the following questions concerning whether one or more of the major processes leading to anaemia may be operative:

- Is the patient bleeding (now or in the past)?
- Is there evidence for increased RBC destruction (haemolysis)?
- Is the bone marrow suppressed?
- Is the patient iron deficient? If so, why?
- Is the patient deficient in folic acid or vitamin B12? If so, why?

Depending on the provisional diagnosis, you may need special investigations like *radiologic tests, bone marrow aspiration, gastrointestinal endoscopies, molecular studies etc.* to arrive at a definite diagnosis.

## 2. History taking

### 2.1 Onset, duration and progress

Insidious onset, long duration and gradual progress of symptoms in a patient with anaemia suggests nutritional anaemia, chronic haemolytic anaemia (congenital or acquired), anaemia of chronic disease and anaemia due to chronic blood loss. Rapid onset, short duration and rapid progress of symptoms indicate acute leukaemia, acute haemolytic anaemia, hemolytic/aplastic crisis in chronic haemolytic anaemia, anaemia secondary to acute blood loss and infiltrative disorders of the bone marrow.
Presence of symptoms other than those due to anaemia is a pointer to underlying disease causing anaemia and provides clues for further work up of the patient. Inquiry should be made to uncover conditions that may cause gastro-intestinal, genito-urinary or any other blood loss.
An anaemic patient who complains of angina or symptoms of cerebral hypoxia urgently needs the oxygen carrying capacity raised by red cell transfusions and inspired oxygen, whatever may be the cause of anaemia.Passage of dark red or brown urine indicates

haemoglobinuria and suggests haemolysis. History of episodes of bone pain, backache, abdominal pain in past suggests the diagnosis of Sickle Cell Disease.

### 2.2 Age & sex

Anaemia is more common in pregnant women, females in reproductive age and children during the phase of rapid growth. A predominantly cereal based diet which is poor in green leafy vegetables and vitamin C containing foods is a common cause of iron deficiency.

In a female patient, a detailed menstrual history and history of reproductive performance (number of deliveries and interval between deliveries), provide information about stress on iron balance and raises the possibility of iron deficiency anaemia.

Self imposed or improperly advised dietary restrictions can contribute to nutritional anaemia.

### 2.3 Drug ingestion

Drug ingestion can cause anaemia in several ways. Long term ingestion of aspirin (in patients of coronary artery disease) can lead to chronic blood loss and iron deficiency anaemia. Certain drugs can cause haemolysis in individuals with G-6-PD deficiency. Rifampicin and alpha methyl dopa can cause autoimmune haemolytic anaemia. Chemotherapeutic drugs can cause marrow depression and pancytopenia.

A past history of cardiac valve surgery can indicate the possibility of haemolysis.

## 3. Physical examination

Clinical examination can provide a wealth of diagnostic information. Although signs are not always present, they can be helpful in making a clinical diagnosis.

A smooth(bald) tongue and nail changes of koilonychia (brittle, flat or concave nails, more common in toe nails than in finger nails), and bilateral, painless parotid enlargement in a patient with anaemia suggests the diagnosis of *iron deficiency anaemia*. Skin pigmentation in the peri-oral region and over the knuckles is suggestive of *megaloblastic anaemia*. The presence of mild jaundice would suggest possibility of *haemolytic anaemia*. A generalized greyish discoloration of skin indicates *iron overload* in anaemic patients who have been given blood transfusions over several years. Skin pigmentation and various skeletal abnormalities may be present in some cases of *constitutional hypoplastic anaemia*. The presence of petechial haemorrhages would indicate a marrow infiltrative disease (leukaemia, lymphoma, myeloma, metastases, etc.), they may also be seen in megaloblastic anaemia.

Fronto-temporal bossing, malar prominence, upper jaw and teeth projecting beyond the lower jaw, flat bridge of the nose - all giving rise to typical facial appearance are characteristic of *Thalassemia syndromes*. Puffiness of lower eye lids, loss of eye brow hair and thick voice would suggest *myxedema* as the cause of anaemia; this can be confirmed by delayed relaxation of muscle after eliciting deep reflexes.

The presence of hypertension should alert the clinician to the possibility of *anaemia secondary to chronic renal failure*.

Tenderness of calf muscles suggests megaloblastic anaemia but could be present even in iron deficiency anaemia. Signs of sub-acute combined degeneration indicate *pernicious anaemia*. Lymphadenopathy suggests the possibility of *leukaemia or lymphoma*.

## 4. Laboratory evaluation

Lab tests in the diagnosis of Anaemia:

| 1.Complete Blood Count(CBC) | 2. Iron supply studies |
|---|---|
| A. Red blood cell count<br>- Haemoglobin<br>- Hematocrit(HCT)<br>- Reticulocyte count | A. Serum Iron<br>B. Total iron binding capacity<br>C. Serum ferritin |
| B. Red blood cell indices<br>- Mean cell volume(MCV)<br>- Mean cell haemoglobin(MCH)<br>- Mean cell haemoglobin Concentration(MCHC)<br>- Red cell distribution width (RDW) | D. Marrow iron stain<br>3. Marrow examination<br>A. Aspirate<br>- M/E ratio*<br>- Cell morphology<br>- Iron stain |
| C. White blood cell count<br>- Cell differential<br>- Nuclear segmentation of Neutrophils | B. Biopsy<br>- Cellularity<br>- Morphology |
| D. Platelet count | |
| E. Cell morphology<br>- Cell size<br>- Haemoglobin content<br>- Anisocytosis<br>- Poikilocytosis<br>- Polychromasia | |

M/E ratio - ratio of myeloid to erythroid precursors.
Source - Harrison's Principles of Internal Medicine, 16th edition.

### 4.1 Mean corpuscular volume

The normal range for MCV is from 80 to 100 femtoliters (fL). Values in excess of 115 fL are almost exclusively seen in vitamin B12 or folic acid deficiency. Even higher values can occur as an artefact when cold agglutinins are present, which causes RBCs to go through the counting aperture in doublets or triplets. Low values usually indicate a microcytic anaemia.

### 4.2 Mean corpuscular haemoglobin

The normal MCH ranges from 27.5 to 33.2 picograms of haemoglobin per RBC. Low values are seen in iron deficiency and thalassemia, while increased values occur in macrocytosis of any cause.

### 4.3 Mean corpuscular haemoglobin concentration

The mean normal value for the MCHC is 34 grams of haemoglobin per dL of RBCs. Low values occur in the same conditions that generate low values for MCV and MCH, while increased values occur almost exclusively in the presence of congenital or acquired spherocytosis or in other congenital haemolytic anaemia in which red cells are abnormally desiccated (eg, sickle cell anaemia, haemoglobin C disease, xerocytosis).

### 4.4 Reticulocyte count

The reticulocyte count, either as a percentage of all RBCs, the absolute reticulocyte count, the corrected absolute reticulocyte count, or as the reticulocyte production index, helps to distinguish among the different types of anaemia:

- Anaemia with a high reticulocyte count reflects an increased erythropoietic response to continued haemolysis or blood loss.
- A stable anaemia with a low reticulocyte count is strong evidence for deficient production of RBCs (ie, a reduced marrow response to the anaemia).
- Haemolysis or blood loss can be associated with a low reticulocyte count if there is a concurrent disorder that impairs RBC production (eg, infection, prior chemotherapy).
- A low reticulocyte percentage accompanied by pancytopenia is suggestive of aplastic anaemia, while a reticulocyte percentage of zero with normal white blood cell and platelet counts suggests a diagnosis of pure red cell aplasia.

### 4.5 White blood cell count and differential

A low total white blood cell (WBC) count (leukopenia) in a patient with anaemia should lead to consideration of bone marrow suppression or replacement, hypersplenism, or deficiencies of cobalamin(B12) or folate. In comparison, a high total WBC count (leukocytosis) may reflect the presence of infection, inflammation, or a hematologic malignancy.

Clues to the specific abnormality present may be obtained from the WBC differential, which, in conjunction with the total WBC may show increased or decreased absolute numbers of the various cell types in the circulation. Examples include:

- An increased absolute neutrophil count in infection or steroid therapy
- An increased absolute monocyte count in myelodysplasia
- An increased absolute eosinophil count in certain infections
- A decreased absolute neutrophil count following chemotherapy
- A decreased absolute lymphocyte count in HIV infection or following treatment with corticosteroids.

### 4.6 Neutrophil hypersegmentation

Neutrophil hypersegmentation (NH) is defined as the presence of >5 percent of neutrophils with five or more lobes and/or the presence of one or more neutrophils with six or more lobes. This peripheral smear finding, along with macro-ovalocytic red cells, is classically associated with impaired DNA synthesis, as seen in disorders of vitamins B12 and folic acid.

### 4.7 Circulating nucleated red blood cells

Nucleated RBCs (NRBCs) are not normally found in the circulation. They may be present in patients with known hematologic disease (eg, sickle cell disease, thalassemia major, various

haemolytic anaemia after splenectomy), or as a part of the leukoerythroblastic pattern seen in patients with bone marrow replacement.
In patients without known hematologic disease, NRBCs may reflect the presence of a life-threatening disease, such as sepsis or severe heart failure.

### 4.8 Platelet count

Abnormalities in the platelet count often provide important diagnostic information. Thrombocytopenia occurs in a variety of disorders associated with anaemia, including hypersplenism, marrow involvement with malignancy, autoimmune platelet destruction (either idiopathic or drug-related), sepsis, or folate or cobalamin deficiency.
High platelet counts, in comparison, may reflect myeloproliferative disease, chronic iron deficiency, and inflammatory, infectious, or neoplastic disorders. Changes in platelet morphology (giant platelets, degranulated platelets) also may be important, suggesting myeloproliferative or myelodysplastic disease.

### 4.9 Pancytopenia

The combination of anaemia, thrombocytopenia, and neutropenia is termed pancytopenia. The presence of severe pancytopenia narrows the differential diagnosis to disorders such as aplastic anaemia, folate or cobalamin deficiency, or hematologic malignancy (eg, acute myeloid leukaemia). Mild degrees of pancytopenia may be seen in patients with splenomegaly and splenic trapping of circulating cellular elements(hypersplenism).

### 4.10 Blood smear

Many clinicians rely on the above RBC parameters and the RDW in evaluating a patient with anaemia. However, the RDW is of limited utility, and examination of the peripheral blood smear provides information not otherwise available.
As examples, the automated counter may miss the red cell fragmentation ("helmet cells", schistocytes) of microangiopathic haemolysis, microspherocytes in autoimmune haemolytic anaemia, teardrop RBCs in myeloid metaplasia, a leukoerythroblastic pattern with bone marrow replacement, the "bite cells" in oxidative haemolysis, or RBC parasites such as malaria or babesiosis.

### 4.11 Serial evaluation of haemoglobin and hematocrit

Measuring the rate of fall of the patient's Hb or HCT often provides helpful diagnostic information. Suppose the Hb concentration has fallen from 15 to 10 g/dL in one week. If this were due to total cessation of RBC production (ie, a reticulocyte count of zero) and if the rate of RBC destruction were normal (1 percent/day), the Hb concentration would have fallen by 7 percent over seven days, resulting a decline of 1.05 g/dL (0.07 x 15). The greater fall in Hb in this patient (5 g/dL) indicates that marrow suppression cannot be the sole cause of the anaemia and that blood loss and/or increased RBC destruction must be present.

### 4.12 Evaluation for iron deficiency

More complete evaluation for iron deficiency is indicated when the history (menometrorrhagia, symptoms of peptic ulcer disease) and preliminary laboratory data (low MCV, low MCH, high RDW, increased platelet count) support this diagnosis. In this setting, the plasma levels of iron, iron binding capacity (transferrin), transferrin saturation, and ferritin should be measured. This is discussed in detail below.

### 4.13 Evaluation for haemolysis

Haemolysis should be considered if the patient has a rapid fall in haemoglobin concentration, reticulocytosis, and/or abnormally shaped RBCs (especially spherocytes or fragmented RBCs) on the peripheral smear. The usual ancillary findings of haemolysis are an increase in the serum lactate dehydrogenase (LDH) and indirect bilirubin concentrations and a reduction in the serum haptoglobin concentration.

The combination of an increased LDH and reduced haptoglobin is 90 percent specific for diagnosing haemolysis, while the combination of a normal LDH and a serum haptoglobin greater than 25 mg/dL is 92 percent sensitive for ruling out haemolysis.

### 4.14 Intravascular haemolysis

Serum or plasma haemoglobin and urinary hemosiderin should be measured if intravascular haemolysis is a consideration, as with paroxysmal nocturnal haemoglobinuria.

### 4.15 Bone marrow examination

Examination of the bone marrow generally offers little additional diagnostic information in the more common forms of anaemia. If erythropoiesis is increased in response to the anaemia, the bone marrow will show erythroid hyperplasia, a nonspecific finding. Similarly, although the absence of stainable iron in the bone marrow had previously been considered the "gold standard" for the diagnosis of iron deficiency, this diagnosis is usually established by laboratory tests alone

Indications for examination of the bone marrow in anaemic patients include pancytopenia or the presence of abnormal cells in the circulation, such as blast forms. Such patients may have aplastic anaemia, myelodysplasia, marrow replacement with malignancy, or a myeloproliferative disease. Other findings that may be seen in the marrow in anaemic patients include megaloblastic erythropoiesis (folate or cobalamin deficiency), absence of recognizable RBC precursors (pure RBC aplasia), vacuolization of RBC precursors (alcohol or drug-induced anaemia), and increased iron-laden RBC precursors (the sideroblastic anaemia).

### 4.16 Multiple causes of anaemia

Multiple causes are frequently present in adults, particularly the elderly. Common examples are:

- A patient with gastrointestinal bleeding secondary to colon cancer may also have the anaemia of chronic disease, leading to a blunted reticulocyte response.
- A patient with a chronic hemolytic anaemia (eg, sickle cell anaemia, hereditary spherocytosis) may develop worsening anaemia following acute infection, particularly with parvovirus B19, which may blunt or temporarily ablate erythropoiesis and the reticulocyte response.
- A patient with autoimmune hemolytic anaemia may develop worsening anaemia from gastrointestinal blood loss following treatment with corticosteroids.
- Anaemia, renal failure, and congestive failure are often found together, a condition that has been termed "cardio-renal anaemia syndrome." Treatment of the anaemia may improve both the renal failure and heart failure.

**Algorithm for diagnosing cause of anaemia**

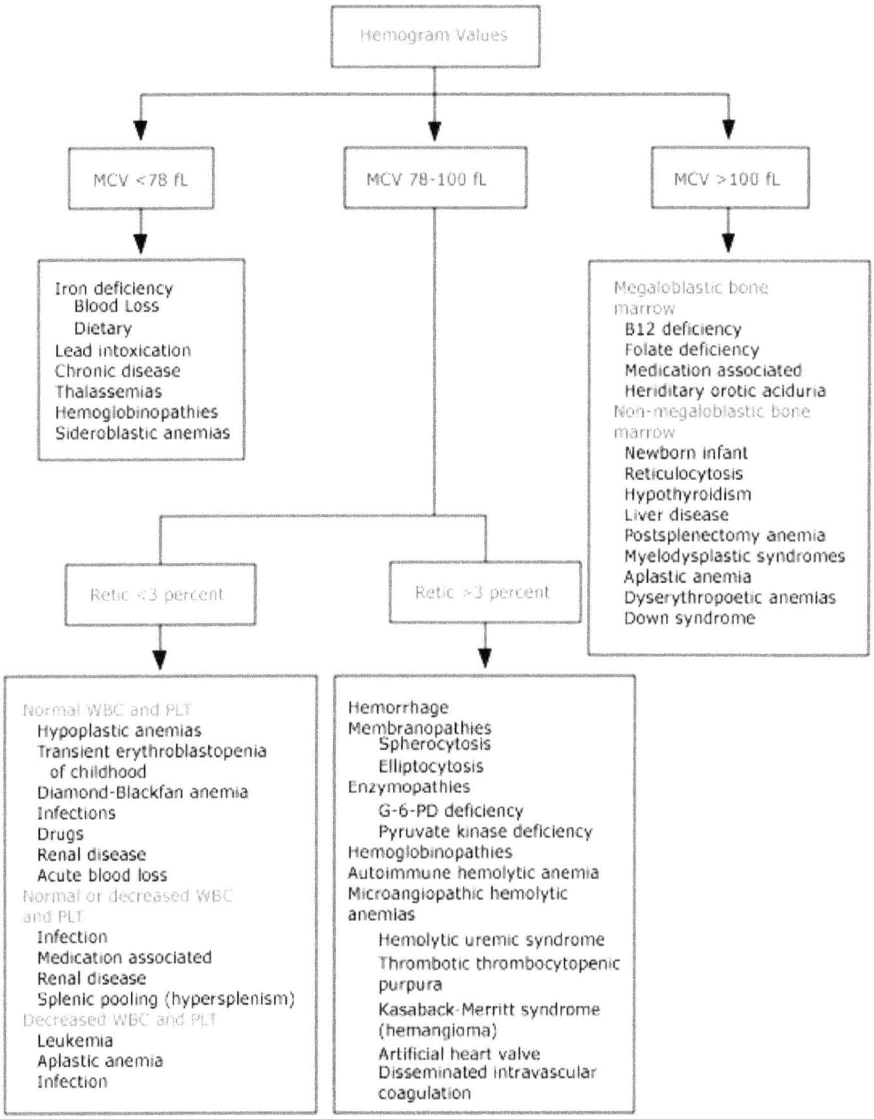


Source : Nathan, DG, Oski, FA. *Hematology of Infancy and Childhood*, 4th ed, WB Saunders, Philadelphia, PA 1993. p. 352.

## 5. Anaemia due to decreased red cell production

A variety of disorders are associated with anaemia due to decreased red cell production (ie, hypoproliferative anaemia). This situation is simplistically identified by the finding of a low corrected absolute reticulocyte count (reticulocytopenia).

The differential diagnosis of a hypoproliferative anaemia can often be narrowed by identification of one of the six specific presenting patterns outlined below.

### 5.1 Normocytic anaemia without leukopenia or thrombocytopenia

The peripheral smear in this setting demonstrates normal red blood cell (RBC) morphology. The red cell indices are normal or slightly hypochromic or microcytic. The white blood cell (WBC) count is usually normal although there may be a neutrophilic leukocytosis. The WBC are not dysplastic and blasts are not seen. The platelet count is usually normal or elevated. The platelets are not dysplastic.

The bone marrow is usually not examined in these cases. If studied, it would show normal cellularity, normal maturation of the several cell lines, and normal iron stores.

This pattern can be induced by a number of disorders-

#### 5.1.1 Anaemia of (chronic) inflammation

This condition is most often associated with infection, inflammation, or malignancy. Initial evaluation with ESR or CRP and then focussed investigations to find a cause should be done.

#### 5.1.2 Mild to moderate iron deficiency

Mild to moderate iron deficiency can be associated with anaemia without the classic findings of hypochromia or microcytosis.

#### 5.1.3 Renal failure

The anaemia associated with renal failure is usually due to a marked reduction in erythropoietin (EPO) production relative to the degree of anaemia. The EPO level usually does not fall until the creatinine clearance drops below 30 mL/minute. Urinalysis for Albumin to Creatinine ratio(ACR) is helpful in detecting renal disease, especially in patients with Diabetes mellitus.

#### 5.1.4 Endocrine disorders

A mild hypoproliferative anaemia can be seen in a number of endocrine disorders, including hypothyroidism, hyperthyroidism, panhypopituitarism, and primary or secondary hyperparathyroidism. How the anaemia occurs in these disorders is not well understood but correction of the endocrine disturbance usually corrects the anaemia.

### 5.2 Normocytic anaemia with low to absent reticulocytes

The presentation in this setting is similar to variant 1 with one important exception: the RBC morphology is normal but the reticulocyte count is very low, usually <10,000/microL, frequently as low as 2,000/microL, and occasionally zero.

This pattern is highly suggestive of pure red cell aplasia. The bone marrow will show normal overall cellularity and morphology except for the virtual absence of all identifiable erythroid precursors. Giant proerythroblasts may be seen in those patients with pure red cell aplasia secondary to infection with parvovirus.

There are many causes of acquired pure red cell aplasia in adults, the most common being idiopathic, drug-induced, myelodysplastic syndrome, T-cell large granular lymphocytic leukaemia, and thymoma. Regardless of the etiology, the final common pathway seems to be an immunologic attack, usually mediated by T cells, on erythroid progenitors at a maturity level between CFU-E (colony-forming units-erythroid) and proerythroblasts.

### 5.3 Normocytic anaemia with pancytopenia

The peripheral smear in these patients usually reveals normal RBC morphology but macrocytosis is occasionally seen. The WBC count is low with prominent neutropenia (absolute neutrophil count below 1000/microL) and, in some cases, lymphopenia (<1000/microL) as well. WBC morphology is normal. The platelet count is reduced; the platelet morphology is generally normal with occasional large platelets.

Bone marrow examination is almost always performed in patients with pancytopenia, usually in conjunction with cytogenetic studies. The marrow in most cases of hypoproliferative anaemia with pancytopenia is either profoundly hypocellular with relatively normal morphology of the remaining elements or hypocellular with dysplasia of red cell, neutrophil, and platelet precursors. In some patients, however, the marrow is totally replaced with malignant cells or fibrosis.

Pancytopenia without prominent morphologic abnormalities has a very different set of clinical implications from isolated anaemia. The major causes of this problem include:

- Aplastic anaemia
- Bone marrow suppression following chemotherapy and/or radiation therapy
- Hypoplastic myelodysplastic syndrome
- Marrow replaced by leukaemia, lymphoma, cancer, or rarely, fibrosis

Although splenomegaly can also cause pancytopenia (ie, hypersplenism), the increased peripheral destruction seen in hypersplenism is associated with enhanced erythropoiesis and a high reticulocyte count, and the bone marrow is normocellular to hypercellular, rather than aplastic or hypocellular.

### 5.4 Macrocytic non-megaloblastic anaemia

The peripheral smear in this disorder shows RBCs that are distinctly macrocytic with very few macroovalocytes. The mean cell volume (MCV) is generally greater than 100 fL. The WBC may be slightly low but there is no dysplasia or blasts. Few, if any, five to six lobed neutrophils are present. The platelet count may be normal or as low as 50,000/microL.

The bone marrow is usually not examined in this setting but, if performed, cellularity and maturation are normal. *Megaloblastosis*, characteristic of cobalamin or folate deficiency, is not seen.

Several disorders can produce a hypoproliferative, macrocytic anaemia without megaloblastosis-

- Alcohol abuse
- Therapy with zidovudine(AZT), other anti-viral agents, hydroxyurea, methotrexate, phenytoin
- Myelodysplastic syndrome, early in its course
- Early in the course of cobalamin or folate deficiency.

### 5.5 Macrocytic megaloblastic anaemia

The peripheral smear in this setting reveals macrocytic RBCs with macroovalocytes. The WBC count is normal or low, but the neutrophils show hypersegmentation with at least 5 percent of the cells having five or more lobes. The platelet count is normal or low.

These findings are highly suggestive of folate or cobalamin (vitamin B12) deficiency. Bone marrow examination is usually not necessary.

### 5.6 Leucoerythroblastic anaemia

The peripheral smear in a patient with a leukoerythroblastic anaemia shows abnormal RBC morphology with tear-drop forms, elliptocytes, macrocytes, and circulating nucleated RBC. The WBC count may be high, low, or normal, but there is myeloid immaturity extending back to the myeloblast stage. The platelet count is usually low with abnormal morphology, including giant platelets and even megakaryocyte fragments.

A leukoerythroblastic picture reflects replacement of the bone marrow by granulomas, cancer, fibrosis, or primary myelofibrosis (PMF). The remaining pluripotent stem cells move to the liver and spleen as they did in fetal life, resulting in extramedullary hematopoiesis. The stromal support system in the liver and spleen is not optimal, as it is in the marrow. As a result, hematopoietic cells are released prematurely or abnormally into the circulation. The reticulocyte count is of limited value in this setting because extramedullary hematopoiesis is associated with both disordered release of reticulocytes into the peripheral blood and disordered maturation of nucleated RBC to reticulocytes in the peripheral circulation.

Having recognized the virtually pathognomonic peripheral smear findings, the differential diagnosis focuses on what is replacing the marrow. Therefore, a bone marrow biopsy (aspiration may result in a dry tap) with appropriate staining (for reticulin and collagen) is necessary. There are two major causes:

-Metastatic cancer.

-Myelofibrosis, as seen in the myeloproliferative syndromes such as PMF or myelofibrosis associated with acute myeloid leukaemia, other cancer, or radiation.

The differential diagnosis of a *hypoproliferative anaemia with microcytosis*, which is most often due to iron deficiency, is discussed below.

## 6. Anaemia due to iron deficiency

The development of iron deficiency, and the rapidity with which it progresses, is dependent upon the individual's initial iron stores which are, in turn, dependent upon age, sex, rate of growth and the balance between iron absorption and loss.

Causes of iron deficiency are discussed below.

### 6.1 Blood loss

The major cause of iron deficiency in affluent countries is blood loss, either overt or occult. Overt blood loss is, by definition, obvious and not difficult for the clinician to recognize, often by history alone. Examples include severe traumatic haemorrhage, haematemesis, malena, haemoptysis, severe menorrhagia and gross haematuria.

Occult bleeding, on the other hand, may be difficult to track down. This usually occurs via the gastrointestinal tract in men. Other causes are repeated voluntary blood donations, the post-operative setting in which blood loss greatly exceeds the amount of blood transfused, or iatrogenic anaemia due to repeated and massive blood drawing in the course of workup of a complicated medical condition. Additional factors are often responsible in women, including underestimating the degree of menometrorrhagia, blood loss during delivery, and direct iron loss to the fetus during pregnancy and to the neonate during lactation.

Although reduced gastrointestinal absorption of iron and a diet deficient in iron can also cause iron deficiency, it is most reasonable to believe, as a first assumption, that *iron deficiency reflects blood loss*, in order to avoiding missing an occult malignancy or other bleeding intestinal lesion.

### 6.2 Decreased iron absorption

Gastrointestinal malabsorption of iron is a relatively uncommon cause of iron deficiency, although it may be observed in certain diseases associated with generalized malabsorption or achlorhydria [5]. However, the use of proton pump inhibitors, which reduce gastric acid secretion, has not been associated with clinical iron deficiency.

### 6.3 Foods and medications

There are a number of foods and medications that impair absorption of iron.

| Absorption of haem iron is affected by: |
|---|
| Amount of haem iron, especially in meat |
| Content of calcium in the meal (calcium impairs iron absorption) |
| Absorption of nonhaem iron is affected by: |
| Iron status |
| Amount of potentially available nonhaem iron |
| Balance between positive and negative factors |
| Positive factors |
| Ascorbic acid |
| Meat or fish (haem iron enhances absorption of nonhaem iron) |
| Negative factors |
| Phytate (in bran, oats, rye fibre) |
| Polyphenols (in tea, some vegetables and cereals) |
| Dietary calcium |
| Soy protein |

### 6.4 Coeliac disease

Iron deficiency anaemia, refractory to oral iron treatment can be seen in patients with coeliac disease, autoimmune atrophic gastritis or Helicobacter pylori infection. It is unclear whether there is a component of blood loss contributing to iron deficiency in this condition, although a component of the anaemia of chronic disease (inflammation) is seen in some individuals.

### 6.5 Other causes

There are several other uncommon causes of iron deficiency:

### 6.5.1 Intravascular haemolysis

Intravascular haemolysis, with its accompanying haemoglobinuria and hemosiderinuria can lead to significant urinary iron losses in patients with paroxysmal nocturnal haemoglobinuria and in cardiac patients with intravascular destruction of red cells secondary to malfunctioning valvular prostheses, patches, or intracardiac myxomas.

### 6.5.2 Pulmonary hemosiderosis

Pulmonary hemosiderosis (eg, chronic pulmonary haemorrhage in anti-glomerular basement membrane antibody disease) can appear as functional iron deficiency.

### 6.5.3 Response to erythropoietin

A response to treatment with erythropoietin (EPO) for the anaemia of chronic renal failure often leads to iron deficiency, since the iron requirements generated by this response can usually not be met by mobilization of the patient's iron stores alone.

### 6.5.4 Gastric bypass for morbid obesity

This form of surgery bypasses the duodenum, the major site of intestinal iron absorption.
As a result, iron deficiency can occur following gastric bypass surgery, not only through the bypassing of the site of major iron absorption, but also as the result of decreased gastric acid availability.

### 6.5.5 Congenital iron deficiency

Rare families with iron deficiency anaemia unresponsive to oral iron therapy, but partially responsive to parenteral iron, have been reported.

## 6.6 Estimation of iron stores

The patient's history, complete blood count, red blood cell indices, and examination of the peripheral blood smear usually allow the clinician to make a presumptive diagnosis of iron deficiency anaemia. This can be followed by a therapeutic trial of iron administration to provide both confirmation of the diagnosis and therapy.

### 6.6.1Therapeutic trial of iron

A presumptive diagnosis of iron deficiency anaemia is made if there is a positive response to a trial of oral iron therapy, characterized by a modest reticulocytosis beginning in about five to seven days, followed by an increase in haemoglobin at a rate of about 2 to 4 g/dL every three weeks until the haemoglobin concentration returns to normal.
The limitation of this approach occurs if there is no response, or the response is modest or incomplete. In this setting, the clinician cannot differentiate among poor patient compliance, inability to absorb the iron preparation, an incorrect diagnosis, continued bleeding, or a coexisting condition such as the anaemia of chronic disease or renal failure that blocks the full reticulocyte response.
For these reasons, laboratory tests (eg, iron studies, iron panel) are often ordered to confirm the diagnosis prior to initiation of therapy

### 6.6.2 Serum or plasma ferritin

The serum or plasma ferritin concentration is an *excellent indicator of iron stores* in otherwise healthy adults and has replaced assessment of bone marrow iron stores as the gold standard for the diagnosis of iron deficiency in most patients. There is no clinical situation other than iron deficiency in which extremely low values of serum ferritin are seen.

### 6.6.3 Pregnancy

Serum ferritin is useful in diagnosing iron deficiency in pregnant women, who often have an elevated serum transferrin in the absence of iron deficiency.

### 6.6.4 Inflammatory states

Ferritin is an acute phase reactant, with plasma levels increasing in liver disease, infection, inflammation, and malignancy.

### 6.6.5 Serum iron and transferrin (TIBC)

In iron deficiency anaemia, the serum iron concentration (SI) is reduced, and the level of transferrin - also measured as total iron binding capacity (TIBC) is elevated; the latter finding reflects the reciprocal relationship between serum iron and transferrin gene expression in most nonerythroid cells.

The accuracy of measurement of transferrin/TIBC for predicting the presence of iron deficiency is second only to the serum or plasma ferritin concentration. Confounding factors are pregnancy and oral contraceptives, which increase the plasma transferrin concentration.

### 6.6.6 Bone marrow iron

Iron in bone marrow macrophages and erythroid precursors (sideroblasts) can be detected with the Prussian Blue stain on marrow spicules. Lack of stainable iron in erythroid precursors as well as marrow macrophages is considered by most clinicians to be the "gold standard" for the diagnosis of iron deficiency. In contrast, in uncomplicated anaemia of chronic disease, iron is present in marrow macrophages but absent or reduced in erythroid precursors.

However, bone marrow sampling and testing for stainable iron is expensive, invasive, and usually unnecessary. It has been replaced in practice by measurement of serum ferritin.

### 6.6.7 Assessment of iron sufficiency

Serum ferritin is often ordered to assess whether the patient is iron sufficient, rather than deficient. Similarly, defining iron sufficiency for the purpose of predicting a response in anaemic patients with chronic renal insufficiency to treatment with erythropoietin requires a relatively high amount of available iron, usually stated as a serum ferritin ≥100 ng/mL and a transferrin saturation ≥20 percent.

### 6.6.8 Red cell morphology and indices

Despite the classic description of iron deficiency as leading to a hypochromic, microcytic anaemia, many iron deficient patients in western countries will have normal red cell morphology. Further, the finding of a hypochromic microcytic anaemia is not pathognomonic of iron deficiency, with thalassemia and, less commonly, the anaemia of chronic inflammation being the other common conditions encountered in daily practice. It is important to rule out these disorders before beginning a trial of iron therapy, since many patients with thalassemia or chronic inflammation are already iron overloaded.

## 7.Evaluation of anaemia due to blood loss

### 7.1 Upper and lower GI evaluation

Upper and lower GI investigations should be considered in all postmenopausal female and all male patients where Iron Deficiency anaemia(IDA) has been confirmed unless there is a history of significant overt non-GI blood loss.

In the absence of suggestive symptoms (which are unreliable), the order of investigations is determined by local availability, although all patients should be screened for coeliac disease with serology. Small-bowel biopsy samples should be taken at OGD if coeliac serology was positive or not performed.

If oesophago-gastro-duodenoscopy (OGD) is performed as the initial GI investigation, only the presence of gastric cancer or coeliac disease, as explained below, should deter lower GI investigation. In particular, the presence of oesophagitis, erosions and peptic ulcer disease should not be accepted as the cause of IDA until lower GI investigations have been carried out.

Colonoscopy has the following advantages over radiology: it allows biopsy of lesions, treatment of adenomas, and identification of superficial pathology such as angiodysplasia and NSAID damage. Performing gastroscopy and colonoscopy at the same session speeds investigation and saves time for both the hospital and the patient, because only one attendance for endoscopy is required.

Radiographic imaging is a sufficient alternative where colonoscopy is contraindicated. The sensitivity of CT colonography for lesions >10 mm in size is over 90%. Barium enema is less reliable, but is still useful if colonoscopy or CT colonography are not readily available.

### 7.2 Screening for and further investigation of coeliac disease

Ideally coeliac serology—tissue transglutaminase (tTG) antibody or endomysial antibody, if tTG antibody testing is not available—should be undertaken at presentation. But if this has not been carried out or if the result is not available, duodenal biopsy specimens should be taken. If coeliac serology is negative, small-bowel biopsies need not be performed at OGD unless there are other features, such as diarrhoea, which make coeliac disease more likely. If the tTG antibody test is negative, the post-test probability of coeliac disease is 0.3%, which is less than in the general population. If coeliac serology is positive, coeliac disease is likely and should be confirmed by small-bowel biopsy.

### 7.3 Further evaluation

Further imaging of the small bowel is probably not necessary unless there is an inadequate response to iron therapy, especially if transfusion dependent. In those with an inadequate response, *video capsule endoscopy or enteroscopy* may be helpful to detect angiodysplasia, Crohn's disease and small-bowel neoplasia.

Video capsule endoscopy has a diagnostic yield of 40-55% in this setting. However, it seldom results in a beneficial subsequent intervention. Many lesions detected by both enteroscopy and video capsule endoscopy are within the reach of a gastroscope, and repeat OGD should be considered before these procedures. Bleeding lesions identified by video capsule endoscopy may be amenable to treatment by push or double-balloon enteroscopy. However, the benefits of these procedures after a normal video capsule endoscopy in the context of IDA are unproven.

Small-bowel imaging (*MRI enteroclysis, CT enterography or barium studies*) should also be considered in patients with symptoms suggestive of small-bowel disease, transfusion-dependent IDA, and rapid recurrence of anaemia after normalisation of Hb concentrations. However, many small intestinal lesions that cause asymptomatic anaemia are mucosal and flat or nearly so and most small intestinal imaging modalities apart from video capsule endoscopy are only efficient at identifying mass lesions. CT has the additional advantage of being able to identify extraintestinal pathology such as renal tumours and lymphomas.

*Helicobacter pylori* colonisation may impair iron uptake and increase iron loss, potentially leading to iron deficiency and IDA. Eradication of *H pylori* appears to reverse anaemia in anecdotal reports and small studies. *H pylori* should be sought by non-invasive testing, if IDA persists or recurs after a normal OGD and colonoscopy, and eradicated if present. *H pylori* urease (CLO) testing of biopsy specimens taken at the initial gastroscopy is an alternative approach.

Autoimmune gastritis has been identified as a potential cause of IDA in up to a quarter of cases, but, although of interest, its diagnosis is currently of little practical value.

*Giardia lamblia* has occasionally been found during the investigation of IDA. If there is associated diarrhoea, then small-bowel biopsy samples will be taken anyway and may detect this. Where giardiasis is suspected, stool should be sent for ELISA, even if histology of duodenal biopsy samples is negative.

Radiological imaging of the mesenteric vessels is of limited use but may be of value in transfusion-dependent IDA for demonstrating vascular malformations or other occult lesions. There is no evidence to recommend labelled red cell imaging or Meckel's scans in patients with IDA. Faecal occult blood testing is of no benefit in the investigation of IDA, being insensitive and non-specific.

## 8. Evaluation of anaemia due to increased destruction

Hemolytic anaemia is defined as anaemia due to a shortened survival of circulating red blood cells (RBCs). Although the time of RBC senescent death in adults is 110 to 120 days, it is convenient to define haemolysis as a shortening of RBC survival to a value of less than 100 days.

While there are no symptoms specific for the diagnosis of hemolytic anaemia, recognizing haemolysis is not difficult in the classic patient, who may have many of the following:

- Rapid onset of pallor and anaemia
- Jaundice with increased indirect bilirubin concentration
- History of pigmented (bilirubin) gallstones
- Splenomegaly
- Presence of circulating spherocytic red cells (eg, autoimmune hemolytic anaemia, congenital spherocytosis)
- Other informative red cell shape changes (see below)
- Increased serum lactate dehydrogenase (LDH) concentration
- Reduced or absent level of serum haptoglobin
- A positive direct antiglobulin test (Coombs test)
- Increased reticulocyte percentage or absolute reticulocyte number, indicating the bone marrow's response to the anaemia

Laboratory findings, including an examination of the peripheral smear, are used to confirm the presence of haemolysis, and, if possible, the underlying cause.

| Extravascular destruction of red blood cells |
|---|
| Intrinsic red blood cell defects |
| Enzyme deficiencies (eg, G6PD or pyruvate kinase deficiencies) |
| Haemoglobinopathies (eg, sickle cell disease, thalassemias, unstable haemoglobins) |
| Membrane defects (eg, hereditary spherocytosis, elliptocytosis) |
| Extrinsic red blood cell defects |
| Liver disease |
| Hypersplenism |
| Infections (eg, bartonella, babesia, malaria) |
| Oxidant agents (eg, dapsone, nitrites, aniline dyes) |
| Other agents (eg, lead, snake and spider bites) |
| Large granular lymphocytic leukaemia |
| Autoimmune hemolytic anaemia (warm- or cold-reacting, drugs) |
| Intravenous immune globulin infusion |
| Intravascular destruction of red blood cells |
| Microangiopathy (eg, aortic stenosis, prosthetic valve) |
| Transfusion reactions (eg, ABO incompatibility) |
| Infection (eg, clostridial sepsis, severe malaria) |
| Paroxysmal cold haemoglobinuria; cold agglutinin disease (on occasion) |
| Paroxysmal nocturnal haemoglobinuria |
| Following intravenous infusion of Rho(D) immune globulin |
| Following intravenous infusion with hypotonic solutions |
| Snake bites |

Common causes of hemolytic anaemia in the adult
Hematologic consultation should be obtained in virtually all patients with a new onset of haemolysis, since sudden and life-threatening worsening of anaemia may occur, requiring urgent coordination between clinicians, clinical pathologists, and blood bank personnel for appropriate management.
Haemolysis may also be the first sign of an underlying systemic disorder (eg, thrombotic thrombocytopenic purpura, lupus erythematosus, chronic lymphocytic leukaemia) and may require urgent intervention to prevent death or disease-related complications.

### 8.1 Peripheral smear

Abnormalities suspicious for the presence of haemolysis include the following:

- Spherocytes, microspherocytes, and elliptocytes.
- Fragmented RBC (schistocytes, helmet cells) indicating the presence of microangiopathic hemolytic anaemia.
- Acanthocytes (spur cells) in patients with liver disease.
- Blister or "bite" cells due to the presence of oxidant-induced damage to the red cell and its membrane.
- RBCs with inclusions, as in Malaria, Babesiosis, and Bartonella infections.
- Teardrop RBCs with circulating nucleated RBC and early white blood cell forms, indicating the presence of marrow involvement, as in primary myelofibrosis or tumor infiltration.
- Red cell "ghosts" indicating the presence of intravascular haemolysis, most often associated with overwhelming bacterial infection (eg, Clostridium perfringens).

### 8.2 Serum LDH and haptoglobin

Two major tests used to diagnose the presence of haemolysis are lactate dehydrogenase (LDH), released from hemolyzed RBCs, and haptoglobin, which binds to haemoglobin released during intravascular or extravascular haemolysis or ineffective erythropoiesis with release of haemoglobin from late erythroid precursors in the bone marrow. Higher haptoglobin values in the presence of haemolysis can reflect either a lesser degree of haemolysis or concurrent inflammation, since haptoglobin is an acute phase reactant.
The combination of an increased serum LDH and a reduced haptoglobin is 90 percent specific for diagnosing haemolysis, while the combination of a normal serum LDH and a serum haptoglobin >25 mg/dL is 92 percent sensitive for ruling out haemolysis.

### 8.3 Reticulocyte count

The normal reticulocyte percentage is 0.5 to 1.5 percent. In patients with an otherwise intact bone marrow, the increase in erythropoietin production induced in a patient with hemolytic anaemia should raise the reticulocyte percentage above 4 to 5 percent. However, when the bone marrow is compromised (eg, following chemotherapy, infection, underlying marrow disease, cobalamin, folate, or iron deficiency), the reticulocyte response may be blunted or ablated.

### 8.4 Other tests

Other tests helpful in determining the presence or absence of haemolysis include:
Increased serum concentrations of indirect bilirubin from the catabolism of haemoglobin haem.

Increased mean corpuscular haemoglobin concentration (MCHC), indicating the presence of spherocytes.
Positive direct antiglobulin (Coombs') test in autoimmune hemolytic anaemia.
Tests for cold agglutinins or the Donath-Landsteiner antibody if symptoms are related to exposure to cold.
Testing for the presence of insoluble globin particles within the red blood cell (ie, Heinz bodies).
Increased blood concentration of carboxyhaemoglobin due to haemoglobin haem catabolism.

### 8.5 Testing for intravascular haemolysis

If intravascular haemolysis is suspected, the following additional tests are of value:

- Measurement of the PLASMA haemoglobin concentration (ie, testing for haemoglobinemia)
- Measurement of free haemoglobin in the urine supernatant (ie, testing for haemoglobinuria)
- Testing for hemosiderin in the urine sediment ≥7 days after the incident, allowing time for hemosiderin-containing tubular cells to be shed into the urine

## 9. Conclusion

Anaemia is a frequent clinical finding, often leading to significant ill health and always requires prompt investigation and selective treatment.
By following a simple escalation pathway from history, examination and targetted investigations, a diagnosis can usually be made and effective treatment applied.

## 10. References

Droogendijk J, et al, *Scand J Gastroenterol.* 2011 Jul 4.
Gehrs BC, Friedberg RC., *Am J Hematol.* 2002 Apr;69(4):258-71.
Goddard AF, James MW, McIntyre AS, Scott BB; on behalf of the British Society of Gastroenterology. *Gut. 2011 Jun 6.*
*Harrison's* Principles of Internal Medicine, 16th Edition.
Mehta BC. Approach to a patient with anaemia. *Indian J Med Sci* 2004;58:26-9
Nathan, DG, Oski, FA. *Hematology of Infancy and Childhood*, 4th ed, WB Saunders, Philadelphia, PA 1993.
Pierce A, Nester T; for the Education Committee of the Academy of Clinical Laboratory Physicians and Scientists. *Am J Clin Pathol.* 2011 Jul;136(1):7-12.
Powell N, McNair A. *Eur J Gastroenterol Hepatol.* 2008 Nov;20(11):1094-100.
Stanley L Schrier, MD, *Uptodate.com,* Approach to the adult patient with anaemia,
Stevens LA, Li S, Kurella Tamura M, et al, *Am J Kidney Dis.* 2011 Mar;57(3 Suppl 2):S9-16.
Trifan A, Singeap AM, et al., *J Gastrointestin Liver Dis.*2010 Mar;19(1):21-5.
Vitale G, Fatti LM, et al. *J Am Geriatr Soc.*2010 Sep;58(9):1825-7.

# 7

# How Can Cancer-Associated Anemia Be Moderated with Nutritional Factors and How Do *Beta Vulgaris* L. Ssp. *Esculenta Var. Rubra* Modify the Transmethylation Reaction in Erythrocytes in Cancerous Patients?

Anna Blázovics[1] et al.*
[1]*Department of Pharmacognosy, and II. Department of Medicine, Semmelweis University, Budapest Hungary*

## 1. Introduction

Genetic predisposition, unhealthy dietary or life habits and heavy social circumstances could result in the changes of redox homeostasis, which is very important for the equilibrium between tissue regeneration and apoptosis. When the balance is disturbed, cancer and/or necrosis may develop (Powis et al., 1997). Moderate dietary habits with natural bioactive agents, antioxidants, methyl donor molecules and metal elements can help restore the normal function of the organism, although the immoderate consumption of nutritive components is contraindicated. Long term antioxidant and/or antioxidant-related treatments as well as metal element owerflow can modify redox-homeostasis because these alimentary components effect signal transduction routes and compensatory effects of altered tissues can be observed (Vanherweghem et al., 1993, Blázovics et al., 2007a,b, Blázovics et al., 2008).

Epidemiological, experimental and clinical investigations have shown that food supplements are not effective in cancer therapy because of inappropriate usage in cases of people suffering from cancers with low vitamin and trace element levels. Significant changes of total scavenger capacity, metal element concentrations, bounded HCHO and

*Péter Nyirády[2], Imre Romics[2], Miklós Szűcs[2], András Horváth[2], Ágnes Szilvás[3], Edit Székely[1], Klára Szentmihályi[4], Gabriella Bekő[5] and Éva Sárdi[6]
[1]Department of Pharmacognosy, and II. Department of Medicine, Semmelweis University, Budapest,
[2]Department of Urology, Semmelweis University,
[3]Saint John Hospital, Budapest,
[4]Institute of Materials and Environmental Chemistry, CRC, Hungarian Academy of Sciences, Budapest,
[5]Central Laboratory Pest, Semmelweis University,
[6]Corvinus University, Budapest

protoporphyrin as well as Zn-protoporphyrin concentrations in erythrocytes can be observed in cancerous processes, which are very important in cancer-associated anemia (Blázovics et al., 2008).

Red blood cells do not get enough oxygen to all parts of the body especially in cancer-related anemia, such as cancer in bone marrow directly or in metastasis, as well as in cisplatin or carboplatin chemotherapy, which lower the erythropoietin production in the kidneys and in radiation therapy caused anemia. It is especially significant if the level of the transmethylation ability is too low in the organism. Alterations in DNA methylation play an important role in neoplasia (Baylin, et al. 1997, Calvisi et al., 2007). DNA hypomethylation leads to elevated mutation rates. (Chen et al. 1998). The most studied mechanisms by epigenetics are DNA and histone methylation and the stable and reversible alterations in the genome that affect gene expression and genome function. The nature and role of the mechanisms of promoter hypermethylation during carcinogenesis were studied worldwide, however the mechanism behind one of the earliest epigenetic observations in cancer nowadays, genome-wide hypomethylation, still remains unclear (Wild, and Flanagan 2010)

Tumor hypermethylation predicts a poor prognosis in patients with earlier stages of prostate cancer, and is commonly found in the plasma DNA of patients with castration-resistant prostate cancer (Rosenbaum et al., 2005, Bastian et al. 2009). Low transmethylation ability can be observed in the erythrocyte in different tumors and in different stages (Blázovics et al., 2008, Nyirády et al., 2010). Hypomethylation seems to be a condition of the system, which can be improved with methyl donating molecules from food ingredients, such as different N-, S- and O- methylated compounds.

## 2. Natural therapy and cancer-related anemia

In spite of an enormous effort and many new excellent experimental data, which come to light in cancer research, cancer therapy is not solved satisfactorily. Several target points are for inhibiting cancerous processes and molecules are developed to modify signal transduction pathways aimed for a better way of using tailored cancer treatment, although the chance of definitive recovery is very different in the various tumors and only half of circa 200 tumor types can be cured nowadays (Blázovics 2011). Therefore new therapeutic solutions are necessary as well as looking for new food ingredients to moderate several problems, such as cancer-related anemia, which improves the erythrocyte function of bone metastatic prostate cancer cases.

It is an endeavor to show attempts of natural therapy with small molecules for inhibiting cancer growth and spreading on the basis of researches. The effectiveness of medicinal therapy can be increased if the therapy is planned for each patient therefore this chapter wants to deal with the importance of the role of transmethylation ability and the question of modification of redox-homeostasis by alimentary supporting therapy.

### 2.1 Transmethylation processes

Bioactive molecule, the small genotoxic and carcinogen formaldehyde is in connection with the redox homeostasis. This molecule plays an important role with free radicals in the biological system (Lichszteld and Kruk 1977, Nieva and Wentworth 2004). Since endogenous transmethylation processes occur via HCHO, this molecule can be considered as an ancient and basic compound of life systems. HCHO can be found in animal tissues in specially-bounded, mainly hydroxymethyl forms. Endogenous HCHO is produced partly by the enzymatic demethylation of different N-, S-, and O- methylated compounds (Huszti et al., 1986, Sárdi et al., 2005, Kovács-Nagy et al., 2009).

S-adenosylmethionine is an important methyl donor in several biological transmethylation reactions such as in the duplication of virus. The product S-adenosylhomocysteine inhibits the transmethylation process because this molecule is hydrolysed to adenosine and L-homocysteine by the action of S-adenosylhomocysteine hydrolase. The accumulation of homocysteine leads to increased cellular oxidative stress (Gersbeck et al., 1989, Stead et al., 2006).

DNA methylation typically occurs at cytosine-phosphate-guanine site. In this process, methylation results in the conversion of the cytosine to 5-methylcytosine. This reaction is catalysed by DNA methyltransferase. The methylation stage of this region can have a major impact on gene (Watson et al., 2003).

Some quaternary ammonium compounds, such as $N^{\varepsilon}$-trimethyl-L-lysine, choline and betaine, are potential HCHO generators as well. Data show the important role of HCHO in proliferative as well as in apoptotic processes. Transmethylation ability is lowered in tumorous processes (Blázovics et al., 2008, Nyirády et al., 2010).

It is also verified, that the arginine (38), methionine (65) and the lysine (72) near the methionine (80) are methylated and coordinated towards the central iron of heme (Stryeer 1988). During moderate transmethylation ability, free protoporphyrin can be found near the Zn-protoporphyrin in the erythrocyte in different cancers and it has pro- and antioxidant forms depending on concentrations. Protoporphyrin concentration is low in cancerous patients, but in metastasis its concentration is significantly high. Oxidized hemoglobin, HbA1c correlates significantly with free radical reactions and with decreased antioxidant status of erythrocytes (Blázovics et al., 2008).

In earlier study, significant changes could be observed in erythrocyte function in patients suffering from colon cancer as well as in metastatic prostate cancer. The erythrocyte mobilized formaldehyde was significantly lower in adult colectomysed patients with no metastasis than in controls. Simultaneously protoporphyrin concentration was low in patients without metastasis, when the diagnosis was Dukes C before operation. HbA1c level correlated significantly with the induced free radical level and decreased antioxidant status of erythrocytes (Blázovics et al., 2008, 2011).

### 2.2 Redox homeostasis

Redox homeostasis can be considered as the cumulative action of free radicals and antioxidant defenses, providing a suitable condition for life. Oxidative stress is a key modulator, which modifies the ligand-receptor interactions extracellularly and intracellularly, and influences gene expression. Free radicals can act as secondary messengers in several transduction pathways, and take part in the activation of chemotactic cytokines and surface adhesion molecules etc. (Abate et al., 1990, Meyer et al., 1993, Polya et al., 2002).

Oxidative stress can induce stress response genes, and moderate oxidative stress by down regulating the gene expression of several genes. DNA synthesis, selective gene expression, enzyme activation and modification of cell proliferation are involved in redoxy signal mechanisms. Moderate free radical production can modify the function of kinases or directly activate the transcription factors, thereby also influencing the gene regulation in the nucleus (Delerive et al., 2000, Kong et al., 2000).

The "antioxidant" concept has meaning only in defense against free radicals for a long period. Its importance is not doubtful in the therapy of diseases in which free radicals are also involved.

Antioxidant consumption is sine qua non for a healthy way of life, but the concentration range is large and dependent on an individual genetic background. Moderate nutritional customs with natural scavengers or antioxidants can help to restore the normal function of tissues and organs, but the immoderate consumption of vitamins and other bioactive agents is contraindicated. The balance between oxidative stress and antioxidant defense is overturned in diseases (Blázovics et al., 1999, Szilvási et al., 1999, Hagymási et al., 2001). Moderate oxidative stress is important in signal transduction pathways and essential for proliferation and apoptosis. The antioxidant overflow as well as oxidative stress mean serious problems. "Janus face" antioxidants can stop protein phosphorylation and the inhibition of activation of transcription factors. They can also therefore stop cell proliferation and injure the adaptation mechanisms against oxidative stress. The direct roles of these antioxidants in original forms are doubtful in transduction therapy (Azzi et al., 2004, Griffiths and Lunec 2001).

Several food-related bioactive agents are important in cancer prevention as well. Metals are also important both in free radical formation and in antioxidant defense in signal transduction.

Four simple redox measurements, H-donating ability, reducing-power property, free SH-group and stimulated chemiluminescent intensity of plasma and erythrocytes can be applied to evaluate the redox homeostasis in several diseases and different treatments compared to the control values. The calculation of total scavenger capacity can be necessary to measure the tissue relative chemiluminescent light. Normal range of healthy peoples is no more 70 RLU%, 80±10% RLU% is the chemiluminescent intensity of erythrocytes in different diseases, e.g. in the severe IBD, where the range is 100±10%, and the range between 100 and 150 RLU% means increased risk for tumors (precancerous stadium and after tumor resection) and >150 RLU% marks the non treated tumors. Very low chemiluminescent intensity - significantly lower than that of healthy control patients - could be observed in metastatic cancerous patients, some weeks before death because of extra high protoporphyrin concentration in the erythrocyte.

Chemiluminescence methods are suitable to differentiate the grade of diseases (Blázovics et al., 1999.) and difference between genders e.g in alcoholic liver diseases (Hagymási et al., 2001), but in both type of IBD and colon cancer gender difference was not observed (Szilvás et al., 1999).

The measured data are in significant correlation with each other and the changes of activity of erythrocyte superoxide dismutase and glutathione peroxidase as well as concentrations of plasma reducing power and H-donating ability. Consequently, erythrocyte total scavenger capacity (inverse of chemiluminescent intensity) is a good predictive factor for neoplasia in early stage (Blázovics et al., 2008). (Figure 1.)

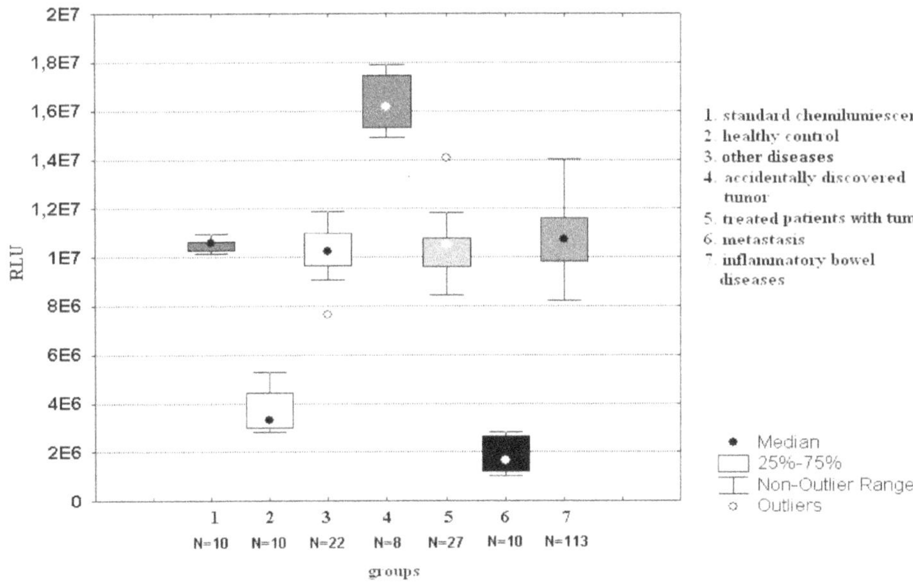


Fig. 1. Chemiluminescent intensity in early state of tumor and metastasis

A significantly higher chemiluminescent intensity of erythrocytes was detected in newly observed tumors. When the patients were operated and treated with chemotherapy and/or irradiation therapy, the erythrocyte chemiluminescence was not altered from that of IBD patients. In severe metastatic stages, before death, the chemiluminescence of erythrocytes was very low, significantly lower than in healthy controls. Plasma chemiluminescence studies rather show only momentary improvement in the course of the therapy of IBD or tumors (Blázovics 2006).

### 2.3 Nutritional factors in tumor

Besides, genetical disposition it was above mentioned, that lifestyle and nutrition with vitamins, polyphenols, flavonoids and quaterner ammonium derivatives play a decisive role in human health care and inhibit the occurrence of many diseases. It is a proven fact that antioxidants have an important role in preventing cancer and improve redox homeostasis (Lugasi and Hóvári 2002, Polya et al., 2002).

Lack of alimentary factors such as iron, vitamin B12, and folic acid, the formation and function of red blood cells is inhibited. These components are available naturally in several vegetables and food items, therefore eating foods with high iron content, such as red meats, dried beans or fruits, almonds, broccoli, and enriched breads and cereals or high folic acid, such as cereals, green leafy vegetables, asparagus, broccoli, spinach, and lima beans can help (Kuramoto et al., 1996).

Bioactive agent as well as metal element-rich vegetables are important in the food chain and play a decisive role in human health care. Table beet is a particularly important vegetable from this supporting alimentary point of view. Table beet is a vegetable that is rich in content of folic acid, iron, betaine, natural coloring agents, polyphenols, metal elements, etc. (Takács-Hájos 1999, Blázovics et al ., 2007, Sárdi et al., 2009).

A healthy system needs antioxidant and metal element supplementation and can tolerate occasional overflow between wide boundaries. Besides this, redox homeostasis and element homeostasis do not change. However, the reactions of sick organisms - e.g. the Fe accumulating porphyria cutanea tarda and haemochromatosis or Cu accumulating Wilson disease as well as the iron-deficiency anemia and the malnutrition of inflammatory bowel diseases - can be different and that is why everybody must be cautious when recommending table beet root supplements. It can be supposed, that the extreme consumption of table beet root can cause several disturbances among others not only in healthy people but in patients suffering from metal accumulating diseases, although moderate consumption may be beneficial in metal-deficiency diseases (Blázovics et al., 2007b).

### 2.4 Table beet

*Beta vulgaris* L. ssp. *esculenta* Gurke var. *rubra* belongs to the *Chenopodiaceae* family and it is in relationship with *Beta vulgaris* L. provar. *altissima, Beta vulgaris* L. convar. *crassa* provar. *crassa* and *Beta vulgaris* L. convar. *cicla*. An ancient form of these species is the wild form of *Beta vulgaris* L. var. *maritime* (Takács-Hájos 1999).

The root of the plant *Beta vulgaris* L. ssp. *esculenta* var. *rubra* is commonly called table beet and has been used for centuries as a traditional and popular food in many national cuisines. The Greek Hypocrates, the Roman, but Greek-born Galenus, the Arabian Avicenna, and the Swiss Paracelsus applied table beet in several gastrointestinal diseases, fevers, anemia, wound-healing etc. Nowadays table beet is also an important component of popular medicine (Frank et al., 2005, Pedreno and Escribano 2000).

The applying of table beet in several diseases can be bordered because the natural colored pigment contents of this vegetable are important food coloring matters, which substitute E123 coloring matter in different creams, substituting soya foods, sweets, gelatin deserts, yogurts, ice- creams, dressings and meats etc. (Takács-Hájos 1999).

Beneficial medical effects are due to bioactive components, such as betaine, betanins, betaxanthins, vulgaxanthine, flavonoids, polyphenols, vitamins (thiamine, riboflavine, piridoxine, ascorbic acid, biotin and folic acid) as well as soluble fibre, pectin and different metal elements (e.g. Al, B, Ba, Ca, Cu, Fe, K, Mg, Mn, Na, Zn), which act on various physiological routes (Wang and Goldman 1996, Rice-Evans et al., 1997, Bobek et al., 2000, Kanner et al., 2001).

The coloring matters in table beet are betalains, as red betacyanins and yellow betaxanthins, and they can be used for human nutrition and prevention of numerous diseases, for example skin and lung cancers (Stintzing and Carle 2004, Schwartz et al., 1983, Frank et al., 2005, Boyd et al., 1982, Kapadia et al., 1996, Kapadia et al. 2003).

According to newer researches, these colored pigments have antioxidant activity and play an important role in the development of antioxidant status in the human organism (Cai et al., 2001, Kanner et al., 2001, Pedreno and Escribano 2000., Wettasinghe et al., 2002, Zakharova and Petrova 1998).

Table beets are mainly characterized by the non high-concentration of sucrose. Glucose and fructose can also be found in the samples but their concentrations are significantly low. With regard to glucose quantity, 51% of the varieties were below 0.2 mg/g, 30% of them belong to the 0.2-0.4 mg/g domain and 19% were characterized by a glucose content above 0.4 mg/g. 52.7% of the varieties were in the 10-15 mg/g domain, 33% were between 15-20 mg/g, while 14.3% contained more that 21 mg/g sucrose.

Among the quarternary ammonium compounds, which have human health significance due to their biological activity, a high concentration of betaine can be found.

In earlier examinations, among the quaternary ammonium compounds, in the table beet samples betaine was found in the highest concentration, carnitine was also detectable but in low concentration (the value was not measurable) and other quaternary ammonium compounds were not detectable. 28.5% of the varieties fall under the 0.6 mg/g level, another 28.5% are above the 0.8 mg/g level and 43% can be characterized by a betaine concentration of 0.6-0.8 mg/g per fresh mass. Betaine was found in significantly higher concentration in the lyophilized samples. Fresh samples contained betaine in a concentration of 0.35-1.3 mg/g, while the concentration of lyophilized ones was between 10.3-18.0 mg/g of dry mass. On the basis of the total phenol concentration of table beet squeezed juice, 23.8% of the compared varieties are under the level of 0.6-0.8 mg/ml in the fresh samples, one-third are 0.80-1.0 mg/ml, another one-third are 1.0-1.20 mg/ml and the phenol concentration of 9.5% of the varieties is between 1.20-2.0 mg/ml (Sárdi et al., 2009). On the basis of the comparison of studied variants, those with a higher concentration of betanine contained a higher amount of phenol as well. The value of betanine is 0.40-1.1 mg/g, total phenol shows significant differences between 0.60-1.90 mg/ml, correlation. Betaine concentrations were different in varieties. Where betaine was higher, betanine and polyphenol were also higher along with antioxidant capacity (Hájos et al., 2004). Between red coloring matter and total polyphenol concentration, significant correlation was calculated (r=0,7577) (Sárdi et al., 2009).

Schiebler already discovered betaine in *Beta vulgaris* in 1869 and since then betaine was observed in several living organisms (Blunden and Gordon 1986, Hougaard et al., 1994) and human cells as well (Lever et al., 1994).

In modern medicine, betaine is an important natural molecule for treating homocysteinuria, alcoholic steatosis, chemically induced liver, lung and skin cancers (Wilcken et al., 1983, Barak et al., 1996, Eikelboom et al., Murakami et al., 1998). This molecule helps to create choline, can help synthesize of carnitine and helps to convert homocysteine into methionine and it takes part in biologic methylation (Finkenstein and Martin 1984, Slow et al., 2004, Awad et al., 1983, Skiba et al., 1982, Evans et al., 2002, Millan and Garrow 1998).

## 2.5 Metal elements in tumor

Metal elements are important in nutrition and prevention of diseases, as anemia could be treated with supplementation of Fe. Concentration of essential metal elements is rigorously regulated in the metabolic pathways in contrary to toxic elements in healthy organisms. Concentration changes of some transition metal elements Cu, Fe, Mn, Zn and non-metal elements S, Se, P can significantly modify the signal transduction. Therefore, their optimal tissue concentrations are not doubtful and daily intake of these elements from natural sources is very important (Szentmihályi et al., 2000a,b, Máday et al., 2000). These elements are ubiquitous in biological systems and play a key role in the catalysis of redox processes. Heavy metals in higher concentrations may inhibit enzyme activities and influence the acute phase protein synthesis and gene expression, as well as the pro-oxidant and antioxidant forms of scavenger molecules. Mainly the free Fe(II) and Cu(I) and Cu(II) redox active metal ions catalyze the formation of reactive oxygen radicals, but they occur in the body in a small amount (Kasprzak et al., 1987). CuZnSOD in the cytoplasm and the nucleus, MnSOD in the mitochondrial matrix, catalase in peroxisomes or in the cytoplasm and glutathione peroxidase in the cytoplasm are known metalloproteins, which take part in the defense mechanism against toxic concentration of free radicals (Yuregir et al., 1994, Schroeder and Cousins 1990, Dinkova-Kostova et al., 2005). Cu occurs in the ceruloplasmin, and it has an oxidase function. It is able to oxidize biogen amines and its phenoxidase activity is also proved (Floris et. al., 2000, Pena, et al., 1999). Zn is a key element in antioxidant superoxide dismutase enzyme as well as Zn-metallothionein, which has hydroxyl scavenging ability (Brando-Neto et al., 1994). Mn also takes part in the enzymatic antioxidant defense system, since the superoxide dismutase enzyme scavenges superoxide anions. In blood, Mn(II) ions take on the forms of free aqua-complexes or are bounded to albumin, α macroglobulin and other glycoproteins (Critchfield and Keen 1992). Mn(II) is an antioxidant, since in fast reaction it exterminates the alkyl peroxyl radicals formed by the peroxidation of fatty acids, while Fe(II) ions generate alkoxy and hydroxyl radicals by splitting the ROOH bond and continue the chain reaction (Siegel and Sigel 1999). Mn(II) ions, similarly to Zn ions, are able to decrease the formation of superoxide radicals by forming $Mn_2$(NADPH) complexes (Schramm 1986). Metal ions are important for the activation of NF-kappaB, AP-1 and in the cases of NF-kappaB proteasome degradation as well as the regulation of IkappaB kinases and other redoxy sytems. The joining of the NF-kappa B to the DNA is the function of the redoxi state of apo 62 cystein in p50 subunit in the DNA-bond domain. This connection is injured by the effect of heavy metals such as As, Cd, Co, Cr, Ni and Pb (Kudrin 2000). The risk of tumor formation is increased in the presence of Ni, Cr and As ions, because DNA repair systems are very sensitive targets of these elements (Hartwig 1998). Divalent cations, such as Zn, Cu, Cd, Mn and Ni can modulate the function of tumor suppressor protein p53 in vitro (Maehle et al., 1992). The excess of Zn and Cd cause inhibition of the apoptosis (Chukhlovin et al., 2001).

In several biochemical pathways Ni, Cr and As toxic metal elements compete with Mg ions. Competition between Ni(II) and Mg(II) may provide an important mechanism for interfering with DNA-protein interactions involved in the repair process, because the inhibition of DNA repair is partly reversible by the addition of Mg(II) (Kasprzak et al., 1987, Hartwig et al., 1994). Presumable Ni(II), Co(II) and As(II) ions displace Zn ion in the zinc-finger structure of DNA repair enzymes (Hartwig 1998). Ni, Cr and As elements are established carcinogens in humans. These heavy metals can induce adhesion molecules and cytokines (Hayat 1996).

Magnesium deficiency alters calcium homeostasis via $Ca^{2+}/Mg^{2+}$ antagonism, leading to transient increase in the concentration of intracellular calcium. Magnesium may act as a physiological „antioxidant", e.g. against lipoprotein oxidation. The transient increase in the intracellular calcium level induced by magnesium deficiency, enhances the production of pro-oxidant cytokines (IL-1, IL-6, IL-8, TNF-α, -β), different growth factors (EGF-α, TGF-β, NFGF, FGF, PDGF), and interferons (IFN-α, -γ) by activation of phosphoinositol diphosphate ($PIP_2$) and MAP kinases (Dolmetsch et al. 1997, Caddell 2000).

The enhanced synthesis of cytokines induces gene expressions of enzymes of reactive oxygen species including NADPH oxidase, xanthine-oxidase/dehydrogenase, cyclooxygenase, lipoxygenase, cytochrome P450, NO synthase, proteins containing iron, and superoxide dismutase, copper zinc and manganase enzymes that are regulated at transcripitional level by phosphorylation of transcription factors. On the contrary, the increase in the intracellular magnesium level inhibits the production of pro-oxidant cytokines via the activation of corresponding protein phosphatases, therefore the generation of reactive oxygen species can be attenuated. Therefore the intake of the right amount of magnesium and magnesium-calcium rations is essential.

### 2.6 Clinical investigation of table beet supplementation

Adenocarcinoma of the prostate is still one of the major reasons of cancer-related mortality in populations of Western countries, but the current understanding of its etiology and pathogenesis is still lacking (Jemal et al., 2008).

Although, prostate cancer is silent and creates no early warning symptoms, after the extensive use of serum prostate specific antigen (PSA) testing, it has increasingly been reported at earlier stages. In case of localized prostate cancer, for a man in good condition, radical prostatectomy is the preferred treatment with more than 10 years life expectancy. Furthermore, radical surgery might provide a therapy for well-selected locally advanced prostate cancer. However, it is still not possible to distinguish who is at a high risk of tumor recurrence after primary local therapy, so will not benefit from surgery. In addition it can not be predicted who will benefit from hormonal therapy and who will become soon hormone resistant in cases of advanced prostate cancer. Nowadays, although using more promising indicators to distinguish between surgically curable and oncologically treatable prostate cancer, there has not still been an optimal factor found which would tell us the prognosis (Barqawi et al., 2004, Nyirády and Romics 2009a,b).

Several papers report effect of table beet supplements in the improvement of quality of life of different diseases, although their physiological investigation is poor. Table beet affects numerous biochemical reaction ways, enzymes and metabolic-synthesis occurring in vivo (Kuramoto et al., 1996, Váli et al., 2007, Blázovics et al., 2007b). In this clinical study 10g natural table beet lyophilized product was given twice daily for 1 month for 24 patients (mean age 68±8 years) with hormone-resistant and metastatic prostate cancer treated with taxan chemotherapy, who reported their complaints themselves first, mean 3.6±2.8 years before. 18 men's data were amenable after treatment for evaluation. (Permission number of clinical study: Semmelweis University 127/2006.) The lyophilized product was purchased from commercial service (Permission number: 1361/004/2003 BFAEE) GPS Powder Kft. Budapest, Hungary) (Nyirády et al., 2010).

In addition to routine laboratory examination values of HbA1c, 9 cytokines and levels of 3 growth factors, the global parameters of redox-homeostasis, few elements, Zn- and level of free protoporphyrin, trans-methylation processes were determined before and one month after treatment.

Results showed that in most of the patients the favorable impact of beet was enforced and significantly high levels of Zn- and free protoporphyrin decreased; furthermore trans-methylation processes fastened which all characterize patients with tumor (Nyirády et al., 2010). Table1. shows the element concentrations of lyophilized table beet powder applied in human study.

The calculated metal element intake concentration, on the basis of daily dose of lyophilized table beet powder, is very low. The essential element concentrations compared to the

| elements | lyophilized table beet powder (µg/g) | daily intake (µg) | percentage of daily needs *, and percentage of average daily intake ** |
|---|---|---|---|
| Al | 21.62 ± 4.60 | 432.4 | 13.1** |
| B | 8.56 ± 4.91 | 171.2 | 7.4* |
| Ba | 3.79 ± 0.16 | 75.8 | 5.1** |
| Ca | 701.0 ± 15.6 | 14020 | 1.4* |
| Co | 0.146 ± 0.003 | 2.92 | 0.5** |
| Cr | 0.311 ± 0.037 | 6.22 | 17.8* |
| Cu | 3.13 ± 0.59 | 62.6 | 6.9* |
| Fe | 17.68 ± 0.03 | 353.6 | 4.4* |
| K | 8057 ± 512 | 161140 | 3.4* |
| Li | < 0.1 | | |
| Mg | 829.9 ± 9.7 | 16598 | 4.0* |
| Mn | 9.99 ± 0.11 | 199.8 | 9.1* |
| Mo | 0.205 ± 0.059 | 4.1 | 9.1* |
| Na | 661.4± 30.9 | 13228 | 0.9* |
| Ni | 0.469 ± 0.125 | 9.38 | 9.4** |
| P | 1545 ±83 | 30900 | 4.4* |
| Se | 0.142 ± 0.011 | 2.84 | 5.2* |
| Si | 53.96 ± 1.48 | 1079.2 | 5.4** |
| Sr | 3.89 ± 0.05 | 77.8 | 1.7** |
| Zn | 6.09 ± 0.21 | 121.8 | 1.1* |

Table 1. Element concentration of lyophilized table beet powder (dose 20g/day) ; (mean±SD).

proposed daily intake (RDA, DRI) and non-essential or toxic element concentrations compared to average daily intake, can be seen in Table 1. The important intake (>15%) can be considered in the case of Cr.

Alteration of metal element homeostasis may elevate the risk of prostate diseases, e.g. intake of high amount of Fe or Zn deficiency may increase the oxidative processes in which NF-kappaB, IL-6 and IL–8 etc. are activated and the incidence of prostate cancer elevates as well as toxic metal elements (Salnikow et al., 2008). Zn depletion in the prostate's peripheral zone is found to correlate with the Gleason score.

Erythrocyte element status of patients with prostate cancer significantly changed versus controls in cases of Al (1.90±1.67 vs 0.537±0.260), Ni (0.722±0.565 vs 0.265±0.195) and Pb (0.309±0.301 vs 0.094±0.053), and these ion concentrations were significantly high in prostate cancer patients with PSA>9 (Nyirády et al., 2009b).

Toxic metal elements and free radicals influence the function of several receptors and genes such as tyrosine kinases, epidermal growth factor (EGF), platelet-derived growth factor (PDGF), vascular endothelial growth factor (VEGF); src and ras genes and signal proteins, nuclear factors - kappaB (NF-kappaB), activated protein-1 (AP-1), p53, nuclear factor of activated cells family (NFAT), hypoxia induced factor (HIF-1) (Suzuki 1997, Atmane 2003).

The plasma concentrations of Ca-, Cu- and Mg in patients did not change significantly during the treatment and they were between the normal range in all cases. Nevertheless, the Fe concentration decreased significantly by the effect of table beet supplementation and moved toward the normal value range. The Se level increased by the effect of treatment, although it reached the normal value only in some cases. The Zn concentration decreased significantly, the mean value was in the normal range. These data show that the metal ion homeostasis begins to restore, the metal ions stay in cells compartments by the effect of table beet consumption (Table 2.).

| groups | Ca normal value:98 | Cu normal value:1.2 | Fe* normal value:1.1 | Mg normal value:22 | Zn* normal value:1.4 | Se* normal value:0.08 |
|---|---|---|---|---|---|---|
| | (mg/kg) | | | | | |
| control (N=9) | 61.38±22.85 | 0.79±0.25 | 4.37±1.47 | 32.09±10.80 | 7.22±3.22 | 0.080±0.026 |
| metastatic postate tumor (N=18) | 77.82±11.03 | 1.25±0.28 | 12.52±9.63 | 21.47±3.51 | 1.46±0.60 | 0.011±0.006 |
| metastatic postate tumor + table beet (N=18) | 77.02±16.44 | 1.17±0.37 | 5.49±3.83 | 20.95±4.93 | 1.03±0.44 | 0.050±0.061 |

significance ($p<0.05$)* ; (mean±SD).

Table 2. Effect of table beet treatment on the plasma element concentrations of metastatic prostate cancer patients with taxan chemotherapy.

IFN-α, β, γ, IL-1α, β, IL-6, IL-10, IL-12, TNF-α, β, MIF and chemokines inflammatory cytokines, which initiate the activation of specific immune cells and regulate their differentiations (Haddad 2002). Chemokines affect the increasing of cell adhesion and chemotaxis, as well as activation of effector leucocytes are increased by them. During leucocyte activation, free radicals and lipid derivatives are liberated (Malaguarnera 2001).

Special components (betaine, folic acid, Fe, flavonoids and vitamins) of table beet could modify the erythrocyte total scavenger capacity and element concentrations as well as improve the transmethylation ability.

The levels of proinflammatory cytokines shown of a declining tendency, but these changes were not significant (IL1a P=0.084; IL6 P=0.154; IL8 P=0.578). The effect was beneficial. Measured parameters of anti-inflammatory cytokines also decreased (IL2 P=0.255; P=0.38; P=0.204). At the same time VEGF was not changed, although EGF was higher (p=0.003), and PSA (P=0.441) was elevated non significantly after supplementation. The levels of IL-6, CRP, IFNG and MCP1 were decreased in small amounts in the sera; these were disadvantageous results (Nyirády et al., 2010).

Consumption of beetroot decreased the proinflammatory cytokines and in some patients (44%) increased the level of IL2. In other patients (52%) we measured lower level of PSA. There were hopeful results, but increased EGF levels draw attention to the fact, that further investigations and correlation analysis must be performed, in which beneficial effects on patients can be observed. Data can be seen in Table 3.

| parameters | patient groups | | | |
|---|---|---|---|---|
| | healthy controls (N=26) | early stage (N=28) | metastatic (N=18) | metastatic+ table beet (N= 8) |
| IL-1 alpha (pg/ml) | 0.64±0.50 | 0.10±0.30 | 0.54±0.42 | 0.35±0.17 |
| IL-1 beta (pg/ml) | 1.57±1.3 | 0.80±2.20 | 1.18±1.60 | 0.42±0.50 |
| IL-2 (pg/ml) | 4.18±2.80 | 4.70±5.60 | 7.80±4.4 | 5.5±7.2 |
| IL-4 (pg/ml) | 4.56±1.84 | 2.30±5.40 | 4.70±2.05 | 4.0±2.01 |
| IL-6 (pg/ml) | 1.51±1.34 | 1.20±2.30 | 14.2±24.20 | 5.6±6.5 |
| IL-8 (pg/ml) | 25.21±16.16 | 9.10±16.30 | 31.20±87.00 | 25.3±29.6 |
| IL-10 (pg/ml) | 1.08±0.69 | 0.20±0.50 | 1.54±1.91 | 0.88±0.99 |
| TNF-alpha (pg/ml) | 7.45±4.23 | 3.00±3.60 | 3.41±1.65 | 3.50±0.98 |
| VEGF (pg/ml) | 190±150 | 183±94 | 272±116 | 282±160 |
| IFNG (pg/ml) | 1.78±1.41 | 0.8±1.50 | 4.28±4.21 | 2.21±1.97 |
| MCP1 (pg/ml) | 346±158 | 306±93 | 347±171 | 323±157 |
| EGF (pg/ml) | 212±81 | 66.8±58.3* | 59.3±40.4* | 110±58.8** |
| CRP (mg/l) | <5 | 5.6±12.8 | 14.4±24.9 | 5.9±4.9 |
| PSA (pg/ml) | <2 | 10.66±7.79* | 93±120** | 133.5±182.5** |

significance ($p<0.05$): control vs *; * vs **; (mean±SD).

Table 3. Immune parameters of prostate cancerous patients with and without table beet treatment in different stages and PSA levels.

Table 4. summarizes the redox parameters of patient groups. Table beet consumption moderated the erythrocyte free radical level in tendency and significant difference was observed in plasma in treated group compared to control. The large SD means that metastatic processes are different in time. There were no differences between HbA1c values.

| groups | plasma (RLU%) | erythrocyte (RLU%) | HbA1c (%) |
|---|---|---|---|
| Control (N=11) | 4.51±1.25 | 73.19±12.09 | <6.1 |
| postate tumor (metastatic) (N=18) | 3,25±4,93 | 71,78±60,07 | 6,1±0,7 |
| postate tumor (metastatic) + table beet (N=10) | 1,69±1,39* | 54,71±43,81 | 6,1±0,9 |

significance ($p<0.05$) control vs*; (mean±SD).

Table 4. Effect of table beet treatment on the redox parameters of prostate cancer patients with taxan chemotherapy.

On the basis of linear regression between chemiluminescent intensity (RLU%) and free protoporphyrin/Zn-protoporphyrin ratio, where y = -237.49x + 156.08 and $R^2$ = 0.6177 were calculated, significance could be observed. If the free protoporphyrin and HCHO ration was analyzed, the linear regression was better: y = -272.77x + 1024.6 and $R^2$ = 0.8331 (Nyirády et al., 2009).

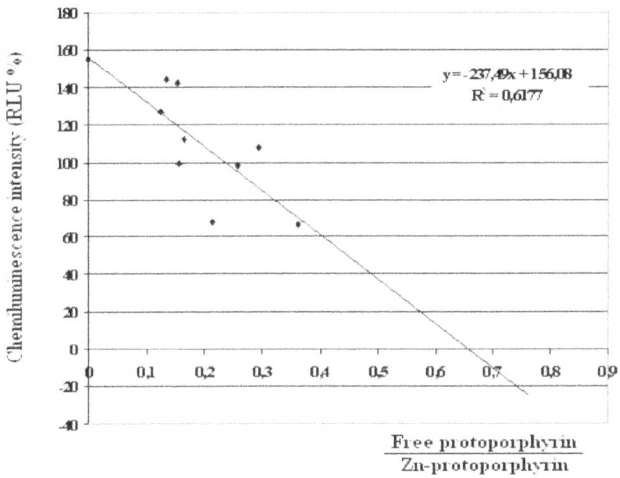


Fig. 2. Correlation between free protoporphyrin/Zn-protoporphyrin and chemiluminescent intensity (RLU%) in erythrocyte of cancerous patients.

Free protoporphyrin is accumulated generally in more cancerous cells than in healthy ones and autofluorescence lifetime is extended in cancer tissues (Chang et al., 2005). The results showed that in cancerous patients protoporphyrin - according to concentration - induces free radicals in small concentration and scavenges in higher concentration.

Accumulation of toxic metal elements and high protoporphyrin and Zn-protoporphyrin concentrations and low bond HCHO in erythrocyte with high PSA level mean wrong diagnosis.

According to the findings it seems that moderate and permanent consumption of table beet product affect favorably the life expectancy of patients, improves the erythrocyte function by the increasing methyl groups and diminishes the Zn-protoporphyrin and free protophorphyrin concentrations, but because of the increasing values of EGF and PSA in 44% of patients with bone metastasis, carefulness is needed. Further examinations are needed in this field.

Table 5. shows the erythrocyte Zn-protoporhyrin-, free- protoporhyrin-, erythrocyte formaldehyde - concentrations and PSA levels of cancerous patients with and without table beet treatment in different stages.

Before the table beet treatment, the HCHO concentration was 1.02 x $10^{-3}$ ± 2,73 x $10^{-4}$ µmol/mg erythrocyte, and after treatment the HCHO concentration was 3.72 x $10^{-3}$ ± 1,08 x $10^{-3}$ µmol/mg erythrocyte. Consequently, the HCHO concentration was elevated and therefore the function of erythrocyte was improved.

| patients | Zn-protoporhyrin (nmol/l ery) | free-protoporhyrin (nmol/l ery) | erythrocyte formaldehyde (μmol/ml) | PSA (ng/ml) |
|---|---|---|---|---|
| healthy control (N=14) | nd | nd | $1.52 \times 10^{-2}$ $\pm$ $1.25 \times 10^{-3}$ | nv |
| prostate tumor (histology -) (N=10) | 1282 ± 513* | 325 ± 50* | $1.06 \times 10^{-2}$* $\pm 1.44 \times 10^{-3}$ | 9.66 ± 5.28* |
| prostate tumor (histology +) (N=30) | 1043 ± 372* | 582 ± 782* | $7.830 \times 10^{-3}$** $\pm$ $2.56 \times 10^{-3}$ | 13.68 ± 21.91* |
| prostate tumor (metastatic) (N=18) | 1470±768* | 334±420* | $1.02 \times 10^{-3}$*** $\pm$ $2.73 \times 10^{-4}$ | 93 ± 120** |
| prostate tumor (metastatic) + table beet (N=18 ) | 857±308* | 301±276* | $3.72 \times 10^{-3} \pm$ *****$1.08 \times 10^{-3}$ | 133.5±182.5** |

nd non detected; nv value is in normal range (normal value of PSA is 0.01-4.00 ng/ml); (mean±SD) significance: control vs *;**;***; * vs **; **vs***, ****.

Table 5. Erythrocyte parameters of cancerous patients with and without table beet treatment in different stages.

## 3. Conclusion

HCHO and protoporphyrin concentrations and the induced free radical level of erythrocytes are very important indexes in cancer. The changes of their concentrations mean changes in tumor stages.

Generally the valuation of beneficial effects of nutrition supplements on patient life quality in tumor is empirical, and clinical studies are very rare. *Beta vulgaris* L. ssp. *esculenta* var. *rubra* is rich in bioactive compounds therefore it affects numerous biochemical reactions, enzyme activities and metabolic pathways. Homeostasis depends on table beet metal ion concentrations. This vegetable can be considered as a functional food, because among others, table beet is a good alimentary factor in cases of fatty liver, it has beneficial lipid lowering effects in obesity. Dietary betaine may need to be factored into the dietary sources of labile methyl groups and increase the methyl-pool. Treatment of betaine lowered plasma homocysteine concentration in homocystinuric patients.

The favorable impact of *Beta vulgaris* is enforced because significantly high levels of Zn- and free protoporphyrin decrease and furthermore trans-methylation processes fasten in cancerous patients. These results clearly verify that iron, folic acid and betaine components as well as colorful compounds with antioxidant activity of table beet extract demand more attention as a preventive therapy in chemotherapy induced anemia. Table beet will have a great impact and application in human cancer, but because of the increasing values of EGF close medical control is necessary for patients especially during chemotherapy.

## 4. Acknowledgements

This study was supported by the Health Sciences Scientific Committee ETT 354/2006, ETT 012/02, ETT 02/02.
Authors express their thanks to Mrs. Sarolta Bárkovits, Mrs. Edina Pintér and Mrs. Judit Sablyán for their excellent technical assistance.

## 5. Abbreviations

CRP = C reactive protein
DNA = deoxy-ribonucleic acid
EGF = epidermal growth factor
HbA1c = glycated hemoglobin
HCHO = formaldehyde
IBD = inflammatory bowel diseases
IFNG = interferon-gamma
IL-1 alpha/beta, IL-2, IL-4, IL-6, IL-8, IL-10, = interleukins
MCP-1 = monocyte chemoattractant protein-1
PSA = prostate-specific antigen
RLU = relative light unit
TNF-α = tumor necrosis factor-alpha

## 6. References

Abate, C., Patel, L., Rauscher, I.F.J., Curran, T. (1990). Redox regulation of Fos and Jun DNA: binding activity in vitro. *Science,* Vol.249, No. 4973, (Sept 1990), pp. 1157–1161, ISSN: 0036-8075

Atmane, N., Dairou, J., Paul, A., Dupret, J.M., Rodrigues-Lima, F. (2003). Redox regulation of the human xenobiotic metabolizing enzyme arylamine N-acetyltransferase 1 (NAT1). Reversible inactivation by hydrogen peroxide. *Journal of Biological Chemistry,* Vol. 278, No. 37, (Jun 2003), pp. 35086-35092, ISSN: 0021-9258

Awad, W.M.J., Whitney, P.L., Skiba, W.E., Mangum, J.H., Wells, M.S. (1983). Evidence for direct methyl transfer in betaine:homocysteine S-methyl-transfrease. *Journal of Biological Chemistry,* Vol. 258, No.258, (1983 Nov 10), pp. 12790-12792, ISSN: 0021-9258

Azzi, A., Gysin, R., Kempná, P., Munteanu, A., Villacorta, L., Visarius, T., Zingg, J,M. (2004). Regulation of gene expression by alpha-tocopherol.. *Biological Chemistry,* Vol.385, No 7, (Jul 2004), pp. 585-591, ISSN: 0021-9258

Barak, A.J., Beckenhauer, H.C., Tuma, D.J. (1996). Betaine, ethanol and the liver: a review. *Alcohol,* Vol.13, No.4, (Jul-Aug 1996), pp. 395-398, ISSN: 0741-8329

Barqawi, A., Thompson, I.M., Crawford, E.D. (2004). Prostate cancer chemoprevention, an overview of United States trials, *Journal of Urology,* Vol.171, No.2, (Febr 2004), pp. S5-8, ISSN: 0022-5347

Baylin, S.B., Herman, J.G., Graff, J.R., Vertino, P.M., Issa, J.P. (1997). Alterations in DNA methylation: a fundamental aspect of neoplasia. *Advances in Cancer Resesearch,* Vol. 72, No.72, pp. 141-196, ISSN: 0065-230X

Bastian, P.J., Palapattu, G.S., Yegnasubramanian, S., et al. (2008). CpG island hypermethylation profile in the serum of men with clinically localized and hormone refractory metastatic prostate cancer. *Journal of Urology,* Vol. 179, No.2, (Febr 2008), pp. 529–534, ISSN: 0022-5347

Blázovics, A. (2011). Small molecules in cancer therapy: cytotoxics and molecularly targeted agents. *Current Signal Transduction Therapy,* Vol.6, No.1, (Jan 2011), pp. 2-19, ISSN: 1574-3624

Blázovics, A., Kovács, Á., Lugasi, A. (2007a). The effect of short and long term antioxidant treatments on redox homeostasis in experimental and clinical studies. In: *Nutritional Research Advances,* (Ed.) Sarah V. Watkins, Nova Science Publisher, ISBN: 978-1-60021-516-2, Chapter 4, pp. 1-34, USA

Blázovics, A., Kovács, A., Szilvás, Á. (2009). Redox homeostasis in gastrointestinal diseases. Acta Biologica. Szegediensis Vol. 53, Suppl. 1, 3-6, pp. 41-45, ISSN: 1588-4082

Blázovics, A., Kovács, Á., Lugasi, A., Hagymási, K., Bíró, L., Fehér, J. (1999). Antioxidant defence in erythrocytes and plasma of patients with active and quiescent Crohn's disease and ulcerative colitis: A chemiluminescence study. *Clinical Chemistry,* Vol.6, No.45, pp. 895-896, ISSN: 0009-9147

Blázovics, A., Nyirády, P., Bekő, G., Székely, E., Szilvás, Á., Kovács-Nagy, E., Horváth, A., Szűcs, M., Romics, I., Sárdi, É. (2011). Changes in erythrocyte transmethylation ability are predictive factors for tumor prognosis in prostate cancer, *Croatica Chemica Acta,* Vol. 84, No.3. pp. 127-131, ISSN: 001-1643

Blázovics, A., Sárdi, E., Szentmihályi, K., Váli, L., Takács-Hájos, M., Stefanovits-Bányai, E. (2007b). Extreme consumption of Beta vulgaris var. rubra can cause metal ion accumulation in the liver. *Acta Biologica Hungarica,* Vol.58, No.3, pp. 281-286, ISSN: 0236-5383

Blázovics, A., Szilvás, Á., Székely, Gy., Tordai, E., Székely, E., Czabai, G., Pallai, Zs., Sárdi É. (2008). Important bioactive molecules of erythrocytes in colorectal cancer patients after colectomy. *The Open Medicinal Chemistry Journal,* No.2, (Febr 2008), pp. 6-10, ISSN: 1874-1045

Blunden, G., Gordon, S.M. (1986). Betaines and their sulphonio analogues in marine algae. *Progress in Phycological Research, Vol.*4, pp. 41-80, ISSN: 0167-8574

Bobek, P., Galbavy, S., Mariássyová M. (2000). The effect of red beet (Beta vulgaris var. rubra) fiber on alimentary hypercholesterolemia and chemically induced colon carcinogenesis in rats. *Nahrung,* Vol.44, No.3 S. (Jul 2000), pp. 184-187, ISSN: 0027-769X

Boyd, J.N., Babish, J.G., Stoewsand, G.S. (1982). Modification by beet and cabbage diets of aflatoxin $B_1$-induced rat plasma α-foetoprotein elevation, hepatic tumorigenesis, and mutagenicity of urine. *Food and Chemical Toxicology,* Vol.20, No.1, (Feb 1982), pp. 47-52, ISSN: 0278-6915

Brando-Neto, J., Stefan, V., Mendoca, B.B. et al. (1995). The essential role of zink in growth, *Nutrition Research,* Vol. 15, No.3, (Marc 1995), pp. 335-338, ISSN: 0271-5317

Caddell, J.L. (2000). Geriatric cachexia: a role for magnesium deficiency as well as for cytokines? *American Society for Clinical Nutrition,* Vol. 71 No.3, (Marc 2000), pp. 851-852, ISSN: 0212-1611

Cai, Y., Sun, M., Corke, H. (2001). Antioxidant activity of betalains from plants the Amaranthaceae. *Journal of Agricultural and Food Chemistry*, Vol.51, No.49, (Apr 2003), pp. 2288-2294, ISSN: 1579-4377

Calvisi, D.F., Ladu, S., Gorden, A., Farina, M., Lee, J.S., Conner, E.A., Schroeder, I., Factor, V.M., Thorgeirsson, S.S. (2007). Mechanistic and prognostic significance of aberrant methylation in the molecular pathogenesis of human hepatocellular carcinoma, *Journal of Clinical Investigation*, Vol. 117, No.9, (Sept 2007), pp. 2713-2722, ISSN: 0895-4356

Chang, C.L., You, C., Chen, H.M., Chiang, C.P., Chen, C.T., Wang, C.Y. (2004). Autofluorescence lifetime measurement on oral carcinogenesis. Conference Publications - IEEE Engineering in Medicine and Biology Society, Vol. 4, pp. 2349-2351. **ISSN:** 1557-170X.

Chen, R.Z., Pettersson, U., Beard, C., Jackson–Grusby, L., Jaenisch, R. (1998). DNA hypomethylation leads to elevated mutation rates. *Nature*. Vol.395, No.6697, (Sept 1989), pp. 89-93, ISSN: 0028-0836

Chukhlovin, A.B., Tokalov, S.V., Yagunov, A.S., Westendorf, J., Reincke, H., Karbe, L. (2001). In vitro suppression of thymocyte apoptosis by metal-rich complex environmental mixtures: potential role of zinc and cadmium excess. *The Science of The Total Environment*, Vol.281, No.1-3, (Dec 2001), pp. 153-163, ISSN: 0048-9697

Critchfield, J.W., Keen, C.L. (1992). Manganese$^{+2}$ exhibits dynamic binding to multiple ligands in human plazma. *Metabolism: Clinical and Experimental*, Vol.41, No10,(Oct 1992), pp. 1087-1092 ISSN: 0026-0495.

Delerive, P., Furman, C., Teissier, E., Fruchart, J., Duriez, P., Staels, B. (2000). Oxidized phospholipids activate PPARα in a phospholipase A2-dependent manner. *FEBS Letters*, Vol. 471, No.1, (Apr 2000), pp. 34-38, ISSN: 0014-5793

Dinkova-Kostova, AT, Holtzclaw, W.D., Wakabayashi, N. (2005). Keap1, the sensor for electrophiles and oxidants that regulates the phase 2 response, is a zinc metalloprotein. *Biochemistry*. Vol.10, No.44, (May 2005), pp. 6889-6899, ISSN: 0001527X

Dolmetsch, R.E., Lewis, R.S., Goodnow, C.C., Healy, J.I. (1997). Differential activation of transcription factors induced by Ca2+ response amplitude and duration. *Nature*, No.386, (Apr 1997), pp. 855-858, ISSN: 0028-0836

Eikelboom, J.W., Lonn, E., Yusuf, S. (1999). Homocysteine and cardiovascular disease: a critical review of the epidemiologic evidence. *Annals of Internal Medicine*, Vol.131, No. 7, (Sept 1999), pp. 363-375, ISSN: 0003-4819

Evans, J.C., Huddler, D.P., Jiracek, J., Castro, C., Millian, N.S., Garrow, T.A., Ludwig, M.L. (2002). Betaine-homocysteine methyltransferase zinc in distorted barrel. *Structure*, Vol.10, No.9, (Sept 2002), pp. 1159-1171, ISSN:0022-2860

Finkenstein, J.D., Martin, J.J. (1984). Inactivation of betaine-homocysteine methyltransferase by adenosylmethionine and adenosylethionine. *Biochemical and Biophysical Research Communication*, Vol.118, No.118, (Jan 1984), pp. 14-19, ISSN: 0006-291X

Floris, G., Medda, R., Padiglia, A., et al., (2000). The physiological significance of ceruloplasmin. A possible therapeutical approach. *Biochemical Pharmacology*, Vol 60, No.12, (Dec 2000), pp. 1735-1741, ISSN: 0006-2952

Frank, T., Stintzing, F.G., Carle, R., Bitsch, I., Quaas, D., Strass, G., Bitsch, R., Netzel, Z. (2005). Urinary pharmacokinetics of betalains following consumption of red beet juice in healthy humans. *Pharmacological Research*, Vol.52 No.4, (Oct 2005), pp. 290-297, ISSN: 1043-6618

Gersbeck, N., Schönbeck, F., Tyihák, E. (1989). Measurement of formaldehyde and its main generators in *Erysiphe graminis* infected barley plants by planar chromatographic techniques. *Journal of Planar Chromatography*, Vol. 2, No.1, pp. 86-89, ISSN:1789-0993

Griffiths, H.R., Lunec, J. (2001). Ascorbic acid in the 21st century: more than a simple antioxidant. *Environmental Toxicology and Pharmacology*, .Vol. 10, No.4, (Sept 2001), pp. 173–182, ISSN: 1382-6689

Haddad, J.J. (2002). Oxygen-sensitive pro-iflammatory cytokines, apoptosis signaling and redox-responsive transcription factors in development and pathophysiology. *Cytokines Cellular and Molecular Therapy*, Vol. 7, No.1, (Marc 2002, pp. 1-14, ISSN: 1368-4736

Hájos, M.T., Varga, I.Sz., Lugasi, A., Fehér, M., Bányai, É.S. (2004): Correlation between pigment contents and FRAP values in beet root (Beta vulgaris ssp. esculenta var. rubra). *International Journal of Horticultural Science*, Vol.10, No.4, pp. 85-89, ISSN: 1585-0404

Hagymási, K., Blázovics, A., Lengyel, G., Kocsis, I., Fehér, J. (2001). Oxidative damage in alcoholic liver disease. *European Journal of Gastroenterology and Hepatology*, Vol.13, No.1, (Jan 2001), pp. 49-53, ISSN: 0954-691X

Hartwig, A. (1998). Carcinogenicity of metal compounds: Possible role of DNA repair inhibition. *Toxicology Letters*, Vol.102-103, (Dec 1998), pp. 235-239 ISSN: 0378-4274

Hartwig, A., Mullenders, L.H.F., Schlepegrell, R., Kasten, U., Beyersmann, D. (1994). Nickel(II) interferes with the incision step in nucleotide excision repair in mammalian cells. *Cancer Research*, Vol. 54, No.15, (Aug 1994), pp. 4045-4051, ISSN: 0008-5472

Hayat, L.(1996). Cations in malignant and benign brain tumors. *Journal. Environmental Science and Health. Part. A* Vol. 31, No.8,(Aug 1996), pp. 1831-1840.ISSN: 1093-4529

Hougaard, L., Anthoni, U., Christophersen, C., Larsen, C., Lever, C., Lever, P.H.N. (1991). Characterization and quantitative estimation of quaternary ammonium compounds in marine demosponges. *Comparative Biochemistry and Physiology Part B: Biochemistry and Molecular Biology*, Vol.99, No.2, (2, 1991), pp. 469-472, ISSN: 1096-4959

Huszti, Z., Tyihák, E. (1986). Formation of formaldehyde from S-adenosyl-L-(mehyl-3H) methionine during enzymatic transmethylation of histamine. *FEBS Letters*. Vol.209, No.2, (Dec 1986), pp. 362-366, ISSN: 0014-5793

Jemal, A., Siegel, R., Ward, E., Hao, Y., Xu, J., Murray, T., Thun, M. (2008). Cancer statistics, *CA: a Cancer Journal for Clinicians*, Vol.58, No.2, pp. 71–96, ISSN:0007-9235

Kanner, J., Harel., S., Granit, R. (2001). Betalains-A New class of Dietary cationized antioxidants. *Journal of Agriculture and Food Chemistry*, Vol. 49, No.11, (2001 Nov), pp. 5178-5185, ISSN: 0021-8561

Kapadia, G.J., Azuine, M.A., Sridhar, R., Okuda, Y., Tsuruta, A., Ichiishi, E., Mukainake, T., Takasaki, M., Konoshima, T., Nishino, H., Tokuda, H. (2003). Chemoprevention of DMBA-induced UV-B promoted, NOR-1-induced TPA promoted skin carcinogenesis, and DEN-induced phenobarbital promoted liver tumors in mice by extract of beetroot. *Pharmacological Research*, Vol.47, No.2, (2003 Feb), pp. 141-148, ISSN: 1043-6618

Kasprzak, K.S., Waalkes, M.P., Poirier, L.A. (1987). Effect of essential divalent metals on carcinogenicity and metabolism of nickel and cadmium. *Biological Trace Element Research*, No.13, (Aug 1987), pp. 253-273, ISSN: 0163-4984

Kapadia, G.J., Tokuda, H., Konoshima, T., Nishino, H. (1996). Chemoprevention of lung and skin cancer by *Beta vulgaris* (beet) root extract. *Cancer Letters,* Vol.100, No.1-2, (Febr 1996), pp. 211-214, ISSN: 0304-3835

Kong, A.N., Yu, R., Chen, C., Mandlekar, S., Primiano, T. (2000). Signal transduction events elicited by natural products: role of MAPK and caspase pathways in homeostatic response and induction of apoptosis. *Archives Pharmacological Research,* Vol.23, No.1, (Febr 2000), pp. 1-16, ISSN:0253-6269

Kovács-Nagy, E., Blázovics, A., Fébel, H., Szentmihályi, K., Sárdi, É. (2009). Chromatographic analytical opportunities on a thin film of mobilizable methyl-groups of different biological objects under the influence of exogenic treatment. *Acta Biologica Szegediensis*, Vol.53, Suppl. 1, pp. 54. ISSN: 1588-385X

Kuramoto, Y., Yamada, K., Tsuruta, O,, Sugano, M. (1996). Effect of natural food colorings on immunoglobulin production in vitro by rat spleen lymphocytes. *Bioscience Biotechnology and Biochemistry*, Vol.60, No.10, (Oct 1996), pp. 1712-1713, ISSN: 0916-8451

Lever, M., Sizeland, P.C., Bason, L.M., Hayman, C.M., Chambers, S.T. (1994). Glycine betaine and proline betaine in human blood and urine. *Biochim Biophys Acta*, Vol. 1200, No.3, (Aug 1994), pp. 259-264, ISSN: 0304-4165

Lichszteld, K., Kruk, L. (1977). Singlet molecular oxygen in formaldehyde oxidation. *Zeitschrift für Physicalische Chemie. (N F)* Vol.108, pp. 167-172, ISBN: 0044-3336

Lugasi, A., Hóvári J. (2002). Flavonoid aglycons in food of plant origin II. Fresh and dried fruits. Acta Alimentaria, Vol. 31, No.1, (Feb 2002), pp. 63-71. ISSN: 0139-3006

Máday, E., Szentmihályi, K., Then, M., Szőke, É. 2000. Mineral element content of chamomile. *Acta Alimentaria,* Vol. 29, No.1, (Febr 2000), pp. 51-57, ISSN:0139-3006

Maehle, L., Metcalf, R.A., Ryberg, D., Bennett, W.P., Harris, C.C., Haugen, A. (1992). Altered p53 gene structure and expression in human epithelial cells after exposure to nickel. Cancer Research, Vol.52, No.1,(Jan 1992), pp. 218-221, ISSN: 0008-5472

Malaguarnera, L., Ferlito, L., Imbesi, R.M, Gulizia, G.S., Di Mauro, S., Maugeri, D., Malaguarnera, M., Messina, S.S. (2001). Immunosenescence: a review. *Archives of Gerontology and Geriatritcs,.* Vol. 32, No.1, (Febr 2001), pp. 1-4, ISSN: 0167-4943

Meyer, M., Schreck, R., Baeuerle, P.A. (1993), $H_2O_2$ and antioxidants have opposite effects on activation of NF-kappa B and AP-1 in intact cells: AP-1 as secondary antioxidant-responsive factor. *EMBO Journal,* Vol.12, No.5, (May 1993), pp. 2005-2015, ISSN: 0261-4189

Millan, N.S., Garrow, T.A. (1998). Human betaine-homocysteine methyltransferase is a zinc metalloenzyme. *Archives of Biochemistry and Biophysics,* Vol.356, No.1 (Aug 1998), pp. 93-98, ISSN: 0003-9861

Murakami, T., Magamura,Y., Hirano, K., (1998). The recovering effect of betaine on carbon tetrachloide indiced liver injury. *Journal of Nutritional Science and Vitamology, (Tokyo), Vol.*44, No.2, (Apr 1998), pp. 249-255, ISSN:0301-4800

Nieva, J., Wentworth, P.Jr. (2004). The antibody-catalyzed water oxidation pathway - a new chemical arm to immune defence? *Trends in Biocheical Science,* Vol.29, No.5, (May 2004), pp. 274-278, ISSN: 0968-0004

Nyirády, P., Blázovics, A., Romics, I., May, Z., Székely, E., Bekő, G., 1 Szentmihályi, K. (2009a). Microelement concentration differences between patients with and without prostate adenocarcinoma. Vol. 3. Deficiency or excess of trace elements in the environment as a risk of health, Eds. Szilágyi M. and Szentmihályi K. Hungarian Academy of Sciences, pp. 26-30. TEFC. Budapest, ISBN:

Nyirády, P., Romics, I. (2009b). Textbook of Urology 2009. Semmelweis Kiadó és Multimédia Stúdió, ISBN: 9789639879232

Nyirády, P., Sárdi, É., Bekő, G., Szűcs, M., Horváth, A., Székely, E., Szentmihályi, K., Romics, I., Blázovics, A. (2010). Effect of bioactive molecules of Beta vulgaris L. ssp. Esculenta var. rubra on metastatic prostate cancer. *Orvosi. Hetilap,* Vol.151, No. 37, (Sept 2010), pp. 1495-1503, ISSN: 0030-6002

Pedreno, M.A., Escribano, J. (2000). Studying the oxidation and the antiradical activity of betalain from beet root. *Journal of Biological Education,* Vol.35, No.1, (Jan 2000), pp. 49-51, ISSN: 0021-9266

Pena, M.M., Lee, J., Thiele D.J. (1999). A delicate balance: homeostatic contol of copper uptake and distribution, *Journal of Nutrition,* Vol.129, No.7, (Jul 1999), pp. 1251-1260, ISSN: 0022-3166

Polya, G.M., Polya, Z., Kweifio-Okai, G. (2002). Biochemical pharmacology of anti-inflammatory plant secondary metabolites. In Recent Progress in Medicinal Plants Vol.8, (Ed) E. Sighn, J.N. Govil, V.K. Sighn, SCI TECH Publishing, Houston, Texas, USA., pp. 1-22. ISBN: 1930813139

Powis, G., Gasdanska, J.R., Baker, A. (1997). Redox signaling and the control of cell growth and death. *Advances in Pharmacology,* Vol.38, pp. 329-358, ISSN: 0009-9236

Rice-Evans, C.A., Miller, N.J., Paganga, G. (1999). Antioxidant properties of phenolic compounds. *Trends Plant Science.* Vol.2, No.4, (April 1997), pp. 152-159, ISSN: 1360-1385

Rosenbaum, E., Hoque, M.O., Cohen, Y., Zahurak, M., Eisenberger, M.A., Epstein, J.I., Partin, A.W., Sidransky, D. (2005). Promoter hypermethylation as an independent prognostic factor for relapse in patients with prostate cancer following radical prostatectomy. *Clinical Cancer Research,* Vol.11, No.23, (Dec 2005), pp. 8321-8525, ISSN: 1078-0432

Salnikow, K., Zhitkovich, A. (2008). Genetic and epigenetic mechanisms in metal carcinogenesis and cocarcinogenesis: nickel, arsenic, and chromium, *Chemical Research in Toxicology,*. Vol.21, No.1, (Jan 2008), pp. 28-44, ISSN: 0893-228X

Sárdi, É., Stefanovits-Bányai, É., Kocsis, I., Takács-Hájos, M., Fébel, H., Blázovics, A. (2009). Effect of bioactive compounds of table beet cultivars on alimenary induced fatty livers of rats. *Acta Alimimentaria,* Vol.38, No.3, (Sept 2009), pp. 267-280, ISSN: 0139-3006

Sárdi, É., Tordai E. (2005). Determination of fully N-methylated compounds in different cabbage and beetroot varieties. *Acta Biologica Szegediensis,* Vol.49. No.1-2, pp. 43-45, ISSN: 1588-385X

Schroeder, J.J., Cousins, R.J. (1990). Interleukin 6 regulates metallothionein gene expression and zinc metabolism in hepatocyte monolayer cultures. *Proceedings of the National Academic of Science U S A.* Vol.87, No.8, (Apr 1990), pp. 3137-3141. ISSN: 0027-8424

Schwartz, S.J., von Elbe, J.H., Pariza, M.W., Goldsworthy, T., Pitot, H.C. (1983). Inability of red beet betalain pigments to initiate or promote hepatocarcinogenesis. *Food and Chemical Toxicology*, Vol.21, No.5, pp. (Oct 1983), 531-535, ISSN: 0278-6915

Sigel, A., Sigel, H. (1999). Interactions between Free Radicals and Metal Ions in Life Processes. Metal Ions in Biological Systems, Marcel Dekker Inc., New York, Vol. No.36, pp. 1-797.

Skiba, W.E., Taylor, M.S., Wells, M.S., Mangum, J.H., Awad, W.M.J. (1982). Human hepatic methionine biosynthesis. Purification and characterization of betaine:homocysteine S/methyltransferase. *Journal of Biological Chemistry*, Vol.257, No.24, (Dec 1982). pp. 14944-14948, ISSN: 0021-9258

Slow, S., Lever, M., Lee, M.B., George, P.M., Chambers, S.T., (2004). Betaine analogues alter homocysteine metabolism in rats. *The International Journal of Biochemistry and Cell Biology*, Vol.36, No.5, (May 2004), pp. 870-880, ISSN: 1357-2725

Stead, L.M., Brosman, J.T., Brosman M.E., Vance D.E., Jacobs, R.L. (2006). Is it time to reevaluate methyl balance in humans? *The American Journal of Clinical Nutrition*, Vol.83, No.1, (Jan 2006), pp. 5–10. ISSN: 0002-9165

Stintzing, F.G., Carle, R. (2004). Functional properties of anthocyanins and betalains in plants food and in human nutrition. *Trends Food Science and Techology*, Vol.15, No.1, (Jan 2004), pp. 19-38, ISSN: 0924-2244

Stryeer, L. Biochemistry 3rd (1988). ed. V.H. Freeman and Co., New York, ISBN: 0716719207

Suzuki, Y.J., Forman, H.J., Sevanian, A. (1997). Oxidants as stimulators of signal transduction. *Free Radical Biology and Medicine*, Vol.22, No.1-2, pp. 269-285, ISSN: 0891-5849

Szentmihályi, K., Blázovics, A., Lugasi, A., Kéry, Á., Lakatos, B., Vinkler, P. (2000a). Effect of natural polyphenol-type antioxidants (Sempervivum tectorum and Raphanus sativus L. var. niger extracts) on metal ion concentrations in rat bile fluid. *Current Topics Biophysics*, Vol. No.24, pp. 203-07, ISSN:

Szentmihályi, K., Csiktusnádi-Kiss, G.A., Keszler, Á., Kótai L., Candeaias, M., Bronze, M.R., Boas, L.V., Spauger, I., Forgács, E. (2000b). Method development for measurement of elements in Hungarian red wines by inductively coupled plasma optical emission spectrmetry (ICP-OES). *Acta Aliment*ary, Vol,29, pp. 105-121, ISSN: 0139-3006

Szilvás, Á., Blázovics, A., Székely, Gy., Fehér, J. (1999). Free radical status and tumor markers in gastrointestinal tumors, European Congress, I.H.P.B.A. Budapest, (Ed) L. Flautner, P.K. Kupcsulik, I. Rózsa, Monduzzi Editore. International Proceeding Divison, pp. 409-412, ISSN: 2039-4632

Takács-Hájos, M. (1999). Color components of different table beet root varieties. *International Journal of Horticulture Science*, Vol. 5, pp. 3-4, ISSN: 1585-04040

Váli, L., Stefanovits-Bányai, E., Szentmihályi, K., Fébel, H., Sárdi, E., Lugasi, A., Kocsis, I., Blázovics, A. (2007). Liver-protecting effects of table beet (Beta vulgaris var. rubra) during ischemia-reperfusion. *Nutrition*, Vol.23, No2, (Feb 2007), pp. 172-178, ISSN: 0899-9007

Wang, M., Goldman, I.L. (1996). Phenotypic variation free folic acid content among F1 hybrids and open-pollinated cultivars of red beet. *Journal of the Amarican Society for Horticultural Science*. Vol.121, No.6, (Nov 1996), pp. 1040-1042, ISSN: 0003-1062

Vanherweghem, J.L., Depierreux, M., Tielemans, C., Abramowicz, D., Dratwa, M., Jadoul, M,, Richard, C., Vandervelde, D., Verbeelen, D., Vanhaelen-Fastre, R, et al. (1993). Rapidly progressive interstitial renal fibrosis in young women: association with slimming regimen including Chinese herbs. *Lancet,* Vol.13, No.341, (Feb 1993), pp. 387-391, ISSN: 0140-6736

Watson, R.E., Curtin, G.M., Doolittle, D.J., Goodman, J.I. (2003). Progressive alterations in global and GC rich DNA methylation during tumorigenesis, *Toxicological Sciences,* Vol.75, No.2, (Oct 2003), pp. 289-299, ISSN: 1096-6080

Wettasinghe, M., Bolling, B., Plhak, L., Xiao, H., Parkin, K. (2002). Phase II enzyme-inducing and antioxidant activities of beetroot (*Beta vulgaris* L.) extracts from phenotypes of different pigmentation. *Journal of Agricultural and Food Chemistry,* Vol.50, No.23, (Nov 2002), pp. 6704-6707, ISSN: 0021-8561

Wilchen, B., Dudman, N., Tyrrell, P.A. (1983). Homocystinuria-the effects of betaine. *New England Journal of Medicine,* Vol. 309, No.8, (Aug 1983), pp. 448-453, ISSN: 0028-4793

Wild, L., Flanagan, J.M. (2010). Genome-wide hypomethylation in cancer may be a passive consequence of transformation. *Biochimica et Biophysica Acta,* Vol.1806, No.1, (Aug 2010), pp. 50-57, ISSN: 0304-419X

Yuregir, G.T., Kayrin, L., Curuk, M.A., Acarturk, E., Unlukurt, I. (1994/1995). Correlation between trace elements and lipid profiles. *Journal of Trace Elements in Experimental Medicine, Vol.7, pp. 113-118, ISSN: 0896-548X*

Zakharova, N.S., Petrova, T.A. (1998). Relationship between the structure and antioxidant activity of various betalains. *Prikladnaya Biocimimija i Mikrobiologiya,* Vol.34, No.2, (March April 1998), pp. 199-202, ISSN: 0555-1099

# 8

# Anaemia in Developing Countries: Burden and Prospects of Prevention and Control

Kayode O. Osungbade[1,2,*] and Adeolu O. Oladunjoye[1,2]

[1]*Department of Health Policy and Management*
*Faculty of Public Health*
*College of Medicine and University College Hospital*
*University of Ibadan and*
[2]*Department of Community Medicine*
*University College Hospital, Ibadan*
*Nigeria*

## 1. Introduction

Anaemia constitutes a public health problem in developing countries. Worldwide, about 2 billion people are estimated to suffer from anaemia and it is reported to account for three-quarters of 1 million deaths a year in Africa and South-East Asia. The underlying causes of anaemia are many, varied and largely preventable; these include nutritional deficiencies, infections and haemoglobin disorders.

Cost-effective interventions against anaemia are well documented in the literature. However, there are constraints to diagnosis, treatment and prevention in resource-poor settings of developing countries. Effective management of anaemia includes treatment of the underlying cause, restoration of the haemoglobin concentration to normal levels, and prevention and treatment of complications, among others. Suggested strategies aimed at preventing anaemia focused on the major underlying causes in developing countries.

## 2. Background

Anaemia is the reduction in the haemoglobin concentration of the peripheral blood below the normal range expected for age and sex of an individual.(1) The World Health Organisation (WHO) defines anaemia as a hemoglobin value below 13 g/dl in men over 15 years of age, below 12 g/dl in non pregnant women over 15 years, and below 11 g/dl in pregnant women.(2) It is a condition in which the number of red blood cells or their oxygen carrying capacity is insufficient to meet physiologic needs and this varies for age, sex, altitude and pregnancy status.(3) However, the determination of hemoglobin concentration should always take the state of hydration and altitude of residence of an individual into consideration.(1)

Anaemia is a global health problem in both developing and developed countries with major consequences on human health as well as social and economic development.(4) Anaemia is

*Correspondence Author

the world's second leading cause of disability.(3) Worldwide, the World Health Organisation (WHO) estimated the number of anaemic persons to be about 2 billion and approximately 50% of all cases can be attributed to iron deficiency.(5) Anaemia is responsible for about 1 million death a year, out of which three-quarters occur in Africa and South-East Asia.(6) Anaemia affects over half of preschool age children and pregnant women in developing countries, and at least 30-40% in industrialized countries.(3) Nevertheless, it is apparent that the prevalence of anaemia in developing countries is about four times more than developed countries.(7) In view of the above, this chapter highlights the burden of anaemia in the population and discusses its causes in developing countries. Furthermore, the chapter reviews the prospects and challenges of diagnosis of underlying causes, treatment and prevention in the developing countries.

## 3. Methods

We reviewed literature using key words of the thrust of the paper; hence, search terms such as prevalence, burden, causes, treatment and prevention of anaemia in developing countries were used. Cross sectional, observational and randomized control trials' literature on the subject published between 2000 and 2010 served as the main sources of information. Commonly used medical databases such as PubMed (Medline), AJOL and Google Scholar were searched as appropriate; in addition, Cochrane Library was used to source for systematic reviews on the subject matter.

## 4. Results

### 4.1 Burden of anaemia in developing countries

The most vulnerable groups in the population are children and pregnant women, while others such as the non pregnant women and the elderly are next affected. An estimated 10-20% of preschool age children in developed countries and 30-80% in developing countries are anaemic at 1 year of age.(8) The consequences of anaemia in children are inimical as it affects their cognitive performance, behaviour and physical growth. Children who suffer from anaemia have delayed psychomotor development and impaired performance of tests; in addition, they experience impaired coordination of language and motor skills, equivalent to a 5 to 10 points deficit in intelligent quotient (IQ).(5)

The World Health Organisation (WHO) estimated that 56% of all pregnant women in developing countries are anaemic.(9) In Southern Asia, the prevalence of anaemia in pregnancy is about 75% in contrast to what obtains in North America and Europe with about 17% prevalence. Furthermore, 5% of pregnant women suffer from severe anaemia in the worst affected parts of the world.(9)

The consequences of anemia in women are enormous as the condition adversely affects both their productive and reproductive capabilities. First, anaemia reduces their energy and capacity for work (10), and can therefore threaten household food security and income. Second, severe anaemia in pregnancy impairs oxygen delivery to the fetus and interferes with normal intra-uterine growth, thereby resulting in intrauterine growth retardation, still birth, low birth weight and neonatal deaths.(10-11) Therefore, anaemia is highly contributory to poor pregnancy and birth outcomes in developing countries as it predisposes to premature delivery, increased perinatal mortality and increased risk of death during delivery and postpartum (10).

Worldwide, it is estimated that about 20% of maternal deaths are caused by anaemia; in addition, anaemia contributes partly to 50% of all maternal deaths.(12) Similar situation is found in sub-Saharan Africa where anaemia is reportedly accounted for about 20% of all maternal deaths brought about through three main mechanisms.(13) First, anaemia resulting from blood loss during or after childbirth makes women more susceptible to deaths by lowering their haematological reserve. Second, severe anaemia is associated with increased susceptibility to infection due to lowered resistance to disease; and third, haemoglobin (Hb) level of less than 4 g/dl is associated with high risk of cardiac failure and death particularly during delivery or soon after, if prompt intervention is not instituted.(14-15)

In terms of lost years of healthy life, iron deficiency anemia causes 25 million cases of Disability Adjusted Life Years (DALYs); this accounts for 2.4% of the total global DALYs.(3) Physical and cognitive losses due to iron deficiency anaemia cost developing countries up to 4.05% losses in gross domestic product per annum(16), thereby stalling social and economic development. In the World Health Organisation (WHO)/World Bank rankings, Iron Deficiency Anaemia (IDA) is the third leading cause of disability-adjusted life years lost for females' aged 15–44 years.(17-18)

### 4.2 Common causes of anaemia in developing countries

Most often, anaemia co-exists with an underlying disease and rarely occurs on its own. The commonest causes of anaemia in developing countries, particularly among the most vulnerable groups (pregnant women and preschool age children) are nutritional disorders and infections.

#### 4.2.1 Iron deficiency

Iron Deficiency Anaemia (IDA) is an underlying risk factor for maternal and perinatal mortality and morbidity; it is estimated to be associated with 115,000 of the 510,000 maternal deaths (i.e. 22%) and 591,000 of the 2,464,000 perinatal deaths (i.e. 24%) occurring annually around the world.(19) Iron is an essential component of haemoglobin (Hb), which is required for basic cellular function in all human tissues, particularly muscle, brain and red blood cells.(20) Therefore, deficiency of iron in the body can lead to anaemia in any age group. Iron deficiency anaemia (IDA) occurs when iron deficiency is sufficiently severe enough to diminish erythropoiesis, thereby leading to a decrease in the number of red cells in the blood and resulting in the development of anaemia.(21) However, mild-to-moderate forms of iron deficiency can occur in which the affected person is yet to become anaemic, but tissues are functionally iron deficient.(5) It is generally assumed that 50% of cases of anaemia are due to iron deficiency(5), but this may vary within population groups or environment.

The risk factors for IDA include a low intake of iron, poor absorption of iron from diets high in phytate or phenolic compounds, and early period of life when iron requirements are expectedly high. (4) Similarly, iron requirements are highest for pregnant women - 1.9 mg/1,000 kcal of dietary energy in the second trimester and 2.7 mg/1,000 kcal in the third trimester. These are followed by iron requirements in infants (1.0 mg), adolescent girls (0.8 mg), adolescent boys (0.6 mg), non pregnant women (0.6 mg), preschool and school age children (0.4mg), and adult men (0.3mg).(22)

Sources of dietary iron include meat, fish and poultry; other sources, though in less quantity, are cereals, dairy products, fruits and vegetables. About 40% of iron content of meat, fish and poultry is in the haem form, out of which about 25% is absorbed;(7) whereas only about 2 - 5% of total iron is absorbed from cereals and legumes. Therefore, these foods have a major influence on iron status.(23) Unfortunately, intakes of these foods especially meat, fish and poultry are low among people of low socio-economic status. Furthermore, some of the foods are avoided or observed as taboos for religious or cultural reasons in certain communities of developing countries.

Inadequate absorption of dietary iron is highly contributory to the high prevalence of anaemia in the developing countries of Asia and other regions, except where it is caused by infections such as hookworm and malaria.(7) Poor absorption of dietary iron can be due to substances which interfere with its absorption such as proton pump inhibitors, calcium supplements and dairy products.(24)

#### 4.2.2 Micronutrient deficiency

Evidence abounds that haemoglobin (Hb) concentration of persons with Vitamin A deficiency (VAD) increases by about 10 g/L when vitamin A supplements are provided.(25) Studies also suggest that vitamin A can improve hematologic indicators and enhance the efficacy of iron supplementation.(26) Thus, it is suggestive that Vitamin A deficiency (VAD) can predispose to anaemia.

It is reported that riboflavin deficiency may be quite common in developing countries where intake of animal products is low, and especially during seasons when there is less intake of vegetables.(7) Vitamin B12 is necessary for the synthesis of red blood cells and its deficiencies have been associated with megaloblastic anemia.(17) Therefore, diets with little or no animal protein, as it is often the case in the developing world, coupled with malabsorption related to parasitic infections of the small intestine, might result in Vitamin B 12 deficiency.(17)

Folic acid is also essential for the formation and maturation of red blood cells and necessary for cell growth and repair. Deficiency of folate reduces the rate of DNA synthesis with consequent impaired cell proliferation and intramedullary death of resulting abnormal cells; this shortens the lifespan of circulating red blood cells and results in anaemia.(27) There is, however, little evidence that folic acid deficiency may be a public health problem in many developing countries.

#### 4.2.3 Infections

##### 4.2.3.1 Malaria

It is now estimated that malaria is responsible for 1.2 million deaths annually and 2.9% of total DALYs in low and middle income countries.(28) About 35% of children with malaria in Africa have anaemia.(29) In sub-Saharan Africa, it is estimated that between 200,000 and 500,000 pregnant women develop severe anemia as a result of malaria.(9) *P. falciparum* malaria in pregnancy is the primary cause of up to 10,000 maternal anaemia related deaths in sub-Saharan Africa annually.(30)

Malaria, especially by the protozoon *Plasmodium falciparum,* causes anaemia by rupturing red blood cells and suppressing production of red blood cells.(31) However, this cannot be explained simply by the direct destruction of parasitized red blood cells at the time of release of meroziotes.(32) Decreased red cell production results from marrow hypoplasia seen in acute infection and dyerythropoiesis.(33) *Plasmodium falciparum* is the primary cause of severe malaria in regions of the world where malaria is endemic, especially sub-Sahara Africa .(7)

#### 4.2.3.2 Parasitic infestation

Helminthes such as flukes, hookworm and whipworm cause chronic blood loss, and consequently iron loss.(34) These parasitic infestations are known to cause chronic haemorrhage and iron deficiency, resulting in the development of anaemia.(35) Blood loss caused by helminthiasis put the mother, fetus and child at risk of iron deficiency, which could lead to anaemia.(36) For example, the trematode, *Schistosomia haematobium* (fluke), predisposes to a significant urinary blood loss in severe infections and infected persons may present with terminal heamaturia, which continues for as long as it is not treated and then results in anaemia. Whereas, *Schistosomia mansoni* eggs can rupture the intestinal lining and result in the leakage of blood, other fluids and nutrients into the lumen.(34)

Hookworm infestation produces a high degree of long-term morbidity by causing iron deficiency anemia.(17) The extent to which this deficiency occurs depends on the host's iron status, the infecting parasites, and the intensity and duration of infection.(36) Blood loss is caused primarily by coagulase released by the parasite and it is responsible for continuous blood loss in the stool.(17) For example, *Ancylostoma duodenale* is estimated to cause up to 0.25 ml of blood loss per worm per day.(30)

A hookworm burden of 40–160 worms (depending on the iron status of the host) is associated with iron deficiency anemia.(37) Several studies in developing countries observed that 51% of anaemic children were iron deficient and if hookworm infection could be reduced by as much as 25%, it would reduce iron deficiency anaemia by 35% and severe anaemia by 73%.(31, 38) The nematode, *Trichuris trichiura* (whipworm) causes anaemia if the worm burden is heavy(31) and colonic lesions are associated with bleeding or there is a chronic reduction in food and micro-nutrient intake caused by anorexia-inducing effects of tumor necrosis factor-α released in response to the infection.(39-40)

#### 4.2.3.3 Human Immuno-deficiency Virus infection (HIV)

Developing countries are the worst hit by the HIV pandemic, which accounts for 22.5 million people (68% of global total) in sub-Saharan Africa and 4.9 million people (15% of global total) in Asia living with HIV/AIDS in 2009.(41) In 2009, 1.3 million Africans died of HIV and this constituted 72% of the global total.(42) Anaemia is a frequent complication among HIV-positive individuals and it has been associated with a rapid HIV disease progression and mortality.(43) The predominant cause of anaemia in the context of HIV is anaemia of inflammation; this is also known as anemia of chronic disease, which is characterized by decreased red blood cell production through a series of mechanisms mediated, in part, by pro-inflammatory cytokines such as tumor necrosis factor-α and interleukin-6.(17)

Studies have also shown that zidovudine (AZT) causes anaemia in pregnant women as early as four weeks of commencing therapy.(44) The cause of anaemia in HIV-positive patients is, therefore, multi-factorial and includes infections, neoplasm, dietary deficiencies, blood loss, medications and antibodies to antiretroviral agents.(45-46) In addition, bone marrow suppression, especially the erythroid lines, by the AIDS virus is also known to cause anaemia in affected persons.(47)

### 4.3 Sickle cell diseases and thalassemia

About 5% of the world's population carries the genes responsible for haemoglobinopathies.(48) Sickle cell disease is an inherited disorder of hemogblobin and it is among the most common genetic diseases in the world.(17) Each year, about 300,000 infants are born with major haemoglobin disorders - including more than 200,000 cases of

sickle-cell anaemia in Africa.(48) It is characterized by lifelong haemolytic anaemia and many other significant morbidities largely related to painful and debilitating vaso-occlusive phenomenon.(49)
Patients present with recurrent anaemia, which sometimes require blood transfusion. *'Sicklers'*, as affected persons are often called, have worsened symptoms of low packed cell volume especially when there is a co-infection or pregnancy. It is a challenge for patients in developing countries, both old and young, in treating their ill conditions as there are usually inadequate supportive measures to restore them back to their stable states.
Thalassemia is the most common single genetic disorder worldwide, resulting from defects in genes producing hemoglobin. (50) It is highly prevalent in many Asian, Mediterranean and Middle Eastern countries.(51) The intermediate clinical forms of thalassemia result in anaemia, with occasional need for transfusions of red blood cells.(17)

## 5. Prospects and challenges of diagnosis of underlying causes of anaemia

Blood test for serum ferritin seems to be a sensitive and an early indicator of iron deficiency. In most developing countries, it is determined by using an immunoassay kit which is readily available, easily done and relatively inexpensive. (52) However, serum iron concentration, total iron-binding capacity and examination of blood films cannot detect the earliest stages of iron deficiency. (52) On the other hand, bone marrow examination showing absence of stainable iron is the definitive method for diagnosing IDA;(53) however, this is a painful and invasive procedure and it is therefore usually used as a last resort.(54)
The World Health Organisation (WHO) recently recommended prompt parasitologic confirmation by microscopy or alternatively, by rapid diagnostic tests (RDTs) in all patients suspected of malaria before treatment is commenced unless parasitological diagnosis is not accessible; this is with a view to reducing cases of resistance to anti malaria treatment. (55) However, many peripheral health facilities in resource-poor settings of developing countries lack the capacity to conduct quality parasitological diagnosis of malaria by microscopy.(56-57) Nonetheless, rapid diagnostic tests (RDTs) for malaria had recently been shown to offer the potential of extending accurate malaria diagnosis to areas when microscopy services are not available, especially in remote locations of the developing countries.(58-59)
In making a diagnosis of any clinical phase of schistosomiasis, the highly sensitive and specific PCR based assays have been developed for the detection of schistosome DNA in faeces or sera and plasma.(60) However, these tests are either not available or very expensive in many developing countries; thus, clinicians often use clinical acumen to make a diagnosis in majority of cases. Furthermore, fresh water bath is common among children in developing countries; thus, children with pruritic reaction or unexplained febrile illness several weeks after a fresh water bath are suspected to have contracted urinary schistosomiasis.(61) Diagnosis is made by finding parasitic eggs in urine sample, which is best taken at midday after exercise when most eggs are being shed.(61) On the other hand, eggs of hookworm are readily isolated from stool samples in developing countries.
Major challenges facing laboratory systems in HIV testing in resource-poor settings include poor infrastructure, lack of human capacity, lack of laboratory policies, and limited synergies between clinical and research laboratories; these factors compromise the quality of test results and patient management.(62) In addition, HIV stigmatization is a major barrier preventing many people from having voluntary counseling and testing done in developing countries. For instance, in the prevention of maternal to child transmission programme

(PMTCT), challenges of diagnosis in developing countries include HIV-associated stigma. This has been reported to pose a barrier to service utilization, including failure of women to return for HIV test results where rapid testing is not available, low acceptance of short-course preventive ARVs offered to HIV-positive women at antenatal clinics, difficulty in tracking and following up of mothers who deliver their infants at home and complexities of infant feeding for HIV-positive mothers in very low-resource settings.(63)

The major challenge in the diagnosis of haemoglobin disorders is detection of the disease conditions during prenatal period. At this period, laboratory confirmation is critically important to enable a couple at risk in making an informed decision about potential termination of pregnancy.(64) With DNA diagnostics, it has become possible to make definitive diagnoses of different haemoglobin disorders during the first trimester of pregnancy by analyzing foetal DNA obtained from chorionic villous biopsy. There is evidence that neonatal screening for sickle-cell anaemia, when linked to timely diagnostic testing, parental education and comprehensive care, markedly reduces morbidity and mortality from the disease condition in infancy and early childhood.(48, 65).

## 6. Management of anaemia

The objectives of management of anaemia include(1):

- Treatment of the underlying cause;
- Restoration of the haemoglobin concentration to normal levels; and
- Prevention and treatment of complications.

### 6.1 Treatment of the underlying cause of anaemia

Iron deficiency anaemia is treated with oral iron supplements as ferrous sulfate, ferrous fumerate or ferrous gluconate given as 200 mg twice or three times daily. Treatment could also be parenteral as iron dextran, especially when there is intolerance to oral iron or anaemia is diagnosed late in pregnancy.

Low birth weight infants are born with low iron stores; therefore, they demand high iron requirements for growth. Furthermore, their iron requirements cannot be readily met from breast milk and it is known that their iron stores are depleted by 2 to 3 months postpartum.(7) The global recommendation is to supply low birth weight infants with supplemental iron drops starting at 2 months of age.(38) A substantial amount of evidence confirms that iron supplementation of anaemic school children improves their school performance, verbal and other skills.(66)

Vitamin A can be given as oral supplementation doses to postpartum mothers irrespective of their breastfeeding options in doses of 200,000 I.U and to less than 5 years of age in doses between 100,000-200,000 I.U. In some countries where vitamin A deficiency is a public health problem, vitamin A supplements in capsule form are administered during National Immunization Days (NIDs) alongside oral polio and measles vaccines.(67) Though, high supplementation dose of vitamin A is of immense benefit to both mother and breast feeding infant, it should be avoided in pregnant women because it can cause miscarriage and birth defects.(68)

Vitamin B 12 is usually given intramuscularly but recent studies have shown that an oral dose is as effective as the injectable administration.(69) The daily requirement of vitamin $B_{12}$ is approximately 2 mcg; the initial oral replacement dosage consists of a single daily dose of 1,000 to 2,000 mcg.

Folic acid supplementation can be given to patients with folate deficiency in doses between 1-5 mg daily. It is routinely given to pregnant women, particularly early in pregnancy, to prevent neural tube defect in the growing foetus in some developing countries. Malaria is treated with a wide range of anti-malaria drugs and most African countries now recommend the Artemisinin-based combination therapy (ACT), which is given to reduce cases of resistance of the parasite to other drugs.

Antihelminthic drugs such as albendazole or mebendale can be given to people infested with hookworm. In addition, iron deficiency aneamia which may co-exist can be treated with iron supplement. Praziquantel is the drug of choice for the treatment of schistosomiasis and it is shown to be effective and safe in pregnancy.(36) Praziquantel can easily be administered according to height using a "dose pole" developed to dispense the drug at 40-60 mg/kg; this is with a view to minimizing under dosage while the "dose pole" helps in identifying five height intervals corresponding to 1½, 2 ,2½, 3 and 4 tablets of praziquantel.(70)

The availability of the highly active antiretroviral therapy (HAART) at no cost has been of immense benefits to people living with HIV and AIDS, especially in developing countries where most affected persons cannot afford the drug treatment. Furthermore, WHO introduced revised treatment guidelines in 2010; these guidelines recommended early initiation of antiretroviral therapy, at a CD4 count of < 350 cells/mm3. This has, therefore, increased the total number of people medically eligible for antiretroviral therapy by about 50% i.e. from 10 million to 15 million in 2009 globally.(42) The main aspect of care for persons affected by sickle cell anaemia involves early treatment intervention of preventable health problems such as analgesics, antibiotics, vitamins, folic acid supplementation and high fluid intake are periodically used.

### 6.2 Restoration of the haemoglobin concentration to normal levels

Generally, blood transfusion is a very important measure in the treatment of anaemia; but it should not be used as a substitute for specific treatment of the underlying cause.(1) Blood can be given as an autologous transfusion, exchange transfusion or direct transfusion with blood products. It is recommended that blood transfusion should be given only if the dangers of failure to transfuse outweigh those of transfusion. (1) In developing countries, problems such as economic constraints may limit blood safety precautions; thus, unsafe blood which ought to have been screed for infections such as HIV, hepatitis B or C and syphilis, is inadvertently transfused.(71)

In addition, many developing countries do not have reliable testing systems because of staff shortage, lack of basic laboratory services, poor quality test kits or their irregular supply.(72) Sometimes, patients receive wrong blood type due to mismatch error and thereafter, develop blood transfusion reaction. These constraints underscore the importance of strengthening blood transfusion services in developing countries; furthermore, the process of obtaining an informed consent from patients, including discussing the risk and benefit of transfusion, except in life-threatening emergencies should be emphasised.(1)

### 6.3 Prevention and treatment of complications

Complications may arise as a result of the underlying disease or anaemia itself. The overall goal is to ensure that anaemia does not re-occur or further deteriorates. Once the underlying cause can be treated, the prognosis is good in most cases. Other supportive measures include a balanced diet with adequate protein and vitamins; bed rest can also go a long way to restore blood levels in the body.

## 7. Strategies to prevent anaemia

Food fortification and dietary diversification with iron are important measures to prevent iron deficiency anaemia(8), especially in the vulnerable groups such as pregnant women and children. A number of strategies are used to deliver additional iron to humans, but food fortification has the greatest potential to improve the iron status of the largest number of people.(7) Ferrous fumarate, ferrous succinate and small particle size iron are suitable iron fortificants for infant cereals.(73) Infant cereals are widely fortified in developed countries and this has resulted in a definite reduction in anaemia. (74) WHO recommends that all pregnant women receive iron supplements of 60 mg daily combined in a pill, which also contains 400 µg folic acid.(75)

In view of the high prevalence of Vitamin A deficiency in developing countries and the potentially high prevalence of deficiencies of other micronutrients required for Hb synthesis and other functions, it is logical to assume that supplementation with multiple micronutrients, rather than just iron or iron plus folate, would be a rational public health strategy.(7) Currently, WHO recommends routine vitamin A supplementation during pregnancy or at any time during lactation in areas with endemic vitamin A deficiency.(76) Vitamin A can be given to children under 5 years of age in doses between 100,000-200,000 I.U as it is practised in some developing countries during national immunization days. Furthermore, absorption of iron from food can be enhanced by increasing intake of vitamin C.

Vector control remains as the most effective measure to prevent transmission of malaria in developing countries; though the methods used may vary considerably in their applicability, cost and sustainability.(77) WHO had recommended a combination of integrated vector management, indoor residual spraying, insecticide treated material and larval control.(78) Insecticide-impregnated bed nets in communities decrease the prevalence of severe anaemia in young children.(7) The home management of malaria (HMM) strategy has been introduced where early recognition, and prompt and appropriate treatment of malaria illness in children under 5 years of age in the home or community can be achieved. If *Plasmodium falciparum* malaria is endemic and transmission of infection is high, women in their first or second pregnancies should be given curative antimalarials at their first prenatal visit followed by locally recommended antimalarial prophylaxis.(7) Malaria control programme is highly necessitated among the highly susceptible group especially in the tropical regions of the world.(7)

In areas endemic with parasitic infections which affect Hb or iron status, the International Nutritional Anemia Consultative Group (INACG), WHO, and United Nations Childrens' Fund (UNICEF) recommended certain complementary control measures.(79) For example, adults and children over 5 years living in hookworm endemic areas (i.e. prevalence of 20-30% and above) are required to be treated with at least an annual dose of albendazole, mebendazole, Levamisole or Pyrantel. These drugs can be given to pregnant and lactating women, but should be avoided in the first trimester of pregnancy.(80)

Other efforts aimed at controlling hookworm infections include sanitary disposal of faeces and educational campaigns on proper use of latrines.(81) Most at risk persons are those who engage in agriculture and fishing, and those who use unsafe water for household chores particularly girls and their mothers.(36) Therefore, primary health care measures such as hand washing and wearing of shoes in hookworm endemic areas can have a major impact on the prevalence of anaemia.(7) All forms of schistosomiasis including intestinal and urinary types can be treated with praziquantel effectively. Prevention is best achieved by eliminating water dwelling snails, which serve as natural reservoirs of the disease.

Effective HIV preventive interventions include condom use, provision of clean injecting equipment, standard precautions, blood safety and post exposure prophylaxis for occupational and non-occupational exposures.(82) Sickle cell anaemia can be prevented if couples at risk of having affected children can be identified by inexpensive and reliable blood test. Periodic prophylaxis against malaria, infections and other factors which may trigger discomfort could improve quality life of affected children.(48)

## 8. Conclusion and recommendations

In developing countries which are usually characterized by resource-limited settings, slow progress has been made toward reducing the prevalence of anemia; this is largely due to persistent micro-nutrient deficiencies, and high prevalence of parasitic diseases, HIV, sickle cell disease and thalassemia.(17) The best approach to preventing IDA in pregnancy is to ensure adequate maternal iron status early in pregnancy or preferably in the pre-conceptional period.(83) Therefore, micronutrient supplements should be given not only to pregnant women but also to non-pregnant women of reproductive age and adolescent girls; this would reduce the prevalence of anaemia in the community and consequently, improve fertility and maternal health.

The apparent failure to reduce the prevalence of anaemia in developing countries may be partly due to existing interventions, which are usually designed with the assumption that iron deficiency is the main cause.(84) Thus, other important causes of anaemia have been underestimated and neglected, and these have been on the increase. Therefore, adequate attention should be given to the emerging causes of anemia in developing countries such as HIV/AIDS and micronutrient deficiency

The involvement of government of developing countries can effectively combine and balance the needs for programme implementation, monitoring and evaluation, research and community involvement. It is expected that the burden of anaemia will drastically reduce if adequate attention is paid to joint participation of all stakeholders in combating the burden in developing countries. Intervention programmes should address iron deficiency with the focus on both dietary quantity and quality of the micronutrient composition. Strategies which are required to improve nutrition knowledge and awareness of mothers and health workers may also be implemented.

Ultimately, treating the underlying causes of anaemia is critical in eliminating anaemia in all age groups, particularly the vulnerable ones. Therefore, it becomes imperative that all stakeholders harmonize and coordinate their efforts in ensuring that the burden and prevalence of anaemia, and its causes are reduced to the barest minimum in all developing countries.

## 9. References

[1] Standard treatment guidelines Nigeria. 2008:Pg 12-4.

[2] World Health Organisation. Nutritional anemia: report of a WHO Scientific Group. Geneva, Switzerland: World Health Organisation1968.

[3] World Health Organisation. WHO Vitamin and Mineral Nutrition/ Anaemia 2011.

[4] World Health Organisation. Worldwide prevalence of anaemia 1993-2005: WHO global database on anaemia2005.

[5] WHO/UNICEF/UNU. Iron deficiency anaemia: assessment, prevention, and control. Geneva: World HealthOrganization2001.

[6] World Bank. Public health at a glance. December 2004.
[7] ACC/SCN. What Works? A Review of the Efficacy and Effectiveness of Nutrition Interventions. Geneva in collaboration with the Asian Development Bank, Manila: ACC/SCN2001.
[8] World Health Organization. WHO Global Database on Iron Deficiency and Anaemia, Micronutrient Deficiency Information System. . Geneva: World Health Organisation2005.
[9] World Health Organization. The Prevalence of Anaemia in Women : A Tabulation of Available Information. Geneva: WHO; 1992.
[10] Axemo P, Liljestrand J, Bergstrom S, Gebre-Medhin M. Aetiology of late fetal death in Maputo. Gynaecol Obstet Invest. 1995;39:103-9.
[11] Brabin BJ, Premji Z, Verhoeff F. An analysis of anaemia and child mortality. J Nutr. 2001;132:636S-45S.
[12] Rae Galloway, Erin Dusch, Leslie Elderet. Women's perceptions of iron deficiency and anemia prevention and control in eight developing countries. Science Direct, Social Science & Medicine August 2002;55( 4):Pages 529-44.
[13] Buseri FI, Uko EK, Jeremiah ZA, Usanga EA. Prevalence and Risk Factors of Anaemia Among Pregnant women in Nigeria. The Open Hematology Journal. 2008;2:14-9.
[14] Ross J, Thomas EL. Iron Deficiency Anaemia and Maternal Mortality. Washington, D.C: Academy for Educational Development; 1996.
[15] UNICEF State of the World's Population 1994. New York: UNFPA1998.
[16] Horton S, Ross J. The economics of iron deficiency. Food Policy. 2003;28:51-75.
[17] Karine Tolentino, Jennifer F. Friedman. An Update on Anemia in Less Developed Countries. Am J Trop Med Hyg. 2007;77(1):44-51.
[18] Yip R, Ramakrishnan U. Supplement: Forging Effective Strategies to Combat Iron Deficiency Experiences and Challenges in Developing Countries. The American Society for Nutritional Sciences J Nutr. 2002 132:827S-30S.
[19] Stoltzfus, Mullany, Black. Iron Deficiency Anemia, "Comparative quantification of health risks: Global and regional burden of disease attributable to selected major risk factors: WHO2004.
[20] World Health Organization. World Health Report. Reducing Risk, Promoting Healthy Life. Geneva: WHO2002.
[21] Stoltzfus R. Update on Issues Related to Iron Deficiency and Anemia Control. Report of the 2003 International Nutritional Anemia Consultive Group: Integrating Programs to Move Iron Deficiency Anaemia Control Forward Symposium. . Marrakech, Morocco: International Life Sciences Institute2003.
[22] Gillespie SR. Major Issues in the Control of Iron Deficiency. Ottawa: The Micronutrient Initiative/UNICEF.1998.
[23] Allen LH, Ahluwalia N. Improving Iron Status through Diet. The Application of Knowledge Concerning Dietary Iron Bioavailability in Human Populations. In: Arlington VA, editor. Management of Social Transformation Programme1997.
[24] Iron Disorders Institute. Iron Disorders. Taylor: Iron Deficiency Anemia; 2009 [cited 2011 24-07].
[25] Sommer A, West KP. Vitamin A Deficiency: Health, Survival and Vision. New York: Oxford University Press.; 1996.

[26] Fishman SM, Christian P, West KP. The role of vitamins in the prevention and control of anaemia. Public Health Nutr. 2000;3:125-50.
[27] Tolentino K, Friedman JF. An Update on Anemia in Less Developed Countries. The American Society of Tropical Medicine. 2007.
[28] Lopez AD, Mathers CD, Ezzati M, Jamison DT, Murray CJ. Global and regional burden of disease and risk factors, 2001: systematic analysis of population health data. Lancet. 2006;367:1747-57.
[29] United Nations Development Programme, World Bank, World health Organisation. The prevention and management of severe anaemia in children in malaria-endemic regions of Africa: A review of research2001.
[30] Steketee RW, Nahlen BL, Parise ME, Menendez C. The burden of malaria in pregnancy in malaria endemic areas. Am J Trop Med Hyg. 2001;64:28-35.
[31] Onyemaobi GA, Onimawo IA. Risk Factors for Iron Deficiency Anaemia in Under-five Children in Imo State, Nigeria. Journal of Applied Sciences Research. 2011;7(1):63-7.
[32] Menendez C, Fleming AF, Alonso PL. Malaria-related Anaemia. Parasitol Today. 2000;16(11):469-76.
[33] Phillips RE, Pasvol G. Anaemia of Plasmodium falciparum malaria. Epidemiology of Haematological Disease: Part II. 1992;5(2):315-30.
[34] Latham MC. Human Nutrition in the Developing World. Rome: FAO1997.
[35] Chitsulo L, Engels D, Montresor A, Savioli L. The global status of schistosomiasis and its control. Acta Trop. 2000;77:41-51.
[36] Hoque M, Hoque E, Kader SB. Risk factors for anaemia in pregnancy in rural KwaZulu-Natal, South Africa: Implication for health education and health promotion. SA Fam Pract. 2009;51(1):68-72.
[37] Hotez PJ, Brooker S, Bethony JM, Bottazzi ME, Loukas A, Xiao S. Hookworm infection. New England Journal of Medicine. 2004;351(8):799-841.
[38] Stoltzfus RJ, Albonico M, Chwaya HM, Tielsch JM, Schulze KJ, Savioli L. Effects of the Zanzibar school-based deworming program on iron status of children. American Journal of Clinical Nutrition 1998;68(1):179-86.
[39] Stephenson LS, Holland CV, Cooper ES. The public health significance of Trichuris trichiura. Parasitology. 2000;121(Suppl):S73-S95.
[40] Duff EM, Anderson NM, Cooper ES. Plasma insulin-like growth factor-1, type 1 procollagen, and serum tumor necrosis factor alpha in children recovering from Trichuris dysentery syndrome. Pediatrics 1999;103:e69.
[41] WHO. Global Health Observatory (GHO)/HIV2011.
[42] Joint United Nations Programme on HIV/AIDS. Overview of the global AIDS epidemic". UN report on the global AIDS epidemic 20102010.
[43] Johannessen A, Naman E, Ngowi BJ, Sandvik L, Matee MI, Aglen HE, et al. Predictors of mortality in HIV-infected patients starting antiretroviral therapy in a rural hospital in Tanzania. BMC Infectious Diseases. 2008;8:52.
[44] Areechokchai D, Bowonwatanuwong C, Phonrat B, Pitisuttithum P, Maek-a-Nantawat W. Pregnancy outcomes among HIV-infected women undergoing antiretroviral therapy. The Open AIDS Journal. 2009;3:8-13.
[45] Moyle G. Anaemia in persons with HIV infection: prognostic marker and contributor to morbidity. AIDS Reviews. 2002;4:13-8.

[46] Omoregie R, Egbeobauwaye A, Ogefere H, Omokaro EU, Ehen CC. Prevalence of antibodies to HAART agents among HIV patient in Benin City, Nigeria. African Journal Biomedical Research. 2008;11:33-7.
[47] Odunukwe N, Idigbe O, Kanki P, Adewale T, Onwujekwe D, Audu R, et al. Haematological and biochemical response to treatment of HIV-1 infection with a combination of nevirapine stavudine + lamivudine in Lagos Nigeria. Turkish Journal of Haematology. 2005;22:125-31.
[48] World Health Organisation. Sickle Cell anaemia. Geneva: Fifty Ninth World Health Assembly, WHO2006.
[49] Mentzer WC, Kan YW. Prospects for research in hematologic disorders: sickle cell disease and thalassemia. JAMA. 2001;285:640-2.
[50] Olivieri NF. The beta-thalassemias. N Engl J Med. 1999;341:99-109.
[51] Greenberg PL, Gordeuk V, Issaragrisil S, Siritanaratkul N, Fucharoen S, Ribeiro RC. Major hematologic diseases in the developing world- new aspects of diagnosis and management of thalassemia, malarial anemia, and acute leukemia. Hematology (Am Soc Hematol Educ Program). 2001:479-98.
[52] Hamedani P, Raza R, Bachand R, Manji M, Hashml K. Laboratory diagnosis of iron deficiency in a developing country, Pakistan. J Int Med Res. 1991;19(1):19-23.
[53] Trost LB, Bergfeld WF, Calogeras E. The diagnosis and treatment of iron deficiency and its potential relationship to hair loss. J Am Acad Dermatol. 2006;54(5):824-44.
[54] Punnonen K, Irjala K, Rajamaki A. Serum transferrin receptor and its ratio to serum ferritin in the diagnosis of iron deficiency. Blood. 1997;89:1052-7.
[55] WHO. Home management of malaria. 2011 [cited 2011 24-07].
[56] Moerman F, Lengeler C, Chimumbwa J, Talisuna A, Erhart A, Coosemans MT. The contribution of the health-care service to a sound and sustainable malaria-control policy. Lancet Infect Dis. 2003;3:99-102.
[57] Bloland P, Kachur S, Williams H. Trends in antimalarial drug deployment in sub-Saharan Africa. J Rxp Biol. 2003;206(3761-3769).
[58] Wongsrichanalai C, Barcus M, Muth S, Sutamihardja A, Wernsdorfer W. A review of malaria diagnostic tools: microscopy and rapid diagnostic test (RDT). Am J Trop Med Hyg. 2007;77:119-27.
[59] Shillcutt S, Morel C, Goodman C, Coleman P, Bell D, Whitty CJ. Bulletin of the World Health OrganizationFeb 2008.
[60] Gray DJ, Ross AG, Li Y-S. Clinical Review: Diagnosis and management of schistosomiasis. British Medical Journal. 2011;342:d2651.
[61] Paul JF, Verma S, Berry K. Urinary schistosomiasis. Emerg Med J. 2002;19:483-4.
[62] Birx D, de Souza M, Nkengasong J. Laboratory challenges in the scaling up of HIV, TB, and malaria programs: The interaction of health and laboratory systems, clinical research, and service delivery. Am J Clin Pathol. 2009;131(6):849-51.
[63] The United States President's emergency plan for AIDS relief. The challenges of HIV/AIDS and children. PEPFAR; 2004 [cited 2011 02-08].
[64] Frenette PS, Atweh GF. Sickle cell disease: old discoveries, new concepts, and future promise. Journal of Clinical Investigation. 2007;117(4):850-8.
[65] WHO. Sickle Cell anaemia 2006.
[66] Draper A. Child Development and Iron Deficiency: the Oxford Brief. Opportunities for Micronutrient Interventions, and Partnership for Child Development. Washington DC: USAID; 1997

[67] WHO. WHO Vitamin A supplementation. 2011 [cited 2011 23-07]; http://www.who.int/vaccines/en/vitamina].

[68] Stoltzfus RJ, Hakimi M, Miller KW. High dose vitamin A supplementation of breast-feeding Indonesian mothers: effects on the vitamin A status of mother and infant. J Nutr. 1993;123(4):666-75.

[69] Robert C, Brown DL. Vitamin B12 Deficiency. Am Fam Physician. 2003 Mar1;67(5):979-86.

[70] WHO expert committee on the control of Schistosomiasis. Prevention and control of schistosomiasis and soil transmitted helminthiasis: report of a WHO expert committee. Geneva: World health Organisation2001.

[71] Wake DJ, Cutting WA. Blood transfusion in developing countries: problems, priorities and practicalities. Tropical Doctor. 1998 Jan;28(1):4-8.

[72] WHO. Blood safety and availability. November 2009 [cited 2011 24-07].

[73] Hurrell RF, Furniss DE, Burri J, Whittaker P, Lynch SR, Cook JD. Iron fortification of infant cereals: a proposal for the use of ferrous fumarate or ferrous succinate. American Journal of Clinical Nutrition. 1989;49:1274-82.

[74] Rush D, Leighton J, Sloan NL, Alvir JM, Garbowski GC. The National WIC Evaluation: Evaluation of the Special Supplemental Food Program for Women, Infants, and Children. II. Review of past studies of WIC. American Journal of Clinical Nutrition. 1988;48:394- 411.

[75] Branca F, Lopriore C, Briesid A, Golden MH. Multi-micronutrient fortified food reverses growth failure and anaemia in 2 - 5 year-old stunted refugee children. Scandinavian Journal of Nutrition. 1999;43(25):51S.

[76] WHO. Safe Vitamin A Dosage During Pregnancy and Lactation. Recommendations and a Report of a Consultation. . Geneva: WHO1998.

[77] WHO. Vector control of malaria. 2011 [cited 2011 24-07]; Available from: www.who.int/malaria/vector_control/en.

[78] WHO. Regional Framework for an Integrated Vector Management Strategy for the South-East Asia Region. New Delhi: World Health Organization Regional Office for South-East AsiaJune 2005.

[79] Stoltzfus RJ, Dreyfuss ML. Guidelines for the Use of Iron Supplements to Prevent and Treat Iron Deficiency Anemia. Geneva: International Nutritional Anemia Consultative Group/ UNICEF/WHO1998.

[80] WHO. Report of the WHO informal consultation on hookworm infection and anaemia in girls and women. Geneva: WHO1996 Contract No.: document WHO/CTD/SIP/96.1.

[81] WHO. Initiative for Vaccine Research: Parasitic disease. 2011 [cited 2011 24-07]; Available from: www.who.int/vaccine_research/disease/soa_parasitic/en.

[82] WHO. HIV/AIDS: Prevention in the health sector. 2011 [cited 2011 24-07]; Available from: www.who.int/hiv/topics/prevention/en.

[83] Okwu GN, Ukoha AI. Studies on the Predisposing Factors of Iron Deficiency Anaemia among Pregnant Women in a Nigeria Community. Pakistan Journal of Nutrition. 2008;7(1):151-6.

[84] Joint World Health Organization/Centers for Disease Control and Prevention. Assessing the iron status of populations : including literature reviews : report of a Joint World Health Organization/Centers for Disease Control and Prevention Technical Consultation on the Assessment of Iron Status at the Population Level. Geneva, Switzerland2004 6–8 April 2004.

9

# Nutritional Anaemia

Alhossain A. Khallafallah[1,2,*] and Muhajir Mohamed[1]
[1]*Launceston General Hospital, Launceston, Tasmania*
[2]*School of Human Life Sciences, University of Tasmania*
*Australia*

## 1. Introduction

Data available in Australia regarding the prevalence of iron deficiency anaemia (IDA) in pregnant women show that about 17.4% of pregnant women suffer from IDA, while the World Health Organization (WHO) global database on anaemia has suggested a prevalence of 14% based on a regression-based analysis.

There is a suggested association between IDA and the following maternal risks: increased fatigue antenatally and postnatally, poor exercise tolerance, impaired thermoregulation, decreased resistance to infection, reduced tolerance of bleeding or surgical intervention at delivery, delayed instigation of lactation and increased risk of postnatal depression. IDA is also a risk factor for preterm delivery and subsequent low birth weight and may be associated with inferior neonatal health. Infants born to women with IDA are more likely to become anaemic themselves which, in turn, is known to have a detrimental effect on an infant's mental and motor development. Although iron supplementation during pregnancy is one of the most widely practiced public health measures, there remain many controversial issues with this practice.

Oral iron supplementation has long been a standard treatment for IDA worldwide. However, patients do not always respond adequately to oral iron therapy due to difficulties associated with ingestion of the tablets and their side effects, which can play a significant role in rates of compliance. The side effects include gastrointestinal disturbances characterized by colicky pain, nausea, vomiting, diarrhoea, and or constipation, and occur in large cohort of patients taking iron preparations. In addition, the presence of bowel disease can affect the absorption of iron and thereby minimize the benefit received from oral iron therapy.

In the past, intravenous iron had been associated with undesirable and sometimes serious side-effects and was therefore limited in use. In recent years, the new type II and III iron complexes have been developed which are better tolerated and can be used for a rapid reversal of iron deficiency anaemia. Despite increasing evidence of the safety of the newer preparations, intravenous iron continues to be underutilized.

### 1.1 Iron deficiency anaemia in the general population

Anaemia occurs in different age groups in a number of clinical situations associated with iron deficiency, iron deficiency anaemia and blood loss. Usually in the presence of intact

*Correspondence Author

erythropoiesis iron therapy is very effective in restoring the depleted iron stores and accordingly improving the haemoglobin. Other treatment strategies that stimulate erythropoiesis such as erythropoietin will also require the presence of iron in order to be an effective treatment. Intravenous iron offers a rapid repletion of iron and is superior to oral iron as proven in many clinical trials.

In this regard, we will describe different clinical scenarios for iron deficiency anaemia in different cohorts of patients and numerate the available management options in the literature.

### 1.2 Other causes for nutritional anaemia

In this part, we are discussing other common nutritional deficiencies apart from iron that result in anaemia such as vitamin B12 and folate deficiencies. Furthermore, we discuss rare nutritional anaemia due to copper and selenium deficiencies and highlighting the most appropriate management approaches and treatment strategies.

## 2. Iron deficiency

Nutritional iron deficiency is the most common deficiency disorder in the world, affecting more than two billion people worldwide, with pregnant women at particular risk.[1-3] World Health Organization (WHO) data show that iron deficiency anaemia (IDA) in pregnancy is a significant problem throughout the world with a prevalence ranging from about 15% of pregnant women in industrialized countries to an average of 56% in developing countries (range 35-75%).[2,3]

Furthermore, IDA is affecting a large number of children and women not only in the developing world, but is also considered the only nutrient deficiency that is significantly prevalent in the developed world too. The numbers of patients with ID and IDA are overwhelming as more than 2 billion people, over 30% of the world's population, are iron deficient with variable prevalence, distribution and contributing factors in different parts of the world.[1-3]

Iron deficiency affects more people than any other condition, constituting an epidemic public health crisis. It is usually present with subtle manifestations and sometimes considered as a chronic slowly progressing disease that is often underestimated and untreated worldwide despite several warnings and awareness efforts of the World Health Organisation.[1-3]

It is worth noting that IDA has a debilitating effect as it reduces the work capacity of individuals and perhaps entire populations, with resultant serious economic consequences and obstacles to national development.[1,4-6]

The high prevalence of IDA has substantial health consequences with subsequent socio-economic hazards, including poor pregnancy outcome, impaired educational performance, and decreased work capacity and productivity.[1,6]

Targeted iron supplementation, iron rich diet, or both, can improve iron deficiency. However, variability of bioavailable iron compounds limit its value against nutritional iron deficiency. Therefore, laboratory measures of iron stores should be utilised to determine iron deficiency and monitor the therapy.[3,4,6]

Iron deficiency anaemia is quite often underestimated despite the high prevalence of iron deficiency. Blood loss is a major cause of anaemia in the general population.[5,6] This review highlights the importance of early diagnosis of IDA and hence offers the most appropriate treatment in order to avoid serious complications of anaemia.

### 2.1 Causes of iron deficiency anaemia

Nutritional iron deficiency generally arises when physiological requirements cannot be met by daily dietary iron ingestion as well as iron absorption. Religious beliefs in some countries and the dietary attitude of individuals may contribute to lack of iron supply when certain populations consume monotonous plant-based diets and hence reduces dietary iron bioavailability.

Women are at particular risk for developing IDA especially in their childbearing period as they have greater iron requirement because of menstrual blood loss and also during the pregnancy and lactation period when they have increased iron demands.[2]

Iron deficiency can also be caused by other types of chronic blood loss including gastro-intestinal blood loss from gastritis, peptic ulcers, inflammatory bowel disease, parasitic infestations (such as *hookworms, Ancylostoma*) as well as haemorrhoids.[7]

The recommended dietary daily iron for men over the age of puberty and women over the age of menopause are 8 mg per day, while for women in the child bearing period the recommended daily dietary iron dose is 18 mg per day.[8] In the typical diet, major sources of iron are meat, poultry, nuts and seeds, legumes and bean products, green leafy vegetables, raisins, whole grains and fortified cereals.[8]

### 2.2 Symptoms of iron deficiency

The presenting symptoms of IDA are variable and usually are the general symptoms of anaemia, including lethargy; unusual fatigue after exertion; signs of iron deficiency including paleness of the skin or eyes, intestinal problems, cognitive problems such as impaired learning ability, spoon nails, easy brittle and fragile nails, leg cramps especially in night time (restless leg syndrome) and sometimes hair loss.[6,7]

### 2.3 Diagnosis of Iron deficiency

Although a study of bone marrow iron stores is an accurate tool for assessing the body stored iron, it remains an impractical, invasive procedure to apply for most patients.

Measurement of both soluble transferrin receptor and serum ferritin provide a tool for accurate diagnosis of IDA. However, transferrin receptor is not a well-standardized test that can be reliably reproduced with high precision in most of laboratories worldwide.

In the meantime, ferritin estimation is an easy automated test to perform in most laboratories in the world; however its use is limited in case of inflammation or infection as it is considered as an acute phase reactant that is affected by many conditions including inflammation or infection and hence negatively influences its value.

Therefore, new technology such as hypochromic reticulocytes and reticulocyte haemoglobin testing, reportedly have higher sensitivity, specificity, reproducibility and cost effectiveness as a screening tool for iron deficiency.[9,10] This may offer a reliable screening test for iron deficiency in the future.

### 2.4 Iron metabolism

The main source of iron in humans comes from the destruction of erythrocytes by macrophages of the reticuloendothelial system including the spleen (recycled internal iron supply), while the daily requirement of external iron remains as little as between 1 to 8 mg daily. However, more external iron is required in case of increased demand for iron such as physiological requirements during growth, pregnancy or in a pathological condition such as bleeding (increase iron loss).[3,4,6,8] Recent studies have shown how the human body up- and down-regulate iron absorption in response to changing iron status via intestinal and hepatic proteins.[6,10]

Transferrin is an important protein synthesized by the liver that provides both a high affinity and high avidity mechanism to increase iron yield required for active erythropoiesis.[11]

Hepcidin is a peptide hormone that is also synthesized by liver that regulates iron and plays a significant role in iron metabolism.[12-15] Hepcidin was first described in January 1998 by Tomas Ganz and colleagues,[12] who sequenced this peptide and found that it contained 25 amino acids and 4 disulfide bonds. This peptide circulates in the plasma and responds to various stimuli that regulate iron stores and serum iron and is usually renally excreted.[13]

Ferroportins are considered as hepcidin receptor/iron exporter in the regulation of iron absorption, recycling, and tissue distribution. Ferroportin 1A (FPN1A) works as an element for translational repression in iron-deficient cells, while FPN1B is expressed in duodenal enterocytes, enabling them to export iron.[12]

Hepcidin, controls ferroportin and hence, the inflows of iron into plasma from main sources; duodenal enterocytes absorbing iron intake and from macrophages involved in the recycling of iron as well as from hepatocytes involved in iron storage.[12-15]

During pregnancy, fetal hepcidin controls the placental transfer of iron from maternal plasma to the fetal circulation. When hepcidin concentrations are low, iron enters blood plasma at a high rate. When hepcidin concentrations are high, ferroportin is internalized, and iron is trapped in enterocytes, macrophages, and hepatocytes.[14,15]

Plasma iron concentrations and transferrin saturation are usually reflecting the difference between the hepcidin and ferroportin-regulated transfer of iron to plasma and iron consumption by the erythropoietic bone marrow tissue and, to a lesser extent, other tissues. Although, plasma transferrin compartment is considered relatively small, its iron content turns over every few hours, allowing iron concentrations to respond rapidly to changes in hepcidin concentrations.[12-15]

The role of hepcidin is mainly to regulate the absorption of dietary haeme, which is the main form of absorbable iron in human. Usually haeme is metabolized to ferrous iron by the enterocytes, however, its transfer to plasma will require ferroportin and hence is subjected to hepcidin-regulation.[12-15]

### 2.5 Treatment of iron deficiency anaemia

Although oral iron therapy is the most widely practiced treatment for iron deficiency anaemia, there are many issues that limit oral iron success in the management of IDA.

For instance, many patients do not respond adequately to oral iron therapy due to difficulties associated with ingestion of the tablets and their side effects, which can play a significant role in rates of compliance.[16-17]

The side effects of oral iron therapy include gastrointestinal disturbances characterized by colicky pain, nausea, vomiting, diarrhoea and or constipation, and occur in about 50% of patients taking iron preparations.[6]

Furthermore, the most widely prescribed oral iron is mainly composed of ferrous salts.[18,19] Ferrous salt is characterized by low and variable absorption rates and also its absorption can be limited in conjunction with ingestion of certain foods as well as mucosal luminal damage.[18-21] Therefore, ferric compounds were introduced to avoid such obstacles. However, these compounds are generally less soluble and have poor bioavailability.[21]

The usual recommended oral iron sulphate dose for the treatment of iron deficiency should be at least 80 mg daily of elemental iron, which is equivalent to 250 mg of oral iron sulphate tablets (Abbott, Australasia Pty Ltd).

In addition to oral iron side effects, patients with chronic bowel disease do not absorb oral iron readily and thereby minimise the benefit received from oral iron treatment.[21]

Although it is debatable whether intravenous iron should be administered or would oral iron have the same effect, many queries remain and are required to be addressed in further research and randomised trials.

The major challenges in the management of IDA are related to the tolerability and side effects of iron therapy in its different forms. Therefore, it is crucial to determine the most appropriate form and dose of iron as well as duration of treatment in order to successfully replenish the iron stores. Traditionally, the oral iron was widely used worldwide, however the effectiveness of oral formulations, due to the several facts mentioned before, is compromised by lack of absorption, poor compliance, adverse effects (up to 56%) and discontinuation of treatment (up to 20%).[6,18,21]

On the other hand, parenteral iron seems to be an attractive alternative to oral iron and is likely to be more popular option due to the introduction of new intravenous iron preparations, which allow high doses of iron to be administered rapidly in a single treatment.

In the past, intravenous iron had been associated with undesirable and sometimes serious side-effects and was therefore limited in use.[22-23] However, in recent years, the new type II and III iron complexes have been developed which are better tolerated and can be used for rapid repletion of iron stores.[24,25] Despite increasing evidence of the safety of the newer preparations, both in pregnant and general populations, intravenous iron continues to be underutilised because of previous concerns with tolerability of older intravenous iron preparations.[26]

Review of infusions of iron dextran among 481 patients revealed that about 25% of patients had mild side effects that have been self-limited. However about 2% experienced severe allergic reactions and about 0.6% were considered as anaphylactic reactions. Most of these reactions occurred immediately during the infusion of the test dose.[27]

On the other hand, iron gluconate is considered to have a lower reaction rate and therefore a test dose is not recommended. During the 1990s, only 3.3 allergic events per million doses per year with iron gluconate were reported.[28] During mid 1970s to mid 1990s There were no life-threatening reactions recorded as a result of iron gluconate infusion.

In contrast, during the same period, there were 31 fatalities among 196 allergic/anaphylactic reactions were reported for iron dextran, with about 16% of case fatality rate.[28]

The high incidence of adverse reactions of iron dextarn including serious adverse events have limited its application in practice.[29-31] Nonetheless, the application of iron gluconate is considered safe, it remains impractical in theory as it requires multiple infusions with huge implications on the often-limited health system resources as well as on patients' compliance.

There are new forms of intravenous iron that have recently been developed and are available in some countries that permit treating physicians to administer safely relatively high doses of iron in a single dose treatment. Furthermore, relatively older and established iron preparation such as intravenous iron polymaltose (Ferrosig, Sigma Pharmaceuticals,

Australia) demonstrated a high safety profile in treatment of IDA in both obstetric and general populations without a maximum dose-limit for treatment of IDA.[26] The total dose of IV iron polymaltose is calculated according to the patient's body weight and entry Hb level according to the product guidelines as following; iron dose in mg (50 mg per 1 ml) = body weight (maximum 90 kg) in kg x (target Hb (120 g/L) - actual Hb in g/L) x constant factor (0.24) + iron depot (500).[26] Recent reports demonstrate the feasibility of rapid infusion over 2 hours.[26,32,33] However, a test-dose of iron polymaltose (100 mg) should be first administered over 30 minutes and premedication is recommended prior to iron treatment for better toleration (antihistamine and or low dose steroids).[2632,33]

Furthermore, in 2009, the United States Food and Drug Administration (FDA) approved ferumoxytol (AMAG Pharmaceuticals, Inc., USA)[34] for the treatment of iron-deficiency anaemia in adult patients with chronic kidney disease (CKD).[34] However, the maximum dose allow only 510 mg of ferumoxytol in a single administration and is limited to use initially in CKD, although with the expected expansion of its spectrum to include other forms of IDA.[35] Another form of iron is ferric carboxymaltose (Vifor Pharma, Glattbrugg, Switzerland), which can be rapidly administered in 15 minutes in doses of 15 mg/kg body weight, with a maximum dose of 1000 mg.[36,37] There is no need for a test-dose of ferric carboxymaltose and its use is not restricted as ferumoxytol. More recently, in July 2010 a new intravenous iron isomaltoside (*MonoFer*, Pharmacosmos A/S, Holbaek, Denmark)[38] is introduced without the requirement of a test dose and it can be administered in 60 minutes at a rate of 20 mg/kg body weight in a single infusion without a maximum dose.[38,39] Iron isomaltoside administration was effective, safe, and was well tolerated when used to replenish iron stores in patients with anaemia of CKD.[39]

Intravenous iron including iron sucrose was employed in randomised controlled trials with improved effectiveness of intravenous iron only or in combination with oral iron compared to oral iron only based on Hb levels.[40,41]

A single IV iron sucrose dose has been reported to produce an increased incidence of thrombosis (9/41; 22%).[42] In contrast, 6 small doses of intravenous iron sucrose were administered over a three-week period without infusion-associated thrombosis as intravenous iron sucrose was administered in 5 daily doses to 45 pregnant women, also well tolerated.[34] In the first study, utilising intravenous iron sucrose, there was no significant difference between intravenous iron sucrose versus oral iron sulphate in the Hb levels at any time as measured at days 8, 15, 21, 30 and at delivery,[42] while in the second trial, with the 6 small doses of iron sucrose, there was a significant difference in Hb levels in favour of the intravenous iron sucrose group as measured at 2 and 4 weeks after administration of IV iron and at delivery.[40]

However, both trials administered IV iron sucrose at the expense of a vastly greater effort from the patients as well as extra demands on hospital resources.[40,41]

Certainly, the new intravenous iron preparations represent a medical revolution in effective, rapid and safe iron repletion in the management of iron deficiency anaemia.[34-39] This will reflect positively in the treatment of IDA in different populations by application of a single high-dose intravenous iron treatment with subsequent repletion of the iron stores effectively and hence, to improve subjective and objective outcomes in IDA.

Although iron deficiency is a precursor of IDA, many clinical studies treat it similarly to IDA. In case of severe IDA, a blood transfusion has been the traditional efficient approach to correct the anaemia, especially if patients did not respond to oral iron therapy or when a rapid correction of anaemia is clinically required.

Currently, the development of new intravenous iron formulations that offer higher doses in a single administration has provided the treating physicians with the opportunity to employ intravenous iron as an effective, rapid and safe treatment for IDA[34-39] avoiding the use of blood transfusion with its known hazards.[43] There are increasing evidence-based research that support the safety and efficacy of IV iron in IDA. There is also increasing evidence for inadequacy of oral iron in terms of adverse effects, lack of compliance as well as lack of absorption and slow and often questionable effect in IDA patients, especially in patients with ongoing blood loss.[44-47]

A common requirement across the range of clinical situations is the need for safe, effective higher, less frequent doses to achieve optimal clinical outcomes. The major goals of such strategy include overall cost reduction, relief to overstretched health system(s), improved patient convenience, improved compliance, preservation of venous access and reduced blood transfusion.[35-41,43,46] This will ultimately reduce the demand for blood transfusions, especially in the case of short supply. Furthermore, some of the new iron preparations such as ferric carboxymaltose and iron isomaltoside, do not require a test dose and therefore, ease the application of intravenous iron in a timely and cost effective fashion. This certainly will enhance the use of intravenous iron in clinical practice.

The WHO identified the problem of IDA as the most debilitating nutritional deficiency worldwide in the twenty first century. Such problem, if left untreated and not addressed properly can have a devastating effect on entire populations with adverse socio-economical consequences. Therefore, the use of intravenous iron should be considered as an effective, rapid and safe treatment option in some clinical scenarios with intravenous iron being employed to avoid or reduce the demand for blood transfusions or when rapid repletion of iron stores are required. Treatment options for IDA should consider the recently developed intravenous iron formulations, which is considered a milestone in the management of IDA.

Overall, the developing world is most vulnerable, especially the poorest and the least educated countries that are disproportionately affected by iron deficiency, and therefore they will gain the most by eradication of IDA. Therefore, awareness of the magnitude and scale of the IDA problem will help in recognising the most appropriate ways of diagnosis and treatment, which is crucial to overcome such devastating health problem. Perhaps consensus guidelines set by world experts in managing IDA incorporating new intravenous iron therapies are warranted.

## 3. Vitamin B12 deficiency anaemia

Cobalamin (vitamin B12) along with folic acid is normally required for DNA synthesis. Deficiency of one or both can cause defect in DNA synthesis, with lesser defect in RNA and protein synthesis, leading to a state of unbalanced cell growth and impaired cell division. The aberrant DNA synthesis causes arrest in S phase of cell cycle, affecting mitosis and cell division. This results in nucleo-cytoplasmic asynchrony and megaloblastic anaemia. [1]

### 3.1 Cobalamin

Cobalamin is a complex organo-metallic compound in which the cobalt atom is situated within a corrin ring. The two active coenzyme forms are methylcobalamin and 5-deoxyadenosyl cobalamin[1].

### 3.2 Main functions of cobalamin[2]

1. Conversion of methyl malonyl coA to succinyl coA in the mitochondria.
2. Methylation of homocysteine to methionine in the cytoplasm.

### 3.3 Effects of cobalamin deficiency

a. Impairment of DNA synthesis

   Cobalamin deficiency causes reduced methionine, which leads to reduced tetrahydrofolate and high methyl tetrahydrofolate in the cells (methyl folate trap hypothesis). This in turn causes low dTMP synthesis with high dUMP levels which results in impairment of DNA synthesis due to uridine for thymidine substitution in base pairing.

b. Defective myelin synthesis and neurological problems.

   Cobalamin and folate have fundamental roles in CNS function at all ages, especially the methionine-synthase mediated conversion of homocysteine to methionine, which is essential for nucleotide synthesis and genomic and non-genomic methylation[3]. Prolonged cobalamin deficiency causes defective conversion of propionate to succinyl coA and also causes high serum methyl malonic acid and homocysteine. Both of these can cause defective myelin synthesis and neurological dysfunction, since methionine is required for synthesis of choline.

c. Venous and arterial thrombosis.

   Plasma homocysteine levels are increased in both folate and cobalamine, which can lead to venous and arterial thrombosis[4].

### 3.4 Sources of cobalamin and dietary requirements

Cobalamin cannot be synthesized in human beings and needs to be supplied in the diet. Animal sources like meat, liver, fish, egg, milk and cheese are good sources of cobalamin. The estimated daily requirement of cobalamin is 1 mcg/day. The recommended daily allowance is 2.4 mcg/day. The daily requirement is so small relative to stores that deficiency typically takes years to develop in adults.[5]

### 3.5 Absorption, transport and cellular uptake

Absorption:

1. Stomach

   Gastric digestion releases cobalamin from the bound proteins. Gastric R-binder (also called haptocorrin) binds with cobalamin forming cobalamin - R binder complex. R-binder is also present in saliva, milk, gastric juice, bile, plasma and phagocytes.

2. Duodenum:

   Cobalamin - R binder complex is digested by pancreatic proteases. Cobalamin binds to Intrinsic Factor (IF). IF is produced by gastric parietal cells and is resistant to proteolytic digestion. IF has two binding sites, one for cobalamin and another for cubulin in Ileal cells.

3. Distal ileum:

   In the Ileal mucosal cell, IF is bound to cubulin. IF is destroyed and cobalamin binds to TCII forming a complex and absorbed into the blood.

4. Blood:

   Cobalamin - TCII complex in the blood is rapidly taken up by liver, bone marrow and other cells. Most cobalamin in the blood is bound to TCI, present in secondary granules of neutrophils, a group closely related to R binder. The function of TCI is not known.

5. Cellular uptake:
Cobalamin - TCII complex is rapidly taken up by liver, bone marrow and other cells. Cobalamin - TCII is released into lysosomes. Lysosomal degradation leads to cobalamin release. Most of the cobalamin (~95%) is bound to two intracellular enzymes.
a. Methyl malonyl coA mutase in the mitochondria catalyses methyl malonyl coA to succinyl coA.
b. Methionine synthase in the cytosol: Methyl cobalamin acts as coenzyme for methionine synthase allowing transfer of methyl group from homocysteine to methionine. 5 methyl tetrahydrofolate donates methyl group to cobalamin thus regenerating methyl cobalamin.

### 3.6 Causes of cobalamin deficiency

a. Nutritional cobalamin deficiency:

Causes: Strict vegans,[6] breast-fed infants of mothers with low cobalamin levels.

b. Cobalamin malabsorption

1. Intrinsic Factor deficiency
   Pernicious anaemia
   Total gastrectomy
2. Food-bound cobalamin malabsorption (FBCM)

Gastritis can cause FBCM. Progression of anaemia is slower than in IF-related malabsorption and may extend beyond a decade.[7]

3. Disorders causing cobalamin malabsorption in small intestine:

- Pancreatic insufficiency
- Blind loop syndrome
- Fish tape worm (Diphyllobothrium latum)
- Mucosal damage :

Causes: Tropical sprue, nontropical sprue, Crohn's disease , Small intestinal tumours like lymphoma, granulomatous disease.

4. Other causes of cobalamin deficiency
   Gastric achlorhydrria
   Partial gastrectomy

- Drugs: H2 receptor antagonists, proton pump inhibitors, Cholestryamine, Neomycin etc.

### 3.7 Perinicious Anaemia (PA)

PA is the most common cause of cobalamin deficiency is intrinsic factor deficiency due to atrophic gastritis or autoimmune destruction of parietal cells. The age of onset is usually after 40 years and more common in Northern European descent.

In autoimmune PA, the gastric parietal cells are affected by cytotoxic T cells. There is an increased incidence of circulating antibodies - antiparietal cell antibodies (90%) & anti-intrinsic factor antibodies (60%). PA can be associated with other autoimmune disorders like Grave's disease, Hashimoto's thyroiditis, Addison's disease and hypo-parathyroidisim.

Gastric atrophy affects acid and pepsin areas of the stomach while the antrum is spared. Atrophic gastritis usually precedes the onset of megaloblastic anaemia by many years. All the cells which have a high proliferation exhibit megaloblastic changes, e.g. epithelial cells lining the gastrointestinal tract (buccal mucosa, tongue and small intestine), cervix, vagina, and uterus. There is a higher risk of gastric cancer and carcinoids in patients with pernicious anaemia.[8]

### 3.8 Clinical features of cobalamin deficiency

Haematologic: Pancytopenia with megaloblastic anaemia
Cardiopulmonary: Congestive heart failure
Gastro-intestinal: Beefy red tongue (glossitis), broad spectrum malabsorption, diarrhoea
Skin: Melanin pigmentation, premature greying of hair
Genitals: Cervical and uterine dysplasia
Reproductive: Infertility or sterility

### 3.9 Central nervous system (CNS)

CNS involvement is unique to cobalamin deficiency. Peripheral nerves, posterolateral columns of spinal cord, cerebrum, optic nerve and rarely autonomous nervous system are affected. Pathological changes are demyelination, axonal degeneration and neuronal death. Symptoms are paraesthesia, numbness in extremities, weakness and ataxia. Psychotic changes can occur in cobalamin deficiency, which can vary from mild irritability and forgetfulness to severe dementia or frank psychosis.

### 3.10 Lab investigation in megaloblastic anaemia

#### 3.10.1 Full blood count & blood film

High MCV usually precedes anaemia. Low red cell count, Hb and reticulocyte counts are common. Low white cell count and low platelet counts can occur in moderate to severe deficiency.

Blood film shows macro-ovalocytes, hypersegmented neutrophils (greater than 5% PMNs with more than five lobes or a single PMN with more than six lobes are pathognomonic). In severe deficiency, leuko-erythroblastic blood picture, tear drop poikilocytes, basophilic stippling, Howell Jolly bodies, nucleated red cells and Cabot's ring can be seen.

#### 3.10.2 Bone marrow analysis

Hypercellularity is prominent in all the three cell lines. Erythroid hyperplasia is more marked than the others. Abnormal erythropoiesis with abnormally large red cell precursors (megaloblasts) with less mature nuclei (nuclear - cytoplasmic asynchrony) is common. Nuclear chromatin is more dispersed with fenestrated pattern, a characteristic feature of megaloblastic anaemia.

In severe megaloblastic anaemia up to 90% of RBC precursors are destroyed before they become mature, when compared to 10 % in normal marrow (ineffective erythropoiesis).

Abnormal leucopoiesis - giant metamyelocytes and band forms are characteristic. Hypersegmented neutrophils are also seen in bone marrow. Abnormal megakaryocytes can be seen (pseudohyperdiploidy).

#### 3.10.3 Serum cobalamin levels[9]

Normal levels : 120 - 680 pmol/L measured using Immunoassay.
The limitations of serum cobalamin levels are

Falsely low levels (in patients with normal cobalamin)
Severe folate deficiency (in 30% of patients)
Low TC- I levels
Physiologically low levels in pregnancy
Intake of large doses of Vitamin C
Falsely normal or high levels (in patients with low cobalamin)
Myeloproliferative disorders (Cobalamin binders like TC-I &TC-II are increased)
Acute liver disease (release of cobalamin from hepatocytes).

### 3.10.4 Other tests

#### 3.10.4.1 Schilling test

The Schilling test measures cobalamin absorption by assessing increased urine radioactivity after an oral dose of radioactive cobalamin. Malabsorption due to any cause produces low radioactivity in urine. The test is useful in demonstrating that the anaemia is caused by an absence of IF. Schilling test helps to identify abnormal IF-related absorption and also to distinguish between gastric and intestinal defects.
If the Schilling test result is normal, non-malabsorptive disorders and FBCM are considered. A modified absorption test, in which the test dose of cobalamin is bound to food, was created specifically to identify FBCM.[10]

#### 3.10.4.2 Serum homocysteine and methyl malonic acid

Elevated serum methylmalonic acid and homocysteine levels are found in patients with cobalamin deficiency. Clinical deficiency often features serum MMA above 1000 nmol/L and homocysteine above 25 uM. In folate deficiency, serum methylmalonic acid levels are normal and homocysteine levels are high.[11, 12,13]

| Patient Condition | Homocysteine | Methylmalonic Acid |
|---|---|---|
| Healthy | Normal | Normal |
| Vitamin B-12 deficiency | Increased | Increased |
| Folate deficiency | Increased | Normal |

Table 1. Serum homocysteine and methylmalonic acid values in healthy persons, cobalamin and folic acid deficiency

The advantage of these tests is they measure tissue vitamin stores and may diagnose the deficiency even when the serum cobalamin and folate levels are borderline or normal.

#### 3.10.4.3 Other tests

1. The indirect bilirubin level may be elevated because pernicious anaemia causes haemolysis associated with increased turnover of bilirubin. The serum lactic dehydrogenase (LDH) concentration usually is markedly increased.
2. Intrinsic Factor (IF) antibodies in serum by Immunoassay.[14]
3. Type 1 (blocking) antibody prevents the attachment of vitamin B12 to intrinsic factor: present in 50-60% of patients with pernicious anaemia. Type 2 (precipitating) antibody

prevents attachment of the vitamin B12-intrinsic factor complex to ileal receptors: present in 30% of patients with pernicious anaemia, and only in those who also have Type 1 antibodies. IF antibody has high specificity for PA (>95%). It is used to help diagnose when pernicious anaemia is suspected. As recent vitamin B12 administration is associated with a high rate of false positive results the sample must be collected prior to commencing therapy or at least one week after vitamin B12 administration. This test shows rarely false positivity in diabetes and thyroid disorders.

4. Parietal cell antibodies

Parietal cell antibodies can be measured using indirect IF. Antibodies react with sub-units of the gastric parietal cell proton pump. Antibodies are positive in 80% of patients with pernicious anaemia and in 40-50% of patients with other organ specific autoimmune diseases.[15]

## 4. Treatment

### 4.1 Cobalamin deficiency

#### 4.1.1 Specific replacement therapy

The 1000-mcg intramuscular dose begins repletion of stores (up to 150 mcg is retained from that injection by most patients).[5] Cyanocobalamin and hydroxocobalamin are commonly available preparations. 8 to 10 injections are given over the first 2 to 3 months followed by monthly injections.[16] Hydroxocobalamin injections can be spaced at twice the interval for cyanocobalamin.[17] The toxicity of cobalamin is minimal with rare allergic reactions which can be anaphylactic.[18]

In a randomized study with cobalamin deficiency, 2 mg of cyanocobalamin administered orally on a daily basis was as effective as 1 mg administered intramuscularly on a monthly basis.[19] For patients who refuse monthly parenteral therapy or prefer daily oral therapy or in those with disorders of haemostasis, cobalamin (1–2 mg/day as tablets) can be recommended for patients with cobalamin malabsorption (where cobalamin is passively absorbed at high doses).[1]

Patients with FBCM may need to take cobalamin supplements on an empty stomach to prevent in vitro binding of cobalamin to food. 1000 mcg oral doses may be necessary in many cases of FBCM, but the undesirable effects of long term high doses, if any, are not known.[20]

#### 4.1.2 Response to treatment

The response to treatment is generally predictable and can be used as a therapeutic trial. Patients have a sense of well-being within 12 to 24 hours, which is an early feature of response. In bone marrow the megaloblastic erythropoiesis starts changing to normoblastic within 12 hours and complete resolution by 48 hours. Brisk reticulocytosis starts at 3 to 4 days and peaks at 5 to 7 days. Hypersegmented neutrophils continue to remain in the blood for 10 to 14 days. Mean corpuscular volume (MCV) will take eight weeks or more to normalize.[1] All these responses will be impaired if there is associated iron deficiency, anaemia of chronic disease or hypothyroidism.

Neurologic improvement also begins within the first week and is typically complete in 6 weeks to 3 months. Its course is not as predictable as a haematologic response. Severe hypokalemia can occur after cobalamin therapy, which requires careful monitoring and management.

### 4.1.3 Causes of non-responsiveness of megaloblastosis to medication

1. Wrong diagnosis (eg: Myelodysplastic syndrome)
2. Combined cobalamin + Folate deficiency ,medication with one vitamin
3. Drugs eg: Hydroxyurea, azathioprine
4. Factors associated with B12 deficiency causing impaired response

c. Iron deficiency
d. Haemoglobinopathy
e. Hypothyroidism

### 4.2 Transfusions

Complications can occur during transfusions, particularly congestive heart failure in elderly. Transfusion should be restricted to symptomatic anaemia, rather than by low haemoglobin values. In severe anaemia, exchange transfusion after removing 250- 300ml of anaemic blood and replacing packed red cells may be beneficial.

### 4.3 Maintenance regimens

High dose cobalamin tablets (1000 mcg) can be used for maintenance therapy. Despite the advantages of ease, cost, and comfort, oral therapy has its own limitations. Oral cobalamin is less effectively absorbed after a meal than when fasted.[21] Monthly parenteral cobalamin injections are a better alternative in patients who are non-compliant with oral therapy.

### 4.4 Cobalamin prophylaxis in clinical practice

The value of general supplementation or dietary fortification with cobalamin are not proven.[22] In some situations, like strict vegetarians, patients with gastric surgery and in elderly persons, life-long supplementation with cobalamin will be essential.

## 5. Folate deficiency anaemia

Folic acid is also known as pteroyl-monoglutamic acid. Fruits and vegetables constitute the main dietary source of the vitamin. Dietary folic acid is heat labile and may be destroyed by cooking. The daily requirement is usually about 50 mcg. The requirement may be increased to many folds during pregnancy.

Folates in various foodstuffs are largely conjugated as polyglutamates. Conjugases in the lumen of the gut convert polyglutamates to mono- and diglutamates, which are readily absorbed in the proximal jejunum. Plasma folate is primarily in the form of *N*5-methyltetrahydrofolate which is a monoglutamate and is transported into cells by a carrier. In the cell, the *N*5-methyl group is removed and the folate is then converted again to the polyglutamate form. Conjugation to polyglutamate may be useful for retention of folate within the cell.

The normal body store of folic acid is 5 to 20 mg. Nearly 50% of the body stores are present in the liver. Folate deficiency usually occurs within 4 to 5 months with dietary deficiency, in contrast to cobalamin deficiency which takes many years.

### 5.1 Role of folate in DNA synthesis

Folate serves as an intermediate carrier of 1 carbon fragment and is essential for denovo synthesis of purines, dTMP and methionine. Its active form is tetrahydrofolate, which acquires 1 carbon from serine and converted to glycine.

For purine synthesis, the 1 carbon is oxidised to formic acid, then transferred to substrate. For methionine synthesis, cobalamin is required and 1 carbon fragment is reduced to the level of methyl group, which is then transferred to homocysteine. In these reactions, the cofactor is released as tetrahydrofolate which can immediately participate in another 1-carbon transfer cycle.

Conversion of dUMP to dTMP is catalysed by thymidylate synthase and dihydrofolate is released. To participate in further 1- carbon transfer cycle, the dihydrofolate is catalysed by dihydrofolate reductase to tetrahydrofolate.

## 5.2 Folate deficiency

### 5.2.1 Causes

1. Inadequate intake
   Alcoholics, infants, anorexia nervosa, malnutrition, prolonged cooking of vegetables.
2. Increased requirements
   a. Pregnancy and lactation
   b. Infancy and childhood
   c. Haemolytic anaemias
   d. Cancers
   e. Exfoliative dermatitis
3. Malabsorption
   a. Tropical sprue and non-tropical sprue
   b. Partial gastrectomy
   c. Crohn's disease
   d. Intestinal Lymphoma
4. Impaired Metabolism
   a. Alcoholism
   b. Dihydrofolate reductase inhibitors: Methotrexate, pentamidine, trimethoprim
5. Reduced hepatic stores
   a. Alcoholism
   b. Chronic liver disease and cirrhosis
   c. Hepatic malignancy

## 5.3 Alcoholism

The common cause of Folate deficiency is alcohol intake. Folate deficiency in alcoholics can be attributed to multiple factors.

a. Dietary malabsorption
b. Reduced food intake
c. Depletion of liver stores of folate
d. Impaired intracellular folate utilization

Prolonged and excessive alcohol can lead to megaloblastic changes in the bone marrow.

## 5.4 Tropical sprue / coeliac disease

In tropical sprue and coeliac disease, low folate levels are caused by folate malabsorption. Steatorrhoea is the major symptom.

In tropical sprue there will be high foecal fat and jejunal biopsy shows subtotal or total villous atrophy. In coeliac disease, d- xylose test is positive.

In coeliac disease, a gluten free diet can correct folate malabsorption.

### 5.5 Anti convulsant drugs

Drugs like phenytoin and phenobarbitone can cause folate deficiency. This is usually due to inhibition of dietary folate absorption caused by reduced levels of small intestinal conjugases.

### 5.6 Pregnancy

Since the foetus accumulates folate, the demand is high during pregnancy.

### 5.7 Haemolytic states

Haemolytic states like hereditary spherocytosis, auto-immune haemolytic anaemia, sickle cell anaemia, thalassaemias and paroxysmal nocturnal haemoglobinuria cause erythroid hyperplasia. Increased erythroid turnover causes an increase in folate demand, thus causing folate deficiency.

### 5.8 Exfoliative disorders

Patients can lose folate in exfoliated skin. In exfoliative skin disorders, folate deficiency can occur.

### 5.9 Neoplastic disorders

In acute leukaemias, myeloproliferative disorders, myeloma and metastatic carcinomas, the neoplastic tissue utilize folate more rapidly than the host tissue.

### 5.10 Clinical features of folate deficiency

Clinical features of folate deficiency are similar to cobalamin deficiency, except that neurological manifestations are not common in folate deficiency.
Haematological - pancytopenia with megaloblastic anaemia
Cardiopulmonary - congestive heart failure
Gastrointestinal - glossitis, broad spectrum malabsorption and diarrhoea
Folate deficiency can also be implicated in:

1. Increased arteriosclerosis risks due to elevated homocysteine[1]
2. Foetal neural tube defects[2]
3. Cancer pathogenesis[3]

### 5.11 Laboratory investigations

#### 5.11.1 Full blood count & blood film

The features are similar to cobalamin deficiency. Macrocytic anaemia with ovalocytes and tear drop cells are seen in the blood film. Hypersegmented neutrophils are commonly seen. Neutropenia and thrombocytopenia are less common. In rare cases, the absolute neutrophil count can drop below $1.0 \times 10^9/L$ and the platelet count below $50 \times 10^9/L$.

#### 5.11.2 Bone marrow analysis

Bone marrow features are also similar to that seen in cobalamin deficiency. Hypercellularity is prominent in all the three cell lines. Erythroid hyperplasia is more marked than the others.

Abnormal erythropoiesis with abnormally large red cell precursors (megaloblasts) with less mature nuclei (nuclear - cytoplasmic asynchrony) is common.

#### 5.11.3 Serum folate levels

Normal serum folate levels are 7-45 nmol/L measured by immunoassay.

Limitations of serum folate assay:

Levels vary with levels of folate in the recent diet. Falsely high values of serum folate can occur in haemolysis (in vivo and in vitro) and in cobalamin deficiency.

#### 5.11.4 Red cell folate levels

Normal serum folate levels are 360-1400 nmol/L, measured by immunoassa. Red cell folate is a good index of folate stores and not affected by dietary folate intake. Low red cell folate levels are a better predictor for folate deficiency than low serum folate levels.

However, there are few limitations in this assay. Low to subnormal range occurs only after all the stores are depleted. In two-thirds of patients with severe cobalamin deficiency, falsely low red cell folate levels are common. Since reticulocytes have increased folate concentrations, haemolytic states may produce falsely normal or high red cell folate despite folate deficiency.

#### 5.11.5 Serum homocysteine and methyl malonic acid

In folate deficiency, serum methyl malonic acid levels are normal and homocysteine levels are high.[4]

## 6. Treatment of folate deficiency

The usual treatment dose of folic acid tablets is 1mg/day. Sometimes up to 5mg/day may be required as in haemolytic anaemias. Adequate absorption with such doses usually occurs even in chronic folate malabsorption. Therapy should be continued until complete hematologic recovery. If the underlying cause is not correctable, folate should be continued. Folinic acid (leucovorin) can be used to rescue drugs with antifolate activity e.g. antimetabolites (methotrexate or 5-fluorouracil) or other drugs like sulfamethoxazole- trimethoprim and pentamidine. Haematological response after folate is similar to cobalamin deficiency.

### 6.1 Prophylaxis

Folic acid prophylaxis is essential in the following situations

a. Pregnancy and lactation: The dose is usually 400mcg daily.
b. Mothers at risk of delivery of neural tube defects: The dose of folic acid is 4mg/day during the peri-conception period and throughout the first trimester.
c. Haemolytic anemias and hyperproliferative haematological states: The dose is usually between 1mg to 5mg daily.
d. Patients with rheumatoid arthritis or psoriasis on medication with methotrexate.[6]

## 7. Other rare nutritional deficiencies that can cause anaemia

Deficiencies of trace elements like copper and selenium can cause anaemia.

Copper is present in legumes, meats, and nuts with a very low daily requirement.[1] It is absorbed through the mucosa of the stomach and proximal duodenum.[2]

Copper is an essential trace metal acting as a ligand to many proteins and enzymes.[2] Dopamine ß-hydroxylase is a copper containing enzyme responsible for conversion of dopamine to norepinephrine, which mediates many neurologic functions. Copper also acts as a ligand to ferroxidase II, which oxidizes iron, helping in the mobilization and transport from hepatic stores to the bone marrow for erythropoiesis.[3] Thus, copper deficiency results in excessive iron in the liver but defective transport of iron to the marrow for effective erythropoiesis.[4]

### 7.1 Causes of copper deficiency

Acquired copper deficiency is rare. The few potential causes are

1. Gastric and bariatric surgery causing malabsorption[5,6]
2. Intravenous hyperalimentation without copper supplementation
3. Hyperzincaemia
4. Menkes disease, an inherited copper deficiency disorder, in which there is a failure of transporting absorbed copper to the rest of the body from mucosal cells.

### 7.2 Haematological manifestations of copper deficiency

Copper deficiency can cause anaemia and leukopenia. Sideroblastic changes and nuclear maturation defects in erythroid precursors leading to anaemia have been observed in patients with copper deficiency.[1] Peripheral smear often reveals sideroblastic anaemia with hypochromic microcytic red cells. Leucopenia and thrombocytopenia are less common.[7] The MCV is normal or increased in anaemia of copper deficiency.

### 7.3 Other manifestations

Copper deficiency is known to cause neurologic deficits due to demyelination. Manifestations include myelopathy, polyneuropathy, ataxia and optic neuritis.[8] The combination of myelopathy, polyneuropathy and anaemia in copper deficiency can mimic the deficits seen with vitamin B12 deficiency.

### 7.4 Treatment

Copper deficiency can be treated with either oral copper supplementation or intravenous copper.[9] If zinc intoxication is present, discontinuation of zinc may be sufficient to restore copper levels back to normal, but this is usually a very slow process.[9] They will also need to take copper supplements in addition to stopping zinc consumption. Haematological manifestations are often quickly restored back to normal.[9] The neurological symptoms will often cease, but the symptoms are not always restored back to normal.

### 7.5 Selenium

Selenium is a vital trace element for efficient and effective operation of many functions of the human immune system.[10,11] Selenium is a mineral that is required by the body in trace amounts. Daily requirement of selenium is 50 micrograms. It is present in most organs of the body like kidneys, spleen, liver, pancreas. Selenium is a component of glutathione peroxidase and can be used as an antioxidant and also plays a large role in cell metabolism and cancer prevention.

### 7.5.1 Selenium deficiency

Selenium deficiency is relatively rare in healthy well-nourished individuals.

Causes of selenium deficiency

1. Eating foods predominantly grown in selenium-deficient soil.
2. Severely compromised intestinal function
3. Total parenteral nutrition
4. Gastrointestinal bypass surgery

Manifestations of a selenium deficiency include cardiovascular disease, nerve degeneration, hypothyroidism, arthritis and anaemia. A selenium deficiency may even increase the chances of developing some forms of cancer.

Selenium deficiency may play a role in causing or aggravating anaemia as glutathione peroxidase protects red blood cells from free radical damage and destruction. In a prevalence study there was low serum selenium found independently associated with anaemia among older men and women.[12] Mean serum selenium among non-anaemic and anaemic adults was 1.60 and 1.51 umol / L (P=0.0003). The prevalence of anaemia among adults in the lowest to highest quartiles of serum selenium was 18.3, 9.5, 9.7 and 6.9%, respectively (P=0.0005).[12]

### 7.5.2 Supplements

There are many forms of selenium supplements including organic selenium rich yeast, selenium in the form of selenomethionine, and inorganic sodium selenite. Selenium yeast increases the blood selenium levels and sodium selenite helps to increase the activity of glutathione peroxidase. Organic selenium is better absorbed and less toxic than the inorganic forms. People who are at risk of selenium deficiency will benefit from supplements.

## 8. References

### 8.1 References part 1 (1-2)

[1] Worldwide prevalence of anaemia 1993-2005 (2008) Editors: Bruno de Benoist, Erin McLean, Ines Egli, Mary Cogswell, 2008. ISBN: 978 92 4 159665 7.

[2] World Health Organization [WHO], Division of Family Health, Maternal Health and Safe Motherhood Programme, Division of Health Protection and Promotion, Nutrition Programme; WHO. The Prevalence of Anaemia in Women: a tabulation of available information. 2nd ed. Geneva, Switzerland, World Health Organization. 1992.

[3] ACC/SCN (United Nations Administrative Committee on Coordination/Standing Committee on Nutrition). 2004. Fifth report on the world nutrition situation: Nutrition for improved development outcomes. Geneva, 2004, available at accscn@who.org.

[4] Maberly GF, Trowbridge FL, Yip R, Sullivan KM, West CE. programs against micronutrient malnutrition: Ending hidden hunger. Annu Rev Public Health 1994; 15:277-301.

[5] Iron deficiency anaemia: assessment, prevention and control. 2001. World Health Organization Publication WHO/NHD/01.3.

[6] Zimmermann MB, Hurrell RF. Nutritional iron deficiency. Lancet 2007; 370, 9586, 511-520. doi:10.1016/S0140-6736.

[7] Looker AC, Dallman PR, Carrol MD, Gunter EW, Johnson CL. Prevalence of Iron Deficiency in the United States. JAMA. 1997;277:973-976.

[8] Institute of Medicine. Dietary Reference Intakes (DRIs) for Vitamin A, Vitamin K, Arsenic, Boron, Chromium, Copper, Iodine, Iron, Manganese, Molybdenum, Nickel, Silicon, Vanadium, and Zinc. Washington, DC: National Academy Press; 2002, 18-19.
[9] Zini G, Di Mario A, Garzia M, Bianchi M, d'Onofrio G.Reticulocyte population data in different erythropoietic states J. Clin. Pathol. 2011 64:159-163.
[10] Goddard AF, James MW, McIntyre AS, Scott BB; on behalf of the British Society of Gastroenterology. Guidelines for the management of iron deficiency anaemia. Gut. 2011 Jun 6. [Epub ahead of print]
[11] Andrews NC. Disorders of iron metabolism. N Engl J Med. 1999;341:1986–1995.
[12] Tomas Ganz. Hepcidin and iron regulation, 10 years later. BLOOD, 2011; 117, 4425-4433.
[13] Park CH, Valore EV, Waring AJ, Ganz T. Hepcidin, a urinary antimicrobial peptide synthesized in the liver. J Biol Chem. 2001;276:7806–7810.
[14] Weinstein DA, Roy CN, Fleming MD, Loda MF, Wolfsdorf JI, Andrews NC. Inappropriate expression of hepcidin is associated with iron refractory anemia: implications for the anemia of chronic disease. Blood. 2002;100:3776–3781.
[15] Nemeth E, Ganz T. The role of hepcidin in iron metabolism. Acta Hematol. 2009; 122: 78-86.
[16] Auerbach M, Ballard H, Glaspy J. Clinical update: intravenous iron for anaemia. Lancet 2007; 369: 1502-4.
[17] Kumar A, Jain S, Singh NP, Singh T. Oral versus high dose parenteral iron supplementation in pregnancy. Int J Gynaecol Obstet 2005; 89:7-13.
[18] Jacobs P, Johnson G, Wood L. Oral iron therapy in human subjects, comparative absorption between ferrous salts and iron polymaltose. J Med. 1984;15:367-377.
[19] Maxton DG, Thompson RP, Hinder RC. Absorption of iron from ferric hydroxypyranone complexes. Br J Nutr. 1994;71:203-207.
[20] Sharma N. Iron absorption: IPC therapy is superior to conventional iron salts. Obstet Gynecol. 2001;515-19.
[21] Geisser P. In vitro studies on interactions of iron salts and complexes with food stuffs and medicaments. Arzneimittelforschung 1990;40:754-760.
[22] Jenkins A. Using iron dextran to treat iron-deficiency anemia. Hospital Pharmacist. 2005; 12: 224-225.
[23] Lawrence R. Development and comparison of iron dextran products. PDA J Pharm Sci Technol. 1998; 52:190-7.
[24] Auerbach M, Goodnough LT, Picard D, Maniatis A. The role of intravenous iron in anemia management and transfusion avoidance. Transfusion 2008; 48:988-1000.
[25] Auerbach M, Rodgers GM. Intravenous iron. N Engl J Med 2007; 357:93-4.
[26] Khalafallah A, Dennis A, Bates J, Bates G, Robertson IK, Smith L, Ball MJ, Seaton D, Brain T, Rasko JE. A prospective randomized, controlled trial of intravenous versus oral iron for moderate iron deficiency anaemia of pregnancy. J Intern Med. 2010; 268:286-95. Epub 2010 May 19.
[27] Hamstra RD, Block MH, Schokert AL. Intravenous iron dextran in clinical medicine. JAMA. 1980; 2;243:1726-31.
[28] Faich G, Strobos J. Sodium ferric gluconate complex in sucrose: safer intravenous iron therapy than iron dextrans. Am J Kidney Dis. 1999;33:464-70.

[29] Burns DL, Pomposelli JJ. Toxicity of parenteral iron dextran therapy. Kidney Int Suppl. 1999; 69:S119-24.

[30] Michael B, Coyne DW, Fishbane S. et al. Sodium ferric gluconate complex in hemodialysis patients: adverse reactions compared to placebo and iron dextran. Kidney Int. 2002; 61:1830-9.

[31] Fishbane S, Kowalski EA. Comparative safety of intravenous iron dextran, iron saccharate and sodium ferric gluconate. Semin Dial. 2000;13:381-4.

[32] Garg M, Morrison G, Friedman A, Lau A, Lau D, Gibson PR. A rapid infusion protocol is safe for total dose iron polymaltose: time for change. Intern Med J. 2011;41:548-54. doi: 10.1111/j.1445-5994.2010.02356.x.

[33] Manoharan A, Ramakrishna R, Pereira B. Delayed adverse reactions to total-dose intravenous iron polymaltose. Intern Med J. 2009;39:857.

[34] Monograph ferumoxytol (Feraheme). (2009) AMAG Pharmaceuticals Inc.

[35] Rosner MH, Auerbach M. Ferumoxytol for the treatment of iron deficiency. Expert Rev Hematol. 2011;4:399-406.

[36] Kulnigg S, Stoinov S, Simanenkov V et al. A novel intravenous iron formulation for treatment of anemia in inflammatory bowel disease: the ferric carboxymaltose (FERINJECT) randomized controlled trial. Am J Gastroenterol. 2008; 103:1182-1192.

[37] Qunibi W, Dinh Q, Benjamin J. Safety and Tolerability Profile of Ferric Carboxymaltose (FCM) a New High Dose Intravenous Iron, across Ten Multi-Center Trials. J Am Soc Nephrol. 2007; 18: SU-PO1029.

[38] Kalra PA. Introducing iron isomaltoside 1000 (Monofer®)-development rationale and clinical experience. NDT Plus; 2011; 4 (s1): doi: 10.1093/ndtplus/sfr042

[39] Jahn MR, Andreasen HB, Fütterer S, Nawroth T, Schünemann V, Kolb U, Hofmeister W, Muñoz M, Bock K, Meldal M, Langguth P. A comparative study of the physicochemical properties of iron isomaltoside 1000 (Monofer®), a new intravenous iron preparation and its clinical implications. Eur J Pharm Biopharm. 2011;78:480-91. Epub 2011 Mar 23.

[40] Al RA, Unlubilgin E, Kandemir O, Yalvac S, Cakir L, Haberal A. intravenous versus oral iron for treatment of anemia in pregnancy: a randomized trial. Obstet Gynecol 2005; 106:1335-40.

[41] Bayoumeu F, Subiran-Buisset C, Baka NE, Legagneur H, Monnier-Barbarino P, Laxenaire MC. Iron therapy in iron deficiency anemia in pregnancy: intravenous route versus oral route. Am J Obstet Gynecol 2002; 186:518-22.

[42] Reveiz L, Gyte GML, Cuervo LG. Treatments for iron-deficiency anaemia in pregnancy. Cochrane Database Syst Rev. 2007; Issue 2. Art. No.: CD003094. DOI: 10.1002/14651858.CD003094.pub2.

[43] Isbister JP, Shander A, Spahn DR, Erhard J, Farmer SL, Hofmann A. Adverse blood transfusion outcomes: establishing causation. Transfus Med Rev. 2011;25:89-101. Epub 2011 Feb 23.

[44] Aickin M, Gensler H. Adjusting for multiple testing when reporting research results: the Bonferroni vs Holm methods. Am J Public Health 1996; 86:726-8.

[45] Reveiz L, Gyte GML, Cuervo LG. Treatments for iron-deficiency anaemia in pregnancy. Cochrane Database Syst Rev. 2007; Issue 2. Art. No.: CD003094. DOI: 10.1002/14651858.CD003094.pub2.

[46] Auerbach M, Goodnough LT, Picard D, Maniatis A. The role of intravenous iron in anemia management and transfusion avoidance. Transfusion 2008; 48:988-1000.
[47] Auerbach M, Rodgers GM. Intravenous iron. N Engl J Med 2007; 357:93-4.

### 8.2 References part 2 (3-4)

[1] Antony AC: Megaloblastic anemias. In: Hoffman R, Benz Jr EJ, Shattil SJ, et al ed. Hematology: Basic Principles and Practice, 5th ed. Churchill-Livingstone; 2008, chapter 39.
[2] Stover P: Physiology of folate and vitamin B12 in health and disease. Nutr Rev 2004; 62:S3.
[3] Reynolds E, Vitamin B12, folic acid, and the nervous system. Lancet Neurol. 2006 Nov;5(11):949-60. Review.
[4] Remacha AF, Vitamin B12 deficiency, hyperhomocysteinemia and thrombosis: a case and control study, Int J Hematol. 2011 Apr;93(4):458-64. Epub 2011 Apr 8.
[5] Chanarin I. The Megaloblastic Anaemias, 1st ed. Blackwell Scientific; 1979.
[6] Antony AC. Vegetarianism and vitamin B-12 (cobalamin) deficiency. Am J Clin Nutr. 2003;78:3-6.
[7] Carmel R. Malabsorption of food cobalamin. Baillieres Clin Haematol. 1995;8:639-655.
[8] Kokkola A, Sjoblom S-M, Haapiainen R, et al.. The risk of gastric carcinoma and carcinoid tumours in patients with pernicious anaemia. Scand J Gastroenterol. 1998;33:88-92.
[9] Curtis AD et al. Clin Lab Haematol 1986; 8: 135-140.
[10] Doscherholmen A, Swaim WR. Impaired assimilation of egg Co57 vitamin B12 in patients with hypochlorhydria and achlorhydria and after gastric resection. Gastroenterology. 1973;64:913-919.
[11] Savage DG, Lindenbaum J, Stabler SP, Allen RH. Sensitivity of serum methylmalonic acid and total homocysteine determinations for diagnosing cobalamin and folate deficiencies. Am J Med. 1994; 96:239-246.
[12] Allen RH, Stabler SP, Savage DG, Lindenbaum J. Diagnosis of cobalamin deficiency: usefulness of serum methylmalonic acid and total homocysteine concentrations. Am J Hematol. 1990;34:90-98.
[13] Lindenbaum J, Savage DG, Stabler SP, Allen RH. Diagnosis of cobalamin deficiency: II. Relative sensitivities of serum cobalamin, methylmalonic acid, and total homocysteine concentrations. Am J Hematol. 1990;34:99-107.
[14] Yao Y et al. J Fam Pract 1992; 35: 524-528.
[15] Oh R et al. Am Fam Physician 2003; 67(5): 993-994.
[16] Savage D, Lindenbaum J. Relapses after interruption of cyanocobalamin therapy in patients with pernicious anemia. Am J Med. 1983;74:765-772.
[17] Tudhope GR, Swan HT, Spray GH. Patient variation in pernicious anaemia, as shown in a clinical trial of cyanocobalamin, hydroxocobalamin, and cyanocobalamin-zinc tannate. Br J Haematol.1967;13:216-228.
[18] Tordjman R, Genereau T, Guinnepain MT, et al. Reintroduction of vitamin B12 in 2 patients with prior B12-induced anaphylaxis. Eur J Haematol. 1998;60:269-270.
[19] Antoinette M. Kuzminski, et al. Effective treatment of cobalamin deficiency with oral cobalamin. Blood, 1998 92: 1191-1198.
[20] Carmel R: How I treat cobalamin (vitamin B12) deficiency, Blood, 2008, Volume 112,6

[21] Berlin H, Berlin R, Brante G. Oral treatment of pernicious anemia with high doses of vitamin B12 without intrinsic factor. Acta Med Scand. 1968;184:247-258.

[22] Carmel R. Efficacy and safety of fortification and supplementation with vitamin B12: biochemical and physiologic effects. Food Nutr Bull. 2008;29(suppl):S177-S187.

### 8.3 References part 3(5-6)

[1] Varela-Moreiras G, Murphy MM, Scott JM. Cobalamin, folic acid, and homocysteine. Nutr Rev. May 2009;67 Suppl 1:S69-72.

[2] Wolff T, Witkop CT, Miller T, Syed SB. Folic acid supplementation for the prevention of neural tube defects: an update of the evidence for the U.S. Preventive Services Task Force. Ann Intern Med. May 52009;150(9):632-9.

[3] Blount BC, Mack MM, Wehr CM, et al. Folate deficiency causes uracil misincorporation into human DNA and chromosome breakage: implications for cancer and neuronal damage. Proc Natl Acad Sci U S A. Apr 1 1997;94(7):3290-5

[4] Savage DG, Lindenbaum J, Stabler SP, Allen RH. Sensitivity of serum methylmalonic acid and total homocysteine determinations for diagnosing cobalamin and folate deficiencies. Am J Med. 1994; 96:239-246.

[5] Herbert V. Development of Human Folate Deficiency. In: Picciano MF, Stokstool ELR, Gregory, JF, eds.Folic Acid Metabolism in Health and Disease (Contemporary Issues in Clinical Nutrition). 13. New York,NY: 1990:195-210.

[6] Whittle S, Hughes R: Folate supplementation and methotrexate treatment in rheumatoid arthritis: A review. *Rheumatology* 2004; 43:267.

### 8.4 References part 4 (7)

[1] Williams DM. Copper deficiency in humans. Semin Hematol 1983; 20: 118–28.

[2] Wu J et al, Copper Deficiency as Cause of Unexplained Hematologic and Neurologic Deficits in Patient with Prior Gastrointestinal Surgery, *JABFM,* 19:191-194 (2006)

[3] Turnlund J. Copper. In: Shils M, Olson J, Shike M, editors. Modern nutrition in health and disease. Philadelphia: Lippincott; 1998. p. 241.

[4] Fields M, Bureau I, Lewis CG. Ferritin is not an indicator of available hepatic iron stores in anemia of copper deficiency in rats. Clin Chem 1997; 43(8 Pt 1): 1457–9.

[5] Kumar N, Ahlskog JE, Gross JB, Jr. Acquired hypocupremia after gastric surgery. Clin Gastroenterol Hepatol 2004; 2: 1074–9.

[6] Thaisetthawatkul P, Collazo-Clavell ML, Sarr MG, Norell JE, Dyck PJ. A controlled study of peripheral neuropathy after bariatric surgery. Neurology 2004; 63: 1462–70.

[7] Hayton BA, Broome HE, Lilenbaum RC. Copper deficiency-induced anemia and neutropenia secondary to intestinal malabsorption. Am J Hematol 1995; 48: 45–7.

[8] Kumar N, Crum B, Petersen RC, Vernino SA, Ahlskog JE. Copper deficiency myelopathy. Arch Neurol 2004; 61: 762–6.

[9] Kumar, N. Copper deficiency myelopathy (human swayback). Mayo Clinic Proceedings. 2006; 81, 1371-1384.

[10] Rayman MP. The importance of selenium to human health. Lancet. 2000;356:233-241.

[11] 14. Arthur JR, McKenzie RC, Beckett GJ. Selenium in the immune system. J Nutr. 2003;133:1457-1459.

[12] Semba RD, Low serum selenium is associated with anemia among older adults in the United States, Eur J Clin Nutr. 2009;63:93-9. Epub 2007 Sep 5.

# 10

# Nutritional Anemia in Developing Countries

Frank T. Wieringa, Jacques Berger and Marjoleine A. Dijkhuizen
[1]*NutriPass - UMR204, Institute for Research for Development (IRD), IRD-UM2-UM1, Montpellier*
[2]*Department of Human Nutrition, Copenhagen University*
[1]*France*
[2]*Denmark*

## 1. Introduction

As described in earlier chapters, anemia is characterized by an insufficient concentration of the protein hemoglobin in the circulation, causing a lack of oxygen transporting capacity. Hemoglobin is the principal component of red blood cells, erythrocytes, and is synthesised in the bone marrow with iron as the key oxygen binding site. Before discussing causes and consequences of nutritional anemia in developing countries, it is important to consider briefly how anemia is diagnosed.

Anemia can be diagnosed clinically, for example by looking at the paleness of the skin or mucosa or by a history of weakness and dizziness. This clinical assessment is often the only method available in resource-poor settings, but unfortunately has a low sensitivity and specificity (Critchley and Bates 2005). A more direct and thus more sensitive and specific approach is to measure hemoglobin concentrations in the blood, using one of many different techniques in blood samples obtained by either finger prick or vena-puncture. The obtained values are then compared to those from a matching, normal population, using pre-defined cut-offs for anemia. It is important to realize that different cut-off thresholds are used for different situations. For example, there are different cut-off points for young children, pregnant women, non-pregnant women and men, as well as ethnic differences and differences between smokers and non-smokers. Moreover, altitude affects hemoglobin concentrations and hence cut-offs for anemia. Therefore, it is very important to select the correct reference population for the subjects studied. Cut-off thresholds are normally chosen as the point at which 2.5% of the normal population (or 2 standard deviations) has a value that is lower. Hence, in a normal population, 2.5% of the people will be anemic according to this definition. From an epidemiological viewpoint, this means that if a survey finds a prevalence of anemia close to 2.5%, the studied population can be regarded as normal. From an individual viewpoint however, if a subject from that same population was diagnosed with anemia, s/he would not regard this as normal, would like to know the cause, and if indicated, s/he would like to be treated! Moreover, cut-offs are certainly not absolute or unequivocal, rather, they should be regarded as a proposed value that is accepted by consensus, and are sometimes challenged if found insufficiently accurate. For example, there is currently discussion regarding the cut-off for anemia in infants. Domellof et al. have proposed more precise, stratified cut-off thresholds for anemia at hemoglobin concentrations of <105 g/L for infants 4 - 6 months of age and <100 g/L for infants 9 mo of age (Domellof et al. 2002a), but as shown in Table 1, these revised cut-offs have not been implemented by the public health community yet.

| Reference group | cut-off (g/L) | Categories of anemia (g/L) | | |
|---|---|---|---|---|
| | | Mild | Moderate | Severe |
| Pregnant women | 110 | 100-110 | 70-99 | <70 |
| Non-pregnant women | 120 | 110-119 | 80-109 | <80 |
| Children 6 - 59 months of age | 110 | 100-109 | 70-99 | <70 |
| Children 5 - 11 years of age | 115 | 110-114 | 80-1-9 | <80 |
| Children 12 - 14 years of age | 120 | 110-119 | 80-109 | <80 |
| Men | 130 | 110-129 | 80-109 | <80 |

Table 1. Cut-off values used by the World Health Organization to define anemia in different population groups (WHO 2001).

There are many different causes of anemia. Pathophysiologically speaking, anemia occurs either through a) blood loss in quantities higher than the body can replete through synthesis, b) an increased breakdown in the body of erythrocytes or c) a defect in the synthesis of hemoglobin protein or of new erythrocytes. An increased breakdown of erythrocytes occurs for example in sickle cell disease (sickle cell anemia) and in malaria. However, almost all anemias caused by nutritional deficiencies affect the production of new erythrocytes or hemoglobin, thereby causing anemia.

A large part of the human population is affected by anemia, with an estimated 1.6 billion people being anemic. Iron deficiency (ID) is most often, but certainly not the only cause of nutritional anemia. Indeed, many studies have shown that iron deficiency accounts roughly for only half of the anemia cases (Wieringa et al. 2007a), meaning that improving iron status in an anemic population will only reduce the prevalence of anemia to a certain extent. On the other hand, more people have insufficient iron stores than anemia, as anemia only occurs at the end stage, when iron deficiency eventually leads to so-called iron-deficiency anemia (IDA). Indeed, the World Health Organization (WHO) estimates that roughly twice as many people are affected by iron deficiency than by iron deficiency anemia (WHO 2001).

Prevalences of anemia and iron deficiency are much higher in developing countries than in affluent countries. However, large differences in anemia prevalence exist among different continents and among different countries on the same continent. Reasons for these differences are many and include differences in basic health and nutrition characteristics (such as diet, prevelance of nutritional deficiencies, prevalence of anemia-causing illnesses such as intestinal parasites or malaria) and other factors affecting hemoglobin and erythrocyte concentrations such as sickle cell anemia or other hemoglobinopathies and altitude. To appreciate the extent of anemia as a public health problem, one only has to review the data on anemia prevalence around the world.

The highest burden of anemia and ID is found in Africa and South Asia, with many studies showing the significant public health impact of anemia in these populations. In India, the prevalence of anemia is >50% in both pregnant and non-pregnant women (WHO 2008). Low birth weight and perinatal mortality increase two-fold when hemoglobin concentrations are <80 g/L during pregnancy. Not surprisingly, anemia is estimated to be responsible for 40% of maternal deaths in India (Kalaivani 2009). In rural Bangladesh, more than 30% of nulliparous married women were anemic when entering pregnancy, with 15% being iron deficient and 11% having IDA (Khambalia et al. 2009). And already more than 80% had inadequate iron stores, which was defined as <500 mg of iron. In Pakistan, anemia prevalence was even higher: in a large prospective observational study in ~1400 pregnant women, 90.5% were anemic (Hb<110 g/L) (Baig-Ansari et al. 2008). In Africa, the prevalence of anemia in women of reproductive age (WRA) is estimated to be ~47% and in pregnant women ~57% (WHO 2008), although prevalence rates differ widely from country to country (Lartey 2008). In Mali, anemia was present in 47% of pregnant women (Hb<110 g/L), but only 13% of the women had ID (serum ferritin <12 μg/l) (Ayoya et al. 2006). Infectious diseases were a major contributor to anemia in this study. Among pregnant women in northern Nigeria, 30% was classified as anemic (Hb< 105 g/l); Here, the major contributing factor to anemia was ID (ferritin<10 μg/L) (Vanderjagt et al. 2007). Besides ID, vitamin B12 and folic acid deficiencies were probably prevalent also. In Ghana, anemia (Hb < 110 g/L) was observed in 34 % of the pregnant women from urban areas, with 16% of the women having ID (ferritin≤ 16 μg/l) and only 7.5% having IDA (Engmann et al. 2008). Malaria was a greater risk factor than ID for being anemic in this study. Hence, in Sub-Saharan Africa ID is prevalent, but not as strongly related to anemia, as other causes of anemia such as malaria infection are also prevalent in vulnerable groups. Other areas in the world are affected by a high prevalence of anemia also. In Vietnam, more than half of 900 women investigated in a representative community survey in healthy women of reproductive age were anemic (Trinh and Dibley 2007). In contrast, in Thailand in a similar survey only 14.1 % of 590 women was found to be anemic (Hb< 11g/dl), and 6.0% had IDA, according to the WHO criteria (Sukrat et al.). These last figures are more typical for developed countries. IDA was found in 4% of French children <2 yrs (Hercberg et al. 2001), and in the USA iron deficiency was found in 14.4% of children between 1 and 2 yrs, and in 9.2% of women of reproductive age (Cogswell et al. 2009). Worryingly, there appears to be no decrease in the prevalence of iron deficiency in young children over the last decades, with especially overweight children at risk for ID (Cogswell et al. 2009).

From above data, it is clear that anemia is widespread throughout the world, and given the negative effects of anemia on health and development, a world-wide public health concern. Indeed, for decades the urgent need for interventions to reduce the prevalence of anemia has been recognized, but most interventions have had little impact (Stoltzfus 2008; Yip 2002). From the above studies, it is also clear that the distinction between anemia, IDA and ID is important, not only because of differences in prevalence and health effects of these entities, but also because the etiology and underlying determinants are distinct and call for different intervention strategies. Anemia, IDA and ID are of course interrelated and overlapping diagnoses but do not constitute a complete continuum, and specific factors, causes and determinants play a different role in each entity. Furthermore, the above studies also show that prevalence patterns of anemia and iron deficiency indicators can vary widely among populations, depending on baseline health and nutritional determinants. Below, some key aspects of the etiology, the measurement and the public health impact of anemia will be reviewed, before discussing what can be done to reduce the global burden of anemia.

## 2. Nutritional causes of anemia with special reference to developing countries

For some micronutrients, such as iron and vitamin $B_{12}$, there is a clear understanding on why deficiency leads to anemia. For others, such as selenium or vitamin A, the underlying mechanisms are less clear. Moreover, it appears that some nutrients act synergistically, where deficiency of one micronutrient might either aggravate or mask the effects of deficiency of another micronutrient, such as is the case for Vitamin $B_{12}$ and folic acid. Furthermore, anemia is the end result of a long process, often with a multi-factorial etiology, with other health determinants often also playing a role. Therefore, anemia has been difficult to address from a public health point of view, and remains present in many populations despite countless intervention efforts.

As the etiology of anemia has been covered extensively in previous chapters and in other books, this chapter will focus mainly on strategies to prevent anemia from nutritional causes and reduce the prevalence in various populations, especially in those vulnerable groups that have the largest burden or the largest health impact of anemia. For more detailed information on the etiology of nutritional anemia, interested readers can freely download the book 'Nutritional Anemia' from the Sight and Life website (Sight_and_Life 2007). However, as some nutritional aspects of the etiology of anemia are important for understanding the ratio behind certain interventions, these are highlighted in this chapter when necessary.

Anemia is often considered a synonym for iron deficiency. However, as described above, anemia and iron deficiency are distinct, albeit overlapping, conditions. Anemia occurs in the later stages of iron deficiency, when iron stores are completely depleted. However, before anemia occurs, iron deficiency is already affecting other functions, such as the immune system and the nervous system, leading to reduced immunocompetence, decreased physical activity and cognitive impairment (Beard 2001). Physiologically, iron deficiency occurs when requirements exceed the amount of iron absorbed from the diet. Requirements are increased by rapid increases in body mass (such as in pregnant women, young children) or by high losses of iron (menstruation, hookworm infection). This explains in part the high prevalence in vulnerable groups such as children and pregnant women, and on the other hand, the association of anemia with poverty and poor health. A special situation is sequestration of iron in the body, making it less available for utilisation for e.g. hemoglobin synthesis, such as happens in (chronic) infection by the acute phase response or in massive erythrocyte breakdown (such as in malaria). Looking at the uptake of iron, it is found that in general iron absorption is low (~5%) from plant-based diets (developing countries) because of iron-uptake inhibiting factors (phytates, polyphenols) and iron absorption is higher (~15%) from diets containing more meat and fish (developed countries) because iron in animal products is often bound in heme protein structures that greatly facilitates absorption. This explains in part the much higher prevalence of ID in developing countries.

Other nutrients in the diet are also important, and deficiencies of other nutrients can directly or indirectly contribute to anemia and sometimes even to ID. The role of vitamin A in iron metabolism was recognized already in the 1980's (Mejia and Chew 1988), when studies showed that the effect of iron supplementation on hemoglobin concentrations could be enhanced by the addition of vitamin A (Suharno et al. 1993). The mechanisms by which vitamin A enhances hemoglobin formation are not completely understood, but vitamin A is thought to play a role in the absorption of iron and/or in the utilization of iron stores for new heme production (Zimmermann et al. 2006). Because interactions are probably on the level of gene expression and protein synthesis, it is an intricate and finely balanced interplay and deficiencies or excess can have indirect and sometimes unanticipated effects. In the latter case, this means that providing vitamin A to subjects with a marginal iron status would make these subjects more iron deficient, as extra iron would be used for the production of hemoglobin, and is no longer available for other tissues such as the brain. Indeed, we showed in a large multi-country trial in SE Asia that vitamin A supplementation in infancy, without interventions to improve iron status, was associated with anemia (Wieringa et al. 2007a). This is an important reminder that understanding of the underlying mechanisms is important, even though the final public health effect is the objective of an intervention.

| Nutrient | (proposed) mechanism leading to anemia | Ref |
|---|---|---|
| Iron | Essential part of heme. Deficiency: reduced production of hemoglobin | (Bates et al. 1989) |
| Folic Acid | Deficiency: Impaired DNA synthesis leading to reduced number of erythrocytes | (Koury and Ponka 2004) |
| Vitamin $B_{12}$ (Cobalamin) | Deficiency: Interference with folic acid metabolism (see above) | (Koury and Ponka 2004) |
| Vitamin $B_2$ (Riboflavin) | Likely involved in iron absorption in gut mucosa | (Powers 2003) |
| Vitamin $B_6$ (Pyridoxal) | Possibly involved in heme biosynthesis | (Sight_and_Life 2007) |
| Vitamin A | Possibly involved in heme biosynthesis, perhaps also involved in regulating availability of iron from liver stores | (Roodenburg et al. 1996; Zimmermann et al. 2006) |
| Vitamin E | Deficiency: Oxidative stress of the erythrocytes leading to increased hemolysis | (Sight_and_Life 2007) |
| Vitamin C | Availability in gut enhances conversion Fe3+ to Fe2+ , increasing iron bioavailability. | (Bates et al. 1989) |
| Selenium | Deficiency: Possibly oxidative stress or increased inflammation | (Van Nhien et al. 2008) |
| Copper | Deficiency: Interference with red cell maturation and iron absorption | (Sight_and_Life 2007) |

Table 2. Nutrients associated with anemia in developing countries.

Other deficiencies clearly related to the development of anemia are vitamin $B_{12}$ and folic acid deficiency. Deficiency will lead to a characteristic megaloblastic anemia, meaning larger than normal erythrocytes, with poorly differentiated nuclei (Sight_and_Life 2007). Neither vitamin $B_{12}$ nor folic acid deficiency is a rare condition in developing countries, and both contribute to the overall high rates of anemia seen in developing countries. Folic acid is also involved in the neural development of the fetus, and deficiency can result in very distinct malformations. Indeed, flour fortification with folic acid in the USA has resulted in a dramatic decrease in neural tube defects (Berry et al. 2010), making it a very cost-effective intervention (Grosse et al. 2005). The role of vitamin E and selenium in the etiology of anemia is less clear. Suggested mechanisms involve increased oxidative stress, leading to earlier breakdown of erythrocytes or increased inflammation.

Inflammation itself is associated with anemia, and this is often referred to as the 'anemia of chronic disease'. Immune activation leads to a decrease in erythropoiesis (synthesis of new erythrocytes), which eventually will lead to lower hemoglobin concentrations and anemia. Immune activation, and especially the so-called acute-phase response, which is the generalized reaction of the body to infection or trauma, also results in a re-distribution of many nutrients in the human body. This re-distribution makes it more difficult for pathogens to replicate, and has been termed 'nutritional immunity' (Weinberg 1975). However, this re-distribution of nutrients such as iron, vitamin A and zinc by the acute phase response also distorts the measurement of micronutrient status by changing the plasma concentration of indicators commonly used to assess status. We and others have been trying to quantify the extent of this distortion by the acute phase response on several indicators (Wieringa et al. 2002), and have proposed factors (Table 3) to correct for the effects of inflammation (Thurnham et al. 2010; Thurnham et al. 2003). This is important for the estimation of the prevalence of micronutrient deficiencies in populations. If inflammation prevalence is high, e.g. in areas with endemic malaria, the perceived prevalence of vitamin A and zinc deficiencies will be significantly higher, as plasma retinol and zinc concentrations are reduced by inflammation. On the other hand, the perceived prevalence of ID and IDA will be significantly lower, as ferritin concentrations are increased in inflammation. Hence, the acute phase response should be taken into account when using indicators of micronutrient status sensitive to it by concomitantly measuring concentrations of acute phase proteins such as C-reactive protein (CRP) and α1-acid glycoprotein (AGP).

| | Incubation phase (only CRP elevated) | Early convalescence phase (CRP and AGP raised) | Late convalescence phase (only AGP raised) |
|---|---|---|---|
| Ferritin ratios compared to no inflammation | 1.30 | 1.90 | 1.36 |
| Proposed correction factors for ferritin concentrations | 0.77 | 0.53 | 0.75 |

Table 3. Effect of different phases of inflammation on ferritin concentration, and proposed factors to correct for the effect of inflammation on ferritin concentrations. Adapted from (Thurnham et al. 2010).

## 3. Interventions to reduce the prevalence of anemia

Unfortunately, efforts in the last decades to reduce the prevalence of anemia and iron deficiency have not been too successful. As anemia has a multi-factorial etiology, reasons for success or failure of interventions are also many. One striking feature of all public health interventions is the huge difference between the efficacy of studies done in a controlled research setting and the effectiveness of strategies implemented on a national scale. Unfortunately, anemia and iron deficiency interventions also demonstrate this difference compellingly. Whereas there are many studies published showing excellent efficacy of interventions to improve iron status in pregnant women or other risk groups, the few studies reporting effectiveness of large-scale iron interventions show little or no impact. Indeed, even the INACG (International Nutritional Anemia Consultative Group) was forced to conclude that although both daily and weekly iron supplementation regimens have been demonstrated to be efficacious in vulnerable population groups, existing data do not demonstrate that large-scale programs with iron supplementation are generally effective (INACG 2004).

### 3.1 Evidence-based intervention development and implementation: Moving policy forward

Globally, most efforts to reduce anemia have focused on pregnant women, with millions of iron and folic acid tablets being provided to pregnant women all over the world annually. There are several reasons for this specific attention during pregnancy. Looking more closely at the reasons shows how science, health care and policy interact together resulting in the development and implementation of interventions. First of all, iron requirements during pregnancy increase by more than two-fold, to >4 mg Fe/day (Steer 2000), an amount that is almost impossible to meet with a diet with low available iron (Yip 1996). Indeed, it is even difficult to meet this requirement with a Western-style diet (with meat) with high iron-availability. Thus interventions would be useful in this situation, and direct effects can be expected. Furthermore by targeting pregnant women, one hopes to break the negative inter-generational vicious circle of poor intra-uterine growth leading to low adult height predisposing to poor intra-uterine growth. . So interventions in this target group can also contribute more indirect, long-term effects. Thirdly, during pregnancy women are encouraged to access health services, offering opportunities for targeted interventions such as iron supplementation. Often, health care access for pregnant women is already part of national public health policy, with encouraging antenatal care programs and registration in place. Finally, most published studies have been done in pregnant women; hence most evidence on impact of interventions such as iron supplementation is available for pregnant women, driving policy towards strategies focusing on pregnant women. The available evidence informs and focuses policy interests, and as policy prefers predictable results this encourages policy development in this field. However, other closely linked groups also at risk for anemia such as young infants and children or women of reproductive age (WRA) are thereby often sidelined, as the available evidence for these groups is less complete and less clear, and effects less well documented. This results in less interest from policy, and less momentum to advocate and develop interventions for these groups. In this way, policy interests may drive science but science also steers policy interests. To remain updated on latest policy developments, specific sites such as eLENA from the WHO (www.who.int/elena/en) are available.

### 3.2 Interventions for pregnant women

A meta-analysis on the effects of iron and folic acid supplementation in pregnancy was recently done by Pena-Rosas and Viteri (Pena-Rosas and Viteri 2009). Their meta-analyses comprises 49 trials with >23,000 women. Data on anemia and IDA was available for 1108 women from 6 trials. In women taking iron supplements, 30.7% were still anemic at term, whereas only 4.9% had IDA. For women not receiving iron these figures were 54.8% and 15.5%. These findings clearly demonstrate the multi-factorial etiology of anemia. Iron deficiency and folic acid deficiency are only part of the problem. Hence, providing only iron and folic acid can only be expected to give a partial improvement in anemia prevalence, depending on the extent of the pre-existing deficiency of iron. Despite this remaining prevalence of anemia, the intervention significantly increased hemoglobin concentrations in the pregnant women, and thereby reduced the risk at term for anemia (RR 0.27 CI 0.17 - 0.42). Surprisingly, the authors found no significant effects on important health outcomes such as premature delivery, low birth weight (RR 0.79 CI 0.61 - 1.03), birth weight (+36.1 g CI -4.8 - 77.0), perinatal death or infant hemoglobin concentrations at 6 mo of age. It is important to consider these conclusions. Currently, blanket iron and folic acid supplementation programs for pregnant women are in place in many countries, with the expectation that it will substantially improve maternal and infant health (Bhutta et al. 2008). But apparently, the benefits of only iron and folate supplementation during pregnancy are less substantial and not as clear-cut as hoped for.

One explanation for the lack of improvement in maternal and infant health outcomes could be that the number of studies providing data on outcomes such as perinatal mortality was too low to draw consistent conclusions. Dibley and colleagues examined Indonesian demographic data with >40,000 pregnancies and showed that the iron and folic acid supplementation program protected against neonatal death in the first week after birth (RR: 0.53; 95% CI: 0.36–0.77) (Titaley et al. 2010b). And this beneficial effect also holds true in countries with endemic malaria, provided that it is combined with intermittent malaria treatment (Titaley et al. 2010a). Another explanation could be that other nutritional deficiencies, such as vitamin A deficiency or zinc deficiency, hampered a beneficial effect of the intervention. Perhaps, providing only iron (and folic acid) is not enough. Are multiple micronutrient supplements during pregnancy more effective? It is known that multiple micronutrient deficiencies often coexist (Dijkhuizen et al. 2001). Indeed, deficiency of multiple micronutrients in one individual is more common than single micronutrient deficiency (Thurlow et al. 2006). And given the multi-factorial etiology of anemia, a greater benefit might be expected from multiple micronutrient supplementation than from supplementation with iron and folic acid alone.

In the last decade, several large studies on the efficacy of multiple micronutrient supplementation during pregnancy on improving anemia and health outcomes have been conducted. However, results have been conflicting or confusing, partly because studies used different combinations of micronutrients, different amounts of micronutrients or different outcomes. An 2006 Cochrane review of 9 trials with >15,000 women showed that multiple micronutrient supplementation decreased the prevalence of low birth weight and maternal anemia (RR 0.61 CI 0.52 - 0.71) (Haider and Bhutta 2006). However, the effect of multiple micronutrient supplementation was not different from iron (+folic acid) supplementation alone and there was no effect on preterm births or peri-natal mortality. Hence, from this review, there appears to be no additional benefit of multiple micronutrient supplementation over only iron + folic acid during pregnancy. However, more recently, another meta-analysis using different criteria and inclusion of 2 recently published large trials, concluded that prenatal multi-micronutrient supplementation was associated with a significantly reduced risk of low birth weight and improved birth weight per se when compared with iron–folic acid supplementation (Shah and Ohlsson 2009). Some studies suggest that different combinations of micronutrients have different effects on the birth weight distribution curve, with iron and folic acid affecting the lower end of the distribution curve, meaning that there is only a specific effect on low-birth weight, without a change in overall birth weight. In contrast, supplementation with multiple micronutrients appears to shift the whole distribution curve to higher birth weights (Katz et al. 2006). Although this seems more beneficial, this could also have a downside. The shift towards higher birth weights after multiple micronutrient supplementation could possibly also increase the number of obstructed deliveries. Hence, the potential benefits on infant survival by reducing the number of low birth weight infants, might be nullified by increasing the number of large-for-gestational age infants (Katz et al. 2006). Also, there are indications that supplementation with micronutrients (especially zinc and vitamin A) during pregnancy might affect the immune system of the newborn, and that these effects might be long-lasting and may not be only beneficial (Raqib et al. 2007; Wieringa et al. 2010; Wieringa et al. 2008). It is unclear at present whether these concerns also hold true with a weekly multiple micronutrient supplement given during pregnancy, with supplements given before conception, or with food-based interventions such as fortification, but these strategies, by being more physiological, could well have less negative or nullifying effects and therefore be more effective overall. However, results of such interventions are scarce and not very clear yet at this moment.

Besides safety concerns, there are other aspects of supplementation programs which need to be taken into account. In a study in China, effects of micronutrient supplementation during pregnancy on outcomes such as birth weight were only significant when supplementation started *before 12 weeks* of gestation (Zeng et al. 2009). Neither iron + folic acid nor multiple micronutrient supplementation started after 12 weeks of gestational age had an effect on birth weight. Other studies confirm that hemoglobin concentrations early in pregnancy are related to low birth weight in a U-shaped curve. Women between 4 and 8 weeks of pregnancy with hemoglobin concentration between 90 and 99 g/L had a 3.27 (CI 1.09 - 9.77) higher risk for a low birth weight baby than the reference category (110 - 119 g/L), whereas risks for low birth weight and preterm birth also increased with hemoglobin concentrations >130 g/L (Zhou et al. 1998). However, it is unlikely that the conditions of the study (high compliance, very early start of supplementation) can be met by standard national programs, where women are more likely to report to the health system for the first time at around 16 weeks of pregnancy. Based on the above observations, it can be expected that the effects of supplementation programs for pregnant women, whether providing iron, iron + folic acid or multiple micronutrients, will be disappointingly small or absent.

### 3.3 Interventions for women of reproductive age

Surprisingly, only few studies have investigated the effects of pre-conception supplementation with iron or multiple micronutrients on maternal or neonatal health, even though improving micronutrient status before or early in pregnancy seems to be most effective, and nutritional status around conception is a very important determinant of pregnancy health and outcome. This is especially clear for folic acid, where pre-conceptual increases in status have a strong effect on the reduction of neural tube defects, with possibly >70% of neural tube defects prevented by adequate intakes of folic acid. For other micronutrients such as iron, the exact effect of pre-conception status on maternal and child health is less clear, mainly due a lack of studies in humans. To meet iron needs during gestation, women need an iron reserve of at least 300 - 500 mg prior to conception so as not to become iron deficient after the first trimester (Milman et al. 2005; Viteri and Berger 2005). Many women in developing countries will have much lower iron reserves than this and hence are at risk of becoming iron deficient during pregnancy. Indeed, even many women in affluent countries fail to enter pregnancy with adequate iron stores. Studies suggest that

56% of non-pregnant women in the USA had iron stores <300 mg (Viteri and Berger 2005) and <20% of Danish women were estimated to have adequate (>500 mg) iron stores before pregnancy (Milman et al. 2005). A multi-country trial in SE-Asia examined long-term effects of supplementing women of reproductive age with iron and folic acid by following the women through pregnancy and delivery (Cavalli-Sforza et al. 2005). In the non-pregnant women, iron status significantly improved over the intervention period. In Vietnam for example, anemia prevalence decreased from 45% at baseline to <20% after 9 months to 1 year. Moreover, longer pre-pregnancy supplementation was associated with less anemia and better iron status during the first and second trimester of pregnancy. Indeed, there was no IDA in the first and second trimester of pregnancy in women who started taking supplements >3 months before conception (Berger et al. 2005). Another important observation was that although anemia prevalence rose in the 3rd trimester of pregnancy, there was almost no severe anemia (Hb< 95 g/L). Severe anemia is directly associated with increased perinatal risk for mothers and newborns, whereas mild anemia is often physiological in the third trimester and is a sign of the hemodilution normally seen in pregnancy. Unfortunately, data on birth weight was available for only 200 infants, but there was a tendency towards higher birth weights per se (+81 g) in the weekly supplementation group (P=0.15) and towards lower prevalence of low birth weight (<2500 g; 3% and 9% respectively, P=0.08) (Berger et al. 2005). In Vietnam, weekly supplementation of iron and folic acid in combination with deworming has been continued as pilot to improve iron status of WRA and has been shown to be successful as such: provision of weekly iron and folic acid for free has resulted in significant reductions in anemia (from 38% to 19%) and ID (ferritin<15 μg/L) (23% to 9%) prevalence in Vietnamese WRA (Casey et al. 2009). Nowadays, the World Health Organization (WHO 2009) recommends weekly iron and folic acid in WRA as one of the strategies to reduce anemia during pregnancy.

Similar to pregnant women, deficiencies of more than one micronutrient are also likely in women of reproductive age. However, until now no studies have documented the long-term effects of providing women of reproductive age with multiple micronutrients.

### 3.4 Interventions for young children

Infants and young children are especially at risk of anemia and iron deficiency as growth increases nutrient requirements. Iron deficiency not only leads to anemia, but may, even before the onset of anemia, cause impairment of psycho-motor development which is in part irreversible (Beard 2001; Black 2003). In many developing countries, over 50% of infants are anemic by 1 year of age (Dijkhuizen et al. 2001). Although blanket iron supplementation for young children has being considered as an option to reduce anemia prevalence in childhood, studies comparing the effects of iron supplementation on infants in Sweden and Honduras suggested that iron supplementation in iron-replete infants may not be beneficial, and can cause growth faltering (Dewey et al. 2002). Furthermore iron supplementation in children living in malarious areas increased morbidity and mortality (Sazawal et al. 2006), iron supplementation may negatively influence zinc uptake and zinc status (Wieringa et al. 2007a), and iron supplementation in infancy may cause a redistribution of vitamin A (Wieringa et al. 2003) . Therefore, as public health interventions must operate from the '*Non Nocere*' (Do No Harm) principle, these potential adverse effects make global blanket iron supplementation for under-five children unfeasible.

Four parallel studies on iron and zinc supplementation in infants were conducted in South-East Asia (Thailand, Vietnam and Indonesia) to investigate effects on micronutrient status and growth. These studies showed that although iron status and anemia prevalence were significantly improved, no overall effect on growth could be found (Dijkhuizen et al. 2008). Also, despite iron supplementation for 6 mo, at least 25% of the infants remained anemic in the iron-supplemented groups. The prevalence of iron deficiency anemia, however, was less than 2.5% after iron supplementation. Hence, the anemia remaining after supplementation may be due to unresolved deficiencies of other nutrients such as vitamin $B_{12}$ or folic acid, to chronic inflammation, or to hereditary hemoglobinopathies. Estimates of for example α-thalassemia prevalence in the region ranges from 3 to 11% (Weatherall and Clegg 2001) and could explain at least part of the remaining anemia. However the data itself could also be interpreted differently perhaps. As discussed earlier, cut-off values for anemia in infancy are being reconsidered, and using other newly proposed (lower) cut-offs on these study results will give lower estimates of the prevalence of anemia. This is an important consideration whenever cut-off thresholds are used, the threshold that is used determines the prevalence found. Cut-off values for anemia that are currently used may not be appropriate for infants and may thus lead to an overestimation of anemia prevalence in this age group (Domellof et al. 2002a). Another interesting finding in the 4 studies in SE Asia, is that the effect of iron supplementation on hemoglobin concentrations was almost twice as large in boys than in girls (Wieringa et al. 2007b). Although hemoglobin concentrations differed between genders at recruitment, the differences were not as large as at the end of the study. Hence the largest part of the difference in hemoglobin concentrations between boy and girl infants developed during the second half of infancy. One possible explanation for these gender differences may be the higher growth rate of boy infants, leading to increased iron requirements. An important implication is that boy infants are more at risk for anemia and iron deficiency (Table 4), a finding that has been reported elsewhere also (Domellof et al. 2002b). We estimated that daily iron intake of boy infants should be almost 1 mg/d higher than that of girl infants to achieve similar iron body stores (Wieringa et al. 2007b). These considerations on age and gender related differences in iron status complicate the development of interventions, and together with the potential adverse effects of iron, make appropriate dosing and targeting important aspects to consider in intervention strategies for infants and under-five children. Also, approaches with lower, more physiological dosing such as weekly dosing and food based interventions such as fortification may have significant advantages here, as will be discussed below.

| | Relative Risk for Boy infants |
|---|---|
| Anemia | 1.6 (1.3 - 2.1) |
| Iron Deficiency Anemia | 3.3 (2.1 - 5.0) |

Table 4. Relative risk for boy infants to be anemic or have iron deficiency anemia at 11 months of age when not receiving iron supplements. Table adapted from (Wieringa et al. 2007b).

Besides supplementation, other strategies to improve anemia prevalence and micronutrient status of young children need to be considered. One noteworthy strategy is the provision of complementary foods fortified with micronutrients. In a series of studies in Vietnam, we showed that micronutrient-fortified complementary foods significantly improved iron status and reduced the prevalence of anemia (Phu et al. 2010). Importantly, the intervention showed that when infants received fortified complementary food from 5 months of age onwards, iron status remained at the same level, whereas iron status in the control group deteriorated over the 6 month intervention period. Other important strategies are delayed cord-clamping and the promotion of exclusive breastfeeding during the first 6 months of life (Dewey and Chaparro 2007). Indeed, iron stores can be increased by 33% by a 2-minute delay in clamping the umbilical cord (Dewey and Chaparro 2007)! De-worming is probably a less effective strategy in this age-group in Vietnam as the prevalence of parasitic infestation is still low, and only increases rapidly when the child starts to venture outside. However, large differences in the prevalence of parasitic infestation exist among cultures, so this intervention is also worth considering, and often added as an adjuvant measure in older children.

To conclude, although iron supplementation benefits hemoglobin concentrations and reduces the prevalence of anemia in infancy, potential adverse effects such as increased morbidity and mortality and growth-faltering in iron-replete infants make blanket supplementation unfeasible. Therefore, targeting is warranted, e.g. by screening infants prior to implementing iron supplementation. Appropriate and more physiological dosing is another important concern. Provision of high-quality complementary foods improves micronutrient status and reduces the prevalence of anemia, probably without the risk of detrimental effects on health or growth as seen with supplementation.

### 3.5 Interventions for school-aged children

School-age children are a neglected group with regard to interventions to reduce the prevalence of anemia or improve micronutrient status. One of the few interventions widely implemented is deworming. Helminthic infections have been shown to be major contributors to anemia and malnutrition in the developing world through effects on digestion and absorption, chronic inflammation and increased nutrient losses (Stoltzfus et al. 2000; Stoltzfus et al. 1997). However, many children only receive deworming every 6 months, a frequency which might not be enough to bring down parasite infestation if the infection rate is high. And only deworming might not be enough to restore depleted micronutrient stores (Hall 2007). Food provided at school that is fortified with multiple vitamins and minerals, in combination with regular deworming could be a more effective strategy to reduce anemia in school-aged children, and will supply the children with a whole range of nutrients necessary to grow and learn. The school food often also provides an additional motive for school attendance, which is an important concern in many countries. Indeed several studies have shown significant improvements in hemoglobin concentrations and micronutrient status from such combined programs (Faber et al. 2005; Nga et al. 2009; van Stuijvenberg et al. 1999). Besides improvements in micronutrient status, these studies also resulted in important improvements in cognitive function, thus showing also functional benefits of the intervention. Interestingly, in one study in Vietnam there was a high prevalence of anemia, but the prevalence of iron deficiency and iron deficiency anemia was low. Yet, biscuits fortified with multiple micronutrient decreased anemia prevalence by 40%, again highlighting the importance of other nutrients than only iron in the etiology of anemia (Nga et al. 2009). The same study reported an enhanced effect of deworming on Ascaris and Trichuris infection when combined with multi-micronutrient fortified biscuits, suggesting also improvements in immune function in school children who received fortified food (Nga et al. 2011). Given the low cost of food fortification (for example, fortifying a meal of rice per day for 1 school child would cost less than US$1/year), and the potential benefits, food fortification should be given high priority for this age group.

### 3.6 Interventions for adolescent girls

Finally, another often-forgotten age group is that of adolescent girls. Anemia prevalence is often high in adolescents girls due to blood loss through menstruation combined with an increase in growth rate. Reaching adolescent girls through existing health programs has been proven difficult, as often the most vulnerable groups are no longer attending school (Ahluwalia 2002), whereas anemia prevalence in these girls can be extremely high (Bulliyy et al. 2007). Otherwise, programs through schools have been shown to be effective in increasing hemglobin concentrations of adolescent girls (Tee et al. 1999), and as discussed above, multiple micronutrient supplementation is more beneficial than only iron and folic acid supplementation in reducing anemia prevalence as other nutritional causes of anemia are also addressed (Ahmed et al. 2010). The cultural context with regard to education, access to health care and other important aspects of the position of women play a disproportionally important role for this group, making the development and implementation of interventions especially challenging. However, as this group is poised to progress to WRA it is at the same time extremely urgent to reach this group.

There rests a special case for anemia in malaria endemic areas. This anemia is in part due to malaria infection, as there is an increased breakdown of erythrocytes. But as malaria itself is associated with poverty, nutritional deficiencies are also an important cause of anemia in these populations. However, interventions are not so easy, as the malaria infection is fuelled by iron and erythropiesis (Oppenheimer 2001). This makes for a dangerous combination, and indeed, many studies have found that iron supplementation increased morbibity and mortality in malaria endemic populations. The consensus for the moment is that iron supplementation interventions need to be combined with adequate bed-net usage and intermittent anti-malarial therapy (WHO/UNICEF 2007). Surprisingly, the increase in morbidity and mortality after iron supplementation in the study in Pemba was not only due to malaria but to a whole range of common childhood infections (Sazawal et al. 2006) suggesting a complex interplay between (sub-clinical) malaria infection, immune function and nutritional status. Again, food based interventions to improve iron status such as fortification and dietary diversification also seem to carry less risk to increase morbidity and mortality in malaria endemic areas, perhaps because the more physiological approach does not lead to an increase in the so-called non-transferrin bound iron (NTBI) (Troesch et al. 2011).

## 4. Conclusion

Anemia is major public health problem in many developing countries. Nutritional deficiencies of iron and also of other micronutrients underlie an important part of this, but are certainly not the sole contributor. Anemia is often regarded as nutritional anemia, however other causes of anemia include hemoglobinopathies (such as sickle cell trait and thalassemia), chronic infections (such as malaria and tuberculosis) and intestinal parasites. Anemia is also often equated to iron deficiency. However, WHO estimates that less than half of the anemia in the world is due to iron deficiency. Indeed, as shown by several studies from Vietnam, anemia prevalence remains high in vulnerable population groups whereas the prevalence of iron deficiency has decreased rapidly over the last decade. Other micronutrient deficiencies, such as vitamin $B_{12}$, folic acid or vitamin A deficiency, might underlie this paradox, although parasitic infestation certainly contributed to the anemia observed in this population. Many interventions with the potential to be effective in reducing anemia prevalence in vulnerable groups exist. Iron supplementation has been promoted for decades as a cost-effective strategy. However, care should be taken when implementing this intervention, as interactions with other micronutrients (zinc, copper, vitamin A) and infectious diseases (malaria) might lead to adverse effects, and correct timing of the intervention (early in pregnancy) appears to be of major importance for success. Interventions with multiple micronutrients have the benefit of addressing multiple causes of anemia, and have been shown to be successful in improving hemoglobin and micronutrient status of school children, with the additional benefit of improving cognition and immune function. Additional benefits of multiple micronutrient supplementation during pregnancy are unclear at the moment, with small gains in birth weight reported, but with no benefits for neonatal survival. New strategies such as weekly supplementation of women of reproductive age with multiple micronutrients need to be investigated urgently. For the long-term, food fortification to improve overall micronutrient status of populations is the most cost-effective strategy, with adverse effects less likely to occur, and targeting or differential dosing often automatically incorporated in the choice of food vehicle. Effective interventions directed at all stages of the life cycle are urgently needed and both policy and science should work in concert. Not only to explore new approaches, but also to critically evaluate existing evidence and efforts, and gain understanding in the complex physiological, nutritional and social factors involved in anemia as a public health problem. This will allow the development of evidence-based effective strategies that are tailored to specific populations, vulnerable groups and cultural settings, providing improved and more accurate tools to reduce anemia.

## 5. References

Ahluwalia N. 2002. Intervention strategies for improving iron status of young children and adolescents in India. Nutr Rev 60:S115-117.

Ahmed F, Khan MR, Akhtaruzzaman M, Karim R, Williams G, Torlesse H, Darnton-Hill I, Dalmiya N, Banu CP, and Nahar B. 2010. Long-term intermittent multiple micronutrient supplementation enhances hemoglobin and micronutrient status more than iron + folic acid supplementation in Bangladeshi rural adolescent girls with nutritional anemia. J Nutr 140:1879-1886.

Ayoya MA, Spiekermann-Brouwer GM, Traore AK, Stoltzfus RJ, and Garza C. 2006. Determinants of anemia among pregnant women in Mali. Food Nutr Bull 27:3-11.

Baig-Ansari N, Badruddin SH, Karmaliani R, Harris H, Jehan I, Pasha O, Moss N, McClure EM, and Goldenberg RL. 2008. Anemia prevalence and risk factors in pregnant women in an urban area of Pakistan. Food Nutr Bull 29:132-139.

Bates CJ, Powers HJ, and Thurnham DI. 1989. Vitamins, iron, and physical work. Lancet 2:313-314.

Beard JL. 2001. Iron biology in immune function, muscle metabolism and neuronal functioning. J Nutr 131:568S-579S.

Berger J, Thanh HT, Cavalli-Sforza T, Smitasiri S, Khan NC, Milani S, Hoa PT, Quang ND, and Viteri F. 2005. Community mobilization and social marketing to promote weekly iron-folic acid supplementation in women of reproductive age in Vietnam: impact on anemia and iron status. Nutr Rev 63:S95-108.

Berry RJ, Bailey L, Mulinare J, and Bower C. 2010. Fortification of flour with folic acid. Food Nutr Bull 31:S22-35.

Bhutta ZA, Ahmed T, Black RE, Cousens S, Dewey K, Giugliani E, Haider BA, Kirkwood B, Morris SS, Sachdev HP and others. 2008. What works? Interventions for maternal and child undernutrition and survival. Lancet 371:417-440.

Black MM. 2003. Micronutrient deficiencies and cognitive functioning. J Nutr 133:3927S-3931S.

Bulliyy G, Mallick G, Sethy GS, and Kar SK. 2007. Hemoglobin status of non-school going adolescent girls in three districts of Orissa, India. Int J Adolesc Med Health 19:395-406.

Casey GJ, Phuc TQ, Macgregor L, Montresor A, Mihrshahi S, Thach TD, Tien NT, and Biggs BA. 2009. A free weekly iron-folic acid supplementation and regular deworming program is associated with improved hemoglobin and iron status indicators in Vietnamese women. BMC Publ Health 9:261.

Cavalli-Sforza T, Berger J, Smitasiri S, and Viteri F. 2005. Weekly iron-folic acid supplementation of women of reproductive age: impact overview, lessons learned, expansion plans, and contributions toward achievement of the millennium development goals. Nutr Rev 63:S152-158.

Cogswell ME, Looker AC, Pfeiffer CM, Cook JD, Lacher DA, Beard JL, Lynch SR, and Grummer-Strawn LM. 2009. Assessment of iron deficiency in US preschool children and nonpregnant females of childbearing age: National Health and Nutrition Examination Survey 2003-2006. Am J Clin Nutr 89:1334-1342.

Critchley J, and Bates I. 2005. Haemoglobin colour scale for anaemia diagnosis where there is no laboratory: a systematic review. Int J Epidemiol 34:1425-1434.

Dewey KG, and Chaparro CM. 2007. Iron status of breast-fed infants. Proc Nutr Soc 66:412-2

Dewey KG, Domellof M, Cohen RJ, Landa Rivera L, Hernell O, and Lonnerdal B. 2002. Iron supplementation affects growth and morbidity of breast-fed infants: results of a randomized trial in Sweden and Honduras. J Nutr 132:3249-3255.

Dijkhuizen MA, Wieringa FT, West CE, Muherdiyantiningsih, and Muhilal. 2001. Concurrent micronutrient deficiencies in lactating mothers and their infants in Indonesia. Am J Clin Nutr 73:786-791.

Dijkhuizen MA, Winichagoon P, Wieringa FT, Wasantwisut E, Utomo B, Ninh NX, Hidayat A, and Berger J. 2008. Zinc supplementation improved length growth only in anemic infants in a multi-country trial of iron and zinc supplementation in South-East Asia. J Nutr 138:1969-1975.

Domellof M, Dewey KG, Lonnerdal B, Cohen RJ, and Hernell O. 2002a. The diagnostic criteria for iron deficiency in infants should be reevaluated. J Nutr 132:3680-3686.

Domellof M, Lonnerdal B, Dewey KG, Cohen RJ, Rivera LL, and Hernell O. 2002b. Sex differences in iron status during infancy. Pediatrics 110:545-552.

Engmann C, Adanu R, Lu TS, Bose C, and Lozoff B. 2008. Anemia and iron deficiency in pregnant Ghanaian women from urban areas. Int J Gyn Obst 101:62-66.

Faber M, Kvalsvig JD, Lombard CJ, and Benade AJ. 2005. Effect of a fortified maize-meal porridge on anemia, micronutrient status, and motor development of infants. Am J Clin Nutr 82:1032-1039.

Grosse SD, Waitzman NJ, Romano PS, and Mulinare J. 2005. Reevaluating the benefits of folic acid fortification in the United States: economic analysis, regulation, and public health. Am J Public Health 95:1917-1922.

Haider BA, and Bhutta ZA. 2006. Multiple-micronutrient supplementation for women during pregnancy. Cochrane Database of Systematic Reviews(4):-.

Hall A. 2007. Micronutrient supplements for children after deworming. The Lancet infectious diseases 7:297-302.

Hercberg S, Preziosi P, and Galan P. 2001. Iron deficiency in Europe. Public Health Nutr 4:537-545.

INACG. 2004. Efficacy and effectiveness of interventions to control iron deficiency and iron deficiency anemia.

Kalaivani K. 2009. Prevalence & consequences of anaemia in pregnancy. Ind J Med Res 130:627-633.

Katz J, Christian P, Dominici F, and Zeger SL. 2006. Treatment effects of maternal micronutrient supplementation vary by percentiles of the birth weight distribution in rural Nepal. J Nutr 136:1389-1394.

Khambalia A, O'Connor DL, and Zlotkin S. 2009. Periconceptional iron and folate status is inadequate among married, nulliparous women in rural Bangladesh. J Nutr 139:1179-1184.

Koury MJ, and Ponka P. 2004. New insights into erythropoiesis: the roles of folate, vitamin B12, and iron. Annu Rev Nutr 24:105-131.

Lartey A. 2008. Maternal and child nutrition in Sub-Saharan Africa: challenges and interventions. Proc Nutr Soc 67:105-108.

Mejia LA, and Chew F. 1988. Hematological effect of supplementing anemic children with vitamin A alone and in combination with iron. Am J Clin Nutr 48:595-600.

Milman N, Bergholt T, Eriksen L, Byg KE, Graudal N, Pedersen P, and Hertz J. 2005. Iron prophylaxis during pregnancy -- how much iron is needed? A randomized dose-response study of 20-80 mg ferrous iron daily in pregnant women. Acta Obstet Gyn Scan 84:238-247.

Nga TT, Winichagoon P, Dijkhuizen MA, Khan NC, Wasantwisut E, Furr H, and Wieringa FT. 2009. Multi-micronutrient-fortified biscuits decreased prevalence of anemia and improved micronutrient status and effectiveness of deworming in rural Vietnamese school children. J Nutr 139:1013-1021.

Nga TT, Winichagoon P, Dijkhuizen MA, Khan NC, Wasantwisut E, and Wieringa FT. 2011. Decreased parasite load and improved cognitive outcomes caused by deworming and consumption of multi-micronutrient fortified biscuits in rural vietnamese schoolchildren. Am J Trop Med Hyg 85:333-340.

Oppenheimer SJ. 2001. Iron and its relation to immunity and infectious disease. J Nutr 131:616S-635S.

Pena-Rosas JP, and Viteri FE. 2009. Effects and safety of preventive oral iron or iron+folic acid supplementation for women during pregnancy. Cochrane Database Syst Rev(4):CD004736.

Phu PV, Hoan NV, Salvignol B, Treche S, Wieringa FT, Khan NC, Tuong PD, and Berger J. 2010. Complementary foods fortified with micronutrients prevent iron deficiency and anemia in Vietnamese infants. J Nutr 140:2241-2247.

Powers HJ. 2003. Riboflavin (vitamin B-2) and health. Am J Clin Nutr 77(6):1352-1360.

Raqib R, Hossain MB, Kelleher SL, Stephensen CB, and Lonnerdal B. 2007. Zinc supplementation of pregnant rats with adequate zinc nutriture suppresses immune functions in their offspring. J Nutr 137:1037-1042.

Roodenburg AJ, West CE, Hovenier R, and Beynen AC. 1996. Supplemental vitamin A enhances the recovery from iron deficiency in rats with chronic vitamin A deficiency. Brit J Nutr 75:623-636.

Sazawal S, Black RE, Ramsan M, Chwaya HM, Stoltzfus RJ, Dutta A, Dhingra U, Kabole I, Deb S, Othman MK and others. 2006. Effects of routine prophylactic supplementation with iron and folic acid on admission to hospital and mortality in preschool children in a high malaria transmission setting: community-based, randomised, placebo-controlled trial. Lancet 367:133-143.

Shah PS, and Ohlsson A. 2009. Effects of prenatal multimicronutrient supplementation on pregnancy outcomes: a meta-analysis. Can Med Assoc J 180:E99-108.

Sight_and_Life. 2007. Nutritional Anemia. In: Kraemer R, and Zimmermann M, editors. 1 ed. Basel: Sight and Life Press.

Steer PJ. 2000. Maternal hemoglobin concentration and birth weight. Am J Clin Nutr 71:1285S-1287S.

Stoltzfus RJ. 2008. Research needed to strengthen science and programs for the control of iron deficiency and its consequences in young children. J Nutr 138:2542-2546.

Stoltzfus RJ, Chwaya HM, Montresor A, Albonico M, Savioli L, and Tielsch JM. 2000. Malaria, hookworms and recent fever are related to anemia and iron status indicators in 0- to 5-y old Zanzibari children and these relationships change with age. J Nutr 130:1724-1733.

Stoltzfus RJ, Chwaya HM, Tielsch JM, Schulze KJ, Albonico M, and Savioli L. 1997. Epidemiology of iron deficiency anemia in Zanzibari schoolchildren: the importance of hookworms. Am J Clin Nutr 65:153-159.

Suharno D, West CE, Muhilal, Karyadi D, and Hautvast JG. 1993. Supplementation with vitamin A and iron for nutritional anaemia in pregnant women in West Java, Indonesia. Lancet 342:1325-1328.

Sukrat B, Suwathanapisate P, Siritawee S, Poungthong T, and Phupongpankul K. The prevalence of iron deficiency anemia in pregnant women in Nakhonsawan, Thailand. J Med Assoc Thai 93:765-770.

Tee ES, Kandiah M, Awin N, Chong SM, Satgunasingam N, Kamarudin L, Milani S, Dugdale AE, and Viteri FE. 1999. School-administered weekly iron-folate supplements improve hemoglobin and ferritin concentrations in Malaysian adolescent girls. Am J Clin Nutr 69:1249-1256.

Thurlow RA, Winichagoon P, Pongcharoen T, Gowachirapant S, Boonpraderm A, Manger MS, Bailey KB, Wasantwisut E, and Gibson RS. 2006. Risk of zinc, iodine and other micronutrient deficiencies among school children in North East Thailand. Eur J Clin Nutr 60:623-632.

Thurnham D, McCabe L, Wieringa F, Northrop-Clewes C, and McCabe G. 2010. Adjusting plasma ferritin concentrations to remove effects of sub-clinical inflammation in the assessment of iron deficiency: a meta-analysis. Am J Clin Nutr 92:546-55..

Thurnham DI, McCabe GP, Northrop-Clewes CA, and Nestel P. 2003. Effects of subclinical infection on plasma retinol concentrations and assessment of prevalence of vitamin A deficiency: meta-analysis. Lancet 362:2052-2058.

Titaley CR, Dibley MJ, Roberts CL, and Agho K. 2010a. Combined iron/folic acid supplements and malaria prophylaxis reduce neonatal mortality in 19 sub-Saharan African countries. Am J Clin Nutr 92:235-243.

Titaley CR, Dibley MJ, Roberts CL, Hall J, and Agho K. 2010b. Iron and folic acid supplements and reduced early neonatal deaths in Indonesia. Bull WHO 88:500-8.

Trinh LT, and Dibley M. 2007. Anaemia in pregnant, postpartum and non pregnant women in Lak district, Daklak province of Vietnam. Asia Pacific J Clin Nutr 16:310-315.

Troesch B, Egli I, Zeder C, Hurrell RF, and Zimmermann MB. 2011. Fortification iron as ferrous sulfate plus ascorbic acid is more rapidly absorbed than as sodium iron EDTA but neither increases serum nontransferrin-bound iron in women. J Nutr 141:822-827.

Van Nhien N, Khan NC, Ninh NX, Van Huan P, Hop le T, Lam NT, Ota F, Yabutani T, Hoa VQ, Motonaka J and others. 2008. Micronutrient deficiencies and anemia among preschool children in rural Vietnam. Asia Pacific J Clin Nutr 17:48-55.

van Stuijvenberg ME, Kvalsvig JD, Faber M, Kruger M, Kenoyer DG, and Benade AJ. 1999. Effect of iron-, iodine-, and beta-carotene-fortified biscuits on the micronutrient status of primary school children: a randomized controlled trial. Am J Clin Nutr 69:497-503.

Vanderjagt DJ, Brock HS, Melah GS, El-Nafaty AU, Crossey MJ, and Glew RH. 2007. Nutritional factors associated with anaemia in pregnant women in northern Nigeria. J Health Pop Nutr 25:75-81.

Viteri FE, and Berger J. 2005. Importance of pre-pregnancy and pregnancy iron status: can long-term weekly preventive iron and folic acid supplementation achieve desirable and safe status? Nutr Rev 63:S65-76.

Weatherall DJ, and Clegg JB. 2001. Inherited haemoglobin disorders: an increasing global health problem. Bull WHO 79:704-712.

Weinberg ED. 1975. Nutritional immunity. Host's attempt to withold iron from microbial invaders. JAMA 231:39-41.

WHO. 2001. Iron Deficiency Anaemia Assessment, Prevention and Control. A guide for programme managers. Geneva: World Health Organization.

WHO. 2008. Worldwide prevalence of anaemia 1993–2005 : WHO global database on anaemia. Geneva: World Health Organization.

WHO. 2009. World Health Organization Position Statement. Weekly iron-folic acid supplementation (WIFS) in women of reproductive age: its role in promoting optimal maternal and child health. In: WHO, editor. Geneva: World Health Organization, 2009 (http://www.who.int/nutrition/publications/micronutrients/weekly_iron_folicacid.pdf (last accessed 20/09/2011).

WHO/UNICEF. 2007. Iron supplementation of young children in regions where malaria transmission is intense and infectious disease highly prevalent. p 1-2.

Wieringa FT, Berger J, Dijkhuizen MA, Hidayat A, Ninh NX, Utomo B, Wasantwisut E, and Winichagoon P. 2007a. Combined iron and zinc supplementation in infants improved iron and zinc status, but interactions reduced efficacy in a multicountry trial in southeast Asia. J Nutr 137:466-471.

Wieringa FT, Berger J, Dijkhuizen MA, Hidayat A, Ninh NX, Utomo B, Wasantwisut E, and Winichagoon P. 2007b. Sex differences in prevalence of anaemia and iron deficiency in infancy in a large multi-country trial in South-East Asia. Br J Nutr 98:1070-1076.

Wieringa FT, Dijkhuizen MA, Muhilal, and Van der Meer JW. 2010. Maternal micronutrient supplementation with zinc and beta-carotene affects morbidity and immune function of infants during the first 6 months of life. Eur J Clin Nutr 64:1072-1079.

Wieringa FT, Dijkhuizen MA, and van der Meer JW. 2008. Maternal micronutrient supplementation and child survival. Lancet 371:1751-1752.

Wieringa FT, Dijkhuizen MA, West CE, Northrop-Clewes CA, and Muhilal. 2002. Estimation of the effect of the acute phase response on indicators of micronutrient status in Indonesian infants. J Nutr 132:3061-3066.

Wieringa FT, Dijkhuizen MA, West CE, Thurnham DI, Muhilal, and Van der Meer JW. 2003. Redistribution of vitamin A after iron supplementation in Indonesian infants. Am J Clin Nutr 77:651-657.

Yip R. 1996. Iron supplementation during pregnancy: is it effective? Am J Clin Nutr 63:853-5.

Yip R. 2002. Iron supplementation: country level experiences and lessons learned. J Nutr 132:859S-861S.

Zeng L, Dibley M, Cheng Y, Chang S, and Yan H. 2009. What is the effect of starting micronutrient supplements early in pregnancy on birthweight, duration of gestation & perinatal mortality. Micronutrient Forum. Beijing.

Zhou LM, Yang WW, Hua JZ, Deng CQ, Tao X, and Stoltzfus RJ. 1998. Relation of hemoglobin measured at different times in pregnancy to preterm birth and low birth weight in Shanghai, China. Am J Epidem 148:998-1006.

Zimmermann MB, Biebinger R, Rohner F, Dib A, Zeder C, Hurrell RF, and Chaouki N. 2006. Vitamin A supplementation in children with poor vitamin A and iron status increases erythropoietin and hemoglobin concentrations without changing total body iron. Am J Clin Nutr 84:580-586.

# 11

# Risk Factors for Anemia in Preschool Children in Sub-Saharan Africa

Dia Sanou[1,*] and Ismael Ngnie-Teta[2]
[1]*Interdisciplinary School of Health Sciences, Faculty of Health Sciences, University of Ottawa*
[2]*UNICEF – Haiti and Adjunct Professor, Program of Nutrition, University of Ottawa*
*Canada*

## 1. Introduction

Iron is a mineral that is found in nature and foods. It is involved in many physiological functions in the body, and poor iron intake can lead to iron deficiency and later to anemia. Iron deficiency anemia (IDA) is the most prevalent nutritional disorder in the world despite iron being the fourth most common element on earth. Anemia is amongst the most important contributing factors to the global burden of disease. According to a recent WHO report on the global prevalence of anemia, one in four people is affected by anemia worldwide (McLean et al., 2009; WHO, 2008), with pregnant women and preschool-age children at the greatest risk. Two thirds of preschool-age children are affected in developing regions of Africa and South East-Asia, and about 40% of the world's anaemic preschool-age children reside in South-East Asia (McLean et al., 2009; WHO, 2008). Of the 293.1 million children who suffer from anemia worldwide, 83 million (28%) are in sub-Saharan Africa, representing 67% of the total population of children of this age group in the continent.

Adverse health consequences of anemia in preschool children include altered cognitive function, impaired motor development and growth, poor school performance, poor immune function and susceptibility to infections, decreased in responsiveness and activity, increased in body tension and fatigue. Even before clinical symptoms are visible, iron deficiency that leads to anemia is detrimental to children and may condemn one third of the world population to live permanently below their full mental and physical potential. Indeed, the impact of iron deficiency anemia on psychomotor development and cognitive function in children under the age of two years may be irreversible despite adequate therapy (Lozoff et al., 2000). Horton & Ross (2003) estimated the median productivity lost due to iron deficiency anemia alone to be about US$2.32 per capita or 4.05% of gross domestic product (GDP). The authors estimated an additional US$14.46 per capita lost in cognitive function, for a total annual loss (cognitive & productive) of about $50 billion in GDP worldwide from iron deficiency anemia. Due to its detrimental effects among children, effective interventions

*Corresponding Author

to improve iron status and reduce the burden of anemia will likely promote health and development.
Anemia is preventable, yet it remains the most widespread nutritional deficiency in the world. Countries, which realized significant progresses in the control of the problem have identified contextual risk factors and implement context relevant programs. In sub-Saharan African, conditions which increase the risk for anemia in children are complex and multidimensional. A first step for evidence-based interventions and policies towards the control and elimination of iron deficiency anemia is a better understanding of these risk factors. The current chapter discusses the determinants of iron deficiency anemia in sub-Saharan Africa children.

## 2. Definition and conceptual framework

In the literature, the terms anemia, iron deficiency, and iron-deficiency anemia are often used interchangeably, but are not equivalent. Anemia is defined as a significant reduction in hemoglobin concentration, hematocrit, or the number of circulating red blood cells at a level below that is considered normal for age, sex, physiological state, and altitude, without considering the cause of the deficiency (Nestel et al., 2002). Iron deficiency anemia is a condition in which there is anemia due to lack of available iron to support normal red cell production. It is the third and last stage of iron deficiency which starts with depletion of iron stores as reflected by a reduced serum ferritin concentration. The second stage is iron deficient erythropoiesis, characterized by decreased serum iron, transferrin saturation and serum ferritin concentration but with a normal hemoglobin concentration. Because anemia can arise from nutritional factors and from non-nutritional ones, several terms are used to classify anemia, including nutritional anemia, anemia of infection, anemia of chronic diseases, pernicious anemia. For the purpose of this chapter, we focus on the first three that are the most common in developing countries, have modifiable risk factors and can be prevented through appropriate behavioral tailored intervention.
Several factors contribute concurrently in childhood anemia, but their relationships to the onset of anemia are not identical. Therefore, from an epidemiological perspective, it is important to distinguish between the different factors. A causal factor is linked to the onset of a disease or the condition and precedes the disease. A risk factor is an element linked to a person (biologic or hereditary), a behaviour, lifestyle or environment that increases the likelihood of developing the condition and has been found correlated with the condition in epidemiological studies (Last, 2004). When an intervention targeting a factor can reduce the likelihood of the condition developing, the factor is considered a modifiable risk factor. A factor susceptible to increase the onset of a pathological condition is a determining factor or determinant. For example the major causal factors of iron deficiency that lead to anemia are low dietary iron intake, inadequate iron absorption, chronic blood loss, and increased iron demand. However, there are several other factors (non causal relationship) that contribute to anemia including among others sociocultural factors, poverty, maternal factors, chronic conditions secondary to AIDS, tuberculosis and genetic factors such as sickle cell and thalassemia. There are several levels of stratification of anemia risk factors for children including structural and environmental level factors, community level factors, household level factors and individual health and nutrition related factors. Figure 1 summarizes the

multi-level risk factors of anemia in children in developing countries. There is an anthropological perspective that can be seen as a transverse risk factor.

## 3. Anthropological perspective

Anthropologists believed that agrarian revolution that resulted in changes in dietary behaviours and outbreak of infectious diseases about 10,000 years ago has played an important role in the emergence and spread of iron deficiency and anemia (Denic & Agarwal, 2008; Wander et al., 2009). According to this theory, meat was the main source of energy prior to agrarian revolution. When humans turned from hunting to agriculture, the diet became deficient in bioavailable iron, thus increased the prevalence of iron deficiency and its subsequent anemia. Cultivating plant-based foods has increased calorie intakes, but reduced meat consumption. As a result, iron intake became insufficient to meet individual daily requirements. According to Mann (2007), daily total iron intake decreased from 87 mg in the Palaeolithic age to 15 mg in the twentieth century. In addition, increased consumption of plant-based foods has reduced the intake of absorbable iron because the amount of non-heme iron and inhibitors of iron absorption has increased in the diet, while the amount of heme iron has decreased.

With sedentarization and animal husbandry, carriers of infectious diseases were able to be transmitted from animals to humans leading to emerging or re-emerging human infectious diseases. Thereafter, poor environmental and hygienic conditions, crowding and lifestyle changes have resulted in proliferation and spread of these carriers (Denic & Agarwal, 2007). Several studies suggested that mild to moderate iron deficiency may protect against acute infection (Oppenheimer, 2001; Prentice, 2008; Sazawal *et al.,* 2006). Thus some authors put forward the hypothesis of a potential metabolic adaptation during which the human body self-regulates its iron to a deficiency status, the « iron-deficient phenotype », to prevent the severity of infections when re-infection is a continuous process (Denic & Agarwal, 2007). According to these authors, the important advancement in developed countries to control anemia are more likely due to the successful eradication of infections rather than the quality of diet. In malaria endemic areas such as Africa, the iron deficiency phenotype survived better over time (Denic & Agarwal, 2007; Wander et al., 2009). Therefore, iron substitution therapy in some population groups such as iron supplementation in children with no functional iron deficiency may cause more harm than good (Sazawal et al., 2006; WHO/UNICEF, 2006).

## 4. Dietary factors

The dietary risk factors for childhood anemia in developing countries include single or combined deficiency of micronutrients such as iron, folic acid, vitamin B6, vitamin B12, vitamin A and copper. Association has been found between anemia and deficiency of vitamin A, riboflavin, protein and other nutrients (Gamble *et al.,* 2004, Semba & Bloem 2002; Thorandenya et al. 2006; Rock et al., 1988). Although nutritional factors are thought to be the most important contributing factors to childhood anemia, their exact contribution to the risk of anemia is not well established and may vary with the level of infection and the diet quality. Magalhaes & Clements (2011) estimated that about 37% of Anemia cases in preschool children in three West African countries namely; Burkina Faso, Ghana and Mali could be averted by treating nutrition related factors alone.

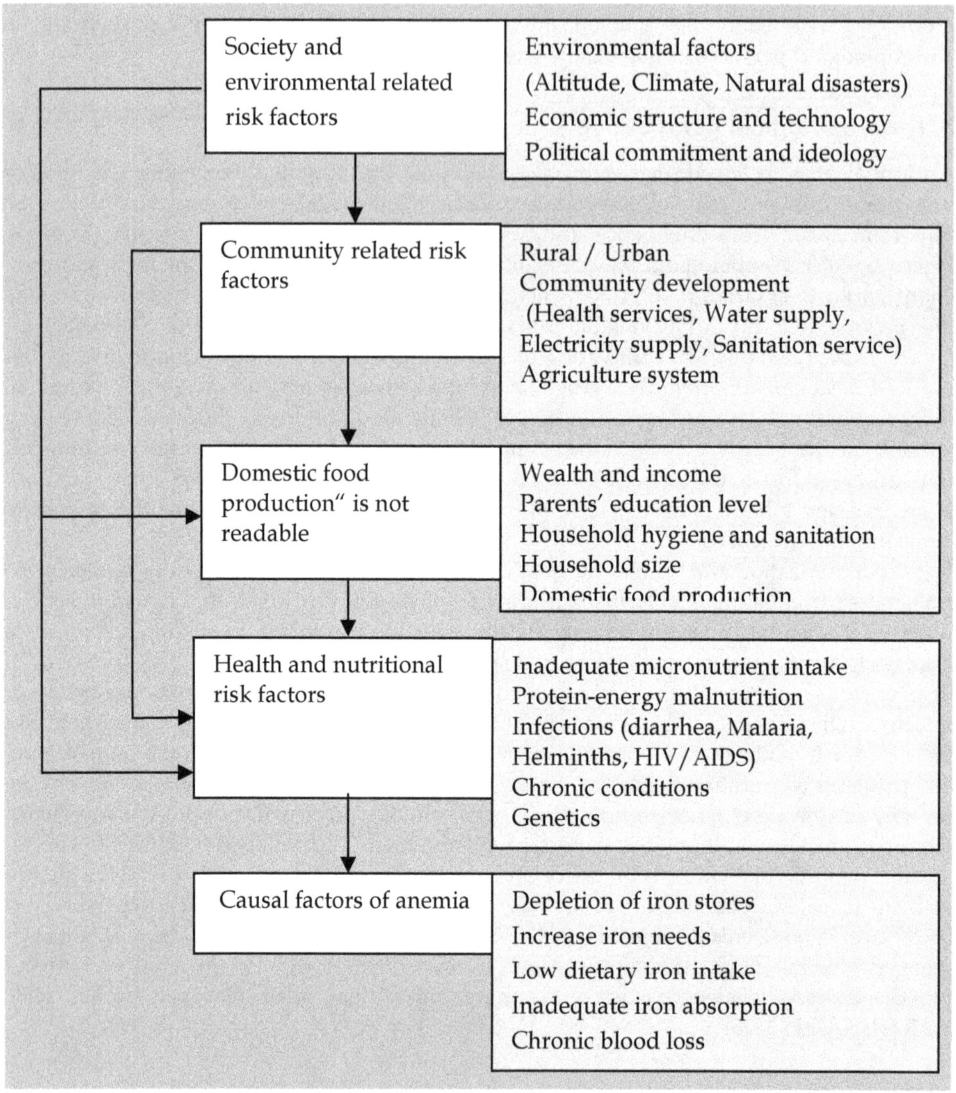


Fig. 1. Simplified conceptual framework for determinants of anemia among children (adapted from Ngnie-Teta et al, 2007).

### 4.1 Iron deficiency

The leading cause of anemia worldwide is iron deficiency due to inadequate intake or malabsorption of dietary iron. The adequacy of dietary iron depends on the intake and the bioavailability, which in turn are contingent to the nature of the food and the composition of the overall diet. In many developing countries, the amount of iron in the diet is usually enough to cover body needs, however because it is mainly provided by plant based food in the form of non-heme iron, its bioavailability is very low (Adish et al., 1998; Sanou et al., 2011; Zimmermann et al., 2005)

Iron is present in food in two forms: heme iron and non-heme iron. Heme is a component of hemoglobin and myoglobin and heme iron is mainly provided by animal tissues such as meat, poultry, fish and shellfish. Heme iron represents about 40% of animal tissue iron and is easily absorbed. However, it contributes to less than 15% of the total dietary iron, and may represent less than 1% in some countries where consumption of animal foods is very low (Monsen *et al.*, 1978). Most of the dietary iron is provided in the form of non-heme iron that is comprised of non-heme iron component of animal tissues, iron from eggs, milk and plant-based foods. The absorption rate of non-heme iron is very low and depends on iron status and combined effects of enhancers and inhibitors of iron absorption (Monsen et al., 1978). Enhancers of iron absorption include animal tissues (meat, poultry, and fish) and vitamin C and organic acids (Diaz *et al.* 2003; Reddy *et al.* 2000). Dietary factors that can reduce the absorption of iron (inhibitors) are phytates and some groups of polyphenols such as tannins (Reddy *et al.*, 2000; Sandberg et al., 1999), high intake of calcium and zinc (Lind *et al.*, 2003; Lynch, 2000), and cow's milk (Kibangou *et al.* 2005). Studies conducted in different regions of the world with high prevalence of anemia showed strong correlation between iron stores and absorbable iron intakes while there is no evidence of association between total iron intake, iron deficiency and anemia (Zimmermann *et al.*, 2005; Talata *et al.* 1998; Adish *et al.*, 1998).

### 4.2 Other micronutrient deficiencies associated with anemia

Other micronutrients are directly or indirectly involved in red blood cell metabolism. Vitamin $B_6$ (pyridoxal phosphate) for example is required for activation of Δ-aminolevulinic acid synthase that is necessary for heme synthesis. Vitamine $B_9$ (folate) and $B_{12}$ (cobalamine) deficiencies result in immature erythrocyte leading to macrocytic anemia (Gropper *et al.*, 2005). Poor vitamin A status has been associated with Anemia (Gamble et al., 2004; Semba & Bloem 2002) and vitamin A supplementation has been shown to reduce the prevalence of Anemia (Semba *et al.*, 2001). Copper is an enzymatic cofactor of ceruloplasmin (ferroxydase) that is involved in iron mobilisation during the hemoglobin synthesis. Therefore, a deficiency of copper may contribute to iron deficiency anemia (Gropper *et al.*, 2005). It has been suggested that because of some similarities metabolic pathways of iron and zinc, high level zinc intake in the form of supplement may reduce the effectiveness of iron supplementation programmes aimed at reducing the burden anemia (Lind *et al.*, 2003).

### 4.3 Severe acute malnutrition

Acute malnutrition resulting from inadequate dietary intake of nutrients and/or from acute infection and disease may also lead to mild to moderate anemia. Several hypotheses have been put forward to explain the relationship between anemia and protein-energy malnutrition; 1) adaptation to lower tissue-metabolic requirements for oxygen transport, 2) the reduction of protein required for hematopoiesis and 3) the reduction of survival time of red blood cells and the maturation of the erythroblasts (MacDougall *et al.*, 1982). Some authors however consider that the anemia of PEM is the outcome of a complex haematological process in which iron and other micronutrient deficiencies interplay (Awasthi *et al.*, 2003).

## 5. Infections

Infections are the second most important cause of anemia after iron deficiency and contribute in some settings to up to 50% of the cases (Asobayire *et al.*, 2001; Stoltzfus *et al.*, 2000). Children are particularly affected by infection-related anemia because of their lower immune response and their frequent exposure to poor sanitation and environmental conditions which favour the transmission and spread of parasites. Infections including malaria, hookworms, schistosomia, etc. are highly prevalent in developing countries and may negatively affect the nutritional status and growth of children. Studies conducted in many regions of Africa found positive associations between the presence and density of infection and chronic undernutrition, anemia and poor cognition (Brooker et al., 1999; Calis et al., 2008a; Friedman et al., 2005; Osazuwa et al. 2011; Sanou et al. 2008; Tolentino & Friedman, 2007). Regardless, the parasites or bacteria causing the anemia are different, all cases of anemia due to infection share some common pathways; 1) resulting iron deficiency through reduction of iron intake due to poor appetite and blood loss; 2) hemolysis i.e increased red blood cell destruction; 3) decreased red cells production and; 4) resulting inflammation. These mechanisms will be discussed later together with some pathways that are specific to each infection.

### 5.1 Malaria

The highest prevalence of childhood Anemia worldwide is found in malaria endemic regions. The WHO recent estimation of the global prevalence of anemia 1993-2005 suggested that between 31% and 90% of children in malaria-endemic areas of Africa suffer from anemia (WHO, 2008). Anemia is a common manifestation of the malaria infection and severe anemia can contribute to malaria mortality through hypoxia and cardiac failure (Memendez et al., 2000). Various *Plasmodium* species cause malaria, yet *P. falciparum* is the most critical for anemia in children. Contrary to iron deficiency anemia that develops slowly, *P. falciparum* causes severe and profound anemia within 48 hours of the onset of the fever. Other Plasmodium that can contribute to malaria include *P. vivax and P malariae.*

Table 1 shows the pathophysiology of malaria induced anemia. Philips and Pasvol (1992) summarized the pathophysiology of malarial anemia as follows, "anemia occurs when red cells are destroyed more rapidly than they can be replaced, or when red cell production falls below the minimal level required to maintain the steady state". Potential causes of increased red blood cell destruction include alteration of the red cell membrane rigidity and deformability, "loss of infected cells by rupture or phagocytosis, removal of uninfected cells due to antibody sensitization or other physico-chemical changes, and increased reticuloendothelial activity, particularly in organs such as the spleen" (Nuchsongsin et al., 2007; Park et al., 2008; Phillips & Pasvol, 1992). Factors leading to decreased red cell production include bone marrow hyploplasia and dyserythropoiesis. The severity of the malaria induced anemia is correlated with the density of the parasitaemia.

Although there is a consensus that clinical malaria causes severe anemia, there is limited evidence on the effect of asymptomatic malaria on severe anemia. While some authors reported that asymptomatic malaria does not significantly impact Haemoglobin level (Nkuo et al. 2002), some studies have demonstrated that asymptomatic malaria can cause homeostatic imbalance and lower Haemoglobin level in children (Kurtzhals et al. 1999); thus contributing to mild to moderate anemia (Price et al. 2001; Sowunmi et al., 2010; Umar et al. 2007). Imbalances of cytokines such as TNF-α, IL-6, IL-10 and IFN-γ resulting from malaria related-inflammation can induce changes in iron absorption and distribution, thus contributing to iron deficiency and subsequent iron deficiency anemia (Cercamondi et al., 2010; Shaw & Friedman, 2011). Bed net use is well documented as effective anemia prevention strategy (Korenromp et al., 2004, TerKuile, 2001). An exhaustive review of impact of malaria control on risk of anemia among children (Korenromp et al., 2004), estimates the protective effect of bed net on severe anemia to be 60%.

| Mechanism | Comments |
|---|---|
| **Increased erythrocyte destruction** | |
| **Non-immune mediated haemolysis** | Rupture of parasitized red blood cells (PRBC) following invasion of RBC by malaria parasites |
| | Phagocytosis of parasitized (PRBC) and unparasitized red blood cells (NPRBC) due to proliferation and hyperactivity of macrophages in the reticuloendothelial system; thus shortening their life span |
| | Premature removal of NPRBC from the circulation due to reduce deformability and membrane binding of parasite components |
| | Increased clearance of parasitaemia due to splenic hypertrophy and hypersplenism (increased activity of the spleen that filters malaria infected RBC from the circulation) |
| **Auto-immune haemolysis** | Increased premature removal and clearance of unparasitized RBC due to immunoglobulin and complement activation leading to an extravascular haemolysis |
| | Hapten induced intravascular haemolysis due to the use of quinine that acts as a hapten combining with RBC protein to become antigenic |
| **Decreased erythrocyte production** | |
| **Morphological abnormalities of the bone marrow** | Aberrations of erythroblast morphology, macrophage hyperplasia, erythroid hypolasia and failure of reticulocyte release following a repeated attacks of malaria |
| **Dyserythropoiesis** | Morphological abnormalities of the eryhtroid series including multinuclearity of the normoblasts, intercytoplasmic bridging, karyorrhexis, incomplete and unequal mitotic nuclear divisions in some individuals with malaria |
| **suppression of erythropoietin (EPO) synthesis** | Suppression of EPO synthesis by inflammatory mediators such as TNF in some adults with malaria |
| **Imbalances of cytokines (Inflammation induced anemia)** | Bone marrow depression, dyserythropoeisis and erythrophagocytosis following low interleukine (IL-10 and IL-12) or excess of T helper cell type 1 (th1), cytokines THF-a et TNF-x, and nitric acid (NO) |
| **Inflammation induced erythroid hypoplasia** | Suppression of normal response to erythropoietin due to an autologous serum factor that may suppress the growth of early precursors of RBC including the burst-forming unit-erythron (BFU-E) and the colony-forming unit erythron (CFU-E). |
| **Concomitant infections** | Increased susceptibility to secondary infections due to reduced immune systems following malaria infection |
| **Anti-malarial drugs** | |
| **Antifolate antimalarial** | Megaloblastic anemia due to overdosing of pyremethamine and/or trimethoprim |
| | Quinine induced intravascular auto-immune haemolysis |

Table 1. Pathophysiology mechanisms of malaria-related anemia (Memendez et al., 2000; Phillips & Pasvol, 1992).

Price et al. (2001) reported that treatment failure in uncomplicated malaria can lead to anemia. It has also been suggested that child undernutrition, particularly stunting modify the associations between malaria and anemia (Verhoef et al. 2002). Verhoef et al (2002) reported that stunting impairs host immunity, increases inflammation, and increases iron demand in developing erythroblasts, thus increasing the malaria-associated anemia.

### 5.2 Hookworms

Helminths are a group of intestinal nematodes that are recognized as a major public health problem in many developing countries. The effects on anemia are well documented for four species, namely trichomonas (*Trichuris trichiura),* ankylostoma (*Necator americanus, Ancylostoma duodenale*), hookworm (*Hymelolepis nana*) and ascaris (*Ascaris lumbricoides*). It is believed that the burden of hookworm is the most important particularly on severe anemia and is mostly due to extracorporeal blood loss in the stools resulting from a parasite release of a coagulase in the blood. *A. duodenale* was found more harmful than *N. americanum* and Skeletee (2003) for example estimated that it can cause approximately 0.25 mL blood loss per parasite per day during pregnancy.

According to a study done in Kenyan preschool children, hookworm contributed to 4% of anemia cases in children and heavy infection with hookworm increases the risk of anemia by 5 (Brooker et al., 1999). However, the authors did not find any association between hookworm and hemoglobin concentration likely due to the relatively low prevalence of the infection. Indeed, the burden of hookworm is directly related to the intensity of infection, the infecting species and the individual's nutritional status.

Calis et al. (2008a) also reported that the likelihood of developing severe anemia was increased by 4.8 in hookworm infected Malawian preschool children. In West Africa, a risk mapping approach using geostatistical models estimated that 4.2% of anemia cases in preschool children could be averted by treating hookworm (Magalhaes & Clements, 2011). *Trichomonas trichiura*, the causal agent of Trichuris Dysentery Syndrome has been associated with growth failure and Anemia. The anaemic effect of *T. trichiura* is thought to be linked to the blood consumption by the worm, inflammation induced anemia and reduced dietary iron intake due to decreased appetite (Shaw & Friedman, 2011).

Intervention studies have shown positive associations between mass deworming and decreased prevalence of anemia, physical performance, cognitive scores, growth and general morbidity among children from developing countries. Further, there is evidence that effectiveness of iron interventions such as supplementation and dietary approaches may be reduced when activities aiming at controlling infections are not part of the strategies (Davidson *et al.*, 2005). Therefore, it is recommended to include deworming in interventions targeting iron status at the community level.

### 5.3 Human schistosomiasis

Three major species of schistosomiasis have been identified as the most prevalent worldwide and cause human disease. These species that are endemic in some rural areas of Africa include *Schistosoma haematobium S. mansoni and S. japonica* (Friedman et al., 2005; Dianou *et al.*, 2004). Although most attention has been on schoolchildren, some studies have examined the relationship between schistosomiasis and anemia in preschool children (Brooker et al., 1999; Magalhaes & Clements, 2011; Talata et al., 1998). Friedman et al. (2005) described four mechanisms underlying the relationship between schistosome infections and anemia: 1) iron deficiency due to extracorporeal blood loss of iron; 2) splenic sequestration iii) auto-immune hemolysis and; 4) anemia of inflammation. It is also important to mention that infection may reduce appetite and disturb the intakes, absorption and metabolism of dietary iron.

### 5.4 HIV/AIDS

Anemia is a common hematological manifestation in Human immunodeficiency (HIV-infection), and has been identified as a marker for disease progression and survival (Calis et al., 2008b). A review of the global literature on HIV-related anemia in children by Calis et al. (2008b) revealed that mild to moderate anemia was more prevalent and hematocrit levels lower in HIV-infected children as compared to uninfected children. The authors also found that Anemia prevalence was higher in children with more advanced disease. However, blood loss and hemolysis are not common in HIV-infection. The suspected pathogenetic mechanisms for HIV-related anemia likely include decreased production of erythrocytes and subsequent inflammation. Further, based on findings from Uganda (Totin et al., 2002) and South Africa (Eley et al., 2002) that have suggested that iron deficiency anemia is equally affecting both HIV-infected and uninfected children, Shaw & Friedman (2011) concluded that HIV-related anemia is an Anemia of inflammation.

### 5.5 Bacteremia

The most common anemia inducing bacteria reported in the literature *is Helicobacter pylori* (Digirolamo *et al.* 2007; Dubois & Kearney 2005). *H. pylori* is thought to cause anemia through three mechanisms: 1) reduced iron absorption due to hypochlorhydria resulting from impaired secretion of gastric acid; 2) inflammation and; 3) competing iron demands of the bacteria and the host (Shaw & Friedman, 2011). Nontyphoid *Salmonella* has been also independently associated with anemia in children (Calis et al. 2008a; Dubois et al., 2005).

Although not investigated, it is possible that other species that can cause bloody dysentery such as *Shigella* and *Enteroinvasive E. coli* contribute to anemia. Comorbid conditions such as fever and respiratory infection often resulting from bacterial infection have been correlated with anemia (Stoltzfus *et al.*, 2000; Howard *et al.*, 2007). Diarrheal illness is associated with loss of iron and decreased absorption of nutrients needed to maintain normal Hb status. It is also likely that as demonstrated for other nutrient deficiencies, diarrhea shares many common causes with anemia (Tomkins, 1986).

Further due to the high susceptibility of HIV-infected children to opportunistic infection, bacteria may also act as synergetic factors in HIV-related anemia. A number of studies have reported biological synergisms between pathogens for disease progression (Ezeamama et al., 2008; Robertson et al., 1992). Ezeamama et al. (2008) investigated the effect of codistribution of schistosomiasis, hookworm and trichuris infection on paediatric anemia and found that hookworm and *S. japonicum* infections were independent risk factors for anemia and that co-infections of hookworm and either *S. japonicum* or *T. trichiura* were associated with higher levels of anemia than would be expected if the effects of these species had only independent effects on anemia. More recently, Magalhaes & Clements (2011) found that hookworm/S. haematobium coinfection significantly increased the likelihood of pediatric anemia as compared to individual infestation with one of these pathogens.

## 6. Inflammation and chronic diseases

Anemia of inflammation also termed the anemia of chronic disease (ACD) is the second most prevalent type of anemia after anemia of iron deficiency. It is observed in patients with chronic infectious disease (tuberculosis, meningitis, pulmonary infection to name a few), non-infectious chronic conditions (rheumatoid arthritis, Crohn disease, burn patients, etc.) or chronic neoplasic conditions (leukemia, carcinoma, Hodgkin disease, etc.) (Weiss & Goodnough, 2005). The pathophysiological mechanisms are not well understood, but it is believed that they are similar to the indirect pathways by which infection causes anemia. Anemia of chronic inflammatory diseases is immune driven and includes several pathways regulated by different immune and inflammatory mediators (Weiss & Goudnough, 2005):

- decreased red blood cell half-life because of dyserythropoiesis, red blood cell damage and increased erythrophagocytosis (TNF-α);
- inadequate erythropoietin responses for the degree of anemia in most, but not all (e.g. systemic-onset of juvenile chronic arthritis) (IL-1 and TNF-α);
- impaired responsiveness of erythroid cells to erythropoietin (IFN-γ, IL-1, and TNF-α);
- inhibited proliferation and differentiation of erythroid cells (IFN-γ, IL-1, TNF-α, and α-1-antitrypsin); and
- pathological iron homeostasis caused by increased DMT-1 (IFN-γ) and TfR (IL-10) expression in macrophages, reduced ferroportin 1 expression (IFN-γ and IL-6-induced high hepcidin levels) in enterocytes (inhibition of iron absorption) and macrophages (inhibition of iron recirculation), and increased ferritin synthesis (TNF-α, IL-1, IL-6, IL-10) (increased iron storage).

In a review published in New England Journal of Medicine, Weiss & Goudnough (2005) carefully discussed these mechanisms and summarized them in a single figure (Figure 2).

Recent studies have identified hepcidin as the main iron regulatory hormone in human (Andrews & Schmidt, 2007, Ganz, 2003). Hepcidin is an antimicrobial hormone that is synthesized in response to liver iron levels, inflammation, hypoxia and anemia. The persistence of inflammation results in excess hepcidin which in the circulation binds ferroportin on enterocytes and macrophages. The excess of hepcidin lowers iron absorption and prevents iron recycling, which results in hypoferremia and iron-restricted erythropoiesis, despite normal iron stores (functional ID), and anemia of chronic disease. In acute inflammation-related anemia (e.g. trauma or surgery), inflammatory responses are mediated by cytokine production mainly IL-6 and IL-8 (Weiss & Goudnough, 2005). Indeed, during inflammation, cytokines such as interleukin IL-6 stimulates the human hepcidin gene (HAMP) which in turns induces hepcidin secretion in the hepatocytes (Nicolas *et al.*, 2002; Nemeth *et al.*, 2004). In contrast, decreased hepcidin expression due to iron deficiency, anemia and hypoxia may lead to hereditary haemochromatosis (HH type I, mutations of the HFE gene) and type II (mutations of the hemojuvelin and hepcidin genes). In persisting iron deficiency due to decreased iron absorption and/or chronic blood loss, anemia of chronic disease evolves to anemia of chronic disease with a true iron deficiency (ACD + ID).

It is also important to keep in mind that the links between anemia and infection are bilateral and may be mutually beneficial. Indeed iron deficiency may protect against adverse effects of infections on iron status (Denic & Agarwal 2007; Sazawal *et al.*, 2006; Oppenheimer, 2001; Weinberg 1984).

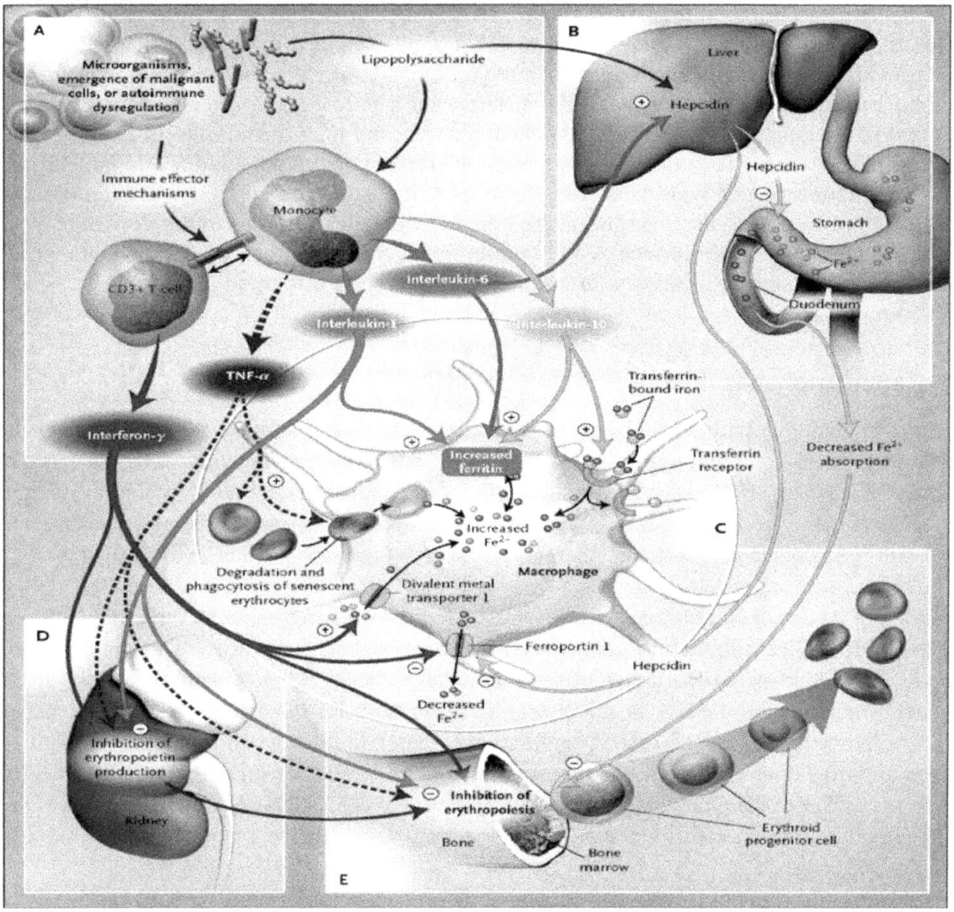


Fig. 2. Pathophysiological mechanisms of anemia of chronic diseases (Weiss & Goudnough, 2005) - reproduced with the permission from the authors and the New England Journal of Medicine -

In Panel A, the invasion of microorganisms, the emergence of malignant cells, or autoimmune dysregulation leads to activation of T cells (CD3+) and monocytes. These cells induce immune effector mechanisms, thereby producing cytokines such as interferon-γ (from T cells) and tumor necrosis factor α (TNF-α), interleukin-1, interleukin-6, and interleukin-10 (from monocytes or macrophages). In Panel B, interleukin-6 and lipopolysaccharide stimulate the hepatic expression of the acute-phase protein hepcidin, which inhibits duodenal absorption of iron. In Panel C, interferon-γ, lipopolysaccharide, or both increase the expression of divalent metal transporter 1 on macrophages and stimulate the uptake of ferrous iron (Fe2+). The antiinflammatory cytokine interleukin-10 up-regulates transferrin receptor expression and increases transferrin-receptor–mediated uptake of transferrin-bound iron into monocytes. In addition, activated macrophages phagocytose and degrade senescent erythrocytes for the recycling of iron, a process that is further induced by TNF-α through damaging of erythrocyte membranes and stimulation of phagocytosis. Interferon-γ and lipopolysaccharide down-regulate the expression of the macrophage iron transporter ferroportin 1, thus inhibiting iron export from macrophages, a process that is also affected by hepcidin. At the same time, TNF-α, interleukin-1, interleukin-6, and interleukin-10 induce ferritin expression and stimulate the storage and retention of iron within macrophages. In summary, these mechanisms lead to a decreased iron concentration in the circulation and thus to a limited availability of iron for erythroid cells. In Panel D, TNF-α and interferon-γ inhibit the production of erythropoietin in the kidney. In Panel E, TNF-α, interferon-γ, and interleukin-1 directly inhibit the differentiation and proliferation of erythroid progenitor cells. In addition, the limited availability of iron and the decreased biologic activity of erythropoietin lead to inhibition of erythropoiesis and the development of anemia. Plus signs represent stimulation, and minus signs inhibition (Weiss & Goudnough, 2005).

## 7. Genetic polymorphisms

Some hemoglobinopathies such as sickle-cell disease, thalassaemias, glucose-6-phosphate deshydrogenase are common in many developing countries (Deyde et al., 2002; Simpore *et al.,* 2003; Thurlow *et al.,* 2005). These disorders are particularly found in malaria endemic areas and have been associated with Anemia. Glucose-6-phosphate deshydrogenase for example is correlated with chronic haemolytic Anemia (Lang *et al.,* 2002; van Bruggen *et al.,* 2002).

Sickle cell Anemia is highly prevalent in West Africa, with a frequency of the trait of 15% to 30% (WHO, 2006). Many studies suggested that these red cell polymorphisms are a human body adaptation against adverse effects of malaria. Sickle cell for example results from genetic mutation of allele A in allele S or C of the β chain to provide resistance against *Plasmodium* effect (Modiano *et al.* 2008; Rihet *et al.* 2004). In Gambia and Burkina Faso, it has been reported that sickle-cell trait is associated with protection against malaria, malaria Anemia and even cerebral Anemia (Hill, 1991; Modiano et al., 2008). In central Burkina Faso, the prevalence is expected to increase if the malaria prevalence does not decrease (Modiano et al., 2008).

Data from the National Health and Nutrition Examination Survey» (NHANES I, II et III) of the USA consistently show hemoglobin levels of Black Americans are usually lower than for their white and hispanic counterparts at all ages, regardless of the iron, health et socioeconomic status (Johnson-Spear & Yip, 1995). This finding has resulted in an adjustment of Haemoglobin cut-off for population origin 1 g/L below the normal cut-off for other population groups (Nestel et al., 2002). Although the causes of this difference is not well established, it is hypothesized that high prevalence of hemoglobinopathies such as thalassaemias and chronic inflammations as well as other genetic disorders may be important contributing factors (Beutler & West, 2005).

## 8. Socio-economic risk factors

The socioeconomic status, commonly measured by household income and/or household assets is a key determinant of anemia. There is strong evidence that that children living in low income household are at greater risk of anemia compared to those with higher income. Limited access to food and poor sanitation are often correlated to low income and to some extent, explain the higher risk of anemia among these children (Osorio et al., 2004). Moreover, the diet of children living in poor families is usually monotonous, even when there is enough food to eat. A study by Ag Bendech et al. (1996) in Burkina Faso showed that even though almost all the family enrolled were having three meals per day, only children from the wealthiest families were taken two or three different meals while their peers from middle income and poor households had the same meals for breakfast, lunch and dinner. The authors also reported that animal source foods which are rich in bioavailable iron were limited, contributing to only 9% of the total protein intake in poor households, 19% in middle income households and up to 41% in wealthiest households (Ag Bendech et al., 1996).

Parent's level of education constitutes another well documented determinant of anemia in children. Educated parents are more likely to have well paid job and also more likely to adopt healthier dietary behavior. In Brazil, Osorio's et al. (2004) found that mean hemoglobin level of children whose mothers attended secondary schools (9 years of schooling) was 11.5 g/dl, 11.2 for mothers with 5-8 years in school and 10.8 g/dl for mothers with less than 4 years of schooling. De Pee et al. (2002) report similar results among Palestinian children with risk of anemia twice higher for children from non-educated mothers. Even in developed countries, low level of education is associated with higher risk of anemia (Sargent et al., 1996; Soh et al., 2004).

Community level factors play an important role in the risk of anemia. Several studies have shown that living in rural areas increases the risk of child malnutrition (Kuate-Defo, 2001 ; Sommerfelt, 1991) and anemia (Bentley 2003; Osorio et al. 2001; Osorio et al., 2004; Ngnie-Teta et al., 2007). Altitude also affects the risk of anemia. Indeed, the amount of oxygen decrease with altitude, hence reducing the saturation ability of hemoglobin to capture oxygen (Cohen & Haas, 1999). This should be counterbalanced by an increased number of red blood cells. Therefore hemoglobin cut-offs have been adjusted for different age groups according to the altitude (Nestel *et al.,* 2002).

Due to increasing use of multilevel, modelling neighbourhood contribution to the risk of disease could now be quantified. A recent study in West Africa reported significant contribution of community factors of 14% to 19% to the prevalence of moderate-to-severe anemia (Ngnie-Teta et al., 2007; 2008). This reflects the variability in the risk of anemia attributable to the differences between communities, regardless of individual and households characteristics.

## 9. Conclusion

Anemia can result from deficiency of one or several micronutrients but also unfavourable environmental conditions and social determinants of health. Although quantitative and qualitative iron deficiency is thought to be the leading cause, infection such as malaria, schistosomiasis, hookworms, HIV and bacteria can contribute to up to 50% of the cases of anemia in developing regions where these conditions are common. Due to the multi-factorial conditions, the complexity of the risk factors of anemia, and potential interactions among them, a single strategy to control anemia in developing countries may have little success. Country level strategies to tackle anemia should include an emergency nutrition programme that will target severe anemia particularly in children under the age of two and children who live in rural areas, but also a broader nutrition and health programme that may to prevent and treat moderate to mild Anemia. Whatever strategy is used, nutrition education to increase animal sources in the diet where possible in order to enhance bioavailability of iron and to improve sanitation and basic hygiene are highly recommended as complementary measures.

## 10. Acknowledgement

We are grateful to Dr Weiss Gunter from the Medical University of Innsbruck, Austria and the Publishing Division of the Massachusetts Medical Society, publisher of the New England Journal of Medicine for granting us the permission to use their illustration. Our colleagues and friends who help with the editing of the earlier version of the manuscript namely Dr Nonsikelelo Mathe from the University of Alberta, Canada, Dr Reginald Annan from the International Malnutrition Task Force, University of Southampton, UK and Mrs Sabra Saleh from the Micronutrient Initiative, Dakar Senegal are kindly thanked.

## 11. References

Adish AA, Esrey ES, Gyorkos TW, Johns T, 1998. Risk factors for iron deficiency anemia in preschool children in northern Ethiopia. *Public Health Nutr* 2(3) : 243–252.

Ag Bendech M, Chauliac M and D Malvy Variability of home dietary habits of families living in Bamako (Mali) according to their socioeconomic status. Sante. 1996;6(5):285-297.

Andrews NC, Schmidt PJ, 2007. Iron Homeostasis. *Ann Rev Physiol* 69 : 69–85.

Awasthi S, Das R, Verma T, 2003. Anemia and undernutrition among preschool children in Uttar Pradesh, India. *Indian Pediatr* 40 : 985-990.

Asobayire FS, Adou P, Davidson L, Cook JD, Hurrell RF, 2001. Prevalence of iron deficiency with and without concurrent anemia in population groups with high prevalence of malaria and infections: a study in Côte d'Ivoire. *Am J Clin Nutr* 74 : 776-782.

Beutler E, West C, 2006. Hematologic differences between African-Americans and whites: the roles of iron deficiency and α-thalassemia on hemoglobin levels and mean corpuscular volume. *Blood* 106(2) : 740–745.

Brooker S, Peshu N, Warn PA, Mosobo M, Guyatt H, Marsh K, Snow RW, 1999. Epidemiology of hookworm infection and its contribution to anemia among pre-school children on the Kenyan coast. *Trans Royal Soc Trop Med Hyg* 93: 240–246.

Calis JCJ, Phiri KS, Faragher EB, Brabin BJ, Bates I, Cuevas LE, et al., 2008a. Severe anemia in Malawian children. *N Engl J Med* 358(9) : 888-899.

Calis JCJ, Boele van Hensbroek MB, de Haan RJ, Moons P, Brabin BJ, Bates I, 2008b. Risk factors and correlates for anemia in HIV treatment-naïve infected patients: a cross-sectional analytical study. *AIDS*. 22(10):1099-112.

Cercamondi CI, Egli IM, Ahouandjinou E, Dossa R, Zeder C, Salami L, Tialsma H, et al. 2010. Afebrile Plasmodium falciparum parasitemia decreases absorption of fortification iron but does not affect systemic iron utilization: a double stable-isotope study in young Beninese women. *Am J Clin Nutr 2010;92:1385–92.*

Chandra J, Jain V, Narayan S, Sharma S, Singh V, Kapoor AK, Batra S, 2002. Folate and cobalamin deficiency in megaloblastic anemia in children. *Indian Pediatr* 39(5):453-7.

Cohen JH, Haas JD, 1999. Hemoglobin correction factors for estimating the prevalence of iron deficiency anemia in pregnant women residing at high altitudes in Bolivia. *Pan Am J Public Health* 6(6) : 392-399.

Davidson L, Nestel P et le comité de pilotage de l'INACG, 2005. *Efficacité et efficience des interventions dans la lutte contre la carence en fer et l'anémie ferriprive.* Washington 6 p.

De Pee S., Bloem M.W., Sari M., Kiess L., Yip R. The high prevalence of low hemoglobin concentration among indonesia infants aged 3-5 months is related to maternal anemia. J. Nutr 2002; 132:2215-21

Denic S, Agarwal MM, 2007. Nutritional iron deficiency: an evolutionary perspective. *Nutrition* 23(7-8) : 603-14.

Deyde V, Lo B, Khalifa I, Ball A, Fattoum S, 2002. Epidemiological profile of hemoglobinopathies in the Mauritanian population. *Ann Hemat* 81 (6): 320-321.

Dianou D, Poda JN, Savadogo LG, Sorgho H, Wango SP, Sondo B,2004. Parasitoses intestinales dans la zone du complexe hydroagricole du Sourou au Burkina Faso. *Vertigo* 5(2) : 1-8.

Diaz M, Rosado JL, Allen LH, Abrams S, García OP, 2003. The efficacy of a local ascorbic acid-rich food in improving iron absorption from Mexican diets: a field study using stable isotopes. *Am J Clin Nutr* 78 : 436–440.

Digirolamo AM, Perry GS, Gold BD, Parkinson A, Provost E, Parvanta I et al., 2007. Helicobacter pylori, anemia, and iron deficiency: relationships explored among Alaska native children. *Pediatr Infect Dis J* 26(10) : 927-934.

Dubois S, Kearney JD, 2005. Iron-deficiency anemia and Helicobacter pylori infection: A review of the evidence. *Am J Gastroent* 100(2) : 453–459.

Eley BS, Sive AA, Shuttleworth M, Hussey GD, 2002. A prospective, cross-sectional study of anemia and peripheral iron status in antiretroviral näive, HIV-1 infected children in Cape Town, South Africa. *BMC Infect Dis* 2(3) Epub 2002

Ezeamama AE, McGarvey ST, Acosta LP, Zierler S, Manalo DL, et al. (2008) The synergistic effect of concomitant schistosomiasis, hookworm, and trichuris infections on children's anemia burden. PLoS Negl Trop Dis 2: e245. doi

Friedman JF, Kanzaria HK, McGarvey ST, 2005. Human schistosomiasis and anemia: the relationship and potential mechanisms *Trends in Parasitology* 21(8):386-92.

Gamble MV, Palafox NA, Dancheck B, Ricks MO, Briand K, Semba RD, 2004. Relationship of vitamin A deficiency, iron deficiency, and inflammation to anemia among preschool children in the Republic of the Marshall Islands. *Eur J Clin Nutr* 58(10) :1396-401.

Ganz T, 2003. Hepcidin, a key regulator of iron metabolism and mediator of anemia of inflammation. *Blood* 102 : 783-788.

Gibson RS, Ashwell M, 2003. The association between red and processed meat consumption and iron intakes and status among British adults. *Public Health Nutr* 6(4) : 341-350.

Gleason GR. Iron deficiency anemia finally reaches the global stage of public health. Nutr Clin Care. 2002 (5):217-9

Gropper SS, Smith JL, Groff JL, 2005. *Advanced nutrition and human metabolism.* 14th ed. Thomson Wadsworth. Belmont CA.

Hill AV, Allsopp CE, Kwiatkowski D, Anstey NM, Twumasi P, Rowe PA, Bennett S, Brewster D, McMichael AJ, Greenwood BM, 1991. Common west African HLA antigens are associated with protection from severe malaria. *Nature* 352(6336):595.

Horton S, Ross J, 2003. The economics of iron deficiency, *Food Policy* 28:51-75.

Howard CT, de Pee S, Sari M, Bloem MW, Semba RD, 2007. Association of diarrhea with anemia among children under age five living in rural areas of Indonesia. *J Trop Pediatr* 53(4) : 238-244.

Jain SK, Williams DM, 1988. Copper deficiency anemia: altered red blood cell lipids and viscosity in rats. Am J Clin Nutr 48(3):637-40.

Johnson-Spear MA, Yip R, 1995. Hemoglobin difference between black and white women with comparable iron status: justification for race-specific anemia criteria. *Am J Clin Nutr* 60 : 117-121.

Kibangou IB, Bouhallab SH, Gwenaele BF, Allouche S, Blais A, Guerin P, Arhan P, Bougle DL, 2005. Milk proteins and iron absorption: contrasting effects of different caseino-phosphopeptides. *Pediatric Res* 58(4) : 731-734.

Korenromp EL, Armstrong-Schellenberg JR, Williams BG, Nahlen BL, Snow RW, 2004. Impact of malaria control on childhood anemia in Africa -- a quantitative review. *Trop Med Int Health* 9:1050-65.

Kuate-Defo B, 2001. Modelling hierarchically clustered longitudinal survival processes with applications to childhood mortality and maternal health. Canadian Studies Population 28 (2)

Kurtzhals JA, Addae M, Akanmori BD, Dunyo S, Koram KA, Appawu MA, Nkrumah FK, Hviid L, 1999. Anemia caused by asymptomatic *Plasmodium falciparum* infection in semi-immune African schoolchildren. *Trans R Soc Trop Med Hyg* 1999;93:623-627..

Lang K, Roll B, Myssina S, Schittenhelm M, Scheel-Walter HG, Kanz L, et al., 2002. Enhanced erythrocyte apoptosis in sickle cell anemia, thalassemia and glucose-6-phosphate dehydrogenase deficiency. *Cell Phys Bioch* 12 : 365-372.

Lind T, Lonnerdal B, Stenlund H, Ismail D, Seswandhana R, Ekstrom EC, Persson LA, 2003. A community-based randomized controlled trial of iron and zinc supplementation in Indonesian infants: interactions between iron and zinc. *Am J Clin Nutr* 77(4) : 883-890.

Lozoff B, Jimenez E, Hagen J, Mollen E, Wolf AW, 2000. Poorer behavioral and developmental outcome more than 10 years after treatment for iron deficiency in infancy. *Pediatrics* 105 : 1-11.

Lynch SR, 2000. The effect of calcium on iron absorption. *Nutr Res Rev* 13 : 141-158.

MacDougall LG, Moodley Gopal, Eyberg C, Quirk M, 1982. Mechanisms of anemia in protein-energy malnutrition in Johannesburg. *Am J Clin Nutr* 35 : 229-235.

Magalhães RJS, Clements ACA, 2011. Mapping the risk of anemia in preschool-age children: the contribution of malnutrition, malaria, and helminth infections in West Africa. PLoS M*edicine*, 8(6): e1000438 doi:10.1371/journal.pmed.1000438

Mann N, 2007. Meat in the human diet: an anthropological perspective. *Nutr Diet* 64 (Suppl. 4) : S102–S107.

Menendez C, Fleming AF, Alonso PL, 2000. Malaria-related anemia. *Parasitol Today 16(11):469-76.*

Mikki N, Abdul-Rahim HF, Stigum H, Holmboe-Ottesen G, 2011. Anemia prevalence and associated sociodemographic and dietary factors among Palestinian adolescents in the West Bank. *East Medit Health J*. 17 (3): 208-217.

McLean E, Coqswell M, Egli I, Wojdyla D, de Benoist B, 2009. Worldwide prevalence of anemia, WHO vitamin and mineral nutrition information system, 1993-2005. *Public Health Nutr*. 12(4):444-54.

Modiano D, Bancone G, Ciminelli BM, Pompei F, Blot I, Simpore J, Modiano G, 2008. Haemoglobin S and haemoglobin C: 'quick but costly' versus 'slow but gratis' genetic adaptations to Plasmodium falciparum malaria. *Hum Mol Genet* 17(6): 789-799.

Monsen ER, Hallberg L, Layrisse M, Hegsted DM, Cook JD, Walter M, Finch CA, 1978. Estimation of available dietary iron. *Am J Clin Nutr* 31 : 134-141.

Sowunmi A, Gbotosho GO, Happi CT, Fateye BA, 2010. Factors contributing to anemia after uncomplicated *Plasmodium falciparum* malaria in children. *Acta Trop 113(2):155-61.*

Nemeth E, Rivera S, Gabayan V, Keller C, Taudorf T, Pedersen BK, Ganz T, 2004. IL-6 mediates hypoferremia of inflammation by inducing the synthesis of the iron regulatory hormone hepcidin. *J Clin Invest* 113 : 1271-1276.

Nestel P et le Comité de pilotage de l'INACG, 2002. *Adjusting hemoglobin values in program surveys.* International Nutritional Anemia Consultative Group (INACG), 6 p.

Ngnie-Teta I, Receveur O, Kuate-Defo B, 2007. Risk factors for moderate to severe anemia among children in Benin and Mali: insights from a multilevel analysis. *Food Nutr Bull* 28(1) : 76-89.

Ngnie-Teta I; Kuate-Defo B; Receveur O, 2009. Multilevel modelling of sociodemographic predictors of various levels of anemia among women in Mali. Public Health Nutrition 12(9):1462-9.

Nicolas G, Chauvet C, Viatte L, Danan JL, Bigard X, Devaux I, et al. 2002. The gene encoding the iron regulatory peptide hepcidin is regulated by anemia, hypoxia, and inflammation. *J Clin Invest* 110 : 1037-1044.

Nkuo-Akenji TK, Ajame EA, Achidi EA, 2002. An investigation of symptomatic malaria parasitaemia and anemia in nursery and primary school children in Buea District Cameroon. Central African journal of medicine. 48 (1-2): 1-4

Nuchsongsin F, Chotivanich K, Charunwatthana P et al. 2007. Effects of Malaria Heme Products on Red Blood Cell Deformability. *Am J Trop Med Hyg* 77(4):617–622.

Oppenheimer SJ, 2001. Iron and its relation to immunity and infectious disease. *J Nutr* 131 : 616S–635S.

Osorio MM, Lira PI, Ashworth A, 2004. Factors associated with Hb concentration in children aged 6–59 months in the State of Pernambuco, Brazil. *Br J Nutr* 91 : 307–315.

Pan WH, Habicht JP, 1991. The non-iron-deficiency-related difference in hemoglobin concentration distribution between blacks and whites and between men and women. *Am J Epidemiol* 134(12) : 1410-1416.

Park YK, Diez-Silva M, Popescu G, Lykotrafitis G, Choi W, Feld MS, Suresh S, 2008. Refractive index maps and membrane dynamics of human red blood cells parasitized by *Plasmodium falciparum PNAS* 105(37):13730–13735

Rock E, Gueux E, Mazur A, Motta C, Rayssiguier Y, 1995. Anemia in copper-deficient rats: role of alterations in erythrocyte membrane fluidity and oxidative damage. *Am J Physiol 269(5 Pt 1):C1245-9.*

Phillips RE & Pasvol G, 1992. Anemia of Plasmodium falciparum malaria. *Baillieres Clin Haematol* 5(2):315-30.

Prentice AM, 2008. Iron metabolism, malaria, and other infections: what is all the fuss about? *J Nutr* 138 (12): 2537-2541.

Price RN, Simpson JA, Nosten F, Luxemburger C, Hkirjaroen L, ter Kuile F, Chongsuphajaisiddhi T, White NJ, 2001. Factors contributing to anemia after uncomplicated falciparum malaria. *Am J Trop Med Hyg* 65:614-622.

Reddy RB, Hurrell RF, Cook RD, 2000. Estimation of nonheme-iron bioavailability from meal composition. *Am J Clin Nutr* 71 : 937–943.

Rihet P, Flori L, Tall F, Traore AS, Fumoux F, 2004. Hemoglobin C is associated with reduced Plasmodium falciparum parasitemia and low risk of mild malaria attack. *Hum Mol Gen* 13(1) : 1–6.

Robertson LJ, Crompton DW, Sanjur D, Nesheim MC (1992) Haemoglobin concentrations and concomitant infections of hookworm and Trichuris trichiura in Panamanian primary schoolchildren. *Trans R Soc Trop Med Hyg* 86: 654–656

Sandberg AS, Brune M, Carlsson NG, Hallberg L, Skoglund E, Rossander-Hulthén L, 1999. Inositol phosphates with different numbers of phosphate groups influence iron absorption in humans. *Am J Clin Nutr* 70 : 240–246.

Sanou D, Turgeon-O'Brien H, Desrosiers T, 2008. Prévalence et déterminants non alimentaires de l'anémie et de la carence en fer chez des orphelins et enfants vulnérables d'âge préscolaire du Burkina-Faso. *Nutr Clin Metab* 22 (1) : 10-19.

Sanou D, Turgeon-O'Brien H, Desrosiers T, 2011. Impact of an integrated nutrition intervention on nutrient intakes, morbidity and growth of rural Burkinabe preschool children. *AJFAND* 11:(4) Epub July 2011. http://www.ajfand.net/Volume11/No4/Sanou9895.pdf

Sargent JD, Stukel TA, Dalton MA, Freeman JL, Brown MJ, 1996. Iron deficiency in Massachusetts communities: Socioeconomic and demographic risk factors among children. *Am J Public Health* 86(4):544-50.

Sazawal S, Black RE, Ramsan M, Chwaya HM, Stoltzfus RJ, Dutta A, et al., 2006. Effects of routine prophylactic supplementation with iron and folic acid on admission to hospital and mortality in preschool children in a high malaria transmission setting: community-based, randomised, placebo-controlled trial. *Lancet* 367 : 133-143.

Semba RD, Bloem MW, 2002. The anemia of vitamin A deficiency: epidemiology and pathogenesis. *Eur J Clin Nutr* 56:271-281

Semba RD, Kumwenda N, Taha TE, Mtimavalye L, Broadhead R, Garrett E, et al., 2001. Impact of vitamin A supplementation on anemia and plasma erythropoietin concentrations in pregnant women: a controlled clinical trial. *Eur J Haematol* 66 : 389-395 .

Shaw FJC, Kuate-Defo B, 2005. Socioeconomic inequalities in early childhood malnutrition and morbidity: modification of the household-level effects by the community SES. Health Place 11:205-25.

Shaw JG, Friedman JF, 2011. Iron deficiency anemia: Focus on infectious diseases in lesser developed countries *Anemia* 260380. Epub 2011 May 15

Simpore J, Nikiema JB, Sawadogo L, Pignatelli S, Blot I, Bere A, et al., 2003. Prévalence des hémoglobinopathies HbS et HbC au Burkina. *Burkina Medical* 32 : 1-13

Skeletee RW, 2003. Pregnancy, nutrition and parasitic diseases. *J Nutr* 133:1661S-1667S

Soh P, Ferguson EL, McKenzie JE, Homs MY, Gibson RS. Iron deficiency and risk factors for lower iron stores in 6-24-month-old New Zealanders. Eur J Clin Nutr. 2004 Jan;58(1):71-9.

Sommerfelt AE. Comparative analysis of the determinants of children's nutritional status. Demographic and Health Surveys World Conference, vol 2, 981-98. 1991 Washington DC, 722-43

Stoltzfus RJ, Chwaya HM, Montresor A, Albonico M, Savioli L, Tielsch JM, 2000. Malaria, hookworms and recent fever are related to anemia and iron status indicators in 0- to 5-y old Zanzibari children and these relationships change with age. *J Nutr* 130 : 1724–1733.

Talata S, Svanberg U, Mduma B, 1998. Low dietary iron availability is a major cause of anemia: a nutrition survey in the Lindi district of Tanzania. *Am J Clin Nutr* 68 : 171–178.

Taylor-Robinson DC, Jones AP, Garner P, 2007. Deworming drugs for treating soil-transmitted intestinal worms in children: effects on growth and school performance. *Cochrane Database of Systematic Reviews Issue* 4. Art. No.: CD000371.

ter Kuile FO, Terlouw DJ, Kariuki SK, et al. Impact of permethrin-treated bed nets on malaria, anemia, and growth in infants in an area of intense perennial malaria transmission in western Kenya. Am J Trop Med Hyg 2003;68:68-77.

Thorandeniya T, Wickremasinghe R, Ramanyake R, Atukorala S, 2006. Low folic acid status and its association with anemia in urban adolescent girls and women of childbearing age in Sri Lanka. *Brit J Nutr.* 95 (3): 511-516.

Thurlow RA, Winichagoon P, Green T, Wasantwisut E, Pongcharoen T, Bailey KB, Gibson RS, 2005. Only a small proportion of anemia in northeast Thai schoolchildren is associated with iron deficiency. *Am J Clin Nutr* 82 : 380–387.

Tolentino K, Friedman JF, 2007. An update on anemia in less developed countries. *Am J Trop Med Hyg* 77: 44–51.

Tomkins AM. Protein-energy malnutrition and risk of infection. Proc Nutr Soc 1986;45:289-304.

Totin D, Ndugwa C, Mmiro F, Perry RT, Brooks Jackson J, Semba RD, 2002. Iron deficiency anemia is highly prevalent among human immunodeficiency virus-infected and uninfected infants in Uganda. *Jf Nutr*132(3):423–429.

Umar RA, Jiya NM, Ladan MJ, Abubakar MK, Hassan SW, Nata`ala U, 2007. low prevalence of anemia in a cohort of pre-school children with acute uncomplicated *falciparum* malaria in Nigeria. *Trends Med Res 2: 95-101.*

van Bruggen R, Bautista JM, Petropoulou T, de Boer M, van Zwieten R, Gomez-Gallego F, et al., 2002. Deletion of leucine 61 in glucose-6-phosphate dehydrogenase leads to chronic nonspherocytic anemia, granulocyte dysfunction, and increased susceptibility to infections. *Blood* 100(3) : 1026 - 1030.

Verhoef H, West C, Veenemans J, Beguin Y, Kok F, 2002. Stunting may determine the severity of malaria-associated anemia in African children. *Pediatrics* 110:E48

Walker FC, Kordas K, Stoltzfus RJ, Black RE, 2005. Interactive effects of iron and zinc on biochemical and functional outcomes in supplementation trials. *Am J Clin Nutr* 82 : 5-12.

Wander K, Shell-Duncan B, McDade TW, 2009. Evaluation of iron deficiency as a nutritional adaptation to infectious disease: An evolutionary medicine perspective. *American Journal of Human Biology*, 2009; 21(2):172-179.

Weinberg, ED. Iron withholding: a defense against infection and neoplasia. *Physiological Reviews*, 1984; 64:65-102.

Weiss G, Goodnough LT, 2005. Anemia of chronic disease. *N Engl J Med* 352 : 1011-1023.

*WHO*, Sickle-cell anemia. Report by the Secretariat of the World Health Organization for the fifty-ninth world health assembly. 24 April 2006.

WHO. 2008. Worldwide prevalence of anemia 1993-2005 : WHO global database on anemia / Edited by Bruno de Benoist,

WHO/UNICEF, 2006. *Iron supplementation of young children in regions where malaria transmission is intense and infectious disease highly prevalent.* Joint statement by the World Health Organization and the United Nations Children's Fund. Geneva. 2 p.

WHO/UNICEF, 2006. *Iron supplementation of young children in regions where malaria transmission is intense and infectious disease highly prevalent.* WHO/UNICEF Joint statement. Geneva.

WHO/UNICEF/UNU. *Iron deficiency anemia assessment, prevention and control: a guide for programme managers.* World Health Organization. (WHO/NHD/01.3) Geneva, 2001.

Zimmermann MB, Chaouki N, Hurrell RF, 2005a. Iron deficiency due to consumption of a habitual diet low in bioavailable iron: a longitudinal cohort study in Moroccan children. *Am J Clin Nutr* 81: 115-121.

# 12

# Acceptance and Effect of Ferrous Fumarate Containing Micronutrient Sprinkles on Anemia, Iron Deficiency and Anthropometrics in Honduran Children

Teresa M. Kemmer[1], Preston S. Omer[2], Vinod K. Gidvani-Diaz[3] and Miguel Coello[4]

*[1]Health and Nutritional Sciences, SDSU Extension and Agricultural Experiment Station South Dakota State University, Brookings,*

*[2]U.S. Army, U.S. Army Medical Command, Fort Riley,*

*[3]U.S. Air Force San Antonio Uniformed Services Health Education Consortium, Pediatric Residency San Antonio,*

*[4]U.S. Medical Element, Joint Task Force-Bravo, Soto Cano Air Base*

*[1,2,3]USA*

*[4]Honduras*

## 1. Introduction

Anemia is reflective of global inequalities between developing and developed countries and is an endemic problem (Balarajan et al., 2011). Global Iron deficiency anemia (IDA) is one of the top ten risk factors contributing to the global burden of disease and economic costs are estimated at 4.05% of gross domestic product per capita from loss in productivity and $14.46 (U.S.) per capital in lost cognitive function (World Bank, 2004). One-quarter of the world's population is affected by anemia (McLean et al., 2009). Using data from the World Health Organization (WHO) Vitamin and Mineral Nutrition Information System for 1993-2005 (WHO, 2008), McLean et al. estimated an anemia prevalence of 47.4% (293 million) in preschool-aged children (2009). Iron deficiency (ID) is attributed annually to 20,854 global deaths in children under 5 years of age (Black et al., 2008), anemia affects 1.62 billion people (24.8% of the population) and anemia prevalence is highest in preschool-age children (47.4%) (WHO, 2008). The WHO categorizes the prevalence of anemia as a public health problem as follows: <5% - no problem, 5-19% - mild public health problem, 20-39% - moderate public health problem, and >40% - severe public health (Badham, 2007). According to the 2011 World Bank World Development Indicators, in children less five years of age, the prevalence of anemia is greatest in South Asia at 71% and is estimated at

66% in low income areas of the world (World Bank, 2011). The average prevalence of anemia in Europe and Central Asia is 30%, Latin America and the Caribbean is 38%, and Middle East and North Africa is 48% (World Bank, 2011).

Iron deficiency anemia contributes to poor growth and cognitive impairment which in turn has a negative effect on learning potential and productivity (Lozoff et al., 2006; Grantham-McGregor & Ani, 2001). At school entry, children that had chronic, severe ID during infancy are at a behavioral disadvantage as compared to their peers (Corapci et al., 2006). Hemoglobin has been shown to be associated with a decrease in verbal short-term memory and the severity of anemia has an impact on neurocognitive deficits, indicating reduced oxygen delivery to the brain as an etiological mechanism (Hijmans et al., 2011). Iron deficiency anemia in infancy results in children and young adults with poorer inhibitory control and executive functioning as well as other negative effects on neurotransmitters, myelination, dendritogenesis, neurometabolism in hippocampus and striatum, gene and protein profiles, and there associated behaviors (Lozoff, 2011). The long term affects of iron deficiency during infancy on poorer cognitive, motor, affective, and sensory system functioning highlight the requirement to focus on early intervention strategies that minimize the long-term effects (Lozoff, 2011). In a review by Madan, et al. (2011) ID resulted in negative developmental and neurophysiologic deficits and lower scholastic achievement. Results from an inner-city study revealed poorer object permanence and short-term memory problems in infants with IDA at 9 months and concluded that these cognitive effects were partially due to IDA related deficits in socioemotional function (Carter et al., 2010). Analysis of multiple trials found 1.73 lower IQ points per 1 g/dL decrease in hemoglobin (Stoltzfus et al., 2004). The predicted rate of mental retardation in a population with hemoglobin distribution shifted 1 g/dL downward due to iron deficiency is estimated at 2.94% (Stoltzfus et al., 2004).

Indirectly, ID negatively impacts the earning potential and entire economy of third world countries throughout the world. It was estimated that 0.2% of deaths and 0.5% of disability-adjusted life-years (DALYs) in children under 5 years of age are attributed to ID (Black et al., 2008). Iron deficiency results in 0.5%of maternal and child deaths in the world and 1.3% of DALYs and are higher in low income countries at 0.8% and 1.6% respectively. Estimated attributable DALYs to maternal and child iron deficiency are 19.7 million (WHO, 2009).

Approximately a quarter of children under five years of age in the developing world are undernourished based on the Millennium Development Goals (MGD) Report (United Nations, 2011), and progress in reducing the proportion of people suffering from hunger is insufficient to reach the target goal by 2015. If this MDG is to be achieved, nutrition must be given higher priority and should include simple, cost-effective measures delivered particularly from conception to two years after birth such as improved maternal nutrition and care, breastfeeding within one hour of birth, exclusive breastfeeding for the first 6 months of life, and timely, adequate, safe, and appropriate complementary feeding and micronutrient intake between 6 and 24 months of age (United Nations, 2011).

According to the Oxford Poverty and Human Development Initiative for Honduras (2010), 18% of the population are poor according to the $1.25 a day poverty line and 51% are poor according to the national poverty line. Inequities in under-5 mortality rate exist within Honduras where the mortality rate spans from 20 deaths per 1000 live births in the wealthiest to 50 per 1000 in the poorest (WHO, 2011). Anemia is very prevalent in

Honduras. A study by Nestel et al. (1999) showed that the prevalence of anemia in Honduran children ages 12 to 71 months was approximately 30%. Albalak and colleagues reported anemia prevalence in Honduran children at 40% in ages 12 to 36 months and 18% in children 36 to 60 months (Albalak et al., 2000). As a developing country, Honduras suffers from the negative impact anemia has on health, growth, and cognitive development, which indirectly decreases the productivity of the country. The estimate of economic loss from IDA as a percent of gross domestic product in Honduras is 2% (Horton & Ross, 2003). Programs within Honduras have tried to decrease the prevalence of anemia through different methods that include fortification of staples as well as supplementation (Dewey et al., 1998, 2004; Darnton-Hill et al., 1999; Darnton-Hill, 1998; Venkatesh Mannar, 2006). In addition, studies by Dewey et al. support the Honduran Ministry of Health's efforts to improve the iron status of breast-fed infants (Dewey et al., 1998, 2004).

The prevalence of ID can be reduced by increasing the consumption of iron-containing foods in the diet, supplementation with iron, or fortification of foods with iron (Finch & Cook, 1984; Provan, 1999; Trowbridge, 2002). The International Nutritional Anemia Consultative Group (INACG), WHO, and United Nations International Children's Emergency Fund (UNICEF) recommend introducing iron supplementation to healthy term infants with normal birth weight at 6 to 12 mo of age if the prevalence of anemia is less than 40% in the population, and supplementing the infants onward until 24 mo of age if the prevalence of anemia is 40% or higher in the population (Zlotkin & Tondeur, 2007). Ferrous sulfate is mainly used to supplement food stuffs (Dary, 2007). An alternative supplement method is adding iron into the diet with "Micronutrient Sprinkles" which were developed at the Hospital for Sick Children (Schauer & Zlotkin, 2003). Sprinkles refer to a blend of micronutrients in powder form that are added to foods to target susceptible populations at higher risk of anemia and micronutrient deficiencies (Sprinkles Global Health Initiative, 2008). Sprinkles may contain any combination of micronutrients and are packaged in a small sachet, the contents of which can be added to any semi-solid food. Sprinkles can be designed and produced based on the population needs and allow susceptible populations to fortify home cooked foods.

The objectives of this randomized case-control study in non-anemic rural Honduran children ages 6 to 60 months were to determine if micronutrient sprinkles 1) are an effective method of preventing anemia and reducing ID, 2) result in improved growth parameters, and 3) are acceptable to the population.

## 2. Methods

This randomized case-control nutritional assessment study in rural Honduras was conducted in collaboration with the Honduran Ministry of Health (MoH); medical liaison officers at Joint Task Force Bravo, Medical Element, Soto Cano, Honduras; the San Antonio Military Pediatric Center; and South Dakota State University in 2006-2007. Immunization records obtained from the local health centers of children within the age range of 6 to 60 months were used for randomization of the household. Immunization records were used for the randomization since 98% of 1-year-old children in Honduras are immunized against Hepatitus B; measles; diphtheria, pertussis and tetanus (DPT); and tuberculosis (TB) and 94% of newborns are protected against tetanus (UNICEF, 2010). A minimum of 10% of the children within each health center were randomly selected for participation. Each child's household was visited with the assistance of local volunteers from the MoH clinics and community. Data collection included anthropometrics, survey data, blood collection, and altitude. Written consent was obtained from one of the primary care providers prior to participation. Completion of the survey required approximately 15 to 20 minutes and was administrated by a fluent Spanish speaker. The household was excluded if consent was not obtained or the household did not have children within the specified age range. No eligible family refused study participation. Officials of the Honduran Ministry of Health approved and supported this project and the protocol was approved through Wilford Hall Medical Center, San Antonio, TX; and the Office of Research/Human Subjects Committee, South Dakota State University, Brookings, SD. Research was conducted in compliance with the Declaration of Helsinki guidelines.

### 2.1 Anthropometric measurements

Weight and height/length were recorded during home visits using standardized equipment and procedures (WHO, 2006). Child weight was measured without clothing to the nearest $10^{th}$ of a kilogram of body weight using a Seca® scale (Seca, Vogel & Halke, Germany). A child who was unable to stand on the scale was held and weight was obtained using the tare weight function. Child length was measured without shoes to the nearest 0.1 cm if the child was younger than 2 years using the infant/child Shorrboard® (Shorr Productions, Olney, MD). Height was obtained for children $\geq$ 2 years of age. World Health Organization Anthro program (WHO, 2005) was used to calculate anthropometrics. The cut-off values used to identify children as stunted was length/height-for-age < -2 z-scores (HAZ), underweight was weight-for-age < -2 z-scores (WAZ), and wasted was weight-for- length/height < -2 z-scores (WHZ) using the WHO standards (WHO, 2006). Following anthropometric data analysis, there were no outliers based on the following definitions: height-for-age < -6.0 and > +6.0, weight-for-age < -6.0 and > +5.0, and weight for height < -5.0 and > +5.0 (WHO, 2006).

### 2.2 Blood analysis

On-the-spot hemoglobin (Hb) was used to determine study eligibility. Hemoglobin was measured using the HemoCue Hemoglobin Photometer (HemoCue US, Mission Viejo, CA) and was adjusted for altitude (Ruiz-Arguelles, 2006). Altitude adjusted age-specific cutoff Hb values of <11.0 g/dL were used to determine anemia (WHO, 2001). The households of non-anemic children were randomly assigned to the sprinkles or non-sprinkles arm. All non-anemic children of the household in the target range were enrolled. All eligible children in one household were randomized to the same arm of the study. Anemic children were not enrolled in the study, were treated with ferrous sulfate, and their names were provided to the local MoH clinic personnel for follow-up.

Finger prick blood samples were obtained from the children. A global positioning system (GPS) was used at the household to determine altitude.

Analysis of transferrin receptor (TfR) to determine iron status was obtained using dried blood spot (DBS) samples on filter paper. The use of DBS is a convenient way of collecting samples in the field compared to venous blood sampling that would require a phlebotomist, centrifugation of samples, and immediate cold storage (Flowers & Cook, 1999). Care was taken not to touch the pre-printed circles on the filter paper before, during, and after blood collection and to avoid having one blood spot flow into another spot. Following blood spot collection, filter papers were exposed to air for a short period of time to allow drying, were placed in an airtight/watertight container with a desiccant, were stored away from light and heat, and were dried overnight in the drying box. Following the drying process, the filter papers were stored in a zip-closure plastic freezer bag with desiccant and were kept at refrigerator or freezer temperature until analysis. The analysis of TfR from DBS was completed by The Craft Technologies, Inc., Wilson, NC, using the quantitative sandwich enzyme linked immunoassay (ELISA) (Erhardt et al., 2004). Iron deficiency was defined based on the manufacture's TfR assay reference. Iron deficiency anemia was defined as anemia in combination with ID.

Participants were enrolled during three separate trips to Honduras over the span of 12 months. A four month supply of sprinkles packets and pictorial and verbal instructions for use were provided for each child assigned to the sprinkles arm. The micronutrient sprinkle formula for this study contained iron (12.5 mg), zinc (5 mg), folic acid (150 μg), vitamin A (1600 I.U.), vitamin C (50 mg), and vitamin D (300 I.U.) and cost $0.025 (U.S.) per packet. Parents were asked to save the empty sachets and to return the empty and unused sachets during the four month follow-up visit as a measure of usage compliance. Measurements of Hb and TfR as well as anthropometric measurements were obtained at the initial visit and at the four and eight month intervals. Enrollees were provided Albendazol for helminthes infestation at each visit. Children found to be anemic at 4 months were started on supplemental iron therapy and were not included in the 8 month follow-up. A survey was administered at the four month follow-up visit to assess compliance, acceptability, side effects, and any logistical problems.

Statistical analysis was performed using SPSS computer software. Differences between the groups were assessed by independent samples t-test. Paired t-test was used to analyze change within groups. Chi-square test was used to compare the proportion of change in prevalence. The acceptable level of statistical significance was $P<0.05$.

## 3. Results

In the households visited, there were 220 children. Of these, 21 were diagnosed with anemia and were ineligible for the study. Those found to be anemic were treated and referred directly to the MoH clinic. The remaining 199 children were enrolled in the study and randomized into the sprinkles (n=114) and non-sprinkles (n=85) groups.

### 3.1 Baseline characteristics

The mean age was 34.66 months (± 15.31 SD), mean Hb was 12.47 g/dL (± 0.81 SD), mean TfR was 7.02 mg/L (± 2.52), mean altitude was 5,023.98 ft (± 558.57 SD) and 55% were male. The groups did not differ significantly at base-line in age, gender, Hb, TfR, weight or height; however, average altitude was significantly different ($P < 0.001$). Children within the sprinkles group were at a higher mean altitude (5134 ft vs 4876 ft). Within this study population, Hb and TfR were not significantly correlated with altitude. Of the 199 children enrolled in the study, four children (2%) did not return for the four month follow-up visit, an additional 3 children did not provide a blood sample to evaluate Hb. At the 4 month follow-up visit 20.3% of participants were anemic, treated with iron, referred to the MoH clinic and were removed from the study. At the 8 month follow-up, an additional 15.2% were anemic.

### 3.2 Primary outcome measures

There was no significant difference seen in mean Hb between the sprinkles and non-sprinkles groups between visits (Table 1). At the 4 and 8 month visits, 4.4% and 2.4%

respectively had IDA. The prevalence of anemia and IDA by visit for the sprinkles and non-sprinkles groups is presented in Table 2. There was no significant difference between groups for ID or IDA at 4 or 8 months.

At baseline, 23.8% of the sprinkles group and 22.8% of the non-sprinkles group were iron deficient (ID). Within children that were ID at baseline, 58.3% of the sprinkles group and 55.6% of the non-sprinkles group were no longer ID at 4 months and 60.9% of the sprinkles group and 77.8% of the non-sprinkles group were no longer ID at 8 months. There was no significant difference in TfR change from baseline to 4 or 8 months between groups (Table 1). At 8 months, 24.5% of the sprinkles group and 20.0% of the non-sprinkles group were ID. Paired T-test results for change in Hb from baseline to 4 months was 0.20 ($p=0.13$) for the sprinkles group and 0.31 ($p<0.05$) for the non-sprinkles group respectively. From baseline to 4 months there were significant paired T-test differences in TfR of -1.37 within the sprinkles group ($p< 0.001$) and -.076 within the non-sprinkles group ($p< 0.05$).

| | Sprinkles (SD) | Non-Sprinkles (SD) | P-value* |
|---|---|---|---|
| Initial Hb (gm/dL) | 12.45 (0.80) | 12.55 (0.83) | |
| 4 months | 12.13 (1.19) | 12.22 (1.26) | 0.63 |
| 8 months | 12.46 (1.35) | 12.47 (1.17) | 0.73 |
| Overall change | | | 0.56 |
| Initial TfR | 7.02 (2.07) | 7.02 (2.39) | |
| 4 months | 8.39 (2.93) | 7.78 (2.29) | 0.98 |
| 8 months | 7.19 (1.64) | 7.02 (1.81) | 0.12 |
| Overall change | | | 0.52 |

* Significance determined at P <0.05.

Table 1. Change in Mean Hemoglobin (Hb) and Serum Transferrin Receptor (TfR) between Visits for Sprinkles vs Non-Sprinkles.

| | Anemia (%)* | IDA (%)* |
|---|---|---|
| Initial | n=199 | n=182 |
| Sprinkles | 0 | 0 |
| Non-Sprinkles | 0 | 0 |
| 4 Months | n=192 | n=180 |
| Sprinkles | 16.5 | 4.0 |
| Non-Sprinkles | 25.3 | 5.0 |
| 8 Months | n=132 | n=123 |
| Sprinkles | 17.5 | 4.1 |
| Non-Sprinkles | 11.5 | 0 |

* No significant differences was seen in prevalence between Sprinkles and non-Sprinkles groups. Significance determined at P <0.05.

Note: No anemic children were enrolled in the study. If children were anemic at 4 months, they were treated and removed from the study.

Table 2. Prevalence of Anemia and Iron Deficiency Anemia (IDA) by visit for Sprinkles vs. non-Sprinkles groups.

### 3.3 Anthropometric measurements

There was no significant difference between baseline and 4 and 8 months in the sprinkles group compared to the non-sprinkles group when comparing change in mean height, weight, weight-for-age Z-score, height-for-age Z-score, or weight-for-height Z-score (Tables 3 & 4). There was also no significant change between groups in the prevalence of stunting, underweight or wasting (Table 5).

| | Sprinkles | Non-Sprinkles | P-value* |
|---|---|---|---|
| Initial weight (kg) | 11.74 | 12.25 | |
| 4 months | 12.54 | 12.89 | 0.63 |
| 8 months | 13.01 | 13.59 | 0.27 |
| Overall change | | | 0.25 |
| Initial height (cm) | 84.45 | 85.94 | |
| 4 months | 87.05 | 88.65 | 0.62 |
| 8 months | 89.82 | 91.07 | 0.35 |
| Overall change | | | 0.35 |

*Significance determined at P <0.05.

Table 3. Change in Mean Weight and Height between Visits for Sprinkles vs Non-Sprinkles.

| | Sprinkles | Non-Sprinkles | P-value* |
|---|---|---|---|
| Initial weight-for-age Z-score | -0.99 | -0.91 | |
| 4 months | -0.98 | -1.0 | 0.89 |
| 8 months | -1.09 | -0.98 | 0.73 |
| Overall change | | | 0.68 |
| Initial height-for-age Z-score | -2.04 | -1.99 | |
| 4 months | -2.09 | -2.05 | 0.75 |
| 8 months | -2.07 | -2.09 | 0.94 |
| Overall change | | | 0.96 |
| Initial weight-for-height Z-score | 0.20 | 0.31 | |
| 4 months | 0.29 | 0.25 | 0.84 |
| 8 months | 0.17 | 0.34 | 0.66 |
| Overall change | | | 0.48 |

*Significance in mean change between time intervals for Sprinkles vs non-Sprinkles. Significance determined at P<0.05.

Table 4. Change in Mean Weight-for-Age Z-score, Height-for-Age Z-score, and Weight-for-Height Z-score by Visit.

| | Stunting (%)* | Underweight (%)* | Wasting (%)* |
|---|---|---|---|
| Initial (n=195) | | | |
| Sprinkles | 48.6 | 16.2 | 0.9 |
| Non-Sprinkles | 54.8 | 14.3 | 0 |
| All | 51.3 | 15.4 | 0.5 |
| 4 Months (n=187) | | | |
| Sprinkles | 51.9 | 13.5 | 0 |
| Non-Sprinkles | 54.2 | 10.8 | 0 |
| 8 Months (n=168) | | | |
| Sprinkles | 46.3 | 14.7 | 0 |
| Non-Sprinkles | 58.9 | 9.6 | 1.4 |

* No significant difference was seen in prevalence between Sprinkles and non-Sprinkles groups. Significance determined at P<0.05.

Table 5. Prevalence of Stunting, Underweight and Wasting by Visit for Sprinkles vs. Non-Sprinkles groups
Stunting = height-for-age Z-score <-2; Underweight = weight-for-age <-2 Z-scores; wasting = weight-for-age <-2 Z-scores.

### 3.4 Sprinkles use and acceptability

Based on parental responses and counting of the returned empty sprinkles packets, children who received sprinkles used an average 108 of 120 (90%) packets. The number of packets consumed ranged from 24 to 120. Of children who received sprinkles, 55% used all 120 packets, and 86% used more than 100 packets. The majority of families, 92%, used seven packets per week with a range from 3 to 7 packets per week. Parents reported that only 3 children (2.75%) disliked food with sprinkles added, 1 child had diarrhea, and one had difficulty in administering sprinkles. Rice, beans and soup were the foods most commonly mixed with the sprinkles. Sprinkles in food were not noticed by 54.1% of the children, 32.1% liked the food better with the sprinkles and 13.8% did not like the food with sprinkles. They were found easy to use in food preparation by 98.2% of the families and one parent reported that it was difficult to use daily and another reported that it took added time. All of the participants reported that they would continue to use the sprinkles if they were delivered free through the MoH clinic.

## 4. Discussion

### 4.1 Anemia and iron status

Only three other studies were located that reported information on sprinkles trials in subjects that were not anemic at the beginning of the study (Lundeen et al., 2010; Giovannini et al., 2006; Zlotkin et al., 2003a). Daily use of sprinkles for 2 months in anemic (72%) and non-anemic children ages 6 to 36 months revealed that within the non-anemic children receiving sprinkles 28% became anemic compared to 50% in the non-sprinkles group (Lundeen et al., 2010).

A 12 month double-blind, placebo-controlled trial in children aged 6 months by Giovannini et al. (2006) included both anemic and non-anemic children within the analysis (mean baseline Hb $\geq$ 10.1 g/dL) and did not report results for non-anemic children only. Prevalence of anemia was significantly reduced in infants receiving either of the sprinkles supplements (Giovannini et al., 2006). A 6 month study performed by Zlotkin et al. looked at the effectiveness of microencapsulated iron (II) fumarate sprinkles with and without vitamin A, iron (II) sulfate drops or placebo sprinkles in preventing the recurrence of anemia in non-anemic (Hb $\geq$ 10.0 g/dL) children between the ages of 8-20 months (2003a). From baseline to the end of the supplementation period, there were no significant changes seen in the mean Hb or ferritin within the four groups and the children that became anemic were equally distributed among groups (Zlotkin et al., 2003a). Within the study, 82.4% of the children from all four groups remained in their non-anemic status, while 77.1% of children maintained their non-anemic status during the post-supplementation period (Zlotkin et al., 2003a). Zlotkin et al. (2003a) concluded that their findings do not support the continued use of long-term prophylactic iron supplementation to maintain iron status in children treated previously for IDA. Within the current study, there were also no significant changes in Hb or iron status between the sprinkles or non-sprinkles groups. Though the change in Hb over the study and the anemia prevalence was not significantly different between groups, a decrease in Hb is a late finding in IDA (Provan, 1999). An additional study being conducted by Bilenko et al. (2010) is similar to the current study in that the objective is to evaluate the efficacy of sprinkles in primary prevention of iron and other micronutrient deficiencies; however, results of the study are pending.

Studies performed in several countries have shown that sprinkles are effective in treating IDA, and that sprinkles are more effective and more easily administered than iron drops due to less side effects (Hirve et al., 2007; Schauer & Zlotkin, 2003; Zlotkin et al., 2004). Efficacy has been shown with sprinkles including formulations containing relatively low amounts of iron, and better results were achieved with daily dosing versus weekly dosing (Christofides et al., 2006; Giovannini et al., 2006; Menon et al., 2007; Shareiff et al., 2006). An analysis of studies that used dispersion of micronutrients in sachets completed by Horton et al. (2010) resulted in an increase in Hb concentration of 0.057 g/dL and IDA was reduced as compared to controls. When allowing flexible administration of micronutrient sprinkles compared to daily administration Hb was significantly higher in the group allowed flexible administration and resulted in an anemia prevalence decrease by 65% vs. 51% (Ip et al., 2009).

In comparison with other studies (Adu-Afarwuah et al., 2008; Giovannini et al., 2006; Zlotkin et al., 2003a), this study attempted to determine the utility of sprinkles to prevent anemia in non-anemic children. The prevention of anemia within children can lower the risk of developing cognitive and physical impairments (Grantham-McGregor & Ani, 2001). Giovannini et al. compared the efficacy of iron plus folic acid and zinc, iron plus folic acid alone, or a placebo and within the two sprinkle supplement groups there was no significant change in the rate of ID; however, the occurrence of ID increased in the placebo group (Giovannini et al., 2006).

A study completed by Adu-Afarwuah et al. compared the effectiveness of sprinkles, crushable Nutritabs, fat-based Nutributter, or a placebo on Ghanaina infants from 6 to 12 months of age (2008). This study showed that the risk of ID or anemia was significantly lower in the three intervention groups compared to the control group (Adu-Afarwuah et al., 2008). A meta-analysis evaluating the effect of multiple micronutrients in micronutrient deficient children, resulted in small but significant improvements in Hb (effect size=0.39) (Allen et al., 2009). In a randomized comparison of the effects of sprinkles, foodlets and iron drops, iron status improved in all treatment groups though there was no difference in change in anemia prevalence; however, drops resulted in significantly greater changes in Hb and serum ferritin (Samadpour et al., 2011).

Other studies determined the effectiveness chewable tablets in the prevention of iron deficiency (Smuts et al., 2005; Lopez de Romaña et al., 2005). Children from South Africa, Peru, Vietnam, and Indonesia were randomly assigned to one of four intervention groups: a daily placebo, a weekly multiple micronutrient supplement, a daily multiple micronutrient supplement, or a daily iron supplement and results showed that the overall prevalence of anemia decreased over the course of the study in all four intervention groups (Smuts et al., 2005). Iron deficiency increased in the placebo and weekly micronutrient supplement groups while decreasing in the daily iron and daily micronutrient supplement groups (Smuts et al., 2005). Lopez de Romaña et al. determined the efficacy of different micronutrient supplements in preventing growth failure, anemia, and other micronutrient deficiencies in Peruvian infants (2005). Infants between the ages of 6 to 12 months were randomly assigned to receive a placebo, a weekly dose of multiple micronutrients, a daily dose of multiple micronutrients, or a daily dose of iron (Lopez de Romaña et al., 2005). The prevalence of anemia decreased in all intervention groups; however, the decrease was not significant in the placebo group and anemia was best controlled by daily micronutrient supplements containing iron (Lopez de Romaña et al., 2005).

Additional studies have included treatment for anemic children (Rosado et al., 2010; Christofides et al., 2006; Menon et al., 2007; Zlotkin et al., 2004; Zlotkin et al., 2001). The use of sprinkles in the treatment of anemia has been shown to be successful within children and infants (De-Regil et al., 2011; Zlotkin et al., 2001; Zlotkin et al., 2003b). In a compilation of six studies, home fortification with sprinkles resulted in anemia reduction by 31% (RR 0.69) and in four studies, iron deficiency was reduced by 51% (RR 0.49) (De-Regil et al., 2011). In an efficacy study of different strategies to treat anemia in children, all treatments significantly increased Hb and total iron concentration; however, ferritin did not change significantly (Rosado et al., 2010). A study by Zlotkin et al. looked at the treatment of anemic children ages between 6 months to 18 months in Ghana and demonstrated that over 50% of children treated with sprinkles were successfully cured (Zlotkin et al., 2001). Menon et al. showed a drop in anemia prevalence from 52.3% to 28.3% in children receiving sprinkles with the fortified wheat-soy blend (WSB) compared to the WSB only, which showed an increase in anemia prevalence from 37% to 45% (2007). Christofides et al. found that various doses of sprinkles and iron drops garnered significant changes in Hb concentration and the prevalence of IDA decreased significantly over the course of the study (2006).

### 4.2 Anthropometric measurements

Higher rates of stunting are seen in Honduras than in its neighboring countries and income peers (World Bank, 2010). Within Honduran children under five years of age, 29% suffer from stunting, 11% from underweight and 1% from wasting (UNICEF, 2010). Growth parameters measured in Honduran children ages 12 to 71 months during the 1996 National Micronutrient Survey revealed that 38% were stunted, 24% were underweight, and 1% were wasted (Nestel et al., 1999). The prevalence of stunting, underweight and wasting within rural Honduran children ages 6 to 60 months was 57%, 33%, and 3.5% respectively (Tolson et al., 2010). Analysis of the 2006 Honduran Demographic and Health Survey data revealed that children that were wanted and had adequate parental care resulted in significant effects on children's height-for-age growth status (Sparks, 2011).

In a pooled analysis of 55 studies completed by Horton et al. (2010) they noted no benefit of iron supplementation on growth. Multi-micronutrient fortified energy-dense, fat-based Nutributter resulted in significantly greater WAZ and HAZ, than the use of micronutrient home fortification in either sprinkles or crushed tablets (Adu-Afarwuah et al., 2007). Even though sprinkles was successful in treating anemia in infants and young children, it did not promote catch-up growth in a stunted and wasted population in Ghana (Zlotkin et al., 2003a). Prevention of growth faltering was not noted in a double-blind, masked, controlled trial in infants provided iron or multiple micronutrients as compared to placebo (Lopez de Romana et al., 2005). When pooling data from four countries, a daily micronutrient supplement proved the most effective in promoting significant weight gain; however, there was no difference in height gain (Smuts et al., 2005). A compilation of eight trials (3748 participants) on the use of micronutrient powders in home fortification of foods showed no effect on growth (De-Regil et al., 2011). A four month evaluation of iron supplements in varying forms provided to anemic children also resulted in no difference in growth parameters (Rosado et al, 2010). In a meta-analysis evaluating the effect of multiple micronutrients on child growth, the intervention resulted in small but significant improvements in height/length (effect size=0.13) and weight (effect size= 0.14) (Allen et al., 2009). In a 4 month trial comparing efficacy of sprinkles, foodlets and drops, there was no significant difference in anthropometric measurements, or change in prevalence of underweight, stunting and wasting between treatment groups (Samadpour et al, 2011).

### 4.3 Sprinkles use and acceptability

The overall use of sprinkles within this study was well accepted with 55% of participants using all of the packets provided for the 4 month intervention. Lundeen et al. (2010) found that on average 45 of 60 sprinkles packets were consumed with 38.8% of participants consuming all 60 packets and 83.1% of children eating the entire portion of food mixed with the sprinkles. In a study conducted by Loechl et al. (2009), 63% of mothers reported using the sprinkles every day based on survey results and 86% based on exit interview results.

Other studies have compared alternative treatments of anemia to sprinkles (Christofides et al., 2006). One study showed that 92.9% of children had a strong dislike for the iron drops while only 6.5% objected to the consumption of sprinkles (Zlotkin et al., 2003a). Hirve et al. (2007) found that the side effects such as diarrhea, vomiting, staining of teeth, and stool discoloration were all significantly higher in the iron drops group than compared to sprinkles. In a study conducted by Adu-Afarwuah et al. (2008), 96.9% of mothers thought it was easy to give the sprinkles supplement, 89.6% said that the child accepted the food well, 95.9% did not have any major problems feeding the sprinkles to the child and 100% had a good impression of the sprinkles supplement. Allowing flexible administration vs. daily administration of micronutrient sprinkles improved adherence and was more acceptable (Ip et al., 2009). In an evaluation of iron drops vs. sprinkles, both groups had generally pour adherence and overall, there was no significant difference between groups (Geltman et al., 2009). Eighty percent of respondents in the sprinkles group vs. 69% in the drops group would use them again; however, the difference was not significant. There was a significant difference between the sprinkles vs. the drops group of respondents being concerned about using a new products and about the product's safety (Geltman et al., 2009).

### 4.4 Use of anti-parasitic medication

At each home visited anti-parasitic medication for children > 2 years of age was provided per MoH protocol. Because helminth infection is common in Honduras (Smith et al., 2001) and is a significant contributing factor to anemia (Bethony et al., 2006; Brooker et al., 2006), this intervention itself likely impacted the prevalence and severity of anemia in both groups (Stoltzfus et al., 1998) thus confounding results focused on the effect of sprinkles. It is important to note that at end of the study, the percentage of children with anemia in each group was less than the general prevalence of anemia among Honduran children.

Study strengths included the large number of participants in this randomized design used to determine efficacy of sprinkle supplements for the prevention of anemia in children ages 6 to 60 months. The large number of participants helps to prove the reliability of the effectiveness of the sprinkles compared to no treatment (Brooker et al., 2006). Altitude was collected at the household for accurate determination of the participants altitude adjusted Hb. Household data collection was convenient for participants. As a measure of compliance, participants were required to turn in empty and leftover sprinkle packets at the 4 month follow-up visit. The field friendly DBS method allowed measurement of iron status and eliminated the requirements for venipucture, a highly trained phlebotomist, centrifugation, and immediate ultra cold storage. Limitations of the study include the DBS were obtained in a field environment and they were not available for all participants due to parental refusal or inadequate blood sample size for analysis. Regarding sprinkle acceptability, parent reports were relied upon and may not be entirely accurate. The areas where the study was conducted were assigned by the Honduran MoH and included rural homes with low socioeconomic status. While this may be a representative sample for much of the population in Honduras, our results may not be applicable to children in different settings.

## 5. Strategies to address anemia and iron deficiency

If the MDG of reducing the proportion of people suffering from hunger is to be achieved by 2015, nutrition must be given higher priority and should include simple, cost-effective measures delivered particularly from conception to two years after birth (United Nations, 2011). These measures should incorporate improved maternal nutrition and care, breastfeeding within one hour of birth, exclusive breastfeeding for the first 6 months of life, and timely, adequate, safe, and appropriate complementary feeding and micronutrient intake between 6 and 24 months of age (United Nations, 2011).

A lifecycle approach to the problem is required to control iron deficiency and should include effective public health programs that consider the whole reproductive cycle and create a combination of strategies that are complementary and comprehensive across vulnerable periods (Stoltzfus, 2011). Anemia prevention and control strategies include: 1) increased food diversity with increased iron bioavailability and improved dietary quality and quantity; 2) biofortification, fortification of staples with iron, open market fortification of processed food, targeted fortification; 3) iron and folic acid supplementation to high-risk groups; 4) disease control; and 5) improved knowledge and education on anemia prevention and control for policy makers and the general public (Balarajan et al., 2011).

When implementing large-scale programs it is essential to assess the coverage, compliance and effectiveness and the programs should promote a food-based approach, including fortification of staple foods and condiments for the general population as well as home fortificants for specific target groups, since they are more sustainable, less perceived as treatment of a condition and are applicable for use in malaria-endemic areas (Badham et al., 2007). Prevention of ID requires policy and program guidance and working closely with decision makers about the what, when and how to implement and manage the program (Lutter, 2008). The widespread endemic of iron deficiency can be approached through a number of options which include dietary measures, fortification, supplementation, and treatment of infections/infestations and it is essential to consider that an effective resolution may vary by population subgroups, region and country (Milman, 2011). Using existing maternal and child health and nutrition programs to distribute micronutrient sprinkles and educate parents on their use is feasible and acceptable (Loechl et al., 2009).

Several recommendations from the World Bank Scaling up Nutrition paper (Horton et al., 2010) that can be implemented in partnership with the health sector in support of reducing the prevalence of anemia and iron deficiency include: 1) the use of multiple micronutrient powders and deworming drugs in children under the age of five years of age; 2) complimentary and therapeutic feeding interventions that provide micronutrient fortified and/or enhanced complementary foods for the prevention and treatment of moderate malnutrition among children 6-23 months of age; 3) promotion of breastfeeding, appropriate complementary feeding practices, and proper hygiene; and 4) iron fortification of staple foods for the general population.

Public health interventions addressing iron deficiency are one of the most cost effective with a cost-benefits ratio for iron programs estimated at 200:1 (Badham et al., 2007). On a worldwide scale, it would take an additional $10.3 billion (U.S.) in public resource support to begin successfully alleviating undernutrition on a worldwide scale benefiting over 360 million (Horton et al., 2010). On a nationwide basis in Honduras, it is estimated that it would take $6 million (U.S.) per year to scale up core micronutrient nutrition interventions and the costs are as low as $0.05-8.46 per person annually with a return on investment as high as 6-30 times the cost (World Bank, 2010; Horton et al., 2010). To alleviate much of iron deficiency's burden, iron fortification of staple foods would cost $0.20 (U.S.) per person per year, deworming cost would be $0.25 (U.S.) per child 24–59 month per round per year, and iron-folic acid supplements for pregnant women would cost approximately $2.00 (U.S.) per pregnancy (Horton et al., 2010). For sprinkles supplementation targeted to children 6–12 mo, it is estimated that cost per DALY saved could be as low as $12 with a benefit: cost ratio of 37:1 (Horton, et al., 2006). When determining the cost effectiveness of home-fortification programs in a low income country with a high infant mortality rate and high prevalence of anemia, it is estimated that cost per DALY saved is $12.2 and the present value of the gain in earnings is $37 for each dollar spent on the micronutrient sprinkles program (Sharieff et al., 2006).

Iron fortification continues to be evaluated in a variety of food stuffs for efficacy and acceptance (Karn et al., 2011; Angeles-Agdeppa et al., 2011; Varma et al., 2007; Andersson et al., 2008; Adu-Afarwuah et al., 2008; Wegmuller et al., 2006; Hurrell et al., 2010; Faber et al., 2005; Torrejon et al., 2004); however, it is essential that the fortification efforts are supported politically, adequately marketed, cost effective and have long-term commercial commitment (Angeles-Agdeppa et al., 2011). Iron supplementation and fortification are effective in controlling iron deficiency in populations and bioavailability of the iron is an important factor, iron status should be used and monitored to assess fortification requirements and efficacy (Zimmermann & Hurrell, 2007).

When implementing anemia prevention strategies the focus should be on preschoolers and adolescent women and on integrated public health programs (Boy et al., 2009). Lutter (2008) recommends iron prevention programs targeted during pregnancy, at birth, the immediate postnatal period and during the first 24 months of life and to not underestimate the challenges of delivery through the public health systems. Recommended practices for children ages 6-24 months include iron rich complementary foods, micronutrient supplements (medicinal iron supplements, micronutrient sachets, fortified complementary foods, lipid-based spreads) and deworming (Lutter, 2008).

National decision makers in each country are responsible to select the type and quantity of micronutrients added to foodstuffs and their decision should be based on their country's situation. The WHO recommends designing flour fortification programs based on four average wheat flour consumption ranges, the type of iron fortification compound (NaFeEDTA, ferrous sulfate, ferrous fumarate, or electrolytic iron) and flour extraction rate (low or high) (Hurrell et al., 2010). Wheat flour fortification programs were evaluated in 78 countries and only nine of the national programs could potentially result in a significant positive impact on iron status and that updated legislation is required to maximize the potential of meeting iron needs through fortification of wheat flour (Hurrell et al., 2010).

Genetic engineering of grains to increase iron content and bioavailability and selective plant breeding are also avenues being explored to combat iron deficiency (Zimmermann & Hurrell, 2007; Lucca et al., 2001 & 2006). Biofortified crops complement fortification and supplementation programs and are an option that provides a rural-based intervention that reaches more remote populations and then transfers into urban populations as production surpluses are marketed (Bouis et al., 2011). New iron fortification technologies that eliminate detrimental effects on taste, appearance, and product stability and that do not interfere with iron bioavailability show promising results (Mehansho, 2006).

Sustainable strategies for the prevention and control of iron deficiency require food based and non food based approaches incorporating agriculture, health, commerce, industry, education, communication and local nongovernmental organizations (Lokeshwar et al., 2011). Barriers to effective implementation of anemia prevention and control strategies include insufficient political priority, lack of resource commitment, lack of institutional and operational capacity, restricted financial access, poor awareness of the magnitude of disease burden, and lack of knowledge and education (Balarajan et al., 2011).

Strategic research is required to address the effective prevention and control of iron deficiency and its consequences in young children living in low-income countries and should address: 1) scaling up known effective interventions, 2) evaluating cost-effective alternatives that are likely to work, 3) efficacy research to discover promising practices that lack proven interventions, and 4) determining physiological processes and mechanisms underlying the risks and benefits of supplemental iron for children exposed to infectious diseases (Stoltzfus, 2008).

## 6. Conclusions

Within this study of non-anemic rural Honduran children ages 6 to 60 months, there were no statistically significant differences between the sprinkles and non-sprinkles groups when comparing change in mean Hb, TfR, and anthropometric measurements or prevalence in anemia, iron deficiency, stunting, underweight and wasting. However, at the end of the study, prevalence of anemia in each study group was less than the general prevalence of anemia for Honduran children. Sprinkle compliance was good; they were well tolerated by children and were accepted among the participating families. Additional research is required to determine efficacy of sprinkles for anemia prevention in larger populations and over longer periods of time.

## 7. Acknowledgements

Funding was provided by Wilford Hall Medical Center, San Antonio, TX; South Dakota State University Agricultural Experiment Station, Brookings, SD; and the Center for Disaster and Humanitarian Assistance Medicine, Uniformed Services University of the Health Sciences, Bethesda, MD. Micronutrient sprinkles were provided by Heinz Company, Canada.

## 8. References

Adu-Afarwuah S, Lartey A, Brown, KH, Zlotkin S, Briend A, Dewey K. (2008). Home fortification of complementary foods with micronutrient supplements is well accepted and has positive effects on infant iron status in Ghana, *Am J Clin Nutr*, 87:929-38

Adu-Afarwuah S, Lartey A, Brown, KH, Zlotkin S, Briend A, Dewey K. (2007). Randomized comparison of 3 types of micronutrient supplements for home fortification of complementary foods in Ghana: Effects on growth and motor development, *Am J Clini Nutr*, 87:929-38

Albalak R, Ramakrishnan U, Stein AD, Van der Haar F, Haber MJ, Schroeder D, Martorell R. (2000). Co-Occurrence of Nutrition Problems in Honduran Children, *J Nutr*, 130:2271-2273

Allen LH, Peerson JM, Olney DK. (2009). Provision of multiple rather than two or fewer micronutrients more effectively improves growth and other outcomes in micronutrient-deficient children and adults, *J Nutr*, 139(5):1022-30

Andersson M, Thankachan P, Muthayya S, Goud RB, Kurpad AV, Hurrell RH, Zimmermann MB. (2008). Dual fortification of salt with iodine and iron: a randomized, double-blind, controlled trial of micronized ferric pyrophosphate and encapsulated ferrous fumarate in southern India, *Am J Clin Nutr*, 88(5):1378-1387

Angeles-Agdeppa I, Saises M, Capanzana M, Juneja LR, Sakaguchi N. (2011). Pilot-scale commercialization of iron-fortified rice: effects on anemia status, *Food Nutr Bull*, 32(1):3-12

Badham J, Zimmermann MB, Kraemer K (ed). (2007). *The Guidebook Nutritional Anemia*. Sight and Life Press, Basel, Switzerland. (51 pages)

Balarajan Y, Ramakrishnan U, Ozaltin E, Shankar AH, Subramanian S. (2011). Anaemia in low-income and middle-income countries, *Lancet*. 2011 Aug 1, [Epub ahead of print]

Bethony J, Brooker S, Albonico M, Geiger SM, Loukas A, Diemert D, Hotez PJ. (2006). Soil-transmitted helminth infections: ascariasis, trichuriasis, and hookworm, *Lancet*, 367:1521-32

Bilenko N, Belmaker I, Vardi H, Fraser D. (2010). Efficacy of multiple micronutrient supplementations on child health: study design and baseline characteristics, *Isr Med Assoc J*, 12(6):342-7

Black RE, Allen LH, Bhutta ZA, Caulfield LE, de Onis M, Ezzati M, Mathers C, Rivera J. (2008) Maternal and child undernutrition: global and regional exposures and health consequences, *Lancet*, 371:243-60

Bouis HE, Hotz C, McClafferty B, Meenakshi JV, Pfeiffer WH. (2011). Biofortification: a new tool to reduce micronutrient malnutrition, *Food Nutr Bull*, 32(1 Suppl):S31-40

Boy E, Mannar V, Pandav C, de Benoist B, Viteri F, Fontaine O, Hotz C. (2009). Achievements, challenges, and promising new approaches in vitamin and mineral deficiency control, *Nutr Rev*, 67:S24-30

Brooker S, Clements ACA, Hotez PJ, Hay SI, Tatem AJ, Bundy DAP, Snow RW. (Nov 2006). The co-distribution of Plasmodium falciparum and hookworm among African schoolchildren, *Malaria Journal*, 5(99), Accessed July 7, 2009, Available at http:www.malaria journal.com/ content/5/1/99

Carter RC, Jacobson JL, Burden MJ, Armony-Sivan R, Dodge NC, Angelilli ML, Lozoff B, Jacobson SW. (2010). Iron deficiency anemia and cognitive function in infancy, *Pediatrics*, 126(2):e427-34. Epub 2010 Jul 26

Christofides A, Asante KP, Schauer C, Sharieff W, Owusu-Agyei S, Zlotkin S. (2006). Multi-micronutrient sprinkles including a low dose of iron provided as microencapsulated ferrous fumarate improves haematologic indices in anaemic children: a randomized clinical trial, *Matern Child Nutr*, 2(3):169-80

Corapci F, Radan A, Lozoff B. (2006). Iron deficiency in infancy and mother-child intereaction at 5 years, *J Dev Behav Pediatr*, 27(5):371-378

Darnton-Hill I, Mora JO, Weinstein H, Wilbur S, Ritu Nalubola P. (1999). Iron and folate fortification in the Americas to prevent and control micronutrient malnutrition: An analysis, *Nutrition Reviews*, 57(1): 25-31

Darnton-Hill I. (1998). Overview: Rationale and elements of a successful food-fortification programme, *Food Nutr Bull*, 19(2):92-100

Dary O. (2007). The importance and limitations of food fortification for the management of nutritional anemia. In: Badham J, Zimmermann MB, Kraemer K (eds). *The Guidebook Nutritional Anemia*. Sight and Life Press, (pages 42-43)

De-Regil LM, Suchdev PS, Vist GE, Walleser S, Peña-Rosas JP. (2011). Home fortification of foods with multiple micronutrient powders for health and nutrition in children under two years of age, *Cochrane Database Syst Rev*, Sep 7;9:CD008959 (83 pages)

Dewey KG, Cohen RJ, Rivera LL, Brown KH. (1998). Effects of age of introduction of complementary foods on iron status of breast-fed infants in Honduras, *Am J Clin Nutr*, 67: 878-84

Dewey KG, Cohen RJ, Brown KH. (2004). Exclusive breast-feeding for 6 months, with iron supplementation, maintains adequate micronutrient status among term, low-birthweight, breast-fed infants in Honduras, *J Nutr*, 134:1091-98

Erhardt, JG, Estes, JE, Pfeifer, CM, Biesalski, HK, Craft, NE. (2004). Combined measurement of ferritin, soluble transferrin receptor, retinol binding protein, and C-reactive protein by an inexpensive, sensitive, and simple sandwich enzyme-linked immunosorbent assay technique, *J Nutr*, 134: 3127-32

Faber M, Kvalsvig JD, Lombard CJ, AJ Spinnler Benadé. (2005). Effect of a fortified maize-meal porridge on anemia, micronutrient status, and motor development of infants, *Am J Clin Nutr*, 82(5):1032-1039

Finch CA, Cook JD. (1984). Iron Deficiency, *Am J Clini Nutr*, 39:471-77

Flowers CH, Cook JD. (1999). Dried plasma spot measurements of ferritin and transferrin receptor for assessing iron status, *Clini Chem*, 45(10):1826-32

Geltman PL, Hironaka LK, Mehta SD, Padilla P, Rodrigues P, Meyers AF, Bauchner H. (2009). Iron supplementation of low-income infants: a randomized clinical trial of adherence with ferrous fumarate sprinkles versus ferrous sulfate drops, *J Pediatr*, 154(5):738-43

Giovannini M, Sala D, Usuelli M, Livio L, Francescato G, Braga M, Radaelli G, Riva E. (2006). Double-blind, placebo-controlled trial comparing effects of supplementation with two different combinations of micronutrients delivered as sprinkles on growth, anemia, and iron deficiency in cambodian infants, *J Pediatr Gastroenterol Nutr*, 42(3):306-12

Grantham-McGregor S, Ani C. (Feb 2001). A review of studies on the effect of iron deficiency on cognitive development in children, *J Nutr*, 131(2S-2):649S-666S; discussion 666S-668S

Hijmans CT, Grootenhuis MA, Oosterlaan J, Heijboer H, Peters M, Fijnvandraat K. (2011). Neurocognitive deficits in children with sickle cell disease are associated with the severity of anemia, *Pediatr Blood Cancer*, 57(2):297-302

Hirve S, Bhave S, Bavdekar A, Naik S, Pandit A, Schauer C, Christofides A, Hyder Z, Zlotkin S. (2007). Low dose 'Sprinkles'-- an innovative approach to treat iron deficiency anemia in infants and young children, *Indian Pediatr*, 44(2):91-100

Horton S, Shekar M, McDonald C, Mahal A, Brooks JK. (2010). *Scaling Up Nutrition: What Will it Cost?* World Bank (136 pages)

Horton S. (2006). The economics of food fortification, *J Nutr*, 136:1068–1071

Horton S, Ross J. (2003). The economics of iron deficiency, *Food Policy*, 28:51-75

Hurrell R, Ranum P, De Pee S, Biebinger R, Hulthen L, Johnson Q, Lynch S. (2010). Revised recommendations for iron fortification of wheat flour and an evaluation of the expected impact of current national wheat flour fortification programs, *Food Nutr Bull*, 31(1) S7-S21

Ip H, Hyder SM, Haseen F, Rahman M, Zlotkin SH. (2009). Improved adherence and anaemia cure rates with flexible administration of micronutrient sprinkles: a new public health approach to anaemia control, *Eur J Clin Nutr*, 63(2):165-72

Karn SK, Chavasit V, Kongkachuichai R, Tangsuphoom N. (2011). Shelf stability, sensory qualities, and bioavailability of iron-fortified Nepalese curry powder, *Food Nutr Bull*, 32(1):13-22

Loechl CU, Menon P, Arimond M, Ruel MT, Pelto G, Habicht JP, Michaud L. (2009). Using programme theory to assess the feasibility of delivering micronutrient Sprinkles through a food-assisted maternal and child health and nutrition programme in rural Haiti, *Maternal Child Nutr*, 5:33-48

Lokeshwar MR, Mehta M, Mehta N, Shelke P, Babar N. (2011). Prevention of iron deficiency anemia (IDA): How far have we reached? *Indian J Pediatr*, 78(5):593-602

López de Romaña G, Cusirramos S, López de Romaña D, Gross R. (2005). Efficacy of multiple micronutrient supplementation for improving anemia, micronutrient status, growth, and morbidity of Peruvian infants, *J Nutr*, 135(3):646S-652S

Lozoff B. (2011). Early iron deficiency has brain and behavior effects consistent with dopaminergic dysfunction, *J Nutr*, 141: 740S–746S

Lozoff B, Beard J, Connor J, Barbara F, Georgieff M, Schallert T. (2006). Long-lasting neural and behavioral effects of iron deficiency in infancy, *Nutr Rev*, 64(5 Pt 2):S34-43; discussion S72-91

Lucca P, Hurrell R, Potrykus I. (2001). Genetic engineering approaches to improve the bioavailability and the level of iron in rice grains, *Theor Appl Genet*, 102:392–397

Lucca P, Poletti S, Sautter C. (2006). Genetic engineering approaches to enrich rice with iron and vitamin A. *Physiologia Plantarum*, 126: 291-303

Lundeen E, Schueth T, Toktobaev N, Zlotkin S, Ziauddin Hyder SM, Houser R. (2010). Daily use of Sprinkles micronutrient powder for 2 months reduces anemia among children 6 to 36 months of age in the Kyrgyz Republic: a cluster-randomized trial, *Food Nutr Bull*, 31:446-460

Lutter CK. (2008). Iron deficiency in young children in low-income countries and new approaches for its prevention, *J Nutr*, 138:2523-2528

Madan N, Rusia U, Sikka M, Sharma S, Shankar N. (2011). Developmental and neurophysiologic deficits in iron deficiency in children, *Indian J Pediatr*, 78(1):58-64

McLean E, Cogswell M, Egli I, Wojdyla D, de Benoist B. (2009). Worldwide prevalence of anaemia, WHO vitamin and mineral nutrition information system, 1993–2005, *Public Health Nutr*, 12: 444–54

Mehansho H. (2006). Iron fortification technology development: New approaches, J Nutr, 136:1059-1063

Menon P, Ruel MT, Loechl CU, Arimond M, Habicht JP, Pelto G, Michaud L. (2007). Micronutrient sprinkles reduce anemia among 9- to 24-mo-old children when delivered through an integrated health and nutrition program in rural Haiti, *J Nutr*, 137(4):1023-30

Milman N. (2011). Anemia- still a major health problem in many parts of the world! *Ann Hematol*, 90:369-377

Nestel P, Melara A, Rosado J, Mora JO. (1999). Vitamin A deficiency and anemia among children 12-71 months old in Honduras, *Pan Am J Public Health*, 6(1): 34-43

Oxford Department of International Development. (2010). Oxford Poverty and Human Development Initiative (OPHI). Country Briefing: Honduras

Provan D. (1999). Mechanisms and management of iron deficiency anemia, *Br J Haem*, 105:19-26

Rosado JL, González KE, Caamaño Mdel C, García OP, Preciado R, Odio M. (2010). Efficacy of different strategies to treat anemia in children: a randomized clinical trial, *Nutr J*, 9:40

Ruiz-Arguelles G (2006). Altitude above sea level as a variable for definition of anemia. *Blood*, 108, 2131-2132

Samadpour K, Long KZ, Hayatbakhsh R, Marks GC. (2011). Randomised comparison of the effects of Sprinkles and Foodlets with the currently recommended supplement (Drops) on micronutrient status and growth in Iranian children, *Eur J Clin Nutr*, doi: 10.1038/ejcn.2011.124. [Epub ahead of print]

Schauer C, Zlotkin SH. (2003). "Home-fortification" with micronutrient sprinkles—A new approach for the prevention and treatment of nutritional anemias, *J Paediatr Child Health*, 8:87–90

Sharieff W, Yin SA, Wu M, Yang Q, Schauer C, Tomlinson G, Zlotkin S. (2006). Short-term daily or weekly administration of micronutrient sprinkles has high compliance and does not cause iron overload in Chinese schoolchildren: a cluster-randomized trial, *Public Health Nutr*, 9(3):336-44

Sharieff W, Horton SE, Zlotkin S. (2006). Economic gains of a home fortification program: evaluation of "Sprinkles" from the provider's perspective, *Canadian J Pub Health*, 97:20-23

Smith HM, DeKaminsky RG, Niwas S, Soto RJ, Jolly PE. (Apr 2001). Prevalence and intensity of infections of Ascaris lumbricoides and Trichuris trichiura and associated socio-demographic variables in four rural Honduran communities, Mem Inst Oswaldo Cruz, Rio de Janeiro, 96(3):303-14

Smuts CM, Lombard CJ, Spinnler Benade AJ, Dhansay MA, Berger J, Hop LT, Lopez de Romaña G, Untoro J, Karyadi E, Erhardt J, Gross R. (2005). Efficacy of a foodlet-based multiple micronutrient supplement for preventing growth faltering, anemia, and micronutrient deficiency of infants: the four country IRIS trial pooled data analysis, *J Nutr*, 135:631S-638S

Sparks CS. (2011). Parental investment and socioeconomic status influences on children's height in Honduras: an analysis of national data, *Am J Hum Biol*, 23:80-88

Sprinkles Global Health Initiative. (2008). Micronutrient sprinkles for use in infants and young children: guidelines on recommendations for use and program monitoring and evaluation. Accessed Sept 20, 2011, Available from: http://sghi.org/resource_centre/GuidelinesGen2008.pdf

Stoltzfus RJ, Albonico M, Chwaya HM, Tielsch JM, Schulze KJ, Savioli L. (1998). Effects of the Zanzibar school-based deworming on iron status of children, *Am J Clin Nutr*, 68:179-86

Stoltzfus RJ, Mullany L, Black RE. (2004). Iron deficiency anaemia. In: Ezzati M, Lopez AD, Rodgers A, Murray CLJ, eds. Comparative quantification of health risks: global and regional burden of disease attributable to selected major risk factors. Geneva: World Health Organization, 163–209

Stoltzfus RJ. (2008). Research needed to strengthen science and programs for the control of iron deficiency and its consequences in young children, *J Nutr*, 138:2542-2546

Stoltzfus RJ. (2011). Iron interventions for women and children in low-income countries, *J Nutr*, 141:756S-762S

Tolson DJ, Kemmer TM , Lynch J, Lougee D, Aviles R, Amador WE, Duron CA, Guifarro Fino RO. (2010). Identifying children at risk for nutritional crisis in rural Honduras, *J Hunger Env Nutr*, 5:1, 13-22

Torrejon CS, Duran-Castillo C, Hertrampf E, Ruz M. (2004). Zinc and iron nutrition in Chilean children fed fortified milk provided by the Complementary National Food Program, *Nutrition*, 20:177-80

Trowbridge, F. (2002). Prevention and control of iron deficiency: priorities and action steps, *J Nutr*, 132:880S-882S

United Nations. (2011). *Millennium Development Goals Report*. New York (72 pages). Accessed Sept 10, 2011, Available from: http://www.un.org/millenniumgoals/pdf/(2011_E)%20MDG%20Report%202011_Book%20LR.pdf

UNICEF. (2010). *UNICEF Honduras Statistics*. Accessed Sept 10, 2011, Available from: <http://www.unicef.org/infobycountry/honduras_statistics.html>

Varma JL, Das S, Sankar R, Venkatesh Mannar MG, Levinson FJ, Hamer DH. (2007). Community-level micronutrient fortification of a food supplement in India: a controlled trial in preschool children aged 36-66 mo, *Am J Clin Nutr*, 85:1127-1133

Venkatesh Mannar MG. (2006). Successful food-based programmes, supplementation and fortification, *J Ped Gastro and Nutr*, 43:S47–S53

Wegmüller R, Camara F, Zimmermann MB, Adou P, Hurrell RF. (2006). Salt dual-fortified with iodine and micronized ground ferric pyrophosphate affects iron status but not hemoglobin in children in Côte d'Ivoire, *J Nutr.* 136:1814-1820

World Bank. (2011). *2011 World Development Indicators*, Accessed Sept 1, 2011, Available from: <http://data.worldbank.org/data-catalog/world-development-indicators>

World Bank. (2010). *Nutrition at a Glance: Honduras.* Accessed September 20, 2011, Available from: <http://siteresources.worldbank.org/NUTRITION/Resources/281846-1271963823772/Honduras.pdf>

World Bank. (2004). *Public Health at a Glance: Anemia-World Bank Group.* Accessed September 17, 2011, Available from: <http://siteresources.worldbank.org/INTPHAAG/Resources/anemiaAAG.pdf>

World Health Organization. (2001). *Iron deficiency anaemia: assessment, prevention and control. A guide for programme managers.* (114 pages)

World Health Organization. (2005). WHO Anthro, Accessed June 20, 2011, Available from: http://www.who.int/childgrowth/software/en/

World Health Organization Multicentre Growth Reference Study Group. (2006). WHO Child Growth Standards: Length/height-for-age, weight-for-age, weight-for-length, weight-for-height and body mass index-for-age: Methods and development. Geneva: World Health Organization (312 pages)

World Health Organization. (2008). *Worldwide Prevalence of Anemia 1993-2005: WHO Global Data Base on Anemia*

World Heath Organization. (2009). *Global Health Risks: Mortality and burden of disease attributable to selected major risks.* (62 pages)

World Heath Organization. (2009). *Recommendations on Wheat and Maize Flour Fortification Meeting Report: Interim Consensus Statement* (3 pages)

World Heath Organization. (2011). *Honduras: health profile.* Accessed September 9, 2011, Available from http://www.who.int/gho/countries/hnd.pdf

Zimmermann MB, Hurrell RF. (2007). Nutritional iron deficiency, *Lancet*, 370:511-520

Zlotkin S, Arthur P, Antwi K, Yeung G. (2001). Treatment of anemia with microencapsulated ferrous fumerate plus ascorbic acid supplied as sprinkles to complementary (weaning) foods, *Am J Clin Nutr*, 74:791-5

Zlotkin S, Antwi KY, Schauer C, Yeung G. (2003a). Use of microencapsulated iron (II) fumarate sprinkles to prevent recurrence of anaemia in infants and young children at high risk, *Bull WHO*, 81:108-15

Zlotkin S, Arthur P, Schauer C, Antwi KY, Yeung G, Piekarz A. (2003b). Home-fortification with iron and zinc sprinkles or iron sprinkles alone successfully treats anemia in infants and young children, *J Nutr*, 133:1075-80

Zlotkin SH, Christofides AL, Hyder SM, Schauer CS, Tondeur MC, Sharieff W. (2004). Controlling iron deficiency anemia through the use of home-fortified complementary foods, *Indian J Pediatr*, 71(11):1015-9

Zlotkin S, Tondeur M. (2007). The importance and limitations of food fortification for the management of nutritional anemia: in Badham J, Zimmermann MB, Kraemer K, (eds). *The Guidebook Nutritional Anemia.* Sight and Life Press, 2007 (pages 36-37)

# 13

# Supplementation and Change of Nutritional Habits for the Prevention and Treatment of Iron Deficiency Anaemia in Gaza Children: A Case Study

Michele Magoni, Ghassam Zaqout, Omar Ahmmed Mady, Reema Ibraheem Al Haj Abed and Davide Amurri
*Terre des Hommes*
*Italy*

## 1. Introduction

Iron deficiency anaemia (IDA) is one of the most severe and widespread nutritional disorders in the world. Children and pregnant women in resource-poor areas represent the most vulnerable groups. Iron deficiency impairs the cognitive development of children from infancy through to adolescence. It damages immune mechanisms and is associated with increased morbidity rates. Iron deficiency commonly develops after six months of age if complementary foods do not provide sufficient absorbable iron, even for exclusively breastfed infants (World Health Organization [WHO] et al, 2001). The WHO recommends universal iron supplementation when prevalence of anaemia is more than 40% (WHO, 2004).

In the Eastern Mediterranean regions there is an endemic high prevalence of iron-deficiency anaemia (Verster, 1996) due to low total iron intake, low bioavailability (in many diets over 80% of iron is of non-haem origin) and high intake of inhibitors of iron absorption (unleavened bread and tea are severe inhibitors of iron absorption and are consumed in large amounts everywhere). Anaemia and stunting prevalence in Gaza have always been found to be very high in recent years (Abdeen, 2002; Rahim et al 2009).

### 1.1 Emergency situation

In the Gaza Strip the basic living conditions of all the inhabitants have deteriorated constantly in recent years, particularly after the "Cast Lead" operation in January 2009: the blockade and the closure of terminals for the movement of goods and people created a very tense situation which severely affected the wellbeing of all the inhabitants: 98% of private businesses closed and the unemployment rate increased to 48.8%, while 80% of the population lives below the poverty line and 79% is aid-dependent. The rate of food insecure households in Gaza has also increased to 75%, up from 56% before the Cast Lead operation. Furthermore, the growing inability of the population to consume iron-rich animal proteins and fresh fruit and vegetables, which contain the vitamins required for iron absorption, is bound to have a critical impact on the already high prevalence of mild and moderate iron deficiency anaemia in the Gaza Strip, habitually already about 20% higher than in the West Bank (WHO, 2009; World Bank, 2009).

The National Nutrition Surveillance System Report (PNA, MOH, 2010) has confirmed a worsening level of anaemia and chronic malnutrition in the Gaza Strip, with an overall anaemia prevalence of 76.2% (45.5% in the West Bank) among children 9-12 months old and 58.6% (9.5% in the West Bank) among school children. Stunting prevalence in school children was 7.9% in the Gaza Strip and 4.4% in the West Bank. The national survey does not provide any data for children between the ages of 12 months and 5 years.

### 1.2 Present humanitarian intervention

Terre des Hommes Italy[1] (Tdh-It) and its Palestinian partner Palestinian Medical Relief Society[2] (PMRS) started operating with several humanitarian projects in Gaza in 2009, targeting pre-school children in a holistic way, where the prevention and treatment of anaemia have played a fundamental role. The projects were supported by the Italian Cooperation and other European donors.

It is worth pointing out that the Tdh-It and PMRS projects were designed and implemented as (and in the framework of) humanitarian interventions and not study; nevertheless, the projects have also been supported by a strong monitoring and evaluation system that has provided us with a massive and structured quantity of information allowing us to present the projects' impact and data as a case study, although the possibility of bias in the sample selections has to be borne in mind.

There is a strong need for a more evidence-based approach in humanitarian medical work and although a substantial body of knowledge has been accumulated regarding the effectiveness of interventions in acute emergencies, especially in refugee settings, the evidence base is much weaker for situations of protracted conflict with longer-term programmes in less controlled settings. (Banatvala and Zwi, 2000; Robertson et al, 2002; Roberts and Hofmann, 2004)

## 2. Method

### 2.1 Nutritional health projects

The interventions that Tdh-It and PMRS implemented included the following components:

- screening for IDA and malnutrition in 22 kindergartens (South Gaza: Rafah and Khan Younis Governorates) and 4 paediatric clinics (North Gaza: Northern Governorate);
- iron and vitamin supplementation based on therapeutic or preventive WHO protocols for all children contacted;
- medical follow-up for anaemic and malnourished children;
- provision of a home visit service for anaemic and malnourished children in order to:
    - assess families' and children's nutritional habits (24-hour recall questionnaire)

---

[1] Terre des Hommes Italia (Tdh-It) was founded in 1989 in Milan (Italy) and is part of the Terre des Hommes International Federation. It is a non profit non-governmental organisation (ONLUS) whose mission it is to carry out humanitarian relief and international development projects for the benefit of children, their families and communities.

[2] Palestinian Medical Relief Society (PMRS) is a grassroots, community- based Palestinian health organization founded in 1979. PMRS operates with 4 Primary Health Care Centres (PHCCs) in the Gaza Strip, providing preventive and curative services, and specialized health care for women and children.

- provide family nutritional counselling
- support behavioural health change;

- health education sessions for mothers and fathers - held at the clinics, in kindergarten and during home visits.

Children who were still anaemic after intervention underwent further clinical investigation, treatment and longer follow-up.

The following table summarizes the activities and treatment protocols for the different projects.

| Period | Area | Target | Intervention for anaemics | Treatment for anaemics* |
|---|---|---|---|---|
| September 2009 - June 2010 | South Gaza (1) | Children in 12 kindergartens and their siblings | Screening and treatment, monthly follow-up with haemoglobin control after 4 months, health education, home visit for anaemic children | Iron polymaltose complex 5mg/kg and multivitamins daily for 4 months, followed by preventive iron (1mg/kg daily) |
| January 2010 - December 2010 | North Gaza | Children from 3 local communities invited to local clinics | Screening, treatment, follow-up after 3 months with haemoglobin test, health education, home visit only for some anaemic children | Iron polymaltose complex 3-6mg/kg and multivitamins daily for at least 3 months, followed by multivitamin including iron (1mg/kg daily) |
| September 2010 - June 2011 | South Gaza (2) | Children in 11 kindergartens and their siblings | Screening and treatment, monthly follow-up with haemoglobin control after 4 months, health education, home visit for anaemic children | Iron polymaltose complex 5mg/kg and multivitamins daily for 4 months, followed by preventive iron (1mg/kg daily) |

**A paediatrician or medical doctor changed the dosage and length of treatment when required by the child's clinical condition.*

Table 1. Summary of Tdh-It/ PMRS nutritional projects in Gaza.

### 2.2 Data collection

Data were collected using two questionnaires, which were also used during the monitoring process:

1. *CHILD FILE (annex-1)*: basic information about family and screened children gathered in the kindergarten during screening and follow-up visits. 10,445 children were screened for anaemia (blood test), including the main anthropometric indicators (height, weight), between October 2009 and March 2011: 3,941 (37.7%) children were screened at 3 paediatric clinics in northern Gaza (Izbet Beit Hanoun, Umm El Nasser, Jabalia/Beit Lahia) while the other 6,504 were screened in the kindergartens (including siblings aged less than 6 years) in southern Gaza (eastern areas of Khan Younis and western areas of Rafah City).

## FAMILY INFORMATION

1) Name of the family's head (four names) ____________

a. Name in Arabic ____________

2) ID number of the family's head ____________ **Family code** _ _/_ _ _ _

3) Full Address: ____________ 4) Telephone n.____________

**5) Number of family's members**: _ _; below 5 years: _ _; 5-18 years: _ _;

**6) Mother's personal status:** Living with husband divorced Widow Married but living alone Married but living with her family Dead mother

**7) Mother's education:** Illiterate can read & write elementary Preparatory secondary lower diploma bachelor and more

**8) Father's education:** Illiterate can read & write elementary Preparatory secondary lower diploma bachelor and more

**9) Father Job:**
(1) Worker (2) Government/Municipality employee (3) Self employee
(4) Business (employing others) (5) Peasant (6) Shepherd
(7) Driver (8) Unemployed (9) Other

**10) Mother age** _____ **11) n. of pregnancy**_____ **12) n. of deliveries** ______

**13) Pregnant now** Yes Not **N° of death children**

| | <1 year | 1-5 years |
|---|---|---|
| M | | |
| F | | |

## CHILD FILE

**14) Date of visit** _ _/_ _/_ _ _ _ Family code_ _/_ _ _ CODE of the Child _ _ _

**15) Name of the Child** .................................................. **16) Date of birth** _ _/_ _/_ _ _ _

**17) ID number of the child**: .................................... **18) attending KG** Yes Not

**19) Sex:** M F **20) Weight (kg)** _ _. _ _ **21) Height (cm)** _ _ _

**22) Percentile weight for age** ______ **23) Hb level** _ _. _

**24) Referred for doctor visit** Yes Not **25) Referred to clinic** Yes Not

**Reason** .................................................. **Reason** ..................................................

**25b) does the child suffer from a chronic disease?** Thalassaemia G6PD Other ....................

**26) Already receiving fortified food?** Yes Not **comments**....................

**27) N° of iron bottles given:** _ _ **(ml/day**_____**)** **28) N° of MULTIVITAMIN given:** _ _

## FOLLOW UP FILE

**CODE of the Child** Date of follow up _ _/_ _/_ _ _ _ visit N° 1

**Medication taken:** regularly (>=5days/week) irregularly (4-2days/week) not taken (<=1)

**Have drugs given been finished?** YES NO why? ____________

Weight (kg) _ _. _ _ Height (cm) _ _ _ C° weight for age _____ Hb level _ _. _

N° of iron bottles given: _ _ **N° of MULTIVITAMIN given:** _ _

ANNEX 1. Extract from the CHILD FILE.

2. *HOME VISIT (annex-2)*: details of the families of anaemic children were collected twice during home visits (coinciding roughly with the start and end of treatment) and concerned mother's knowledge, nutritional habits of all the children, iron treatment compliance and adoption of healthy life styles.

In the project implemented in northern Gaza only some families received home visits and there was also a problem with coding of the children, so the link between data collected during screening and the home visit was not available; for this reason we analysed only data from the kindergarten visits carried out in southern Gaza. A total of 1,733 families of anaemic children screened in kindergartens were visited at home.

## NUTRITIONAL QUESTIONNAIRE

Is the child presently breastfed?

| Child 1 | Child 2 | Child 3 | Child 4 |
|---|---|---|---|
| Yes No<br>if yes no. of times________ | Yes No<br>if yes no. of times________ | Yes No<br>if yes no. of times________ | Yes No<br>if yes no. of times________ |

How many meals the child has on average per day? Child 1______ Child 2______ Child 3______ Child 3______

| | Child 1 | Child 2 | Child 3 | Child 4 | | Child 1 | Child 2 | Child 3 | Child 4 |
|---|---|---|---|---|---|---|---|---|---|
| Indicate number of "portion" of the following food *(or number of items where indicated)* that the CHILD has eaten in the last <u>24 h</u>? (One portion is big as the person's fist) | | | | | | | | | |
| Vegetables | | | | | Cheese and dairy products | | | | |
| Fruits | | | | | Bread | | | | |
| Legumes | | | | | Rice | | | | |
| Nuts and Seeds | | | | | Pasta | | | | |
| Meat | | | | | Potatoes | | | | |
| Chicken | | | | | Biscuits/cake | | | | |
| Fish | | | | | Chocolate bars (n.) | | | | |
| Eggs (n.) | | | | | Sweets and candies (n) | | | | |
| Chips (n. of sachet) | | | | | Jam/ cream (n. of big spoon) | | | | |
| Indicates how many cups/glasses the CHILD had of the following drinks in the last 24 h? (mark with X) | | | | | | | | | |
| Milk (with sugar) | | | | | Tea (outside meal) | | | | |
| Milk (without sugar) | | | | | Tea (with main meal) | | | | |
| Water | | | | | Fresh Juice | | | | |
| Soft drink | | | | | Packed Juice | | | | |

How many times is the child eating junk food outside main meals? Child 1______ Child 2______

**KNOWLEDGE OF THE MOTHER ASSESSMENT** (don't prompt the mother before she has finished to answer the all questions)

- **Why anaemia is bad for the child?** Doesn't know____; mental retard ____; weakness____; infection vulnerability_____; poor school performance____; other answers____; AHA.....?????
- **What are the causes of anaemia is bad for the child?** Doesn't know____; tea___; Tea with meal____; lack of meat/chicken /fish ____, lack of rich iron vegetable (she can mention one) ____; some diseases _____; poverty_____; other answers_____;
- **What can be done to prevent or treat anaemia?** Doesn't know____; good diet___; iron supplementation _____, food fortification ______, wrong answer_____;
- **What is the GOOD food for the child growth?** doesn't know____; Breast feeding___; Vegetables____; Legumes____; Fruits____; Meat____; Chicken ____; Fish____; Eggs____; Milk___; Cheese and milk products____; fresh juice _____; other answers_____;
- **What are the food BAD for the child growth?** doesn't know____; Sugar____; Soft drinks___; Chips____; Salted biscuits___; Butter___; Biscuits___; Cakes ____; Chocolate bars ___; Sweets and candies ____; ice cream_____; jam and cream _____; other answers_____;

ANNEX 2. Extract from the HOME VIST FILE (nutritional questionnaire and mother's knowledge assessment).

Data were collected for 3,619 children (2,024 anaemics and 1,595 non-anaemic siblings) of these families concerning:

- drug adherence, tolerance, storage and administration
- mother's knowledge of anaemia and nutrition
- nutritional habit (24-hour recall nutritional questionnaire)

The second visit took place on average 111 days (SD=46) after the first visit.
The home visit data included children on iron preventive treatment, not only anaemics.

### 2.3 Haemoglobin assessment

Blood samples taken at kindergarten were analysed using the Haemocue rapid test.
Blood samples in clinics were tested using an aXE-2100D automated haematology analyser (Sysmex).

### 2.4 Definition of anaemia and malnutrition

*Anaemia.* Children with a haemoglobin level below 11g/dl were considered anaemic. Anaemia was defined as mild for a haemoglobin level of 10-11g/dl, moderate for 7-9.9 gm/dl and severe for less than 7gm/dl.
*Malnutrition.* The software used to calculate Z score was "WHO ANTHRO, Software for Calculating Anthropometry, Version 2.0" and "WHO ANTHROPLUS". Segments of the population below -2 Z score (2SD) were considered as suffering from wasting (acute malnutrition, weight/height), underweight (weight/age) and stunting (chronic malnutrition, height/age). Segments of the population above 2Z of body mass index for age were considered as overweight (WHO, 2009).

### 2.5 Statistical analyses

Statistical analyses were performed using STATA software (Stata Statistical Software release 9.2, 2007; Stata Corporation, College Station, Texas). Uni- and multivariate binary regression and chi square test were used where appropriate. All statistical tests were two sided, and P values of < 0.05 were considered significant.

### 2.6 Main objectives

As already mentioned, the intervention was not conceived or performed as a study, thus the monitoring and evaluation (M&E) system was a tool for correct activity management and for evaluating the impact of the project, but it did allowed us to gather useful information:

- for comparing the prevalence of anaemia and malnutrition before and after the project in the pre-school child population;
- for identifying risk factors for anaemia;
- for assessing compliance and tolerability of treatment and their association with lack of improvement;
- for assessing change in the families' knowledge of anaemia and nutrition (mothers);
- for assessing nutritional habits and evaluating changes promoted by intervention;
- for evaluating anaemia prevalence 1 year after intervention (long-lasting impact);
- for monitoring and evaluating anaemic children who did not improve during the first phase of the project, including identification of non-iron deficiency anaemia (e.g. thalassaemia).

### 2.7 Ethical approval

The Helsinki Committee of Palestinian Ministry of Health gave approval for publication of present paper.

## 3. RESULTS

### 3.1 Anaemia prevalence at screening

10,445 children were screened for anaemia between October 2009 and March 2011: 3,941 (37.7%) of them were screened at the PMRS paediatric clinics in northern Gaza, while the other 6,504 (including siblings) were screened at the 22 kindergartens in southern Gaza.

51.6% (5,391) of the screened children were male. The mean age of the screened children was 39.7 months (SD=18.0), with no difference between the sexes.

5.877 (56.3%) of the tested children were not anaemic and 4,568 (43.7%) were anaemic (HB level <11g/dl); 421 of the anaemics (4.1%) had a haemoglobin level below 9g/dl.

The prevalence of anaemia was similar in males (44.0%) and females (43.4%, p=0.5) and strongly and inversely associated with age, as shown in Figure 1 and Table 1: anaemia had a very high prevalence in children below 24 months, peaking at 6-11 months (76.2%) and 12-23 months (72.2%). The percentage was much lower in older children (17.0% for children > 5 years old).

When considering only the under-5 population, the prevalence of anaemia was 49% (4,271/8,709), but it should be noted that children below 12 months of age were under-represented and our sample did not adequately represent the under-5 population of Gaza.

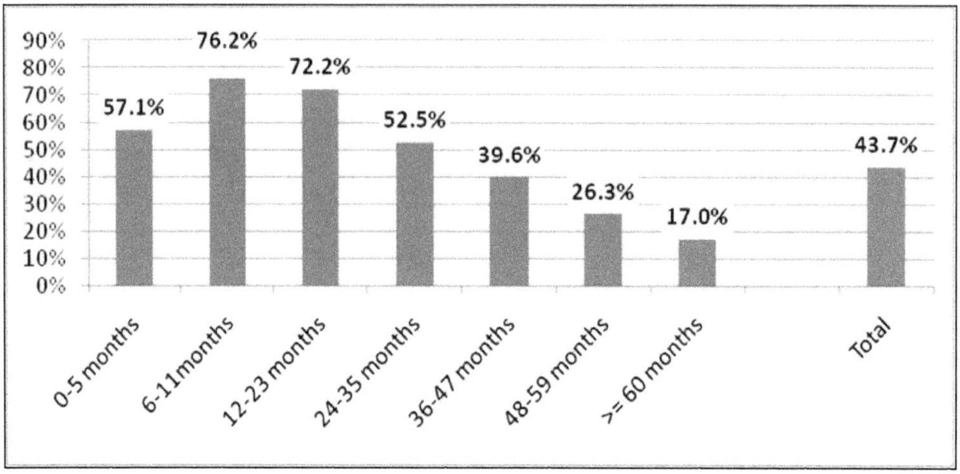


Fig. 1. Prevalence of anaemia by age group.

| Age groups | N° of screened | N° of anaemics | % of anaemics | % of stunting | % of underweight | % of wasting | % of overweight |
|---|---|---|---|---|---|---|---|
| 0-5 months | 56 | 32 | 57.1% | 0.0% | 3.6% | 8.9% | 5.4% |
| 6-11 months | 513 | 391 | 76.2% | 6.9% | 2.7% | 5.5% | 5.7% |
| 12-23 months | 2,026 | 1,462 | 72.2% | 10.7% | 2.9% | 2.9% | 7.2% |
| 24-35 months | 1,973 | 1,036 | 52.5% | 10.8% | 2.2% | 3.6% | 8.2% |
| 36-47 months | 1,967 | 778 | 39.6% | 9.6% | 2.5% | 3.2% | 6.3% |
| 48-59 months | 2,174 | 572 | 26.3% | 6.6% | 2.6% | 2.7% | 5.3% |
| ≥ 60 months | 1,726 | 294 | 17.0% | 6.2% | 2.1% | 1.8% | 3.0% |
| Total | 10,435 | 4,565 | 43.7% | 8.7% | 2.5% | 3.1% | 6.2% |

Table 2. Prevalence of anaemia and malnutrition by age group.

As shown in Table 3, anaemia was also associated with:

- mother's poor education, regardless of child's age (p<0.0001)
- stunting in children over 24 months of age
- not having received fortified food (data collected for kindergarten children only).

| | | Children below 24 months (2,595) | Children over 24 months (7,850) |
|---|---|---|---|
| Mother's education | No education (278) | 88% | 54% |
| | Primary (1,380) | 82% | 49% |
| | High school (5,887) | 71% | 31% |
| | University (2,423) | 69% | 30% |
| Stunting | No (9,495) | 73% | 33% |
| | Yes (901) | 73% | 45% |
| Received fortified food *(only children screened at kindergarten)* | No (2,172) | 73% | 30% |
| | Yes (4,312) | 60% | 24% |

Table 3. Anaemia prevalence by age group and other variables.

A multivariate logistic analysis showed that being anaemic was associated with:

- child's younger age (odds ratio=0.95 for every month of age, p<0.0001)
- mother's education (OR=0.73 for each level, p<0.0001)
- stunting (OR=1.36, p<0.0001)
- not having received fortified food (OR=1.35, p<0.0001).

No association was found between anaemia and: mother's age, number of pregnancies, father unemployment or sex of the child.

Prevalence of underweight and wasting (acute malnutrition) were low (around 2-3%), similar to the level registered in the normal healthy population according to WHO standards; prevalence of stunting was high (8.7%), and overweight was moderately higher (6.2%) than in the healthy population.

### 3.2 Anaemia improvement after intervention

4,077 of the anaemic children were monitored until a second haemoglobin test was performed, on average after 175 days (SD=43) of treatment. Table 4 below shows that:

- of 4,077 children anaemic at enrolment 2,690 (66.0%) were no longer anaemic and 1,387 (34.0%) were still anaemic after 4-6 months of treatment;
- severe and moderate anaemia was reduced from 9.4% to only 1.7%;
- of the 1,387 children still anaemic 360 (26.0%) had an improvement in haemoglobin $\geq$1g/dl, a clinically significant result, bringing to 74.8% the percentage of anaemic children with improved status;
- the mean haemoglobin level increased from 9.99 g/dl to 11.0 g/dl.

| Type of anaemia | Admission n. | Admission % | Last follow-up n. | Last follow-up % | p value |
|---|---|---|---|---|---|
| Severe and moderate anaemia <9g | 383 | 9.4% | 71 | 1.7% | <0.0001 |
| Mild anaemia | 3,694 | 90.6% | 1,316 | 32.3% | |
| No anaemia | 0 | | 2,690 | 66.0% | |
| | | | | | |
| Mean haemoglobin level among 1,211 | 9.99 g/dl | | 11.09 g/dl | | <0.0001 |

Table 4. Anaemia status before and after treatment.

Anaemic children at screening were classified as "improved" if they recovered from anaemia or if they had at least a >1g/dl increase in haemoglobin level. A strong link between improvement and child age was noticed: improvement was much lower for younger children (less than 60%) compared to older ones (around 80%), as shown in Figure 2.

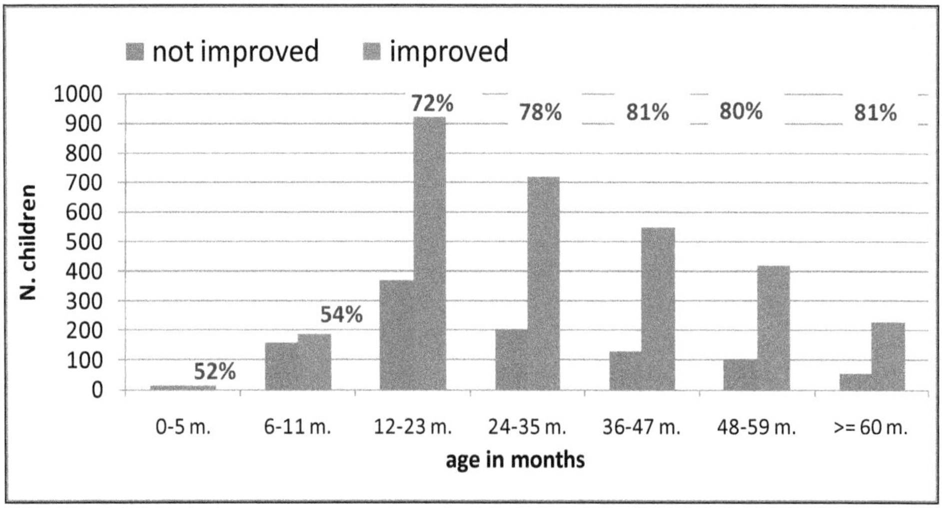


Fig. 2. Anaemia improvement after treatment by age group (number of children and % of improved).

Improvement was not associated with mother's education or other family variables collected.
In order to investigate the reasons for not improving we linked data collected via the CHILD FILE and HOME VISIT file to establish whether improvement was associated with:

- drug adherence
- drug tolerance
- mother's level of knowledge
- change in nutritional habits.

The above information was not available for all the children enrolled and is presented in detail in the following subsections (3.3 to 3.6).

### 3.3 Adherence to iron supplementation

In the first two phases of the project (South Gaza-1 and North Gaza) we were unable to associate improvement with good adherence to iron supplementation; this was due to the fact that almost all the mothers reported having given the iron as prescribed. A more careful investigation in a subsample of still anaemic children showed that in order to obtain more reliable answers:

- the questions on adherence had to be more precise and more specific
- the investigator was not to blame the mothers.

For this reason a more precise and more sensitive data collection method was introduced in SOUTH GAZA-2; therefore, with regard to drug adherence, we present data limited to this project. Information on drug adherence was collected for all the 2,804 children enrolled, during each distribution at the kindergarten and during the home visit. Specific questions were asked, such as whether the drugs had been taken regularly (≥5 days/week), irregularly (4-2 days/week) or not at all (≤ 1/week) during the previous week. Figure 3 below shows that:

- drugs were taken regularly by 57% of the children after one month, the percentage decreasing constantly to 45.7%;
- the percentage of children who took drugs irregularly rose with time from 21.7% to 32.8%;
- the percentage of children not taking drugs or not showing for follow-up increased with time.

The major reason mentioned for not taking drugs regularly were careless mother and/or child's refusal.

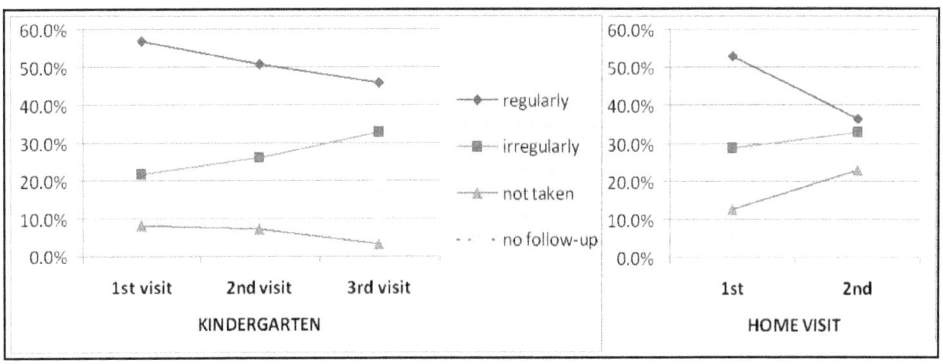


Fig. 3. Reported adherence among anaemic children.

To allow a better comparison we created a comprehensive index of drug adherence by combining all assessments performed, giving a score of 2 when the drugs were taken regularly, 1 when taken irregularly and 0 when not taken or the follow-up was missed. As shown in Table 5, there were 136 children who always took the drugs regularly, (score=10) and 31 who never took the medicine. We can further classify in 3 categories the level of adherence

| Adherence category | Adherence score | No. | % | Cumulative % |
|---|---|---|---|---|
| POOR | 0 | 31 | 3.6% | 3.6% |
| | 1 | 35 | 4.1% | 7.7% |
| | 2 | 49 | 5.7% | 13.5% |
| | 3 | 39 | 4.6% | 18.1% |
| | 4 | 72 | 8.4% | 26.5% |
| FAIR | 5 | 77 | 9.0% | 35.5% |
| | 6 | 99 | 11.6% | 47.1% |
| | 7 | 93 | 10.9% | 58.0% |
| GOOD | 8 | 116 | 13.6% | 71.6% |
| | 9 | 106 | 12.4% | 84.1% |
| | 10 | 136 | 15.9% | 100.0% |

Table 5. Adherence scores for anaemic children.

*We found a significant association ($p<0.0001$) between improvement of anaemia and the treatment adherence score (as previously described). The percentage of improvement after adjustment for age was:*

- *68.0% for children with good adherence (score 8-10)*
- *64.2% for children with fair adherence (score 5-7)*
- *60.5% for children with poor adherence (score <5)*

### 3.4 Drug tolerance, storage and administration

In the previous subsection we presented data on drug adherence recorded for anaemic children; the data here include non-anaemic children undergoing preventive treatment (prophylaxis).

There were very few reported complaints related to drug intake: around 2% in children with anaemia who received a higher dosage of iron and less than 1% for children on preventive treatment.

Vomiting and diarrhoea were the most common symptoms reported.

Drug storage was adequate in more than 90% of the cases during the first visit, the figure dropping slightly declined at the second visit. A similar pattern was noticed with regard to correct drug administration.

| | | 1st visit | 2nd visit |
|---|---|---|---|
| Drug-related complaints | anaemics | 1.8% (38 cases) | 1.8% (37 cases) |
| | non-anaemics | 0.7% (11 cases) | 0.4% (7 cases) |
| | | | |
| Adequate drug storage | anaemics | 94.32% | 93.08% |
| | non-anaemics | 92.75% | 89.33% |
| | | | |
| Correct drug administration | anaemics | 89.65% | 87.54% |
| | non-anaemics | 86.26% | 81.89% |

Table 6. Drug tolerance, storage and administration among anaemic and non-anaemic children.

### 3.5 Mother's knowledge of anaemia and nutrition

A total of 1,724 mothers answered a questionnaire on anaemia and nutrition (annex-2) twice during the two home visits. The questions were open-ended and the social workers did not prompt any answers to them.

Considering the average number of good/correct answers given by mothers, it is clear for each section that there was a significant increase in knowledge (p-value paired t-test was always <0.0001).

The average number of good answers increased by 35%, from 7.7 to 10.4. The number of mothers improving their score was 1,205 (70%), while 247 showed the same and 272 a lower score.

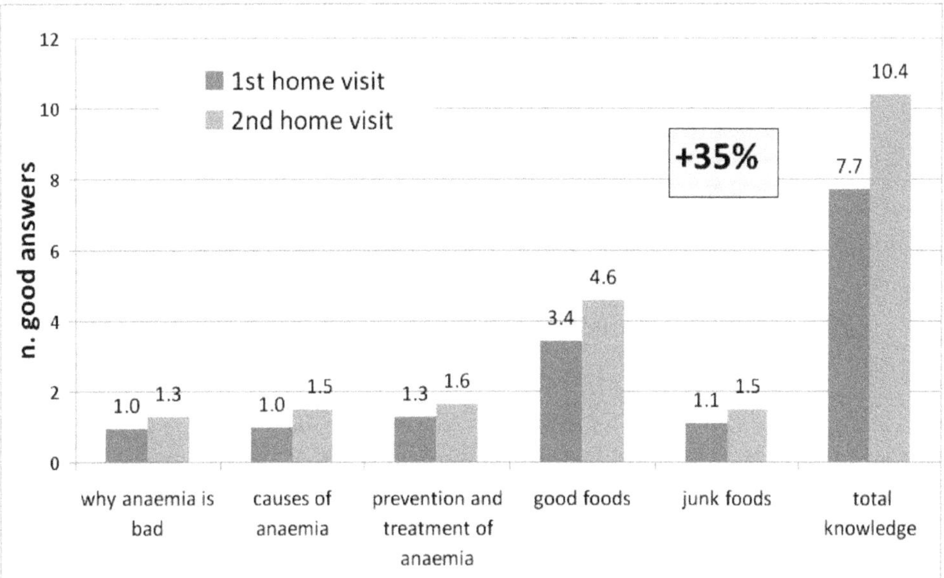


Fig. 4. Mother's knowledge of anaemia and nutrition at the first and second home visit.

When we considered as having a "good basic knowledge" women with a score of $\geq 10$ with at least one good answer for every section, we found that the percentage of mothers with a good basic knowledge was only 20.2% at the first home visit, rising to 51.6% at the second home visit (p<0.0001).

The level of "good basic knowledge" was strongly related to mother's education at the first home visit, ranging from 10% in women with primary education to 28% for the highly educated (p>0.0001). At the second visit no difference in good basic nutritional knowledge was seen between mothers with different standards of education (apart from the 12 illiterate subjects).

This is particularly important since:

- less educated mothers displayed a proportionally higher increase in knowledge than highly educated ones;
- disparity was reduced at the end of the project;
- we proved that the nutritional messages given were well understood even by the less advantaged, who are more in need,

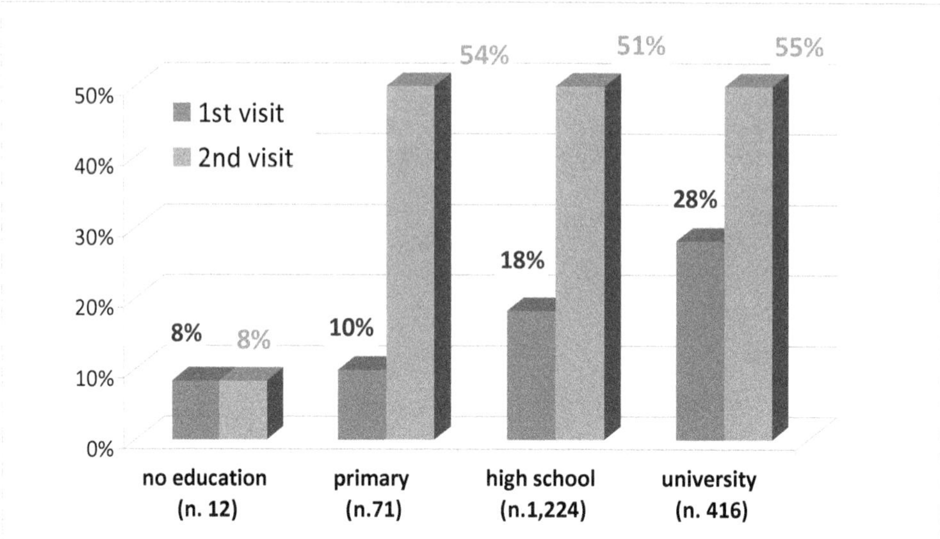


Fig. 5. Good-basic knowledge at the first and second home visit by mother's education level.

*We found an association between improvement in anaemic status and mother's good basic knowledge at the second home visit: after adjustment for child's age, mothers with a good-basic knowledge were 24% more likely to have a child with improved status than mothers without a good basic knowledge (odds ratio=1.24, p=0.013).*

Furthermore, in a sub-sample of children with available data, we found a significant association (p=0.016) between improvement of anaemia with mothers' and fathers' participation in awareness sessions at the kindergarten. The percentages of improvement stratified for participation were:

- 78.3% for the 69 children whose mother and father both participated in the awareness session
- 69.1% for the 162 children whose mother participated in the awareness session
- 62.3% for the 533 children whose parents did not participate in the awareness session.

### 3.6 Change in children's nutritional habits

In order to appreciate a possible impact in nutritional habit we compared the results of the 24-hour recall nutritional survey done during the first home visit with those of the same survey repeated 3-4 months later.

Since children below 2 years of age, who are at the weaning stage, can have a substantial change in their nutritional habit independently of the project, we analysed in a stratified way the results for children below 24 months of age (where considerable change is naturally expected) and those for older children (where changes can reflect project impact).

The specific messages of nutritional counselling were:

- stop tea consumption during meals;
- increase vegetable and fruit consumption;
- increase haem-rich animal food consumption (meat, fish, chicken);
- reduce junk food consumption.

### 3.6.1 Children over 24 months of age at screening

The overwhelming majority of children were having an average of 3 meals a day before and after the project.

When considering the average number of portions consumed the previous day, we noticed a 25% increase in the consumption of fruit and vegetables, +29% for staple food, +19% for animal products and +25% for haem-rich animal food.

| Table 7a | | Anaemic children ≥ 24 months | | | |
|---|---|---|---|---|---|
| | | 1st visit | 2nd visit | change | p value paired t-test |
| Number of children | | 1,251 | | | |
| Average no. of meals | | 2.93 | 2.96 | | |
| **% of children having fewer than 3 meals** | | **10.27%** | **6.59%** | **-36%** | **0.0001** |
| | | | | | |
| Average number of portions* consumed the previous day | Vegetables, fruits and legumes | 2.26 | 2.83 | **25%** | <0.0001 |
| | Staple food | 2.11 | 2.73 | **29%** | <0.0001 |
| | Animal foods | 2.42 | 2.88 | **19%** | <0.0001 |
| | *Of which haem-rich food* | *0.56* | *0.71* | **25%** | <0.0001 |
| | Junk food | 2.24 | 2.01 | **-10%** | <0.0001 |
| | *Of which chips* | 0.82 | 0.57 | **-30%** | <0.0001 |
| | *Of which candies* | 0.21 | 0.24 | **18%** | 0.03 |
| | *Of which soft drinks* | 0.11 | 0.08 | **-28%** | 0.026 |
| Average number of times child eats junk food between meals | | 2.04 | 1.93 | **-6%** | 0.0001 |
| | | | | | |
| Average cups/glasses consumed the previous day | Water | 4.17 | 5.07 | **22%** | <0.0001 |
| | Tea — No. of cups | 1.18 | 0.76 | **-35%** | <0.0001 |
| | (Percentage drinking tea) | (67%) | (54%) | **-19%** | <0.0001 |
| | *Of which tea outside meals* | 0.90 | 0.61 | **-33%** | <0.0001 |
| | *Of which tea with meals* | 0.28<br>(16.3%) | 0.15<br>(10.6%) | **-45%**<br>**-35%** | <0.0001<br><0.0001 |
| **Table 7b** | | Non-anaemic children ≥24 months | | | |
| | | 1st visit | 2nd visit | change | p value paired t-test |
| Number of children | | 1451 | | | |
| Average no. of meals | | 2.95 | 2.99 | | |
| **% of children having fewer than 3 meals** | | **6.72%** | **4.56%** | **-32%** | |
| | | | | | |
| Average number of portions* consumed in the previous day | Vegetables, fruit and legumes | 2.26 | 2.77 | **23%** | <0.0001 |
| | Staple food | 2.21 | 2.79 | **26%** | <0.0001 |
| | Animal foods | 2.44 | 2.89 | **19%** | <0.0001 |
| | *Of which haem-rich food* | *0.58* | *0.69* | **19%** | <0.0001 |
| | Junk food | 2.26 | 2.12 | **-6%** | 0.003 |
| | *Of which chips* | 0.87 | 0.63 | **-27%** | <0.0001 |
| | *Of which candies* | 0.21 | 0.29 | **37%** | <0.0001 |
| | *Of which soft drinks* | 0.10 | 0.11 | **16%** | 0.13 |
| Average number of times child eats junk food between meals | | 2.04 | 2.01 | **2%** | **-3%** |
| | | | | | |
| Average cups/glasses consumed the previous day | Water | 4.53 | 5.30 | **17%** | <0.0001 |
| | Tea — No. of cups | 1.18 | 0.78 | **-34%** | <0.0001 |
| | (Percentage drinking tea) | (65%) | (53%) | **-18%** | <0.0001 |
| | *Of which tea outside meals* | 0.92 | 0.64 | **-30%** | <0.0001 |
| | *Of which tea with meals* | 0.26<br>(14.9%) | 0.14<br>(10.2%) | **-46%**<br>**-32%** | <0.0001<br><0.0001 |

Table 7. Food consumption during previous 24 hours as recorded during first and second home visit for children over 24 months of age, anaemic (7a) and not anaemic (7b).

The increase in fruit and vegetable consumption may not be an effect of the project since we recorded at the same time an increase in staple food that the project did not promote.
Junk food consumption declined slightly, with chips and soft drinks up and candies down.
Tea consumption decreased by 35%, and tea with meals decreased even more (-45%). At the same time water consumption increased. Similar results were recorded in the non-anaemic population.
As shown in Table 8, the children of parents who participated in awareness sessions seem to have had a better improvement of nutritional habits, particularly in terms of reducing tea consumption during meals: -72% versus -32% when considering cups; -55% versus -10% when considering the percentage of children drinking tea.

| | | 843 children with parents who did not attended awareness sessions | | | 362 children with parents who attended awareness sessions | | |
|---|---|---|---|---|---|---|---|
| | | 1st visit | 2nd visit | Change | 1st visit | 2nd visit | Change |
| Average number of portions consumed the previous day | Vegetables, fruit and legumes | 2.66 | 2.94 | 11% | 2.77 | 3.48 | 26% |
| | Staple food | 2.54 | 3.16 | 24% | 2.49 | 3.34 | 34% |
| | Animal foods | 2.60 | 2.76 | 6% | 2.45 | 2.92 | 19% |
| | *Of which haem-rich food* | *0.61* | *0.69* | 13% | *0.48* | *0.64* | 33% |
| | Junk food | 2.67 | 2.79 | 4% | 2.29 | 2.26 | -1% |
| Average number of times child eats junk food between meals | | 2.02 | 2.16 | 7% | 1.94 | 1.86 | -4% |
| Average cups/glasses consumed the previous day | Tea | 1.37 | 0.87 | -36% | 1.43 | 0.89 | -38% |
| | *Of which tea with meals* No. of cups | 0.25 | 0.17 | -32% | 0.25 | 0.07 | -72% |
| | (% drinking tea) | (13.3 %) | (12.0%) | -10% | (14.0 %) | (6.3%) | -55% |

Table 8. Food consumption during previous 24 hours stratified for participation of parents in awareness sessions.

### 3.6.2 Children below 24 months of age at screening

The overwhelming majority of children were having an average of 3 meals a day and the percentage was stable. However, the percentage of children receiving fewer than 3 meals a day was reduced from 15.5% to 8.4.% (breast feeding was not considered).
As expected, the consumption of all types of food increased, with the exception of junk food, which remained stable. The consumption of soft drinks and candies, however, increased significantly
Tea consumption was high, even among small children, half of whom had drunk it the previous day. There was an 18% decrease in quantity, and tea with meals decreased even more (-40%). At the same time water consumption increased.
Similar values were found in the non-anaemic population (144 children).

| | | Anaemic children <24 months | | | |
|---|---|---|---|---|---|
| | | 1st visit | 2nd visit | change | P |
| | N. of children | 773 | | | |
| | Average no. of meals | 2.90 | 2.96 | | |
| | **% of children having fewer than 3 meals** | **15.5%** | **8.4%** | **-46%** | <0.0001 |
| Average number of portions consumed the previous day | Vegetables, fruit and legumes | 2.04 | 2.61 | **28%** | 0.0014 |
| | Staple food | 1.85 | 2.27 | **23%** | <0.0001 |
| | Animal foods | 3.00 | 3.28 | **9%** | 0.0014 |
| | *Of which rich haem food* | *0.53* | *0.64* | **21%** | *0.002* |
| | Junk food | 1.92 | 1.86 | **-3%** | 0.4 |
| | *Of which chips* | 0.62 | 0.50 | **-20%** | <0.0001 |
| | *Of which candies* | 0.17 | 0.23 | **39%** | 0.001 |
| | *Of which soft drinks* | 0.06 | 0.09 | **49%** | 0.07 |
| | Number of times child eats junk food between meals | 1.91 | 1.88 | **-2%** | 0.4 |
| Average cups/glasses consumed the previous day | Water | 3.73 | 4.69 | **26%** | <0.0001 |
| | Tea no. of cups | 0.82 | 0.67 | **-18%** | 0.0008 |
| | (Percentage drinking tea) | (49%) | (47%) | **-4%** | 0.3 |
| | *Of which tea between meals* | 0.63 | 0.55 | **-12%** | 0.06 |
| | *Of which tea with meals* | 0.19 | 0.12 | **-40%** | 0.0007 |
| | | (12.2%) | (8.1%) | **-34%** | 0.002 |

Table 9. Food consumption during previous 24 hours as recorded during first and second home visit for anaemic children below 24 months of age.

*WE COULD NOT FIND ANY ASSOCIATION BETWEEN IMPROVEMENT OF ANAEMIC STATUS AND CHANGE IN NUTRITIONAL HABIT*

### 3.7 Anaemia prevalence after 1 year of intervention: a random sample of Phase 1 KGs children

One of the biggest challenges of any medical intervention is to maintain the benefit obtained in the short term also in the long term. This is particularly important for nutritional supplementation intervention, such as treatment for iron deficiency anaemia: it is reasonable to have an improvement after iron supplementation, but what happens then? It is true that even a temporary improvement in anaemia at a crucial age with regard to growth can have long-lasting benefits, but our task was to assess the level of anaemia 1 year after the end of the intervention.

#### 3.7.1 Methods

We randomly selected 178 children who were anaemic when enrolled in October 2009 during the SOUTH GAZA-1 project and had improved by the end of the project (May 2010), and we re-tested them in May 2011, one year after the end of the project. To evaluate improvement we compared anaemia prevalence and haemoglobin level at the three different time points using the pair t-test (comparison of each subject with himself/herself).

### 3.7.2 Results

It can be seen from Table 10 below and Figure 6 that:

- at the end of phase 1 only 8 children were still anaemic (all of them had an improvement in Hb level ≥1g/dl; none had moderate or severe anaemia);
- 1 year later the vast majority of children (88.2%) were still not anaemic and only 21 had regressed to mild anaemia;
- the level of anaemia increased significantly after 1 year (from 5.5% to 11.8%; p=0.011) but was still much lower than found at baseline;
- none of the 21 anaemic cases in May 2011 had moderate or severe anaemia and only 2 had an Hb level below 10g/dl, meaning that even the children who were still anaemic were at the limit of normality. The average haemoglobin level among the children was lower than in May 2010, yet much higher than the level recorded at the beginning of the SOUTH GAZA 1 project.

| Type of anaemia | October 2009 No. | % | May 2010 No. | % | May 2011 No. | % | P value |
|---|---|---|---|---|---|---|---|
| Severe and moderate anaemia <9g | 18 | 10.1% | 0 | 0% | | | |
| Mild anaemia | 160 | 89.9% | 8 | 5.5% | 21 | 11.8% | <0.0001 |
| No anaemia | 0 | | 170 | 95.5%% | 157 | 88.2% | |
| Mean Hb level among 178 children | 9.94 g/dl | | 11.98 g/dl | | 11.85 g/dl | | <0.0001 |
| Mean Hb level among 21 children still anaemic in May 2011 | 9.89 g/dl | | 11.71 g/dl | | 10.42 g/dl | | <0.0001 |

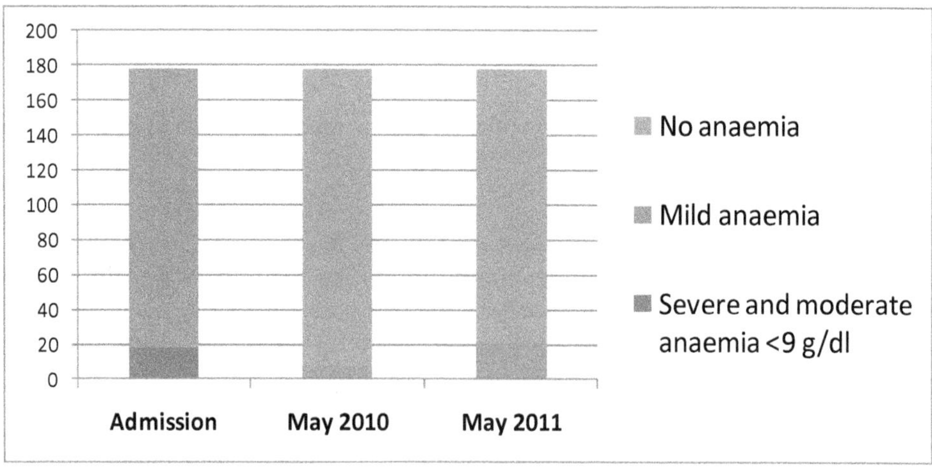


Table 10. and Fig. 6. Anaemia prevalence at three different time points.

Conclusions drawn:

- anaemia improvement achieved during the SOUTH GAZA 1 project persisted after 1 year;
- the overwhelming majority of children were still not anaemic after 1 year;

- there was still a fraction of children who regressed to anaemia after stopping supplementation, but their Hb levels were much higher than before project implementation.

### 3.8 Follow-up of still anaemic children

Children who were still anaemic after intervention underwent a more thorough clinical investigation, treatment and a longer follow-up.
Only 50 were diagnosed as having thalassaemia: the 0.48% of the 10.445 children screened and the 1.01% of the children found to be anaemic.
Out of the 296 children found to be still anaemic during follow-up screening at the end of the SOUTH GAZA-1 project, 159 (from 140 families) were still attending kindergarten in October 2010 and were enrolled in Phase 2 activities; the others had left, mainly to go to school. One hundred and twenty-nine of them were tested again; the other 33 refused to enter the new program.
After intensive counselling, the majority of children with no improvement in anaemic status were found to:

- have had poor drug adherence and/or
- have high tea consumption during meals and/or
- drink large amounts of tea.

Extra counselling was given to the mothers of these children.
The results for the 129 children re-tested in October 2010 showed a substantial change from their previous status (Table 11):

- 50.4% of children were no longer anaemic;
- the number of children with severe/moderate anaemia dropped from 17 to 3;
- 19 children were still anaemic, but improved their Hb value by at least 1g/dl;
- only 45 children did not improve.

| Type of anaemia | June 2010 No. | June 2010 % | October 2010 No. | October 2010 % | p value |
|---|---|---|---|---|---|
| Severe and moderate anaemia <9gr | 17 | 13.2% | 3 | 2.3% | |
| Mild anaemia | 111 | 86.2% | 61 | 47.3% | <0.0001 |
| No anaemia | 1 | 0.8% | 65 | 50.4%% | |
| | | | | | |
| Mean Hb level among 129 children | **9.62 g/dl** | | **10.91 g/dl** | | **<0.0001** |

Table 11. Haemoglobin level and anaemic status of children not improving in the first phase.

## 4. Discussion

### 4.1 Anaemia prevalence

Our sample cannot be considered as fully representative of the under-5 population of the Gaza Strip because they were not randomly selected, and because children below 12 months of age were under-represented. We found an anaemia prevalence at screening of 43.7%, which was strongly associated with children's younger age (from 76.2% at 6-11 months to 17.0% for children over 5 years of age).

The prevalence we found is very similar to that reported by the local Ministry of Health (PNA MOH, 2011) for children below 12 months (prevalence 76.2% among children aged 9-12 months) but much lower for the oldest age group (prevalence 58.6% among school children in 2009). The lower prevalence noticed in our children over 5 years of age could be explained by the fact that there have been several instances in the last 2 years of iron-fortified-food distribution in kindergartens, and we found that children receiving fortified food had a significantly lower level of anaemia. However the fortified food distribution, which was not implemented within a public health scheme, does not seem to be able to tackle completely the problem and several kids were found anaemic despite it.

In addition to child's age and utilisation of fortified food, we found a significant association of anaemia with mother's poor education (an indication that low-social-status subjects are more vulnerable) and with stunting (not surprising since anaemia and stunting both reflect poor quality nutrition).

It is worth noting that children aged between 12 and 48 months, particularly those below 24 months, have very high prevalence of anaemia but are particularly difficult to reach because they do not attend the health clinic regularly (the vaccination program ends in the first year) or go to kindergarten: specific actions to target them should be implemented because anaemia can have very negative consequences for them (Walter, 2003).

Universal growth monitoring at least once a year for all under-5s, including haemoglobin level testing, could be one of the measures to take in the Palestinian context, where medical facilities and health workers are readily available and could easily provide this service. This would also provide the opportunity to monitor and contrast stunting, an age-old chronic problem, at an early stage, and also obesity, the new rampant one.

### 4.2 Anaemia improvement

Overall performance for anaemia was very good. Nearly 70% of the children treated were cured within 4-6 months. A review of the literature shows that this rate is in line, if not better, with what has been achieved in specific studies elsewhere (Rosadoet al, 2010) or in the region where children received iron daily or weekly (Faqih et al, 2006; Tavil et al, 2003), but these were clinical trials with a small number of participants and effectiveness in the field is always more complicated.

One good result seen is an impact of the supportive counselling, including home visits: this is backed up by the fact that mothers who gained a better knowledge had an additional 24% chance of having a child who recovered from anaemia. The effect of well-motivated parents - something rarely studied in trials, where almost all participants are well motivated - is confirmed by the better results achieved when parents participated in awareness sessions.

Of course we have to be careful in considering this difference as a result of the awareness sessions, since it is likely that we had a strong selection bias: parents most interested in "nutritional" topics even before the project probably attended more awareness sessions, and they were also more attentive in monitoring their children's adherence and nutritional habits.

The lower rate of improvement in children below 24 months of age confirms the high vulnerability of this age group.

The use of more palatable iron with fewer side effects, such as that used in our projects (Toblli et al, 2007), can explain the relatively good adherence and impact: and the link between adherence and improvement was clearly proven during our interventions.

As found in another study (Zlotkin et al, 2003), further supplementation is not needed to maintain non-anaemic status in most children previously treated for anaemia: almost all the children who recovered from anaemia were not anaemic 1 year later.

### 4.3 Nutritional habits: knowledge and practice

Knowledge of anaemia and nutrition was quite low, particularly for less educated mothers, but health education achieved a substantial increase in the level of knowledge, particularly in the less educated.

The 24-hour nutritional questionnaire was designed as a tool for diagnosis and family counselling, not for gathering information, but it provided some interesting data on food consumption:

- high prevalence of junk food in the under-5s, as also noticed for school children (PNA MOH, 2011);
- low consumption of fruit and vegetables;
- high consumption of tea, half of the children below 24 months of age having drunk some during the previous day.

During the second home visit we found a consistent decrease in tea consumption in all age categories, particularly during meals, but we were unable to establish a real reduction in junk food consumption and there was only a minimal increase in the intake of fruit and vegetables.

It is important to point out that food consumption was reported by the mothers, so the reported "good change" should be treated with caution because this could in part be the result of the mother's desire to give the (counselling) interviewer a good impression.

Our data confirm that increased knowledge did not immediately result in improved feeding habits, a constraint found in many interventions that try to address chronic nutritional problems such as obesity in children (Branca et al, 2007).

Little change in nutritional habits and the weakness of having only two monitoring measures of habits could explain why we were unable to establish a significant association between change in nutritional habit and anaemia improvement.

## 5. Acknowledgment

*The article preparation was not funded by the donors in any way, and all its contents are published under the responsibility of Terre des Hommes Italia and the Palestinian Medical Relief.*
*Thanks go to the staff of PMRS, Tdh-It and kindergarten who implemented the projects*

## 6. References

Abdeen, Z., Greenough, G., Shahin, M., Tayback M; 2002. Nutritional Assessment of the West Bank and Gaza Strip. Accessed on the internet on the 07/07/2007 at: http://www.usaid.gov/wbg/reports/Nutritional_Assessment.pdf

Azeredo CM, Cotta RM, Sant'Ana LF, Franceschini Sdo C, Ribeiro Rde C, Lamounier JA, Pedron FA. Greater effectiveness of daily iron supplementation scheme in infants. Rev Saude Publica. 2010 Apr;44(2):230-9.

Faqih AM, Kakish SB, Izzat M. Effectiveness of intermittent iron treatment of two- to six-year-old Jordanian children with iron-deficiency anemia. Food Nutr Bull. 2006 Sep;27(3):220-7.

Palestinian National Authority, 2011. National Nutrition Surveillance System. 2010 Report. Ministry of Health, Nutrition Department

Rahim HF, Wick L, Halileh S, Hassan-Bitar S, Chekir H, Watt G, Khawaja M. Maternal and child health in the occupied Palestinian territory. Lancet. 2009 Mar 14;373(9667):967-77. Epub 2009 Mar 4. Erratum in: Lancet. 2009 Jun 27;373(9682):2200.

Roberts, L. and Hofmann, C.A.; 2004. Assessing the impact of humanitarian assistance in the health sector. Emerg Themes Epidemiol. 1:3. Available from: http://www.ete-online.com/content/1/1/3

Robertson, D.W., Bedell, R., Lavery, J.V., Upshur. R.; 2002. What kind of evidence do we need to justify humanitarian medical aid? Lancet. 360, 330-333

Rosado JL, González KE, Caamaño Mdel C, García OP, Preciado R, Odio M. Efficacy of different strategies to treat anemia in children: a randomized clinical trial. Nutr J. 2010 Sep 23;9:40.

Rychetnik, L., Frommer, M., Hawe, P., Shiell, A.; 2002. Criteria for evaluating evidence on public health interventions. J Epidemiol Community Health. 56,119-127.

Tavil B, Sipahi T, Gökçe H, Akar N. Effect of twice weekly versus daily iron treatment in Turkish children with iron deficiency anemia. Pediatr Hematol Oncol. 2003 Jun;20(4):319-26.

Toblli JE, Brignoli R. Iron(III)-hydroxide polymaltose complex in iron deficiency anemia / review and meta-analysis. Arzneimittelforschung. 2007;57(6A):431-8. Review

Verster, A.; 1996. Guidelines for the control of iron deficiency in countries of the Eastern Mediterranean, Middle East and North Africa. World Health Organization, Regional Office for the Eastern Mediterranean. WHO-EM/NUT/177, E/G/11.96/1000.

Walter T. Effect of iron-deficiency anemia on cognitive skills and neuromaturation in infancy and childhood. Food Nutr Bull. 2003 Dec;24(4 Suppl):S104-10. Review.

WHO and UNICEF; 2004. Focusing on anaemia. Towards an integrated approach for effective anaemia control. Accessed on the internet on the 05/10/2011 at: http://www.who.int/medical_devices/publications/en/WHO_UNICEF-anaemiastatement.pdf

Francesco Branca, Haik Nikogosian and Tim Lobstein, 2007. The challenge of obesity in the WHO European Region and the strategies for response. WHO Regional Office for Europe, Copenhagen, Denmark

WHO, 2009. Multicentre Growth Reference Study Group. WHO Child Growth Standards: Growth velocity based on weight, length and head circumference: Methods and development. Geneva: World Health Organization, 2009.

WHO, UNICEF, United Nations University; 2001. Iron deficiency anaemia: assessment, prevention, and control. Geneva, World Health Organization. WHO/NHD/01.3.

WHO; 2009. Health conditions in the occupied Palestinian territory, including east Jerusalem, and in the occupied Syrian Golan. Provisional agenda item 14 A62/24: Provisional agenda item 13 A59/INF.DOC./21 May 2009. Accessed on the internet on the 05/08/2011 at: h http://apps.who.int/gb/ebwha/pdf_files/A62/A62_R2-en.pdf

14

# Management of Anaemia in Pregnancy

Ezechi Oliver[1] and Kalejaiye Olufunto[2]
[1]*Chief Research Fellow and Consultant Obstetrician and Gynaecologist*
*Coordinator, Sexual, Reproductive and Childhood Diseases Research Programme*
*Head of Division, Clinical Sciences Division,*
*Nigerian Institute of Medical Research, Yaba Lagos*
[2]*Senior Research Fellow and Haematologist*
*Unit Head, Laboratory Services Unit ,*
*Clinical Sciences Division, Nigerian Institute of Medical Research, Yaba Lagos*
*Nigeria*

## 1. Introduction

Obstetric practice in developing countries is known for unacceptably high maternal morbidity , mortality and perinatal deaths. Factors contributory to these include poor health care delivery system, cultural beliefs, poor nutrition, illiteracy, gender inequality, teenage pregnancies and high parity. Other factors such as infections and infestations ultimately cause anaemia and increase morbidity and mortality in pregnant women and their offspring. Anaemia during pregnancy is a well-known risk for unfavourable pregnancy outcomes.

Globally, anaemia has been found to be the most common complication in pregnancy. The World Health Organization (WHO) estimates that more than 40% of non-pregnant and over 50% of pregnant women in developing countries are affected. The majority of the cases occur in sub-Saharan Africa and South East Asia. In 1993, the World Bank ranked anaemia as the 8th leading cause of disease in girls and women in the developing world. Apart from maternal morbidity and mortality, neonatal mortality is high among the babies of anaemic mothers.

## 2. Hematological changes in pregnancy

Pregnancy is associated with normal physiological changes that assist fetal survival and prepares the mother for labour, delivery and breastfeeding. The changes start as early as 4 weeks of gestation and are largely as a result of progesterone and oestrogen. The total blood volume increases steadily from as early as 4 weeks of pregnancy to reach a maximum of 35-45 % above the non-pregnant level at 28 to 32 weeks. The plasma volume increases by 40-45 % (1000mls). Red blood cell mass increases by 30- 33 % (approximately 300mg) as a result of the increase in the production of erythropoietin. Erythropoietin levels increase throughout pregnancy, reaching approximately 150% of their prepregnancy levels at term.

The increase is steady until term. The greater increase in plasma volume than the increase in red blood cell mass results in a modest reduction in haematocrit, with peak haemodilution occurring at 24-26 weeks. This is termed physiological anaemia of pregnancy (see Fig 1). This dilution picture is often normochromic and normocytic. Occasionally physiologic anaemia can also be associated with a physiologic macrocytosis, MCV increases to 120fl although average at term is 104 fl.

In pregnancy, there is an additional demand of about 1000 mg iron equivalent to 60 mg elemental iron or 300 mg ferrous sulphate daily. While the transferrin and total iron binding capacity rises, the serum iron falls . Thus women who enter pregnancy in an iron deficient state are then unable to meet the demands of pregnancy by diet alone and require supplementation. It takes approximately 2-3 weeks after delivery for these haematologic changes to revert to pre-pregnancy status.

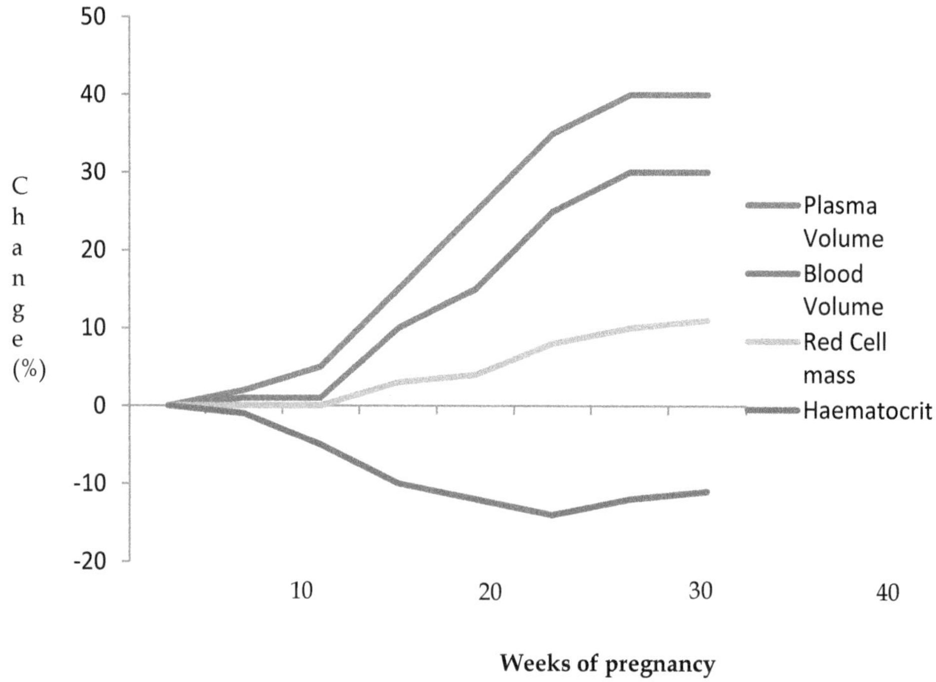


Fig. 1. Graphical representation of haematological changes in pregnancy.

## 3. Epidemiology of anaemia in pregnancy

Anaemia has been found to be associated with poverty and underdevelopment and is one of the most common disorders globally. The incidence of anaemia varies from place to place even within the same country and depends on the socioeconomic status and level of development. The World Health Organization reports anaemia among the top ten most important contributors to global ill health and deaths. It estimated that about a third of the world's population of 7 billion have haemoglobin levels below the WHO criteria for diagnosis of anaemia. The majority of these persons reside in Sub-Saharan Africa and South East Asia.

Pregnant women are particularly considered to be the most vulnerable group because of the additional demands that are made on maternal stores during pregnancy. The average global prevalence of anaemia in pregnancy is reported to be 51%. Like anaemia in the general population the prevalence of anaemia in pregnancy varies from 17% in Europe to 52 % and 60% respectively in Africa and Asia. In sub-Saharan Africa it is estimated that 20% of maternal deaths are associated with anaemia. It is also a major risk factor for infant iron deficiency which has been shown to be associated with adverse behavioural and cognitive development of children and low birth weight, which is one of the main risk factors for infant mortality.

## 4. Definition of anaemia

The term anaemia refers to the reduction in the oxygen-carrying capacity of the blood due to fewer circulating red blood cells than normal or a reduction in the concentration of haemoglobin. The deficiency may occur as a result of a reduction in the production or an increased loss of erythrocytes.

Anaemia is said to occur when the haemoglobin content of blood is below the normal range expected for the age and sex of the individual, provided that the presence of pregnancy, the state of hydration of the individual and the altitude have been taken into account. While several authorities and experts accepts the lower limits of normal haemoglobin concentration as 12g/dl in women and 14g/dl in men, WHO accepts up to 11gm percent as the normal haemoglobin level in pregnancy. Thus any haemoglobin level below 11gm in pregnancy by WHO standard should be considered as anaemia. However in most of the developing countries the lower limit is often accepted as 10 g/dl because a large percentage of pregnant women in this setting with haemoglobin level of 10 g/dl tolerate pregnancy, labour and delivery very well and with good outcome.

The centre for disease control, USA defined anaemia as a hemoglobin (Hgb) or hematocrit (Hct) value less than the fifth percentile of the distribution of Hgb or Hct in a healthy reference population.

## 5. Classification of anaemia

Anaemia can be classified as physiological (eg pregnancy), according to the aetiology (Table 1) and red blood cell morphology (Table 2).

Classification based on red cell morphology classifies anaemia based on the size and shape of the red blood cell,(normocytic MCV80-90fl, macrocytic MCV>100fl, microcytic MCV<80fl), as well as .pigmentation (hypochromic, normochromic, hypochromic) (Table 2).

Blood loss

- a. Acute
  - i. Antepartum haemorrhage (eg placenta praevia , abruptio placenta)
  - ii. Intrapartum haemorrhage
- b. Chronic
  - i. Hookworm infestation
  - ii. Bleeding hemorrhoids
  - iii. Peptic Ulcer Disease

B. Nutritional Anaemia

- i. Iron deficiency
- ii. Folate deficiency
- iii. B12 deficiency

C. Bone marrow failure

- a. Aplastic anaemia
- b. Isolated secondary failure of erythropoiesis
- c. Drugs (eg Chloramphenicol, Zidovudine)

D. Haemolytic

- a. Inherited
  - i. Haemoglobinopathies ( eg Sickle cell disorders, Thalassemia)
  - ii. Red cell Membrane defects ( eg Hereditary spherocytosis, elliptocytosis)
  - iii. Enzyme deficiencies (eg G6PD deficiency, Pyruvate kinase defeciency)
- b. Acquired
  - i. Immune Haemolytic anaemias ( eg autoimmune, alloimmune, drug induced)
  - ii. Non- Immune Haemolytic anaemias
    - a. Acquired membrane defects (eg Paroxysmal nocturnal Haemoglobinuria)

b.Mechanical damage ( eg Microangiopathic haemolytic anaemia)

iii Secondary to systemic disease (eg renal diseases, liver disease)

iv.Infections (Malaria, Sepsis, HIV)

Table 1. Classification of anaemia based on aetiology.

| |
|---|
| A. Hypochromic Microcytic |
| • Iron deficiency |
| • Thalassemia |
| • Sideroblastic anemia |
| • Anaemia of chronic disorders |
| • Lead poisoning |
| B. Macrocytic |
| • Folic acid deficiency |
| • Vitamin B12 deficiency |
| • Liver disease |
| • Myxoedema |
| • Chronic Obstructive Pulmonary Disease |
| • Myelodysplastic syndromes |
| • Blood loss anemia |
| C. Normocytic Normochromic |
| • Autoimmune haemolytic anaemia |
| • Systemic Lupus Erythomatosis |
| • Collagen vascular disorders |
| • Hereditary spherocytosis |
| • Haemoglobinopathies |
| • Bone marrow failure |
| • Malignancies |
| • Myelodysplasia |
| • Blood loss anemia |
| • Anemia of chronic disease |

Table 2. Morphological Classification of Anemia and causes.

The classifications are not necessarily independent of each other as the cause of the anaemia could be multifactorial.

Anaemia can be classified according to severity as mild, moderate, severe and very severe ( Table 3). Following the diagnosis and possible cause(s) of anaemia in the pregnant woman, management as regards the need for blood transfusions or not will depend on the severity as well as rapidity of development of anaemia.

| Degree of Severity | Haemoglobin level (g/dl) |
|---|---|
| Normal haemoglobin level | >11g/dl |
| Mild Anaemia | 9-11g/dl |
| Moderate | 7-9g/dl |
| Severe | 4-7g/dl |
| Very severe | <4g/dl |

Table 3. Classification of Anaemia by degree of severity.

## 6. Aetiology

The causes of anaemia in the general population are generally same for anaemia in pregnancy. The causes of anaemia in pregnancy are often multifactorial. In developing countries, the major causes of anaemia in pregnancy are nutritional deficiencies, infections and infestations, haemorrhage and haemoglobinathies. Anaemia is also seen also in some chronic medical disorders like renal and hepatic diseases.

### 6.1 Nutrition

In many regions of the world nutritional deficiency is the major cause of anaemia in pregnancy. The World health Organization ((WHO) estimates that about half of all pregnant women globally suffer from nutritional anaemia. Nutritional anaemia is mainly due iron and folate deficiency in diet. Diseases that cause poor dietary intake or malabsorption of these nutrients will also result in nutritional anaemia.

Iron deficiency is the commonest cause of nutritional anaemia in both developing and industrialized countries and is usually as a result of poor diet. Sources of iron include meat(liver in particular) vegetables and dairy products. The demand for iron increases in pregnancy as it is required by both mother and fetus for growth and development. In developing countries the already depleted iron stores as a result of poor diet, too early, too many and too frequent pregnancies are unable to cope with the requirement of 1000mg of iron required during a normal pregnancy. The resultant effect is iron deficiency anaemia. Hook worm infestation is another cause of iron deficiency anaemia in the tropics.

The folic acid requirement is also increased two fold in pregnancy. Normal body stores can only last for 3- 4 months. Folate deficiency in pregnancy often develops as a result of poor dietary intake which is often the case in developing countries as well as excess utilization. Sources of folate include liver, egg yolk, and leafy green vegetables. Folate deficiency results in ineffective erythropoesis.

Folate deficiency can be further exacerbated in pregnant women with hemoglobinopathies as well as in those residing in areas of high malaria endemicity as increased haemolysis leads to high red cell turnover and increased folate demand.

Vitamin B12 is rare during pregnancy as the daily requirement is as low as 3- 5μg and liver stores last for as long as 2 years.

### 6.2 Infections

Pregnant women are more prone to infections as a result of depressed immunity. Anaemia due to infections is usually as a result of products from the infecting organisms causing ill health, fever, red cell destruction and/ or reduced red cell production. Bacterial infections used to be a leading cause of anaemia, however in the tropics and developing countries, malaria and more recently, HIV/AIDS are leading contributors to anaemia in pregnancy.

### 6.3 Malaria

Malaria infection is a leading cause of anemia in the tropics both in pregnant and non-pregnant individuals. Malaria induced anaemia is more profound in pregnancy as the susceptibility to malaria is greater in the primigravidae. Anaemia resulting from malarial infection is caused by the destruction of infected and uninfected red blood cells as well as bone marrow suppression. Red blood cells infected with malaria parasites also accumulate and sequester in the placenta. Macrophages and cytokines(e.g.Tumor necrosis factor α, Interferon γ and interleukin 1),enhance red cell destruction, splenic clearance capacity,and depress bone marrow erythropoesis. Concurrent micronutrient deficiencies, infection with HIV , hookworm infestation or other chronic inflammatory states will worsen anaemia in these persons.

### 6.4 HIV/AIDS

Anaemia is the most common haematological complication of the Human Immunodeficiency Virus (HIV) infection and may be consequent upon the effects of the virus itself or treatment with various drugs. The mechanisms of HIV induced anaemia occur through three mechanisms of decreased red blood cell production, increased red cell destruction and ineffective production of red blood cells. The aetiology of HIV associated anaemia is multifactorial and may include the infiltration of the bone marrow by tumour or infection, bone marrow suppression by the virus itself, the use of myelosuppressive drugs like Zidovudine or drugs that prevent the utilization of folate like cotrimoxazole. Other aetiologies include decreased production of erythropoietin , red cell destruction as a result of autoantibodies to red blood cells, and nutritional deficiencies. Nutritional deficiencies could occur as a result of reduced intake due to difficult in swallowing as a result of oropharnygeal thrush, malabsorption or increased catabolism as a result of ill health and associated fever from various infections. Apart from iron and folate deficiency, other reported vitamin deficiencies in HIV infection include vitamin B12, vitamin B6 and vitamin A.

### 6.5 Haemoglobinopathies

Haemoglobinopathies are inherited disorders affecting haemoglobin structure (Sickle cell disorders) or synthesis (thalassemias). They are usually seen in individuals from Africa, the Middle East, the Mediterranean, Asia and the Far East. The haemoglobinopathies that cause anaemia in pregnancy are sickle cell disorders- HbSS, HbSC and HBS-β thalassemia. Haemoglobinopathies cause a chronic haemolytic anaemia. In sickle cell disorders, the abnormal haemoglobin S sickles in hypoxic states, predisposing the structurally damaged cells to early destruction hence affected persons are chronically anaemic. Folate demands are increased and concurrent infections will worsen anaemia.

### 6.6 Haemorrhage

Acute blood loss as result of ectopic pregnancy, antepartum haemorrhage and abortions are common causes of anaemia in pregnancy. Chronic blood loss from worm infestations, gastrointestinal ulcers and hemorrhoids results in depletion of iron stores and ineffective erythropoesis.

### 6.7 Red cell aplasia

This is a rare cause of anaemia in pregnancy and results from a selective failure of erythropoesis. In most cases, the cause is unknown The identified causes of pure red cell aplasia include autoimmune diseases (e.g. SLE,) drugs, and infection with parvovirus B19.

## 7. Risk factors for anaemia in pregnancy

Pregnant women in developing countries of sub-Saharan Africa, South America and South East Asia are at particular risk of anaemia in pregnancy as a result of poverty, malnutrition and depleted iron stores from too early, too many and too frequent pregnancies. Irrespective of race and economic situation, the prevalence of anemia in pregnancy is highest amongst teenage mothers. A recent report by Scholl estimates that in a low income setting, rates of iron deficiency anemia are 1.8% in the first trimester, 8.2% in the second trimester, and 27.4% in the third trimester.

In all regions of the world, the risk factors for iron deficiency anemia include a diet poor in iron-rich foods, a diet poor in iron absorption enhancers, a diet rich in foods that diminish iron absorption, gastrointestinal disease affecting absorption, heavy menstrual bleeding and postpartum bleeding.

## 8. Consequences of anemia in pregnancy

### 8.1 Fetal

The fetal consequences of anaemia in pregnancy are well established and depend not only on the severity of anaemia but also on the duration of the anaemic state. A fall in maternal haemoglobin below 11.0 g/d1 is associated with a significant rise in perinatal mortality rates. The rate of perinatal mortality triples at maternal haemoglobin levels below 8.0 g/d1 and increase by ten fold when anaemia is very severe. Similar findings have also been noted for both infant birth weight and preterm delivery rates. A significant fall in birth weight as a result of increase in preterm rate and intrauterine growth restriction has been reported with maternal haemoglobin levels below 8.0 g/d1 .

### 8.2 Maternal

The presence of, severity and duration of anaemia affect maternal as well as fetal well being. Women whose means of livelihood involve manual labour may find it difficult to earn a living as tolerance and capacity for exercise is reduced. This is worse if the onset of anaemia is acute. When anaemia is of gradual onset and is chronic, adequate compensatory mechanisms enable the women to go through pregnancy and labour without any adverse consequences.

Where anaemia is moderate, there is a substantial reduction in work capacity and she may be unable to cope with household chores and child care. Women with moderate anaemia tend to experience higher rates of morbidity during pregnancy as compared to those with mild anaemia. Evidence has shown that a large percentage of maternal deaths due to antepartum haemorrhage, pre-eclampsia and infections occur in women with moderate anaemia.

The maternal outcomes in severe anaemia depend on level of decompensation. If not recognized early and corrected, the heart is unable to compensate for the severity of anaemia and eventual circulatory failure occurs leading to pulmonary oedema and death. The women are unable to tolerate third stage of labour and blood losses associated with delivery. When the anaemia is very severe, there is a steep rise in maternal deaths.

## 9. Clinical features

The clinical features of anaemia in pregnant or non pregnant states are dependent on rapidity of onset and severity of anaemia. In general, symptoms occur with moderate to severe anaemia and are more severe when anaemia has been rapidly progressive. In presence of anaemia the body initiates a number of compensatory mechanisms. The symptom (s) that is subsequently felt by the individual is dependent on whether the compensation is sufficient or insufficient. As such, a pregnant woman with anaemia may be asymptomatic body systems adjust to reduced haemoglobin mass. Where the patient is symptomatic, symptoms may be those of vague ill health, headaches, light headedness, tinnitus, intermittent claudication, or symptoms of angina. However, as decomposition ensues, there may be palpitations, easy fatigability and patients can present in heart failure.

The signs of anaemia can be general or specific. General signs of anaemia include pallor of the mucous membranes, hyperdynamic circulation with tachycardia, a bounding pulse, cardiomegaly and a apical systolic flow mummur (haemic mummur) . The specific signs are associated with particular types of anaemia e.g painless glossitis, angular stomatitis,ridged or spoon shaped nails, unusual dietary cravings for non-food substances(pica) in iron deficiency, jaundice in haemolytic and megaloblastic anaemias, neuropathy, widespread melanin pigmentation in B12 deficiency. Hepatoslenomegaly (may be difficult to elicit when pregnancy is advanced) may be features of chronic hemolytic disorders, megaloblastic anaemia, or other haematologic pathologies. The findings of anaemia with fever and spontaneous bruising may be indicative of bone marrow failure.

## 10. Diagnosis of cause(s) of anaemia

A detailed history, physical examination and appropriate investigations are necessary for the identification of the cause(s) of anaemia. Except in very severe anaemia where there is an urgent need to treat the pregnant woman to avoid death, the cardinal rule is to establish the cause of anemia before commencing treatment.

### 10.1 History

A detailed history including diet, gynaecological, obstetric,drug and social history should be taken. As nutritional anaemia is common in developing countries, a detailed enquiry into the person's and diet and feeding habits should be made. Knowledge of the dietary and food habits will be necessary to plan strategies to prevent reoccurrence after management of the present anaemic state. It is also important to enquire in detail about duration and symptoms of anaemia (if any), symptoms of decompensation and possible predisposing factors. Other specific symptoms like a beefy red painful tongue, discoloured nails, parasthesias can also be sought. Previous history of postpartum haemorrhage or abortion, drug ingestion should be sought. Ideally, the history should address all possible aetiology of anaemia, features and its complications.

### 10.2 Physical examination

A good physical examination should confirm the presence of anaemia, possible aetiology and signs of decompensation. Where anaemia has been chronic, physical examination may reveal cardiomegaly, bounding pulses and a systolic flow murmur (hemic murmur). In acute blood loss the patient can present in shock. On examination the presence of pallor, jaundice, spleen and liver size should be documented.

### 10.3 Investigations

Investigations for anaemia are general and specific. A full blood count is required as part of the general investigation and includes the haemoglobin levels, packed cell volume, white cell and platelet counts. Red cell indices include mean corpuscular volume (MCV), mean corpuscular haemoglobin (MCH) and mean corpuscular haemoglobin concentration (MCHC). These indices will in the classify anaemia into either microcytic (MCV <80 fL), macrocytic (MCV >100fL) and normocytic (MCV80-100fL) or hypochromic or normochromic (MCH and MCHC)., A peripheral blood smear and reticulocyte count are also mandatory. While peripheral blood smear provides information about red cell morphology , variations in size, and shape, the reticulocyte count provides information on the marrow response. In the presence of anaemia a reticulocyte count less than 2-3 times normal indicates inadequate bone marrow response. Elevated neutrophil counts may suggest an infection.and peripheral smears that reveal a pancytopenia is suggestive of marrow failure. Stools should also be examined for colour, consistency, occult blood, ova and parasites. It is also important to note that in the tropics most of the causes may coexist. Other specific tests are often dictated by suspected cause of the anaemia. In the tropics, it is usual to screen for malaria as it is a well documented cause of anaemia in pregnancy. Some specific tests necessary to confirm some common causes and features of anemia is shown in Table 4.

| | |
|---|---|
| 1. **Iron deficiency**<br>a. **Serum ferritin**<br>b. **Total iron binding capacity**<br>c. **Transferrin saturation**<br>d. **Marrow iron stain** | 2. Haemoglobinopathies<br>a. **Hb electrophoresis**<br>3. HIV infection<br>a. **Detection of antibody to HIV using ELISA or Western blot assays.** |
| 4. **Chronic medical disorders**<br>a. **Liver function tests**<br>b. **Serum electrolyte, urea and creatinine**<br>c. **Screening for autoimmune diseases** | 5. **Antepartum haemorrhage**<br>a. Ultrasonography |

Table 4. Specific investigations for some common causes of anaemia.

## 11. Treatment

It is of utmost importance to establish the cause of anaemia prior to definitive management. However, features of decompensation, very severe anaemia and acute blood loss require immediate red cell transfusion as soon as the required samples have been collected. The only caveat is that we must ensure that all necessary samples have been collected before transfusion.

The goal of treatment of anaemia in pregnancy is therefore to maintain wellbeing, identify and correct the underlying cause(s) and correct anemia within shortest time possible and improve patient quality of life and survival.

The definitive management of anaemia depends on the cause. The identified causes must be treated appropriately otherwise the anaemia becomes recurrent.
By and large, the management of anaemia in a pregnant woman depends on the duration of pregnancy, severity of the anaemia and complication (obstetric, medical or both).
Mild and moderate anaemia in pregnancy as a result of iron deficiency should be carefully assessed for the cause and the patient placed on iron therapy apart from the treatment of the aetiology. The preferred route of iron replacement is oral route as there is no benefit in giving parenteral iron as opposed to oral iron. Ferrous sulphate (200mg per tablet containing 67mg elemental iron) is the least expensive and best absorbed form of Iron. Ferrous glutamate (300mg per tablet containing 37mg elemental iron) and fumarate can also be used where iron sulphate is not tolerated. The optimal doses are 120-200mg daily of elemental iron in divided doses. Oral iron should be given for long enough to correct the anaemia and to replenish iron stores which usually means for at least 6 months. Haemoglobin should rise at the rate of approximately 2g/dl every 3 weeks. Side effects of oral iron include gastrointestinal symptoms such as diarrhea, nausea, constipation, abdominal pain.
Parenteral iron may be indicated in cases of poor adherence, intolerable side effects or malabsorption of oral iron. In such situation parenteral iron such as iron dextran or sorbitol may be administered by the intravenous or intramuscular route. The hematological response to parenteral iron is not faster than adequate dosage of oral iron but the stores are replenished faster. Ferric hydroxide -sucrose (Venofer) is the safest form and is administered by slow intravenous injection or infusion usually 200mg in each infusion. Iron dextran (Cosmofer) can be given as slow injection or infusion in small doses or as a total dose infusion given in one day.
Total dose Intravenous infusion of iron with iron dextran in pregnancy (50mg iron per ml)
Dose (mL) = 0.0442 (Desired Hb - Observed Hb) x Lean Body Weight (45.5 kg + 2.3 kg for each inch of patient's height over 5 feet.) + (0.26 x LBW) + 1g.
The total dose of iron dextran is added to 500ml normal saline and infused over a period of 4 hours. The major drawback of parenteral iron is anaphylaxis which can occur within 30 mins of commencing the infusion and may prove rapidly fatal.
Intramuscular iron therapy can be given as iron sorbitol (Jectofer)(50mg/ml). Injections should be given deep into the gluteal muscle. The drawbacks of intramuscular iron include pain and staining of the skin at the injection site,myalgia, athralgia and injection abscess
Severe or very severe anaemia requires the immediate hospitalization of the woman, management of heart failure and transfusion of packed cells. Once the emergency is averted, the iron replacement is as in mild to moderate anaemia.
Treatment of anaemia from folate deficiency is with folic acid 5mg daily for 4 months and is usually given throughout pregnancy. Vitamin B12 deficiency is rare in pregnancy and is treated with intramuscular injections of hydroxocobalamin 1000ug . Initial doses are 6 injections over 2-3 weeks then 100ug every 3 months.
Erythropoietin is beneficial in patients -with marrow suppression . 100-200U/Kg 3times a week until normalization of the red cell and then once a weekly to maintain haemoglobin of approximately 12g/dl.
Treatment of malaria with artemisin combination therapy, bacterial infections with appropriate antibiotics, hookworm infestation with mebendazole or Albendazole and use of

highly active antiretroviral therapy according to treatment guidelines in HIV infection. Other co-morbidities e.g. diabetes, hypertension should also be managed.

## 12. Prevention

Approximately 1g of iron is required during a normal pregnancy. Up to 600mg of iron is required for the increase in maternal red cell mass, and a further 300mg for the foetus. These requirements exceed the iron storage of most young women and often cannot be met by the diet. Therefore, few women avoid depletion of iron reserves by the end of pregnancy. Folate requirements are increased approximately twofold in pregnancy (800ug/day vs 400ug/day because of transfer of folate to the growing fetus and if diet is insufficient, may exceed the body's stores of folate(5-10mg).

To prevent anaemia in pregnancy the following are necessary. Routine screening for anaemia in adolescence, nutritional education about foods rich in iron(meat, liver, leafy green vegetables, legumes) and folate (liver, egg yolk, yeast and leafy green vegetables) to encourage consumption, early as well as regular antenatal clinic attendances, iron, folate supplementation in pregnancy and early treatment of concomitant infections. In areas of high malaria endemicity, intermittent prophylactic therapy with pyrimethamine-sulphodoxine for malaria should also be given at 16-17 weeks and 4 weeks later. A third dose is given in HIV infection.

## 13. Conclusion

Anaemia in pregnancy is a major public health problem in developing countries and is associated with an increased risk of maternal and perinatal morbidity and mortality. Fortification of foods with iron and folate, routine screening for anaemia from adolescence, health education, and prompt treatment of infections and attendance of antenatal facilities by pregnant women can reduce this burden.

## 14. References


Agarwal KN, Agarwal DK, Mishra KP. Impact of anaemia prophylaxis in pregnancy on maternal hemoglobin, serum ferritin and birth weight. Indian J Med Res 1991;94:277–8

Aimakhu CO, Olayemi O. Maternal haematocrit and pregnancy outcome in Nigerian women. *West Afr J Med.* 2003;22(1):18–21.

Blanc B, Finch CA, Hallberg L, et al. Nutritional anaemias. Report of a WHO Scientific Group. WHO Tech Rep Ser. 1968;405:1-40.

Beutler E, West C. Hematologic differences between African-Americans and whites: the roles of iron deficiency and α_-thalassemia on hemoglobin levels and mean corpuscular volume. Blood.2005;106:740-745.

Breymann C, Iron Deficiency and Anaemia in Pregnancy: Modern Aspects of Diagnosis and Therapy. Blood Cells, Molecules, and Diseases. 2002; 29(3) Nov/Dec: 506 516

Centers of Disease Control . CDC Criteria for Anemia in Children and Childbearing-Aged Women. *Morbidity and Mortality Weekly Report 1989;* 38(22: 400–404.

Ezzati M, Lopez D, Rodgers A, Murray CJL, eds. Comparative quantification of health risk: Global and regional burden of disease attributable to selected major risk factors. Vol 1. Geneva: World Health Organization; 2004:163-208.

Harrison KA. Anaemia in pregnancy. In: Lawson JB, Harrison KA, Bergstrom S, editors. Maternity care in developing countries. RCOG Press. 2001:112-128.

Hemminki E, Rimpela U. Iron supplementation, maternal packed cell volume, and fetal growth. Arch Dis Child 1991;66:422-5.

Hisano M, Suzuki R, Sago H, Murashima A, Yamaguchi K. Vit B6 deficiency and anaemia in pregnancy. *Eur J Clin Nutr*. 2010;64:221-223.

Hoque M, Hader SB, Hoque E. Prevalence of anaemia in pregnancy in th uthungulu health district of KwaZulu- NatalSouth Africa. SAFamPract2007:49(6)16-16d.

Hoque M, Hoque E, Kader SB. Risk factors for anaemia in pregnancy in rural KwaZulu-Natal, South Africa: Implication for health education and health promotion SA Fam Pract 2009;51(1):68-72

Ilobachie GC, Meniru GI. The increasing incidence of anaemia in pregnancy in Nigeria. Orient J Med. 1990;2:194-198.

International Nutritional Anaemia consultative group. The INACG Symposium, "Integrating programs to move Iron Deficiency and Anaemia Control Forward". Marrakech, Morocco, International life Science Institute; 2003.

Iron dextran dosing calculator. Total dose infusion -iron deficiency anaemia. http://www.globalrph.com/irondextran.htm

Komolafe JO, Kuti O, Oni O, Egbewale BE. Sociodemographic characteristics of anaemic gravidae at booking: A preliminary study at Ilesha, western Nigeria. *Nig J Med*. 2005;14(2):151-154.

Lone FW, Qureshi RN, Emanuel F Maternal anaemia and its impact on perinatal outcome. Trop Med Int Health. 2004 Apr;9(4):486-90.

Massawe SN, Urassa En, Nystrom L, Lindmark G. Effectiveness of primary level care in decreasing anemia at term in Tanzania. Acta Obstet Gynecol Scand. 1999;78:573-579.

Martha P. Mims, Josef T. Prchal.Haematology during pregnancy. In Lichtman MA, Beutler E, Kipps TJ, Seligsohn U, KaushanskyK, Prchal JT editors.Williams Haematology 7thed 2006 Mcgraw-Hill publishers pp101-106.

McMullin MF, White R, Lappin T et al. Haemoglobin during pregnancy :Relationship to erythropoietin and haematinic status. Eur J Haematol 71:44,2003

Nduka N, Aneke C, Maxwell Ochukwu S. Comparison of some haematological indices of Africans and Caucasians resident in the same Nigerian environment. Haematologica budap. 1988;21 (1) 57-63

Nokes C, Van Den Bosch C, Bundy DAP. The effect of iron deficiency and anemia on mental and motor performance, educational achievement and behavior in children: An annotated bibliography. Washington,DC, International Nutritional Anaemia Consultative Group; 1998.

Nyuke RB, Letsky EA. Etiology of anaemia in pregnancy in South Malawi. Am J Clin Nutr. 2000;72:247-256

Ogbeide O, Wagbatsoma V, Orhue A. Anaemia in pregnancy. East Afr Med J 1994;71:671-3.

Ogunbode O. Anaemia in Pregnancy. In: Okonofua F, Odunsi K, editors. Contemporary Obstetrics and Gynaecology For Developing Countries. Benin City, Nigeria: Women's Health and Action Research Center; 2003. pp. 514-529.

Omigbodun AO. Recent trends in the management of anaemia inpregnancy. *Trop J Obstet Gynaecol.* 2004;21(1):1-3.

Ross J, Thomas EL. Iron deficiency anaemia and maternal mortality. Profiles 3. Working Notes Series No3.WashingtonDC;Academy for Educational Development;1996.

Rusia U, Madan Sikka M, Sood S. N Effect of maternal iron deficiency anaemia on foetal outcome. Indian J Pathol Microbiol 1995;38:273-9

Sarin AR. Severe anaemia of pregnancy - recent experience. Int J Gynae col Obstet 1995;50:S45-S49.

Scholl TO. Iron status during pregnancy: setting the stage for mother and infant. Am J Clin Nutr 2005;81: 1218S-22S. (Level III)

Singla PN, Tyagi M, Kumar A, Dash D, Shankar R. Fetal growth in maternal anemia. J Trop Pediatr 1997;43:89-92.Stoltzfus RJ. Update on issues related to iron deficiency and anaemia control. Report of the 2003

Sharma A, Patnaik R, Garg S, Ramachandran P. Detection & management of anaemia in pregnancy in an urban primary health care institution. *Indian J Med Res 2008; 128* : 45-51

Society for Gynaecology and Obstetrics of Nigeria (SOGON). Report of the maternal mortality situation in six (6) tertiary hospitals in Nigeria. Needs assessment. 2004:1-65

Uneke CJ, Sunday-Adeoye I, Iyare FE, Ugwuja EI, Duhlinska DD. Impact of maternal Plasmodium falciparum malaria and haematological parameters on pregnancy and its outcome in Southeastern Nigeria. *J Vector Borne Dis.* 2007;44:285-290.

World Health Organization. The prevalence of anaemia in women: A tabulation of available information. Geneva, World Health Organization; 1992 (unpublished document WHO/MCH/MSM/92.2; available upon request from Division of Reproductive Health, World Health Organization, 1211 Geneva 27, Switzerland).

World Health Organization (WHO) The prevalence of Anaemia in women: a tabulation of available information. Geneva, Switzerland: WHO; 1992. WHO/MCH/MSM/92.2 .

World Health Organization (WHO) Prevention and Management of Severe Anaemia in Pregnancy: Report of a Technical Working Group. Geneva, Switzerland: WHO; 1993. WHO/FNE/MSM/93.5.

World Health Organization. Prevention and management of severe anaemia in pregnancy. WHO; 1993

# 15

# Clinical Management of Hemolytic Disease of the Newborn and Fetus

Sebastian Illanes and Rafael Jensen
*Fetal Medicine Unit, University of Los Andes, Santiago Chile*

## 1. Introduction

Hemolytic disease of the fetus and newborn (HDFN) is caused by maternal alloantibodies directed against antigens present in fetal red cells. Paternally inherited antigens of the Rh system, which differ to those from the mother, are present on fetal red cells and when the maternal immune system makes contact with a significant number of these cells create an immune response with antibodies against these antigens. This may happen because of fetomaternal transplacental bleeding (in traumatic events during pregnancy, obstetric procedures, labor, cesarean section) or by events unrelated with pregnancy, such as transfusion, contamination by needle use, etc. Maternal antibodies (IgG) can cross the placenta and activate macrophages in the fetal spleen which cause fetal red cell destruction with subsequent hemolytic anemia. This leads to jaundice and kernicterus in the newborn or hydrops and death in the fetus.

Before the 70's, HDFN was a major obstetric problem, that had a large impact on fetal and neonatal morbidity and mortality. Today, without an appropriate programme, up to 50% of untreated HDFN will result in death or severe brain damage. In developing countries, especially those lacking an efficient prophylactics progamme, this causes an important public health problem. In fact, it has been estimated that more than 50 thousand fetuses could be affected by this condition every year in India (Zipursky and Paul, 2010). With the established use of post-natal anti-D prophylaxis for rhesus (Rh) negative women, together with its increasing use for routine antenatal prophylaxis, the incidence of Rh-D sensitization has dramatically fallen (Hughes RG et al., 1994). Nevertheless, 15-17% of the Caucasian population in Europe and North America is D negative (Ubarkian S, 2002). With the sensitization against other red cell antigens such as Kell RhC/c, RhE/e, this pathology could still affect a large number of pregnancies every year, with significant health and financial implications (Abdel-Fattah SA et al., 2002; Illanes S and Soothill P, 2009). In England and Wales, about 520 fetuses develop HDFN each year, of which about 37 would die in the fetal or neonatal period and 28 would present developmental problems (Daniels G et al., 2004, NICE 2008).

On the other hand, in fetus affected by HDFN, survival rates can exceed 90 percent if anemia is diagnosed and treated with intrauterine blood transfusions in a timely manner (Van Kamp IL et al., 2001). Women with rising red cell antibody levels are usually referred to tertiary fetal medicine units for specialized management. The main challenge facing fetal medicine specialists today is not the skill required for invasive therapy, but rather the non-invasive monitoring of the disease so that its progress can be predicted to guide the need and timing of intrauterine transfusions to minimize unnecessary invasive testing (Ubarkian S, 2002).

## 2. Non-invasive management

### 2.1 Use of cell-free fetal DNA for the determination of fetal RhD genotype

The identification of blood group genes and subsequent detection of the molecular bases of blood group polymorphisms has made it possible to predict blood group phenotypes (Avent ND et al., 2000). The source of DNA used to predict fetal blood groups was initially done invasively by sampling amniotic fluid or chorionic villi (Finning KM et al., 2002). However, the related risk of the obstetric procedures (0.5–1% for fetal loss) (Nanal R et al., 2003) and risk of fetomaternal hemorrhage (amniocentesis 17%) (Tabor A et al., 1987) was associated with an unwanted increase in gestational maternal immunization (Murray JC et al., 1983).

The fact that cell-free fetal DNA (ffDNA) is present in the plasma of pregnant women in sufficient quantities for the determination of fetal RhD genotype (Lo YM, 1999), leads to the possibility of fetal D typing using a non-invasive approach. If the rhesus sequence is present in a D-negative women's blood it is indicative that the fetus is D-positive (Lo YM et al., 1997). Initially, cell-free DNA was studied as a tumor marker (Lo YM et al., 1998), but the presence of Y signals in pregnant women carrying a male fetus was the first evidence that this technique could be used to assess the fetus condition as well as for prenatal diagnosis (Lo YM et al., 1997). In a normal pregnancy, the placental tissue goes through a physiological remodeling via apoptosis and necrosis in the chorionic villus. As a consequence, ffDNA is released to the maternal plasma in increasing amounts as gestation progresses (Wataganara T and Bianchi DW, 2004; Alberry MS et al., 2009; Huppertz B et al., 2006; Fomigli L et al., 2000; Arnholdt H et al., 1991; Illanes S et al., 2009).

Non-invasive prenatal diagnosis using ffDNA is the focus of intense research nowadays because of its many potential uses. It's being evaluated for inherited diseases and genetic disorders such as trisomy 21 (Ehrich M et al., 2011; Deng YH et al., 2011; Sehnert AJ et al, 2011), trisomy 18 (Sehnert AJ et al, 2011), β-thalassaemia (Li Y et al, 2009; Hahn S et al., 2011), hemophilia (Tsui NB et al., 2011), X-linked genetic disorders (Miura K et al., 2011) and achondroplasia (Chitty LS et al., 2011). Genome-wide scanning may be implemented for fetal genetic prenatal non-invasive diagnosis (Lo YM el al., 2010) and quantitative changes in ffDNA blood levels have been proposed as a potential marker for preeclampsia (Hahn S et al., 2011). Finally, the combination of real-time PCR with improved rhesus D (RhD) typing enables a highly accurate prediction of fetal D status from maternal plasma (Finning KM et al., 2002). Moreover, this is now available as a world-wide service (Daniels G et al., 2004; Finning KM et al., 2002; Finning KM et al., 2004; Legler TJ et al., 2002; Rouillac-Le Sciellour C et al., 2004; Van der Schoot CE et al, 2006; Tynan JA et al., 2011; Tounta G et al., 2011)

A recent meta-analysis has been performed to evaluate the diagnostic sensitivity and specificity of fetal Rh genotyping using ffDNA (Geifman-Holtzman O et al., 2006). A total of 3261maternal plasma samples were analyzed in 37 publications and approximately 500 study protocols in order to assess fetal RhD status. Results showed total accuracy of 91.4% (94,8% if studies with small numbers of samples were excluded), with a wide variation, from 31.8 to 100 percent, depending on which protocol, gestational age at testing and study design was applied. Two recent studies have evaluated the feasibility of this testing in the first trimester of pregnancy. Akolekar et al tested patients at 11-13 weeks using a high-throughput robotic technique. They concluded that it was an accurate method with a positive predictive value of 100% and a negative predictive value of 96,5% (Akolekar R et al., 2011). The second study, reported a sensitivity of 100% and a specificity of 93%, with a 97% diagnostic accuracy for RhD genotyping in the first trimester of pregnancy using a quantitave PCR method (Cardo el al., 2010)

Non-invasive fetal RhD genotyping was compared to traditional postnatal serologic assay in a large scale validation study (Müller SP et al., 2008). The authors studied over one thousand samples of RH negative women who gave whole blood specimens at a gestational age of 25 weeks. Tests were drawn up using an innovative automated DNA extraction method using magnetic tips and spin columns that have been recently developed by members of Special Non-Invasive Advances in Fetal and Neonatal Evaluation Network of Excellence (SAFE NoE) (Chitty LS et al., 2008; Legler TJ et al., 2007). The sensitivity of fetal *RHD* genotyping was 99.7% for spin columns and 99.8% for magnetic tips, and these results were comparable to conventional serology (99.5%). In the case of specificity, the serology was slightly better (99.7% versus 99.2% for spin columns and 98.1% for magnetic tips). It has also been established that it is an accurate method in multi-ethnic populations such as Brazil, by using two or three exons for RHD gene (Amaral DR et al, 2011; Chinen PA et al., 2010). This new approach has significantly reduced the number of invasive procedures carried out in different fetal medicine units for fetal D grouping (Finning KM et al., 2004) and has proved that the automated DNA extraction method can be used in a clinical setting.

Non-invasive studies for other blood group antigens have also been flourishing, including Kell antigen, the second most important cause of hemolytic disease (Li Y et al., 2008), RhC/c and RhE/e (Li Y et al., 2008; Van der Schoot CE et al., 2003; Finning K et al., 2007). The International Blood Group Reference Laboratory, at Bristol (Finning K et al., 2007) has developed and tested allele-specific primers for detecting the K allele of KEL and alleles of RhC/c RhE/e (Van der Schoot CE et al., 2003), with great accuracy for each allele. The matrix assisted laser desorption/ionization time-of-flight mass spectrometry or MALDITOF MS (Li Y et al., 2008), is able to detect the fetal KEL1 allele in KEL negative mothers with an accuracy of 94%. In a recent meta-analysis, collective reported diagnostic accuracy of fetal RhCE genotyping, with a combined accuracy for fetal genotyping of 96.3% for RhC/c and 98.2% for RhE/e (Geifman-Holtzman O et al., 2009) was estimated. A recent Dutch report, after 7 years of non-invasive fetal blood group genotyping from maternal blood samples for D, K, c, and E groups, revealed that diagnosis could be achieved in 97% of cases in a medium gestational age of 17 weeks, with no false-positive or false-negative results, implying that it is an accurate and applicable diagnostic tool in clinic (Scheffer P et al., 2011). The use of cell-free fetal DNA in maternal plasma for fetal RhD genotype could eventually enable the screening of all D negative pregnant women, thereby confining the administration of prophylactic anti-D only to those pregnancies in which it is needed (Bianchi DW et al., 2005). Since the accuracy of the actual test is not 100%, there is an ongoing debate about the advantage of introducing such a policy. Some researchers propose that guided prophylaxis should have a lower cost than the routine prophylaxis to all RhD negative women (Daniels G et al., 2009). However, a recent cost benefits study evaluated the implementation of this strategy in England and Wales, and concluded that is unlikely to be sufficiently cost-effective for a large scale introduction. They estimated that only minor savings would be gained and that an increase in maternal sensitization may be unacceptably high due to test inaccuracies in different ethnic minority populations (Szczepura A et al., 2011). It is expected that new technologies should alter this picture. Nevertheless, any policy for the prevention of unnecessary administration of human-derived products, such as prophylactic anti-D, should be taken into account because of the potential contamination of blood products that at the present time cannot be tested, as unidentified viruses or prions (Avent ND. 2008, Avent ND. 2009).

## 3. Detection of fetal anemia non-invasively by ultrasonography

### 3.1 Ultrasound findings

Severe anemia causes tissue hypoxia (Soothill PW et al., 1987), with endothelial damage and increased capillary permeability. This may lead to protein loss into the interstitial space, hypoproteinaemia and consequently ascites (Nicolaides KH et al., 1985). Moreover, in response to red cell haemolysis and fetal anemia, extramedullary haematopoiesis occurs, increasing portal and umbilical venous pressures. This would impair hepatic function and protein synthesis, resulting in worsening hypoproteinaemia which would further deteriorate the hydrops process (Bowman JM, 1978; Socol ML et al., 1987). The ultrasonographic features of hydrops include ascites (the earliest sign), pleural effusions, pericardial effusions, scalp edema, subcutaneous edema and polyhydramnios. These findings are an indication of a hemoglobin deficit of more than 6 standard deviations below the normal mean for gestational age, and will need urgent intrauterine fetal transfusion (Nicolaides KH et al., 1988).

The many attempts to identify sonographic fetal anemia features which occur before the development of fetal hydrops have been unsuccessful (Queenan JT, 1982, De Vore GR et al., 1981,Nicolaides KH et al., 1988), because of their failure to quantify the real degree of the fetal anemia (Nicolaides KH et al., 1988). Moreover, these ultrasound findings, including the evaluation of the liver and spleen, have been abandoned, because when high quality Doppler measurements are used to predict fetal anemia, these anatomic evaluations add little useful independent information. In our practice, we don´t usually look for any structural measurement or appearance, save for the early signs of fetal ascites.

### 3.2 Fetal Doppler ultrasonography

Doppler ultrasonography is a non-invasive method used for studying fetal hemodynamic changes in vessels that supply fetal organs responding to pathological conditions. In anemic fetuses, the Doppler measurement that describes the hemodynamic changes occurring in response to this pathological condition has been attempted in several vessels. However, because of the rapid hemodynamic changes observed in the middle cerebral artery (MCA) (Mari G et al., 2000), have transformed the measurement of its peak systolic velocity (the maximum Doppler shift at the peak of the spectral curve) in the gold standard for anemia fetal prediction. (Campbell S et al., 1995). After Vyas et al in 1990 (Vyas et al., 1990) described an increase in the average MCA time for mean blood velocity in fetal anemia cases, Mari and colleagues reported that the degree of fetal anemia could be accurately detected by Doppler measurement of blood-flow velocity in the MCA, with an inverse relationship between the MCA peak velocity and the fetal hematocrit, with no false negative results for anemic fetuses (Mari G et al., 2000). The statistically significant increase in fetal hematocrit, following intrauterine transfusion, also resulted in a rapid reduction in the middle cerebral artery peak velocity. These results confirm that the traditional management of pregnancies complicated by Rh alloimmunization with serial invasive amniocentesis to determine bilirubin levels is no longer required. Even more, a recent study has shown that Doppler measurement of the peak velocity of systolic blood flow in the MCA can safely replace invasive testing in the management of Rh-alloimmunized pregnancies, avoiding all the complications related with the traditional invasive approach (Oepkes et al., 2006).

Several studies have used the MCA Dopplers in a clinical basis for the prediction of fetal anemia with at-risk cases, without ultrasound evidence of fetal hydrops. These have shown that there is a good correlation with fetal Hemoglobin (Abdel-Fattah SA et al., 2002). This non-invasive investigation can be reliable in predicting anemia in cases in which the need to sample fetal blood is not certain, therefore delaying invasive testing until treatment is likely to be required. The neonatal outcome where invasive testing has been avoided (based on reassuring MCA Doppler velocity results) did not result in life-threatening fetal or neonatal morbidities (Abdel-Fattah SA et al, 2005). Therefore, the routine use of MCA Doppler's can avoid unnecessary invasive procedures on at-risk fetuses. There are several normal reference ranges of fetal blood flow velocity in the middle cerebral artery. However, when compared in terms of discriminatory power, sensitivity and specificity, Mari's curve and its given cut-offs perform better when fetal anemia is predicted. (Mari G et al., 2000; Bartha JL et al., 2005).

## 4. Invasive approach

Intrauterine blood transfusion of anemic fetuses represents one of the great successes of fetal therapy. After the first approach with intraperitoneal blood transfusion introduced in 1963 by Liley (Liley AW, 1963), Rodeck (Rodeck CH et al., 1981) described intravascular fetal blood transfusion (IVT) by the needling of the chorionic plate or umbilical cord vessels via fetoscopy direct vision. In 1982, Bang in Denmark started IVT by umbilical cord puncture under ultrasound guidance. This is now the gold standart (Bang et al., 1982). IVT has produced a marked improvement in the survival rate of the anemic hydropic fetus. This in turn can also prevent complications from developing by treating anemic non-hydropic fetuses, where moderate or severe anemia is detected non-invasively by Doppler ultrasonography, by increased peak velocity of systolic blood flow or time-averaged mean velocity in the MCA in fetuses at risk (Abdel-Fattah SA et al., 2002; Mari G et al., 2000). It is estimated that between 10 and 12% of fetuses of sensitized RHD negative women will require IVT (NICE 2008) with the survival rate exceeding 95% in experienced centers, particularly when opportune IVT treatment is established in a timely manner (Van Kamp IL et al., 2001).

When possible the umbilical vein is sampled because artery puncture may pose a risk for bradycardia (Weiner CP et al., 1991). The hemoglobin concentration (Hb) is measured and interpreted according to gestational age, with the severity classified on the fetal hemoglobin deviation from the normal mean for gestation into mild (hemoglobin deficit less than 2 g/dl), moderate (deficit 2-7 g/dl), and severe (deficit greater than 7 g/dl) (Nicolaides KH et al., 1988). A blood transfusion will be attempted in cases were a moderate or severe anemia is detected. For IVT to be realized, the blood volume required to correct the fetal Hb needs to be calculated, using pre-transfusion fetal Hb, the donor blood Hb (adult blood usually packed to a hematocrit of about 70-80%) and the gestational age (Nicolaides KH et al., 1986). The volume required is given as fast as possible without causing changes to the fetal heart rate and it seems that the feto-placental unit is able to handle the blood volume expansion much more easily than when transfusing neonates without the benefit of a placenta. Infusion of packed blood through a 15-cm long, 20-gauge needle at rates of 1–10 ml/min does not result in significant hemolysis (Nicolaides KH et al., 1986). After the volume calculated to correct the Hb deficit has been given a post-transfusion, Hb is measured to help time the subsequent transfusion. After two or three transfusions, fetal blood production is suppressed and instead adult blood cells become more dominant. The fall of Hb becomes very predictable at about 1% haematocrit point per day (Thein AT and Soothill P, 1998). We aim to complete the last transfusion at 35-36 weeks and then to induce labor at 37 weeks to allow maturation of both the pulmonary and hepatic enzyme systems. With this programme, we hope to avoid neonatal exchange transfusions.

As this management of anemic fetuses is increasing, and the number of cordocentesis and transfusions are decreasing, the problem of maintaining the skills needed is rising too. It has been suggested that operators should perform at least 10 procedures per year to keep competence. (Lindenburg IT et al., 2011). Complications associated with intrauterine procedures such as cord hematoma, hemorrhage, fetal bradycardia and intrauterine death could increase in the future (Illanes S and Soothill PW, 2006). A possible solution would be to introduce a health policy that gave transfusions, via some centers, to all those cases that needed one. This could potentially avoid any complications such as lack of operator training.

## 5. Neonatal outcome

For the neonate, the consequences of HDFN are anemia and hiperbilirrubinemia. Postnatal treatment options include top-up red blood cells transfusions for the former, and phototherapy and exchange transfusions for the latter. Top-up transfusions, even with a minimal risk, carry a theoretical possibility of anaphylactic reaction and transmission of viral disease. In contrast, exchange transfusion carries a high morbidity and mortality rate (5% and <0.3% respectively), but the number of neonates requiring exchange transfusions has reduced due to advances in phototherapy.

Few studies specifically investigate the short-term neonatal outcomes for pregnancies affected by hemolytic red cell alloimmunisation. Two recent retrospective studies have assessed this question. De Boer *et al.* (De Boer *et al* 2008) investigated the short-term morbidity for neonates treated for Rhesus disease with or without IVT. Those treated with IVTs were found to require a higher number of top-up red blood cell transfusions and had less need of phototherapy. However, both groups had a similar need for exchange transfusion. The second study, is a Scottish report of postnatal outcomes following intrauterine transfusion, and showed that 20% of newborn needed exchange transfusion, 50% had top-up transfusion, and most of them needed phototherapy (McGlone L et al., 2009). More studies are needed, to evaluate the neonatal outcomes and associated morbi mortality, related to the number of transfusions, the gestational age at first and last transfusion, and the hemoglobin level at first IVT.

## 6. Conclusion

The management of the HDFN represents one of the genuine successes of fetal therapy. The current aspects of this clinical management have shifted from a long-established invasive approach to a non-invasive one. This applies to the detection of fetuses at risk of HDFN with the use of cell-free fetal DNA in the plasma of pregnant women to determine fetal RhD genotype. If the fetus is D negative, then it is not at risk and no further procedures are required; if it is D positive the appropriate management of the pregnancy can be arranged. On the other hand, maternal plasma testing for fetal RhD genotype could eventually enable the screening of all D negative pregnant women, thereby confining the administration of prophylactic anti-D only to those pregnancies in which it is needed. In addition, when a fetus is antigen positive, the follow up of these fetuses is for the detection of moderate or severe anemia non-invasively by Doppler ultrasonography on the basis of an increase in the peak velocity of systolic blood in the middle cerebral artery. When anemia is suspected, an invasive approach is required in order to perform an intrauterine blood transfusion which should only be attempted when the fetus needs transfusion.

## 7. Summary

Hemolytic disease of the fetus and newborn (HDFN) is caused by maternal alloantibodies directed against paternally inherited antigens on fetal red blood cells. It was also a significant cause of fetal and neonatal morbidity and mortality until the introduction of anti-D immunoglobulin during pregnancy and shortly after delivery. However, it is still a major problem in affected pregnancies. The emphasis of current clinical management of HDFN is a non-invasive approach. This work is carried out on fetuses at risk with HDFN, with the use of cell-free fetal DNA in the plasma of pregnant women, in order to determine the fetal RhD genotype, or to see if the fetus is antigen positive. If the mother is sensitized, for the follow up and detection of moderate or severe anemia - this is done, primarily, non-invasively by Doppler ultrasonography of the middle cerebral artery. If anemia is suspected, an invasive approach is required in order to perform an intrauterine blood transfusion. This management represents one of the genuine successes of fetal therapy.

## 8. References

[1] Abdel-Fattah SA, Shefras J, Kyle PM, Cairns P, Hunter A, Soothill PW. Reassuring fetal middle cerebral artery doppler velocimetry in alloimmunised pregnancies: neonatal outcomes without invasive procedures. Fetal Diagn Ther. 2005 Sep-Oct;20(5):341-5

[2] Abdel-Fattah SA, Soothill PW, Carroll SG, Kyle PM. Middle cerebral artery Doppler for the prediction of fetal anaemia in cases without hydrops: a practical approach. Br J Radiol. 2002 Sep;75(897):726-30

[3] Akolekar R, Finning K, Kuppusamy R, Daniels G, Nicolaides KH. Fetal RHD Genotyping in Maternal Plasma at 11-13 Weeks of Gestation. Fetal Diagn Ther. 2011;29(4):301-6. Epub 2011 Jan 8.

[4] Alberry MS, Maddocks DG, Hadi MA, Metawi H, Hunt LP, Abdel-Fattah SA, Avent ND, Soothill PW. 2009. Quantification of cell free fetal DNA in maternal plasma in normal pregnancies and in pregnancies with placental dysfunction. Am J Obstet Gynecol. 200(1):98.e1-6.

[5] Amaral DR, Credidio DC, Pellegrino J Jr, Castilho L. Fetal RHD genotyping by analysis of maternal plasma in a mixed population. J Clin Lab Anal. 2011;25(2):100-4.

[6] Arnholdt H, Meisel F, Fandrey K, Lohrs U. 1991. Proliferation of villous trophoblast of the human placenta in normal and abnormal pregnancies. Virchows Arch B Cell Pathol Incl Mol Pathol.60: 365-72.

[7] Avent ND. 2008. RHD genotyping from maternal plasma: guidelines and technical challenges. Methods Mol Biol. 444:185-201.

[8] Avent ND. 2009. Large-scale blood group genotyping: clinical implications. Br J Haematol. 144(1):3-13.

[9] Avent ND, Finning KM, Martin PG, Soothill PW. Prenatal determination of fetal blood group status. Vox Sang. 2000;78 Suppl 2:155-62.

[10] Bang J, Bock JE, Trolle D Ultrasound guided fetal intravenous transfusion for severe rehus haemolytic disease. BMJ 1982; 284: 373–374.

[11] Bartha JL, Illanes S, Abdel-Fattah S, Hunter A, Denbow M, Soothill PW. Comparison of different reference values of fetal blood flow velocity in the middle cerebral artery for predicting fetal anemia. Ultrasound Obstet Gynecol. 2005 Apr;25(4):335-40

[12] Bianchi DW, Avent ND, Costa JM, van der Schoot CE.Noninvasive prenatal diagnosis of fetal Rhesus D: ready for Prime(r) Time. Obstet Gynecol. 2005 Oct;106(4):841-4. Review.

[13] Bowman JM. The management of Rh isoimmunization. Obstet Gynecol 1978; 52: 1-16

[14] Campbell S, Harrington K, Hecher K. The fetal arterial circulation. In: A colour atlas of Doppler ultrasonography in obstetrics, Eds Harrington K, Campbell S. Edward Arnold 1995; 59-69

[15] Cardo L, García BP, Alvarez FV. Non-invasive fetal RHD genotyping in the first trimester of pregnancy. Clin Chem Lab Med. 2010 Aug;48(8):1121-6.

[16] Chinen PA, Nardozza LM, Martinhago CD, Camano L, Daher S, Pares DB, Minett T, Araujo Júnior E, Moron AF. Noninvasive determination of fetal rh blood group, D antigen status by cell-free DNA analysis in maternal plasma: experience in a Brazilian population. Am J Perinatol. 2010 Nov;27(10):759-62.

[17] Chitty LS, Griffin DR, Meaney C, Barrett A, Khalil A, Pajkrt E, Cole TJ. New aids for the non-invasive prenatal diagnosis of achondroplasia: dysmorphic features, charts of fetal size and molecular confirmation using cell-free fetal DNA in maternal plasma. Ultrasound Obstet Gynecol. 2011 Mar;37(3):283-9. doi: 10.1002/uog.8893. Epub 2011 Feb 1.

[18] Chitty LS, van der Schoot CE, Hahn S, Avent ND. 2008. SAFE—the Special Non-invasive Advances in Fetal and Neonatal Evaluation Network: aims and achievements. Prenat Diagn.28: 83-8.

[19] Daniels G, Finning K, Martin P, Massey E. 2009. Noninvasive prenatal diagnosis of fetal blood group phenotypes: current practice and future prospects. Prenat Diagn. 29(2): 101-7.

[20] Daniels G, Finning K, Martin P, Soothill P. Fetal blood group genotyping from DNA from maternal plasma: an important advance in the management and prevention of haemolytic disease of the fetus and newborn. Vox Sang. 2004 Nov;87(4):225-32. Review.

[21] De Boer, I.P., Zeestraten, E.C., Lopriore, E., van Kamp, I.L., Kanhai, H.H. & Walther, F.J. Paediatric outcome in Rhesus haemolytic disease treated with and without intrauterine transfusion. *American Journal of Obstetrics & Gynaecology,* 2008: 198(1):54.e1-4.

[22] De Vore GR, Mayden K, Tortora M, Berkowitz RL, Hobbins JC. Dilation of the fetal umbilical vein in rhesus hemolytic anemia: a predictor of severe disease. Am J Obstet Gynecol 1981; 141: 464-66.

[23] Deng YH, Yin AH, He Q, Chen JC, He YS, Wang HQ, Li M, Chen HY. Non-invasive prenatal diagnosis of trisomy 21 by reverse transcriptase multiplex ligation-dependent probe amplification. Clin Chem Lab Med. 2011 Apr;49(4):641-6.

[24] Ehrich M, Deciu C, Zwiefelhofer T, Tynan JA, Cagasan L, Tim R, Lu V, McCullough R, McCarthy E, Nygren AO, Dean J, Tang L, Hutchison D, Lu T, Wang H, Angkachatchai V, Oeth P, Cantor CR, Bombard A, van den Boom D. Noninvasive detection of fetal trisomy 21 by sequencing of DNA in maternal blood: a study in a clinical setting. Am J Obstet Gynecol. 2011 Mar;204(3):205.e1-11. Epub 2011 Feb 18.

[25] Finning K, Martin P, Daniels G. A clinical service in the UK to predict fetal Rh (Rhesus) D blood group using free fetal DNA in maternal plasma. Ann N Y Acad Sci. 2004.Jun;1022:119-23.

[26] Finning KM, Martin PG, Soothill PW and Avent ND, Prediction of fetal D status from maternal plasma: introduction of a new noninvasive fetal RHD genotyping service. Transfusion 42 (2002), pp. 1079–1085.

[27] Finning K, Martin P, Summers J, Daniels G. 2007. Fetal genotyping for the K (Kell) and Rh C, c, and E blood groups on cell-free fetal DNA in maternal plasma. Transfusion. 11: 2126-33.

[28] Formigli L, Papucci L, Tani A, et al. 2000. Aponecrosis: morphological and biochemical exploration of a syncretic process of cell death sharing apoptosis and necrosis. J Cell Physiol. 182:41-9.

[29] Geifman-Holtzman O, Grotegut CA, Gaughan JP. 2006. Diagnostic accuracy of non-invasive fetal Rh genotyping from maternal blood—a meta-analysis. Am J Obstet Gynecol. 2006 4:1163-73.

[30] Geifman-Holtzman O, Grotegut CA, Gaughan JP, Holtzman EJ, Floro C, Hernandez E. 2009. Non-invasive fetal RhCE genotyping from maternal blood. BJOG. 116(2):144-51.

[31] Hahn S, Lapaire O, Tercanli S, Kolla V, Hösli I. Determination of fetal chromosome aberrations from fetal DNA in maternal blood: has the challenge finally been met? Expert Rev Mol Med. 2011 May 4;13:e16.

[32] Hahn S, Rusterholz C, Hösli I, Lapaire O. Cell-free nucleic acids as potential markers for preeclampsia. Placenta. 2011 Feb;32 Suppl:S17-20.

[33] Hughes RG, Craig JIO, Murphy WG, Greer IA. Causes and clinical consequences of Rhesus (D) haemolytic disease of the newborn: a study of Scottish population, 1985–1990. Br J Obstet Gynaecol 1994;101:297–300.

[34] Huppertz B, Kadyrov M, Kingdom JC. 2006. Apoptosis and its role in the trophoblast. Am J Obstet Gynecol. 195:29-39.

[35] Illanes S, Parra M, Serra R, Pino K, Figueroa-Diesel H, Romero C, Arraztoa JA, Michea L, Soothill PW. 2009. Increased free fetal DNA levels in early pregnancy plasma of women who subsequently develop preeclampsia and intrauterine growth restriction. Prenat Diagn. 29(12):1118-2.

[36] Illanes S, Soothill PW. 2006. Fetal therapy. In Progress in Obstetrics and Gynaecology. John Studd (Ed). Elselvier; United Kingdom: 65-78.

[37] Illanes S, Soothill P. 2009. The non-invasive approach for the management of haemolytic disease of the fetus and newborn. Current aspects of the clinical management of haemolytic disease of the newborn and foetus. Expert Review of Hematology 5, 577-582.

[38] Legler TJ, Liu Z, Mavrou A, Finning KM, Hromadnikova I, Galbiati S, Meaney C, Hul; én MA, Crea F, Olsson ML, Maddocks DG, Huang D, Armstrong Fisher S, Sprenger-Haussels M, Soussan AA, van der Schoot CE. 2007. Workshop report on the extraction of foetal DNA from maternal plasma. Prenat Diagn. 27: 824-29.

[39] Legler, T.J., Lynen, R., Maas, J.H., Pindur, G., Kulenkampff, D., Suren, A., Osmers, R. & Kohler, M. Prediction of fetal Rh D and Rh Cc Ee phenotype from maternal plasma with real-time polymerase chain reaction. Transfus Apher Sci, 2002. 27, 217-223.

[40] Li Y, Di Naro E, Vitucci A, Grill S, Zhong XY, Holzgreve W, Hahn S. Size fractionation of cell-free DNA in maternal plasma improves the detection of a paternally inherited beta-thalassemia point mutation by MALDI-TOF mass spectrometry. Fetal Diagn Ther. 2009;25(2):246-9. Epub 2009 Jun 5.

[41] Li Y, Finning K, Daniels G, Hahn S, Zhong X, Holzgreve W. 2008. Noninvasive genotyping fetal Kell blood group (KEL1) using cell-free fetal DNA in maternal plasma by MALDI-TOF mass spectrometry. Prenat Diagn. 28(3): 203-8.

[42] Liley AW Intrauterine transfusion of fetus in haemolytic disease. BMJ II 1963: 1107–1109.

[43] Lindenburg IT, Wolterbeek R, Oepkes D, Klumper FJ, Vandenbussche FP, van Kamp IL. Quality Control for Intravascular Intrauterine Transfusion Using Cumulative Sum (CUSUM) Analysis for the Monitoring of Individual Performance. Fetal Diagn Ther. 2011;29(4):307-14. Epub 2011 Feb 8.

[44] Lo YMD. Fetal RhD genotyping from maternal plasma: Ann Med 1999; 31:308-312

[45] Lo YM, Chan KC, Sun H, Chen EZ, Jiang P, Lun FM, Zheng YW, Leung TY, Lau TK, Cantor CR, Chiu RW. Maternal plasma DNA sequencing reveals the genome-wide genetic and mutational profile of the fetus. Sci Transl Med. 2010 Dec 8;2(61):61ra91.

[46] Lo YM, Corbetta N, Chamberlain PF, Rai V, Sargent IL, Redman CW, Wainscoat JS. 1997. Presence of fetal DNA in maternal plasma and serum. Lancet 350: 485–487.

[47] Lo YM, Tein MSC, Lau TK,Haines CJ, Leung TN, Poon PMK, Wainscoat JS, Johnson PJ, Chang AMZ, Hjelm NM. 1998. Quantitative analysis of fetal DNA in maternal plasma and serum: implications for noninvasive prenatal diagnosis. Am J Hum Genet. 62: 768–775.

[48] Mari G, Deter RL, Carpenter RL, et al. Noninvasive diagnosis by Doppler ultrasonography of fetal anemia due to maternal red-cell alloimmunization. N Engl J Med 2000;342:9-14.

[49] McGlone L, Simpson JH, Scott-Lang C, Cameron AD, Brennand J. 2009. Short term outcomes following intrauterine transfusion in Scotland. Arch Dis Child Fetal Neonatal. 23.

[50] Miura K, Higashijima A, Shimada T, Miura S, Yamasaki K, Abe S, Jo O, Kinoshita A, Yoshida A, Yoshimura S, Niikawa N, Yoshiura K, Masuzaki H. Clinical application of fetal sex determination using cell-free fetal DNA in pregnant carriers of X-linked genetic disorders. J Hum Genet. 2011 Apr;56(4):296-9. Epub 2011 Feb 10.

[51] Müller SP, Bartels I, Stein W, Emons G, Gutensohn K, Köhler M, Legler TJ. 2008. The determination of the fetal D status from maternal plasma for decision making on Rh prophylaxis is feasible. Transfusion, 11: 2292-301.

[52] Murray JC, Karp LE, Williamson RA, Cheng EY, Luthy DA. Rh isoimmunization related to amniocentesis. Am J Med Genet 1983;16:527-34.

[53] Nanal R, Kyle P, Soothill PW. A classification of pregnancy losses after invasive prenatal diagnostic procedures: an approach to allow comparison of units with a different case mix. Prenat Diagn. 2003 Jun;23(6):488-92

[54] National Institute for Clinical Excellence: Technology Appraisal Guidance 156. 2008, review date: may 2011. Routine antenatal anti-D prophylaxis for women who are rhesus D negative. London, NICE.

[55] Nicolaides KH, Fontanarosa M, Gabbe SG, Rodeck CH. Failure of ultrasonographic parameters to predict the severity of fetal anemia in rhesus isoimmunization. Am J Obstet Gynecol 1988; 158: 920-6.

[56] Nicolaides KH, Soothill PW, Clewell WH, Rodeck CH, Mibashan RS, Campbell S. Fetal haemoglobin measurement in the assessment of red cell isoimmunisation. Lancet 1988; 1: 1073-75

[57] Nicolaides KH, Soothill PW, Rodeck CH, Clewell W Rh disease: intravascular fetal blood transfusion by cordocentesis. Fetal Ther. 1986; 1(4): 185-92.

[58] Nicolaides KH, Warenski JC, Rodeck CH. The relationship of fetal plasma protein concentration and Hemoglobin level to the development of hydrops in rhesus isoimmunization. Am J Obstet Gynecol 1985; 152: 341-4

[59] Oepkes D, Seaward PG, Vandenbussche FP, Windrim R, Kingdom J, Beyene J, Kanhai HH, Ohlsson A, Ryan G; DIAMOND Study Group.Doppler ultrasonography versus amniocentesis to predict fetal anemia.N Engl J Med. 2006 Jul 13;355(2):156-64.

[60] Queenan JT. Current management of the Rh-sensitized patient. Clin Obstet Gynecol 1982; 25: 293-301

[61] Rodeck CH, Kemp JR, Holman CA, Whitmore CA, Karnicki J,Austin MA. Direct intravascular fetal blood transfusion by fetoscopy in severe Rhesus isoimmunisation. Lancet I 1981:625- 627.

[62] Rouillac-Le Sciellour, C., Puillandre, P., Gillot, R., Baulard, C., Metral, S., Le Van Kim, C., Cartron, J.P., Colin, Y. & Brossard, Y. Large-scale pre-diagnosis study of fetal RHD genotyping by PCR on plasma DNA from RhD-negative pregnant women. Mol Diagn, 2004. 8, 23-31.

[63] Scheffer P, van der Schoot C, Page-Christiaens G, de Haas M. Noninvasive fetal blood group genotyping of rhesus D, c, E and of K in alloimmunised pregnant women: evaluation of a 7-year clinical experience. BJOG. 2011 Jun 14.

[64] Sehnert AJ, Rhees B, Comstock D, de Feo E, Heilek G, Burke J, Rava RP. Optimal detection of fetal chromosomal abnormalities by massively parallel DNA sequencing of cell-free fetal DNA from maternal blood. Clin Chem. 2011 Jul;57(7):1042-9. Epub 2011 Apr 25.

[65] Socol ML, MacGregor SN, Pielet BW, Tamura RK, Sabbagha RE. Percutaneous umbilical transfusion in severe rhesus isoimmunization: Resolution of fetal hydrops. Am J Obstet Gynecol 1987; 157: 1369-75

[66] Soothill PW, Nicolaides KH, Rodeck CH, Clewell WH, Lindridge J. Relationship of fetal hemoglobin and oxygen content to lactate concentration in Rh isoimmunized pregnancies. Obstet Gynecol 1987; 69: 268-71
[67] Szczepura A, Osipenko L, Freeman K. A new fetal RHD genotyping test: costs and benefits of mass testing to target antenatal anti-D prophylaxis in England and Wales. BMC Pregnancy Childbirth. 2011 Jan 18;11:5.
[68] Tabor A, Bang J, Nørgaard-Pedersen B: Feto-maternal haemorrhage associated with genetic amniocentesis: results of a randomized trial. Br J Obstet Gynecol 1987; 94:528-34
[69] Thein AT, Soothill P. Antenatal invasive therapy. Eur J Pediatr. 1998 Jan; 157 Suppl 1: S2-6
[70] Tounta G, Vrettou C, Kolialexi A, Papantoniou N, Destouni A, Tsangaris GT, Antsaklis A, Kanavakis E, Mavrou A. A multiplex PCR for non-invasive fetal RHD genotyping using cell-free fetal DNA. In Vivo. 2011 May-Jun;25(3):411-7.
[71] Tsui NB, Kadir RA, Chan KC, Chi C, Mellars G, Tuddenham EG, Leung TY, Lau TK, Chiu RW, Lo YM. Noninvasive prenatal diagnosis of hemophilia by microfluidics digital PCR analysis of maternal plasma DNA. Blood. 2011 Mar 31;117(13):3684-91. Epub 2011 Jan 24.
[72] Tynan JA, Mahboubi P, Cagasan LL, van den Boom D, Ehrich M, Oeth P. Restriction enzyme-mediated enhanced detection of circulating cell-free fetal DNA in maternal plasma. J Mol Diagn. 2011 Jul;13(4):382-9. Epub 2011 May 6.
[73] Ubarniak S, 2002. The clinical application of anti-D prophilaxis. In: Alloimmune Disorders of Pregnancy: Anaemia,Thrombocytopenia and Neutropenia in the Fetus and Newborn. Andrew Hadley, Peter Soothill (Ed). Cambridge University Press; Cambridge: 97-121.
[74] Van der Schoot, C.E., Soussan, A.A., Koelewijn, J., Bonsel, G., Paget-Christiaens, L.G. & de Haas, M. Non-invasive antenatal RHD typing. Transfus Clin Biol. 2006.13, 53-57.
[75] Van der Schoot, C.E., Tax, G.H., Rijnders, R.J., de Haas, M. & Christiaens, G.C. 2003. Prenatal typing of Rh and Kell blood group system antigens: the edge of a watershed. Transfus Med Rev. 17: 31-44.
[76] Van Kamp IL, Klumper FJCM, Bakkum RSLA, et al. The severity of immune fetal hydrops is predictive for fetal outcome after intrauterine treatment. Am J Obstet Gynecol 2001;185:668-673.
[77] Vyas S, Nicolaides KH, Campbell S. Doppler examination of the middle cerebral artery in anemic fetuses. Am J Obstet Gynecol 1990; 162: 1066-8
[78] Wataganara T, Bianchi DW. 2004. Fetal cell-free nucleic acids in the maternal circulation: new clinical applications. Ann N Y Acad Sci . 1022: 90–99.
[79] Weiner CP, Wenstrom KD, Sipes SL, Williamson RA. Risk factors for cordocentesis and fetal intravascular transfusion. Am J Obstet Gynecol. 1991 Oct; 165 (4 Pt 1): 1020-5.
[80] Zipursky A, Paul VK The global burden of Rh disease, Arch Dis Child Fetal Neonatal Ed. 2011 Mar;96(2):F84-5. Epub 2010 Oct 30.

# 16

# The Pathogenesis of Anaemia in African Animal Trypanosomosis

Savino Biryomumaisho* and E. Katunguka-Rwakishaya
*Department of Veterinary Medicine, Makerere University, Kampala Uganda*

## 1. Introduction

The pathogenesis and pathology of animal trypanosomosis has been a subject of numerous investigations and anaemia has long been recognized as a significant pathological feature. It is the consensus that this anaemia is haemolytic in origin, occurring intravascularly in the acute phase and also extravascularly in the subacute and chronic stages of the disease. The cause of this anaemia is multifactorial and includes increase in erythrocyte destruction coupled with shortening of erythrocyte lifespan. The destruction of erythrocytes largely occurs in the liver by erythrophagocytosis. The other mechanism that has been suggested is that trypanosomes may exert a direct haemolytic action on erythrocytes by generating potentially haemolytic factors on autolysis, a phenomenon that was first described by Landsteiner & Raubitscheck (1901) who hypothesized that the haemolytic factor is lipid in nature. Other mechanisms that have been suggested are haemodilution, bone marrow dysfunction (dyshaemopoiesis) and immunologically-mediated destruction of erythrocytes. In this chapter, the roles of biochemical changes particularly the lipid sub-fraction, bone marrow dysfunction and haemodilution in Small East African goats experimentally infected with *Trypanosoma congolense* or *T. brucei brucei* shall be examined. The effect of *T. congolense* on the life span of erythrocytes in sheep, inferred from $^{51}Cr$-labelled erythrocytes, will be presented and discussed.

An in-depth knowledge of development of anaemia during trypanosomosis in different animal species is pivotal in instituting appropriate treatment in clinically sick animals and during convalescence. Similarly, the same knowledge can be utilized by animal health workers to manage anaemia derived from causes other than trypanosomosis.

## 2. Free fatty acids and other blood biochemical changes

The subject of blood biochemical changes and the role of individual biochemicals mainly those derived from the protein and lipid sub-fractions have been investigated over decades with the aim of elucidating the mechanisms by which anaemia in trypanosome-infected animals is induced. Of particular significance in the pathogenesis of anaemia in trypanosome-infected animals are free fatty acids (FFAs). Free fatty acids generated from both *T. congolense* (Tizard & Holmes, 1976) and *T. brucei* (Huan et al., 1975) form potent hemolytic material when permitted to autolyse in saline at 20°C. This material contains a mixture of FFAs and to a lesser extent lysophospholipids (Tizard et al., 1977). Massive trypanosome destruction as a result of the hosts' immune responses occurs especially during the acute phase of trypanosome infection. Therefore, the rapid decrease of the erythrocyte mass in this phase may among other factors be mediated by the generation of FFAs from autolysing trypanosomes (Biryomumaisho et al., 2003).

Free fatty acids may be saturated and unsaturated; both groups can significantly modify the host immune response (Berken & Benacerraf, 1968) by either blocking lymphocytic reactivity to mitogens (Mertin & Hughes, 1975) or antigens (Field et al., 1974) or through production of potent immunosuppressive prostaglandins (Quagliata et al., 1972). There is remarkable resemblance between the immunological lesions induced by administration of free fatty acids and those observed in trypanosomosis. The question is: what is the significance of variations of FFAs concentrations that are observed during trypanosomosis infections in different animal species? Observations have shown that relatively large quantities of FFA mostly stearic, linoleic, palmitic and oleic acids are generated by autolysing trypanosomes (Tizard et al., 1976; Assoku et al., 1977). These FFAs are potentially cytotoxic and haemolytic *in vitro*. In both *T. congolense* and *T. brucei* infected Small East African goats (Biryomumaisho et al., 2003), FFAs were significantly higher than those of control uninfected animals. However, the other biochemical parameters showed a different pattern: hypoproteinaemia, hypoalbuminaemia, hypocholestraemia, low and high density hypolipidaemia. These changes suggest that growing trypanosomes require some lipids and proteins to support their growth. At the same time, anaemia developed after goats were challenged with trypanosomes; the pattern of increase of FFAs corresponded to the decrease of packet cell volume (PCV), haemoglobin and erythrocyte counts. These observations re-affirm that FFAs generated from autolysing trypanosomes in goats contribute to anaemia development *in vivo*.

The fatty acids of trypanosomes are mainly esterified as phosphoglycerides or as cholesterol esters though they also exist as FFAs (Dixon et al., 1972). Lipids constitute 15-20% of the dry weight of African trypanosomes with total lipid content of the stumpy forms being substantially higher than that of the slender forms (Vankatesan & Ormerod, 1976). On autolysis, *T. congolense* releases a number of haemolytic FFAs of which the most potent is linoleic acid. These fatty acids can lyse washed rat and bovine erythrocytes *in vitro* (Tizard et al., 1978); autolysis will cause increased erythrocyte fragility in whole rat blood but not in whole bovine blood. Observations in Small East African goats during the first 16 days post infection (Biryomumaisho et al., 2003) showed that total serum lipids decreased from 12.88 mg $dl^{-1}$ three days before infection to 8.84 mg $ml^{-1}$ on day 16 post infection in *T. brucei*-infected goats and to 9.46 mg $ml^{-1}$ in *T. congolense*-infected goats respectively. These findings are in agreement with observations made in rats. Although this mechanism of red cell destruction may not be important in cattle, it may be important in small ruminants. In principal, mechanisms of red cell destruction may differ with different animal species; for instance, infections by *T. brucei* in mice (Igbokwe et al., 1994) and sheep (Taiwo et al., 2003) and *Babesia bigemina* in cattle (Saleh, 2009) render to the animals a reduced ability to peroxidation in the erythrocyte membrane. Furthermore, these oxidative changes in the erythrocytes can accelerate the destruction of these cells in the spleen (Morita et al., 1996). Lipid peroxidation studies in rats infected with *T. evansi* (Wolkmer et al., 2009) showed that these oxidative changes reduce the capacity of erythrocytes in rats to prevent oxidative damage in erythrocyte membrane *in vivo* as is the case *in vitro*.

The understanding of the lipid sub-fraction changes in different trypanosomes and animal species is an ongoing process; their effects could be associated with detrimental effects in affected hosts (Adamu et al., 2009). Many studies have observed decline is serum lipids and cholesterol levels in trypanosomosis infections. These phenomena could aggravate the neurological disorders often associated with trypanosomosis since cholesterol is vital in cell signaling in neuronal synapses formation.

## 3. Dyshaemopoiesis as a mechanism of anaemia development

Studies on the role of dyshaemopoiesis in the pathogenesis of anaemia, done with *T. congolense* infection in cattle (Valli et al., 1978); *T. vivax* infection in calves (Logan et al., 1991); *T. congolense* infection in sheep (Katunguka-Rwakishaya et al., 1992); and in *T. congolense* infection in multimammate rats (Ojok et al., 2001), give conflicting results. In this chapter, the role of dyshaemopoiesis in anaemia development in Small East African goats is presented. Bone marrow biopsies were obtained with a 16-gauge Salah sternal puncture needle positioned at right angles to the bone. All biopsies were collected aseptically after a small sharp incision was made under local analgesia.
Bone marrow function was studied by aspirating bone marrow biopsies once a month lasting four months and determining the myeloid:erythroid ratio (M:E ratio) by making a differential count of a total of 500 cells of nucleated granulocytic precursors divided by the number of precursor cells of the erythrocytic series. Typical bone marrow cells are represented in Figure 1 and the results were recorded in a modified bone marrow tally sheet as described by Schalm et al., (1975). The lowest PCV and mean erythrocyte counts occurred between the 4$^{th}$ and 7$^{th}$ weeks after infection in both groups *T. congolense* and *T. brucei*-infected goats. Concurrently, the M:E ratio progressively decreased as the disease progressed (Table 1).

| Days post infection | *T. congolense* | *T. brucei* | Uninfected controls |
|---|---|---|---|
| -5 | 0.48 ± 0.06 | 0.46 ± 0.07 | 0.41 ± 0.07 |
| 29 | 0.33 ± 0.06 | 0.29 ± 0.03 | 0.36 ± 0.22 |
| 59 | 0.21 ± 0.04* | 0.32 ± 0.05 | 0.37 ± 0.03 |
| 85 | 0.22 ± 0.05* | 0.27 ± 0.05 | 0.38 ± 0.04 |
| 121 | 0.28 ± 0.04 | 0.43 ± 0.10 | 0.44 ± 0.12 |

*$p < 0.05$.

Table 1. Mean myeloid: erythroid ratios (± standard error of the mean) of goats infected with either *T. congolense* or *T. brucei* and of uninfected controls.

The results from the experiment with goats agree with the findings of Valli et al., (1978) in experimental *T. congolense* TREU 112 infection in Holstein calves: the anaemia was of moderate severity and normochromic and macrocytic in the acute phase changing to normochromic, normocytic with chronicity. At the same time, the anaemia was haemolytic and regenerative as was shown by sharply decreased myeloid: erythroid ratio. In the East African goats, however, the anaemia was severe as shown by a sharp decline of haemoglobin concentration by the 7$^{th}$ week from 9.2 ± 0.2 g dl$^{-1}$ pre-infection to 5.4 ± g dl$^{-1}$ in *T. congolense*-infected group and from 9.5 ± 0.2 g dl$^{-1}$ to 5.9 ± 0.1 g dl$^{-1}$ in goats challenged with *T. brucei* (Biryomumaisho et al., 2007). At the same time, the anaemia was regenerative, a parameter that was inferred from decreased M:E ratios. For the parameters observed, *T. congolense* produced more severe effects than *T. brucei*.

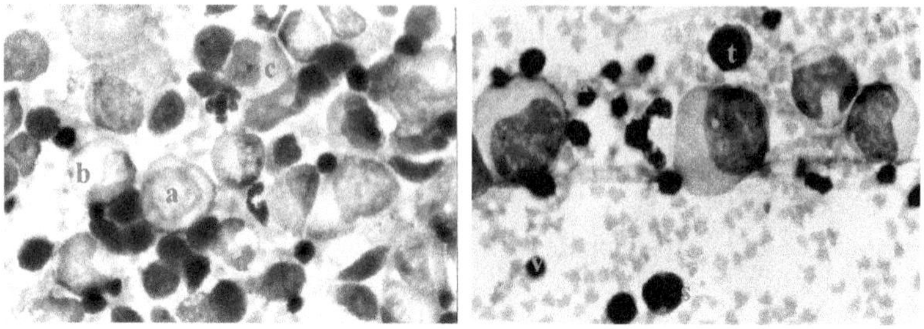


*[Micrographs adopted from Biryomumaisho, 2001].*

Fig. 1. Giemsa-stained sternal bone marrow biopsies from Small East African goats (x 1,000). **Panel 1.** A highly cellular bone marrow micrograph showing precursors of both myelocytic and erythrocytic series at different development stages collected 5 days before infection with trypanosomes in Small East African goats. Cell (a) is progranulocyte; (b) neutrophilic myelocyte; (c) eosinophilic myelocyte and (d) band neutrophil
**Panel 2:** One month after infection, when animals reached the lowest PCV value, it was more difficult to collect marrow smears without contamination with peripheral blood. (s) dividing metarubricyte; (t) rubricyte and (u) late rubricyte; (v) more late rubricytes can be seen in the micrograph. The large nucleated cells are myelocytic cell line precursors.

Ojok et al., (2001) made similar observations in multimammate rats; but in chronic stages, erythropoietic activity reduced while intra and extra-vascular erythrophagocytic activity increased. Also in agreement is *T. vivax* infection in calves where erythroid hyperplasia, evidenced by decrease in the M:E ratio, was observed (Logan et al., 1991).
The interpretation of results of M:E ratio should be viewed within the framework of the ratio of erythrocytic to granulocytic cell precursors: if the ratio is equal to one, the implication is the rate of manufacture of granulocytic precursors equals that of erythrocytic precursors. A decrease in the ratio means erythrogenesis exceeds granulopoiesis, a phenomenon that was observed in the Small East African goats (Biryomumaisho et al., 2007). The expectation, however, is that if erythrogenesis was increased, anaemia development would be halted. Progressive development of anaemia insinuates that the rate of destruction of erythrocytes exceeds the rate of their replenishment by the bone marrow which results in decrease of all parameters indicative of anaemia *viz.* lowered PCV, hypohaemoglobinaemia and decreased erythrocyte counts in peripheral blood. In the goats in this experiment, increased erythrogenesis did not sufficiently compensate for red cell loss. Similar observations in sheep (Katunguka-Rwakishaya et al., 1992) were made and in both instances erythrogenesis was enhanced but did not sufficiently compensate for the accelerated destruction of erythrocytes. The conclusion here is that anaemia state at those stages of trypanosomosis could be attributed to increased destruction of erythrocytes since there was no evidence of dyshaemopoiesis (as observations in sheep and goats suggest)

## 4. Reduced red cell lifespan: Erythrokinetic studies

Knowledge of the normal life span of red cells in different animal species is helpful in understanding the dynamics of red cell production and destruction. Life-span studies in animals indicate that erythrocytes of each animal species have a characteristic mean survival time that is the result of both the potential life span and loss of cells from random destruction irrespective of the age of the animal. Early reports of red blood cells (RBC) survival studies were done in canines using a serological technique as reported by Schalm et al., (1975). Serological techniques involve treating the recipient's blood with specific immune serum to cause RBC autoagglutination leaving the donor or transfused cells unagglutinated. For instance, this method estimated RBC life-span to be 90-100 days in the canine; however, a longer (112-133 days) erythrocyte survival period was estimated by Hawkins & Whipple (1938), using bilirubin production as a measure of the length of red cell life. Tagging or labeling erythrocytes with isotopes is considered to be more accurate. Using isotopes, the mean RBC life span in man with $^{15}N$ is 127 days; 70-133 days in adult sheep by $^{14}C$; 125 days in an adult domestic goat by $^{14}C$ and 150 days in a mature cow by $^{14}C$ (Schalm et al., 1975).

### 4.1 Factors influencing erythrocyte lifespan

Erythrocyte survival may be related to age of the animal; for instance, rapid destruction of erythrocytes has been observed in newborn puppies between birth and 2 weeks of age (Lee et al., 1971). However, erythrocyte survival in new born babies is similar to that of adults (Berlin, 1964) although fetal red cells have a shorter life span of 70 days. Differences in life span (days) with $^{14}C$-labeled erythrocytes for sheep at different ages has been shown to be 75 ± 14.8 days for newborn lambs, 46 days for three-month old lambs; 52 days in lambs one year old while adult sheep have an average of 130 days (Schalm et al., 1975).

Diet has been shown to be a factor in erythrocyte survival: *T. congolense*-infected N'Dama 2-5 year old cattle supplemented with 4 kg hay day$^{-1}$ of a mixture of rice bran, groundnut cake, milled *Andropogon* hay and common salt developed similar degrees of anaemia as animals which were not supplemented but recovered from the anaemia more rapidly. Ferrokinetic measurement in *T. congolense*-infected Blackface Scottish sheep (Katunguka-Rwakishaya et al., 1997) indicated that plasma iron turnover rates and $^{59}Fe$-incorporated rates were higher in the high protein infected group than the low protein infected group. Comparatively, nutritional deficiencies (Vitamin $B_{12}$, folic acid and iron) in man are reported to result in defective red cells having shortened survival time (Harris & Kellermeyer, 1970). However, in pyridoxine (Vitamin $B_6$) deficiency, the erythrocyte survival time has been shown to be normal but in folic acid and copper deficiencies, it was decreased in swine (Bush et al., 1956).

### 4.2 Erythrokinetics during animal trypanosomosis

Studies of animal trypanosomosis have consistently indicated reduced life span of erythrocytes: erythrokinetic studies in N'dama and Zebu cattle experimentally infected with *T. brucei* (Dargie et al., 1979); *T. congolense*-infected calves (Valli et al., 1978; Preston et a., 1979) all showed reduced life span. Erythrokinetic and ferrokinetic studies (Katunguka-Rwakishaya et al., 1992) of sheep after infection with *T. congolense* had lower $^{51}Cr$-red cell half lives and lower red cell life spans than control sheep. Similar observations were made by Mamo & Holmes (1975) in *T. congolense*-infected bovines and Ikede et al., (1977) in *T. congolense*-infected mice that was accompanied by progressive increase in osmotic fragility.

## 5. Blood volume changes and anaemia development

The total volume of circulating blood is a function of lean body weight: in most animals, blood volume occupies approximately 7-8% of the body weight except in the cat (4%) (Radostatis et al., 2000). The blood volume is very important to dynamics of circulation that it is kept relatively constant despite periodic water intake, production of water by metabolism and continuous loss of water through various body organs like the skin, lungs, alimentary tract and kidneys.

### 5.1 Methods of obtaining blood volume

The earliest methods for estimating blood volume consisted of bleeding animals to death followed by washing out the blood vessels and adding the blood contained in the washings to that collected during bleeding (Schalm et al., 1975). Another early method was by injection of known quantity of isotonic solution (NaCl) into the vascular system and shortly noting the extent of dilution of blood as determined by the change in specific gravity, red cell number or haemoglobin concentration.
At present, the most accurate and reliable method for the determination of plasma volume is by measurement of the intravenous dilution of macromolecules labeled with radioisotopes (Mackie, 1976). However, such animals become unfit for human consumption; coupled with the difficulty of maintaining animals treated with radioactive material and disposal of waste from such animals. Basing on these reasons, Evan's blue dye (T-1824) that binds to albumin component of plasma and can rapidly be removed from the body can be used. Plasma and total blood volume in Small East African goats infected with either *T. congolense* or *T. brucei* (Biryomumaisho, 2001) were determined by injecting a 0.03% solution of T-1824 at a dose rate of 0.4 mg $kg^{-1}$ of the goat in the right jugular vein and after 10 minutes, blood was collected from the left jugular and centrifuged to obtain plasma-tagged dye. By using absorbance of the dye in plasma of the standard against a blank (prepared from plasma of individual goats) in a U-1,000 Hitachi spectrophotometer at a wavelength of 620 nm, the concentration of the dye in plasma was calculated as follows:

$$\frac{\text{[T-1824] in Plasma (mg)}}{\text{[T-1824] in Standard}} = \frac{\textbf{Optical density of diluted Plasma}}{\text{Optical density of the Standard}} \quad (1)$$

$$\text{Plasma volume (mls)} = \frac{\textbf{mg of dye injected}}{\text{mg/ml of dye in Plasma}} \quad (2)$$

$$\text{Blood volume (mls)} = \frac{\textbf{Plasma volume} \times 100}{\text{100-PCV} \times 0.98^{*}} \quad (3)$$

**Trapped plasma after centrifugation was corrected for by including a 2% (0.98) factor.*

Plasma volume and total blood volume of individual goats in ml $kg^{-1}$ were determined by dividing the values obtained in (2) and (3) by the body weight of individual goats. Mean values of all 5 measurements taken at 30-day intervals are shown in Table 2 while measurements taken in *T. congolense*-infected Scottish Black Face sheep with $^{125}$I-albumin and $^{51}$Cr-red cells respectively are shown in Table 3 (Katunguka et al., 1992).

#### 5.1.1 Blood volume changes in trypanosomosis

In trypanosomosis infections, anaemia development has been shown to be mainly haemolytic during the acute phase of the disease. In the sub acute and chronic stages of the disease, however, extravascular mechanisms are thought to play a major role. One such mechanism is thought to involve an abnormal retention of large quantities of fluid within the plasma compartment. Results from *T. congolense*-infected N'Dama and Zebu cattle (Dargie et al., 1979) showed that both groups developed significant anaemia. Measurement of plasma and red cell volumes showed that the low PCV of infected cattle was due to reductions in red cell volume and not haemodilution.

The implication of increased plasma here can be explained by a normal homeostatic response for maintenance of blood volume and pressure. Studies using $^{51}$Cr-red cells, $^{125}$I-albumin and $^{59}$Fe as ferric citrate 11 weeks after infection revealed that infected sheep had significantly lower mean circulating red cell volumes but higher plasma and blood volumes than control sheep (Katunguka-Rwakishaya et al., (1992). In *T. congolense* and *T. brucei*-infected goats (Biryomumaisho, 2001), the mean plasma volume and total blood volume values were higher than those of the controls although the differences were not significant (Table 2).

| | *T. congolense* *n* = 10 | *T. brucei* *n* = 10 | Controls *n* = 5 | Significance |
|---|---|---|---|---|
| Plasma volume (mls / kg) ± SEM | 58.3 ± 3.0 | 53.1 ± 6.1 | 44.7 ± 7.0 | P > 0.05 |
| Total blood volume (mls / kg) ± SEM | 72.8 ± 3.9 | 67.9 ± 7.5 | 58.6 ± 7.4 | P > 0.05 |

*[Table adopted from S. Biryomumaisho, 2001].*

Table 2. Mean T-1824-plasma and blood volume in trypanosome-infected goats.

| | Plasma volume mls kg $^{-1}$ ± SEM | Blood volume mls kg $^{-1}$ ± SEM |
|---|---|---|
| Infected, n=5 | 45.1 ± 1.5 | 57.9 ± 1.1 |
| Control, n = 5 | 36.2 ± 1.0 | 52.9 ± 2.2 |
| Significance | P < 0.01 | P < 0.01 |

Table 3. Blood volumes of sheep infected with *T. congolense* (mls kg $^{-1}$ ± SEM).

## 6. Conclusion

Knowledge about the pathogenesis of anaemia can be utilized to manage cases of anaemia caused by trypanosomosis as well as cases of anaemia derived from other causes other than trypanosomosis provided the primary cause is dealt with. The aspects of cross matching the blood of donor and recipient animals and whether to replace whole blood or its components are beyond the scope of this chapter. However, a veterinarian can utilize some aspects of the knowledge of dyshaemopoiesis and blood volume to manage anaemia in routine practice.

Blood volume changes can be estimated at clinical examination: basically, most animals with exception of the cat have blood volumes approximately 7-8% of their body weight. An animal health care worker can estimate the total blood volume of a donor animal that way. However, the amount of blood lost (in the anaemic / recipient animal) can be estimated from measurement of PCV as follows:

$$\text{Blood lost (litres)} = \frac{\textbf{Normal PCV of animal species - patient PCV}}{\text{Normal PCV x 0.08 of patient weight in kg}} \quad (4)$$

*In our opinion and experience, for blood transfusion to be effective, at least 25% of the deficit should be corrected.*

Haemodilution is a state when the fluid content of blood is increased and this results into lowered concentration of the formed elements. For the case of the red cell component, this can result in apparent anaemia. The converse is haemoconcentration, a state in which there is increased concentration of formed elements of blood mainly as a result of loss of water from the body. The clinical importance of both scenarios dictates that the veterinarian should first evaluate the animal as to whether haemoconcentration or haemodilution is pathological or not. In both cases, the primary cause should be dealt with.

The more commonly encountered of the two scenarios is haemoconcentration and subsequent hypovolaemia resulting from loss of fluid such as in diarrhaea / dysentery, vomiting (especially in monogastric animals), skin burns, starvation and thirst, among other causes. In all cases, hypovolaemia leads to reduction in blood plasma and, in severe instances, leads to hypovolaemic shock. A low blood volume leads to multiple organ failure, kidney and brain damage and death. An appropriate fluid for replacement containing electrolytes, metabolic enhancers or plasma expanders should be chosen (selection of suitable fluids for therapy is outside the scope of this chapter).

Basing on presenting clinical signs, the degree of dehydration and hence amount of water lost can be estimated from the percentage of dehydration basing on skin elasticity, demeanor of the animal and sinking of the eyes in the orbit.

## 7. References


Adamu, S., Barde, N., Abenga, J.N., User, J.N., Ibrahim, N.D.G. & Esievo, K.A.N. (2009). Experimental *Trypanosoma brucei* infection-induced changes in the serum profiles of lipids and cholesterol and the clinical implications in pigs. *Journal of Cell and Animal Biology*. Vol.3, No.2, 15-20.

Assoku, R.K.G., Tizard, I.R. & Nielsen, K.H. Free fatty acids, complement activation and polyclonal B-cell stimulation as factors in the immunopathogenesis of African trypanosomiasis. *Lancet II*, 956-959.

Berken, A. & Benacerraf,B.(1968). Depression of reticuloendothelial system phagocytic function by ingested lipids. *Proceedings of the Society for Experimental Biology and Medicine*, pp. 793-795 (1968), Vol.128. No.3

Berlin, N.I. (1964). Life span of the red cell, In: *The Red Blood Cell*, Bishop, C. & Swigenor, D.M., 423-450, Academic Press, New York.

Biryomumaisho, S. & Katunguka-Rwakishaya, E. (2007). The pathogenesis of anaemia in goats experimentally infected with *Trypanosoma congolense* or *Trypanosoma brucei*: use of the myeloid: erythroid ratio. *Veterinary Parasitology*, Vol.143, 354-357.

Biryomumaisho, S. (2001). Comparative Clinical Pathology of *Trypanosoma congolense* and *Trypanosoma brucei* infection in Small East African goats. M.Sc. Thesis, Makerere University, Uganda, pp. 70-74.

Biryomumaisho, S., Katunguka-Rwakishaya, E. & Rubaire-Akiiki, C. (2003). Serum biochemical changes in experimental *Trypanosoma congolense* and *Trypanosoma brucei* infection in Small East African goats. *Veterinary Archives*, Vol.73, No.3, 167-180.

Radostatis, O.M., Gay, C.C., Blood, D.C. & Hinchcliff, K.W. (2000). Diseases of blood and blood-forming organs, In: *Veterinary Medicine,* pp 399-417, ISBN 0-7020-26042, W.B. Saunders, Saskatoon, Canada.

Bush, J.A., Jensen, W.N., Ashenbrucker, H., Cartwright, G.E. & Wintrobe, M.M. (1956). The kinetics of iron metabolism in swine with various experimentally induced anaemias. *Journal of Experimental Medicine,* Vol.103, 161.

Dargie, J.D., Murray, M., Grimshaw, W.R. & McIntrye, W. I. M. (1979). Bovine trypanosomiasis: red cell kinetics of N'dama and Zebu cattle infected with *Trypanosoma congolense. Parasitology,* Vol.78, 271-286.

Dixon, H., Ginger, C.D. & Williamson, J. (1972). Trypanosome sterols and their metabolic origins. *Comparative Biochemical Physiology B,* Vol.41, 1-18.

Field, A. M., Gardner, S. D., Goodbody, R. A., & Wood-House, M. A. (1974). Identity of a newly isolated human polyoma-virus from a patient with progressive multifocal leuko-encephalopathy. *Journal of Clinical Pathology,* Vol. 27, 341–347.

Harris, J.W. & Kellermeyer, R.W. (1970). The red cell, Production, Metabolism, Destruction: Normal and Abnormal. Harvard University Press, Cambridge, Massachusetts, 1970.

Hawkins, W.B. & Whipple, G.H. (1938). The life cycle of the red blood cell in the dog. *American Journal of Physiology,* Vol.122, 418.

Huan, C.N., Webb, L., Lambert, P.H. & Miescher, P.A. (1975). Pathogenesis of the anaemia in African trypanosomiasis: characterization and purification of the haemolytic factor. *Schweizerische Medizinische Wochenschrift.* Vol.105, 1582-1583.

Igbokwe, I.O., Esievo, K.A.N.& Obagaiye, O.K. (1994). Increases susceptibility of erythrocytes to *in vitro* peroxidation in acute *Trypanosoma brucei* infection in mice. *Veterinary Parasitology,* Vol.55, No.4, 279-286.

Ikede, B.O., Lule, M. & Terry, R.J. (1977). Anaemia in trypanosomiasis: mechanisms of erythrocyte destruction in mice infected with *Trypanosoma congolense* or *T. brucei. Acta Tropica,* Vol.34, No.1, 53-60.

Katunguka-Rwakishaya E., McKechnie, D., Parkins, J.J., Murray, M. & Holmes,P.H. (1997). The influence of dietary protein on live bodyweight, degree of anaemia and erythropoietic responses of Scottish blackface sheep infected experimentally with *Trypanosoma congolense. Research in Veterinary Science,* Vol.63, No.3, 273-277.

Katunguka-Rwakishaya, E., Murray, M. & Holmes, P.H. (1992). Pathophysiology of ovine trypanosomiasis: ferrokinetics and erythrocyte survival studies. *Research in Veterinary Science,* Vol.53, 80-86.

Landsteiner & Raubitscheck (1901) *as cited in Firtz Assman (2011).* Beiträge zur Kenntnis pflanzlicher Agglutinine, Pflügers Archiv European Journal of Physiology Volume 137, Numbers 8-10, 489-510, DOI: 10.1007/BF01679970

Lee, P., Brown, M.E. & Hutzler, P.T. (1971). Turnover of red blood cell mass in new-borne puppies. *Federation Proceedings,* Vol.30, 195.

Logan, L.L., Anosa, V.O. & Shaw, M.K. (1991). Haemopoiesis in Ayrshire-Guarnsey calves infected with Galana stock of *Trypanosoma vivax.* OAU/STRC [1991]. Pp 317-322.

Mackie, W.S. (1976). Plasma volume measurements in sheep using Evan's blue and continuous blood sampling. *Research in Veterinary Science,* Vol.21, 108-109.

Mamo, E. & Holmes, P.H. (1975). The erythrokinetics of zebu cattle infected with *Trypanosoma congolense. Research in Veterinary Science,* Vol.18, 105-1

Mertin, J. & Hughes, D. (1975). Specific inhibitory action of polyunsaturated fatty acids on lymphocyte transformation induced by PHA and PPD. International Archives of Allergy and Applied Immunology. Vol. 48, No.2, 203-210.

Morita, T., Saeki, H. & Ishii, T. (1996). Erythrocyte oxidation in artificial *Babesia gibsoni* infection. *Veterinary Parasitology*, Vol.63, Nos.1-2, 1-7.

Ojok, L. & Kacufer-Weiss, E. (2001). Bone marrow response to acute and chronic *Trypanosoma congolense* infection inmultimammate rats *(Mastomys coucha). Journal of Comparative Pathology*, Vol.124, Nos.2-3, 149-158.

Preston, J.M., Wellde, B.T. & Kovatchi, R.M. (1979). *Trypanosoma congolense*: calf erythrocyte survival. *Experimental Parasitology*, Vol.48, 118-125.

Quagliata, F., Lawrence, V.J.W. & Phillips-Quagliata, J.M. (1972). Prostaglandin E as a regulator of lymphocyte function selective action on B lymphocytes and synergy with procarbazine in depression of immune responses. *Cell Immunology, Vol.*6, 457-465.

Saleh, M.A. (2009). Erythrocytic oxidative damage in crossbred cattle naturally infected with *Babesia bigemina. Reseach in Veterinary Science*, Vol. 86, No. 1, 43-48.

Schalm, O.W., Jain, N.C. & Carrol, E.J. (1975). Blood volume and water balance, In: *Veterinary Hematology*, 1-14, Lea and Febiger, IBSN 0-8121-0470-6, Philadelphia.

Schalm, O.W., Jain, N.C. & Carrol, E.J. (1975). The erythrocytes: their production, Function and Destruction, In: *Veterinary Hematology*, 356-404, Lea and Febiger, IBSN 0-8121-0470-6, Philadelphia.

Schalm, O.W., Jain, N.C. & Carrol, E.J. (1975). The Hematopoietic System, In: *Veterinary Hematology*, 301-335, Lea and Febiger, IBSN 0-8121-0470-6, Philadelphia.

Taiwo, V.O., Olaniyi, M.O. & Ogunsanmi, A.O. (2003). Comparative plasma biochemical changes and susceptibility of erythrocytes to *in-vitro* peroxidation during experimental *Trypanosoma congolense* and *T. brucei* infections in sheep. *Israel Journal of Veterinary Medicine*. Vol.58, No.4, 1-7

Tizard, I.R. & Holmes, W.L. (1976). The generation of toxic activity from*Trypanosoma congolense. Experientia*, Vol.32, 1533-1534.

Tizard, I.R., Holmes, W.L., York, DA. & Mellors, A. (1977). The generation and identification of the haemolysin of *Trypanosoma congolense. Experientia*, Vol.33, 901.

Tizard, I.R., Holmes, W.L. & Nielsen, K. (1978). Mechanisms of the anaemia in trypanosomiasis: studies on the role of haemolytic fatty acids derived from *Trypanosoma congolense. Tropenmedicine and Parasitology*, Vol.29, 108-104.

Valli, V.E.O., Forsberg, G.A. & McSherry, B.J. (1978). The pathogenesis of *T. congolense* in calves: Anaemia and erythroid response. *Veterinary Parasitology*, Vol. 15, 733-745.

Vankatesan, S. & Ormerod, W.E. (1976). Lipid content of the slender and stumpy forms of *Trypanosoma brucei rhodesiense*: a comparative study. Comparative Biochemistry and Physiology Part B, Vol. 53, 481-487.

Wolkmer, P., Schafer da Silva, A., Traesel, C.K., Paim, F.C., Cargnelutti, J.F., Pagnoncelli, M., Picada, M.E., Monteiro, S.G. & Terezinha dos Anjos

# 17

# The Mechanisms of Anaemia in Trypanosomosis: A Review

Albert Mbaya[1,*], Hussein Kumshe[2] and Chukwunyere Okwudiri Nwosu[3]
[1]*Department of Veterinary Microbiology and Parasitology, University of Maiduguri,*
[2]*Department of Veterinary Medicine, University of Maiduguri,*
[3]*Department of Veterinary Parasitology and Entomology, University of Nigeria, Nsukka*
*Nigeria*

## 1. Introduction

Trypanosomosis is an important disease of both humans and animals commonly found in most parts of Africa and South America (Swallow, 2000). The tsetse fly (*Glossina*) is responsible for biological (cyclical) transmission while haematophagus arthropod vectors of the family, *Tabanidae, Stomoxynae* and *Hippoboscidae* are responsible for its mechanical transmission (Soulsby, 1982). Transplacental transmission has also been recorded in cattle (Ogwu et al., 1992). *Trypanosoma congolense, T. vivax and T. brucei* have been reported to cause nagana in cattle while *T. evansi* caused surra in camels (*Camelus dromedarieus*) (Mbaya et al., 2010). In humans, *Trypanosoma brucei gambiense* and *Trypanosoma brucei rhodeseinse* are responsible for human sleeping sickness in West and East Africa respectively, while *T. cruzi,* transmitted by triatomid bugs (*Triatoma magista*) is responsible for transmitting chagas diseases to humans in South America (Solano et al., 2003). The *T. brucei* group of trypanosomes (*T. brucei, T. b. gambiense, T. b. rhodesianse* and *T. evansi*) mostly invade tissues (humoral) whereas, *T. congolense* and to a lesser extent *T. vivax* and *T. cruzi* predominantly restrict themselves to the blood circulation (haemic) (Igbokwe, 1994; Mbaya et al., 2011).

The mechanism or pathophysiology of anaemia in trypanosomosis is complex and multifactorial in origin (Naessens et al., 2005). It initiates a cascade of events leading to haemolytic anaemia and cardiovascular collapse (Anosa, 1988). In human trypanosomosis, disseminated intravascular coagulation has been reported (Barret-Connor et al., 1973). Among the complex and multifactorial etiologies associated with the anaemia is haemolysin, a sensory/excretory product of living trypanosomes. This product is known to lyse red blood cells in the absence of antibodies (*in-vitro*) and haemodilution (*in-vivo*). This mechanism has been adequately described in gold fish (*Carassius auratus*) infected with *Trypanosoma dahilewskyi* (Nazrul-Islam and Woo, 1991) and in murine models infected with *T. b. rhodesiense* (Naessens et al., 2005).

## 2. Haemolytic anaemia caused by animal and human trypanosomes

Haemolytic anaemia has been reported in *T. brucei* infection of red fronted gazelles (*Gazella rufifrons*) (Mbaya et al., 2009a), sheep and goats (Edward et al., 1956; Ikede & Losos, 1972), *T.*

*congolense* infection of sheep and goats (Edwards et al., 1956), *T. vivax* infection of sheep and goats (Anosa, 1977). Similarly, it was reported in vervet monkeys (*Cercopethicus aethiopes*) (Abenga & Anosa, 2006), and baboons (*Papio anubis*) (Mbaya et al., 2009c, b) infected with the West African human sleeping sickness trypanosome; *T.b. gambiense.*

### 2.1 Various stages of the anaemia in trypanosomosis

Three phases of anaemia have been reported to occur in trypanosomosis. They are, phase I (acute crises), phase II (chronic) and phase III (recovery) (Anosa, 1988).

#### 2.1.1 Phase I: Acute crises

This phase begins with the initial appearance of trypanosomes in peripheral circulation. The parasitaemia in this case is usually high, fluctuating and evident in most days (Maxie & Losos, 1979; Anosa & Isoun, 1980; Anosa, 1988; Abenga & Anosa, 2006; Mbaya et al., 2009a, b, c; 2010; Mbaya & Ibrahim, 2011; Mbaya et al., 2011). During this phase the anaemia is morphologically classified as macrocytic and normochromic (Maxie & Losos, 1979; Anosa & Isoun, 1980). At this stage death commonly occurs due to severe pancytopoenia and other pathologies (Anosa, 1988). Sub-acute cases have been produced experimentally in rodents infected with *T. congolense* (Isoun & Esuroso, 1972) and with *T. brucei* (Mbaya et al., 2007, 2010, 2011).

#### 2.1.2 Phase II: Chronic

This phase follows the acute crises phase and is characterized by low levels of parasitaemia. The low to moderate erythrocyte value at this point persists with minor fluctuations. This period ranges from several weeks to months. With the *T. brucei* group, which mostly invade tissues, this is the aparasitaemic phase when the parasites establish extravascularly and are less numerous in peripheral circulations (Rabo, 1995) or absent (Mbaya et al., 2007, 2009a, d). In this chronic phase, the morphological classification of the anaemia is normochromic and normocytic (Maxie & Losos, 1979).

#### 2.1.3 Phase III: Recovery

This phase is characterized by the low, infrequent or absence of parasitaemia. At this point, declined erythrocyte values begin to return towards pre-infection values and other pathological changes undergo resolution (Anosa, 1988) leading to self-recovery as commonly encountered in trypanotolerant wildlife (Mbaya et al. 2009a).

## 3. The mechanism of anaemia in trypanosomosis

The interplay of several factors acting either individually or synergistically contributes to the development of haemolytic anaemia in human and animal trypanosomosis (Figure 1).
Most common among these factors are erythrocyte injury caused by lashing action of trypanosome flagella, undulating pyrexia, platelet aggregation, toxins and metabolites from trypanosomes, lipid peroxidation and malnutrition (Murray & Morrison, 1978; Morrison et al., 1981; Saror, 1982; Igbokwe, 1994). Meanwhile, idiopathic (unknown) serum and tumor necrosing factors are responsible for dyserythropoieses (Mabbot & Sternberg, 1995; Lieu & Turner, 1999; Maclean et al., 2001).

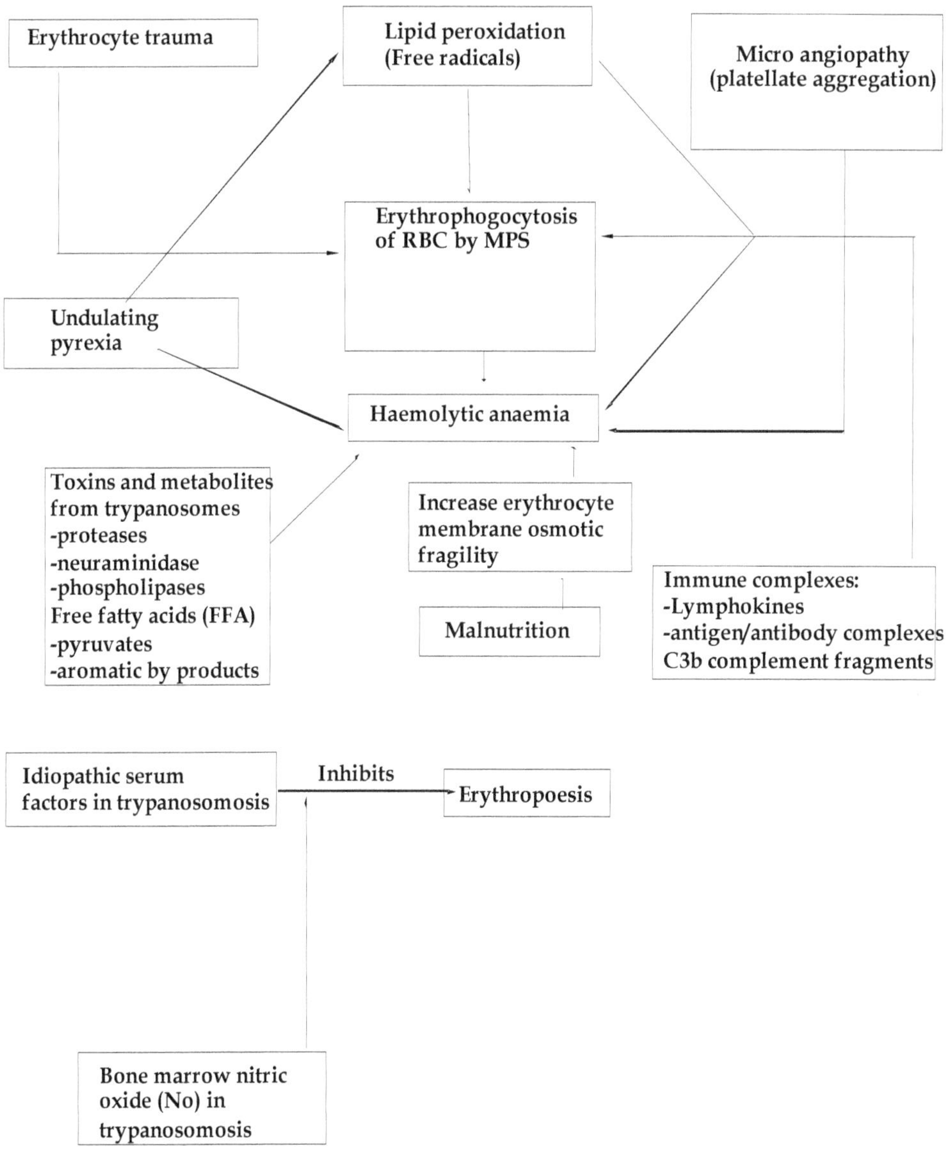


Fig. 1. Pathophysiology of anaemia in African trypanosomosis, Source by Dr. A.W. Mbaya.

## 4. Anaemia through mechanical injury to erythrocytes

Anaemia caused by mechanical injury to erythrocyte occurs by the lashing action of the powerful locomotory flagella and microtubule reinforced bodies of the millions of the organisms during parasitaemia (Vickerman & Tetley, 1978). Erythrocyte membrane damage has also been associated with adhesion of erythrocytes, platelets and reticulocytes to trypanosome surfaces via sialic acid receptors leading to damages to erythrocyte cell membranes (Bungener & Muller, 1976; Banks, 1980; Anosa & Kaneko, 1983; Shehu et al., 2006). As such, several areas of discontinuity occur along the surface of erythrocyte membranes where they adhere to the trypanosomes. Mechanical damage to vascular endothelium has been reported when tissue-invading trypanosomes such as the *T. brucei* group penetrate tissues via the interstices (Anosa & Kaneko, 1983).

## 5. Anaemia through undulating pyrexia

In trypanosomosis, a direct relationship exists between undulating pyrexia and fluctuating parasitaemia (Nwosu & Ikeme, 1992; Igbokwe, 1994; Mbaya et al., 2009a, e). Under laboratory conditions, Karle (1974) exposed erythrocytes to temperatures above the normal body temperature and found out that the osmotic fragility and permeability of erythrocytes were greatly enhanced. It was also reported that increased body temperatures decreased erythrocyte plasticity and longevity *in-vivo* (Woodruff et al., 1972). Consequently, temperature elevation increased the rate of immunochemical reactions thereby initiating lipid peroxidation of erythrocytes (Igbokwe, 1994).

## 6. Anaemia through platelet aggregation (microangiopathy)

Intact trypanosomes or fragments of trypanosomes may cause platelet aggregation commonly called microangiopathy (Davies et al., 1974). This can lead to the release of platelet autoantibodies that in turn releases procoagulants and thereby causing fibrin deposits. Subsequently microthrombi formation or disseminated intravascular coagulation occurs (Igbokwe, 1994). During trypanosomosis, erythrocytes with weak cell membranes become fragmented and lyse as they squeeze through the fibrin deposits of the microthrombi (Anosa & Kaneko, 1983; Murray & Dexter, 1988). Disseminated intravascular coagulation has been reported in *T. b. gambiense* infection of the baboon (*Papio anubis*) (Mbaya et al., 2009b), *T. vivax* infection of cattle (Isoun and Esuroroso, 1972) and in goats (Vanden Inh et al., 1976; Anosa & Isoun, 1983).

## 7. Anaemia caused by trypanosome toxins and metabolites

Living and dead trypanosomes can produce various forms of active chemical substances, which can elicit erythrocyte injury (Tizzard & Holmes, 1976; 1977; Tizzard et al, 1977; 1978a, b, c; Zwart & Veenendal, 1978; Naessens et al., 2005). Common among these chemical substances are proteases, neuraminidase, phospholipase, free fatty acids, pyruvates and aromatic by-products. Neuraminidase has been generated *in-vitro* by *T. vivax* during periods of parasitaemia, making erythrocytes prone to phagocytosis (Esievo, 1979; 1983). One of the factors that make erythrocytes prone to phagocytosis by the expanded mononuclear phagocytic system (MPS) during trypanosomosis is associated with the activity of neuraminidase. This enzyme cleaves off sialic acids on the surface of erythrocytes and thereby disabling them (Verma & Gautam, 1978; Igbokwe, 1994; Adamu et al., 2009) and by damaging erythropoietin (Igbokwe et al., 1989).

Trypanosomes are capable of releasing proteolytic lysosomal enzymes (proteases) from pockets on their flagella and from damaged or dead trypanosomes (Vickermon & Tetley, 1978; Rautenberg et al., 1982; Londsdale-Eccles & Grab, 1986; Igbokwe, 1994). The enzyme, when released into the general circulation is capable of damaging erythrocytes and vascular endothelium by cleaving sialic acid fractions from the cell membrane in the form of glycopeptides (Cook et al., 1966). It was also reported that aromatic amino acids could be metabolized by trypanosome to produce toxic by-products, which acts directly on the erythrocyte cell membrane to cause osmotic fragility and lyses (Igbokwe, 1994). Similarly, phenylalanine could be catabolized to phenylpyruvate, which is proteolytic in nature and inhibitory to mitochondrial gluconeogenesis (Igbokwe, 1994). Tryptophan can also be broken down during trypanosomosis to indole-ethanol, which damages erythrocyte cell membranes (Igbokwe, 1994).

## 8. Lipid peroxidation

The mechanism of aneamia in trypanosomosis is greatly associated with the generation of free radicals and super oxides following lipid peroxidation. These oxidative products generally attack the cellular integrity of erythrocytes during trypanosomosis (Anosa & Kaneko, 1983; Igbokwe, 1994; Umar et al., 2007). They also particularly attack erythrocyte membrane polyunsaturated fatty acids and proteins (Slater, 1984) or red blood cells directly leading to oxidative haemolysis (Ameh, 1984; Igbokwe, et al., 1989; Umar et al., 2007). Sialic acids consist of about four derivatives of nine-carbon sugar neuraminic acids (Varki, 1992; Schauer & Kamerling, 1997). It was therefore concluded that anaemia in trypanosomosis might occur due to erythrophagocytosis (Holmes & Jennings, 1976) and may be associated with the formation of antigen-antibody complexes with sialic acids (Audu et al., 1999).

Esievo et al. (1982) pointed out that trypanosomosis may cause a deficit in the systematic antioxidant capacity of the infected host. This has been demonstrated in acute *T. b. gambiense* infection in rats (Ameh, 1984), *T. evansi* (Wolkmer et al., 2009) and in *T. brucei* infected mice (Igbokwe et al., 1989), where erythrocytes were susceptible to free radical-damage following hydrogen peroxidation. This process in mice led to enhanced oxidative haemolysis. Peroxidation caused the erythrocytes to produce large quantities of lipid peroxidation by-products. This is suggestive therefore that erythrocytes of the infected animals possessed decreased antioxidant ability, leading to its inability to withstand oxidative stress (Igbokwe, 1994). *Trypanosoma vivax* produced neuraminidase enzyme, which had a direct relationship with parasitaemia. It was therefore concluded that neuraminidase produced by trypanosomes *in-vivo,* cleaved off erythrocyte surface sialic acid, making the red cells prone to phagocytosis. Similarly, Nok and Balogun (2003) showed a progressive increase in the level of serum sialic acid corresponding with anaemia and parasitaemia in *T. congolense* infected mice. *Trypanosoma vivax* was observed to be highly erythrogenic in mice, which was probably associated with depressed erythropoietin activity following the cleaving of sialic acid fragments (Igbokwe et al., 1989). It has also been reported that glycolysis in trypanosomosis leads to the accumulation of pyruvate *in-vivo* as parasitaemia increases (Grant & Fulton, 1957; Coleman et al., 1957).

A ten-fold increase of pyruvate has been observed in *T. brucei* infected rabbits (Goodwin & Guy, 1973). In as much as the influence of pyruvate is debatable, it may not reach toxic levels in the blood during trypanosomosis (Igbokwe, 1994) however, Newton (1978) suggested that pyruvate might lead to acidosis and a lowered affinity of haemoglobulin for oxygen. It also inhibited the tricarboxylic acid cycle (TCA) in human mitochondria during *T. b. gambiense* infection (Seed & Hall, 1985). After death and autolysis, trypanosomosis releases large quantities of phospholipase A1 and lysophospholipase A1 (Tizard et al., 1978c). These chemical substances can cause erythrocyte degradation, damage to vascular endothelial cells and haemolysis (Colley et al., 1973). Phospholipase A1 was demonstrated in extreme proportions *in-vitro* in tissue fluids and less in plasma of rabbits infected with *T. brucei* (Hambrey et al., 1980). Tizard et al. (1978a, c) observed that phospholipase released free fatty acids (FFA) from phosphatidylcholine *in-vivo*. Most common of them were palmitic, stearic and linoleic acids (Tizard & Holmes, 1977).

Tizard et al. (1978b) reported that linoleic acid possessed a detergent - like activity, which produced severe haemolysis and cytotoxicity *in-vitro*. It was however believed that free fatty acids are easily bound by albumin and may not cause haemolysis *in-vivo*. The author however pointed out that during high parasitaemia in *T. congolense* infection, the FFA released exceeded the binding capacity of albumin and thereby leading to cytotoxicity and haemolysis. Similarly, it was reported that even the albumin bound FFA may cause haemolysis due to the activities of its oxidized products. Nok et al. (1992a, b) reported that trypanosomes could cause certain alterations that invariably affected erythrocyte membrane fluidity hence a decrease in erythrocyte membrane-bound enzymes (NoK-ATpase and CaMg-ATpase). Lipid peroxidation of membranes has been associated with decrease in membranes fluidity and in the activities of membrane-bound enzyme (McCay & King, 1980; Slater, 1984; Igbokwe, 1994). It was however suggested that a comprehensive study in ruminants is needed to highlight the extent of anti-oxidant deficiency and the degree of susceptibility of red cells to oxidative damage during trypanosomosis (Igbokwe, 1994).

## 9. Idiopathic serum factors

In trypanosomosis, an unknown (idiopathic) serum factor, not of a trypanosome origin but a heat stable-protein has been demonstrated to inhibit activities of erythropoiesis (Kaaya et al., 1979; 1980). It was however reported that serum from cattle infected with *T. congolense* and *T. vivax* did not depress colonies of erythrocytes *in-vitro*. However, an unknown serum factor entirely different from those reported by Kaaya et al. (1979; 1980) had effect on an erythroid colony (Igbokwe et al., 1989).

## 10. Immune complexes

Immunological mechanisms in trypanosomosis have been advanced as a major reason for the removal of erythro autolologous immunoglobulin (IgM and IgG) antibodies and complement (C3) on the surface of red cells (Kobayashi et al., 1976; Facer et al., 1982; Assoku & Gardiner, 1992; Naessens et al., 2005). The mechanism suggested that autoantibodies appeared after the first peak of parasitaemia that correlated with the decline in packed cell volume (PCV). Red cell surfaces may bind auto or poly reactive antibodies, or may be sensitized by absorption of immune complexes (Naessens et al., 2005). Alternatively, erythrocytes may passively absorb trypanosome molecules followed by binding of antitrypanosome antibodies with subsequent removal from the system (Rifkin & Lansberger, 1990; Naessens et al., 2005). Although Naessen et al. (2005) reported that immunological competence is not essential for the development of anaemia, irradiated rats still became anaemic after *T. brucei* infection (Murray & Dexter, 1988) and when cattle were depleted of T-cells. The authors also reported that specific, non-specific antibody production was drastically reduced, delayed, and at the same time, anaemia was consistent. Several authors (Ikede & Losos, 1972; Mackenzie & Cruickshank, 1973; Mackenzie et al., 1978; Anosa & Isoun, 1983; Igbokwe, 1994) reported an overwhelming proliferation of tissue macrophages during trypanosomosis.

The activation of macrophages was through lymphokines, antigen-antibody complexes and C3b complement fragments (Woo & Kobayashi, 1975; Allison, 1978). It was suggested therefore, that cytokines mediated loss of erythrocytes in trypanosomosis (Naessens et al., 2005). Similarly, strong evidence suggested that anaemia in trypanosomosis was mediated by TNF-a, IFN gamma and other inflammatory cytokines (Jelkmann, 1998). However, in more recent studies (Nemeth et al., 2004) suggested that anaemia in trypanosomosis involving hypofferaemia was caused by IL-6 and hepeidin. Although Naessens et al. (2005) concluded that this is unlikely to cause anaemia in trypanosomosis, some weak evidence of the role of THF-a-in the severity of anaemia in trypanosome-infected cattle (Silegham et al., 1994), mice infected with *T. brucei* (Magez et al., 1999) and in *T. brucei gambiense* infected mice (Naesens et al., 2005) was documented.

## 11. Malnutrition

Trypanosomosis may cause a drop in feed intake hence there is energy deficit and loss of tissue associated with catabolism of body fat, deficiencies of vitamin C, B and essential amino acids (Igbokwe, 1994). Inadequate energy supply to erythrocytes may alter the erythrocyte membrane surface therefore leading to weakening of the cell membrane, increased osmotic fragility and haemolysis (Jennings, 1976).

## 12. Tumor necrosis factor/Bone marrow nitric oxide (NO)

It has been reported that tumor necrosis factor (TNF) production by monocytes from cattle infected with *Trypanosoma (Duttonella) vivax* and *T. (Nannomonas) congolense,* was found to play in concert in the severity of anaemia associated with trypanosomosis (Sileghem et al., 1994). Bone marrow cell population from *T. brucei* infected mice exhibited levels of bone marrow nitric oxide production. This was found to coincide with suppressed bone marrow T-cell proliferation in response to stimulation with mitogen concanavalin *in-vivo* and *in-vitro*. It was therefore concluded that nitric oxide might inhibit proliferation of haemopoitic precursors leading to anaemia in trypanosomosis (Mabbot & Sternberg, 1995; Liew & Turner, 1999). A similar synthesis of nitric oxide and cytokines leading to anaemia in human trypanosomosis has been reported (MacLean et al., 2001).

## 13. Conclusion

The mechanism of anaemia in trypanosomosis was caused mainly by extra vascular haemolysis in the expanded active mononuclear phagocytic system of the host. This was followed by a drastic reduction of all red blood cell indices during successive waves of parasitaemia. The pattern of anaemia varied, depending on whether the specie of trypanosome was "humoral" or "haemic". Although the mechanism of anaemia is complex and multifactorial, it primarily compromised the cellular integrity of erythrocytes leading to either haemolytic anaemia or enhanced erythrophagocytosis. Injuries sustained by red blood cell (RBC) membranes caused by the flagella and microtubule reinforced body of the organisms greatly enhanced erythrophagocyosis of damaged RBC by the MPS. Similarly, erythrocytes, reticulocytes and platelets that adhered to trypanosomes via sialic acid receptors, caused injuries to erythrocyte membrane at the point of contact. Other factors that promoted haemolytic anaemia in trypanosomosis were trypanosome autolysates, immunochemical reactions, platelet aggregation, undulating pyrexia, oxidative stress, lipid peroxidation, nutritional and hormonal imbalances, disseminated intravascular coagulation, idiopathic and tumor necrosis factors (TNF) and bone marrow nitric oxide (NO) activity.

## 14. Acknowledgement

The authors highly appreciate the efforts of Professor I.O. Igbokwe in providing some of the literature used in this chapter.

## 15. References

Abenga. J.N. & Anosa, V.O. (2006). Clinical studies on experimental Gambian trypanosomosis in vervet monkeys, *Veternarski Arhiv* 76(1): (February 2008), 11-18, ISSN 0372-5480

Adamu, S., Maashin Useh, N., Ibrahim, D.N., Nok, A.J. & Esievo, K.A.N. (2009). Erythrocyte surface sialic acid depletion as predisposing factor to erythrocyte destruction in sheep experimental model of African trypanosomosis: A preliminary Report, *Slovenian Veterinary Research* 46(1): (March 2009), 19-28, ISSN 1580-4003

Allison, A.C. (1978). Mechanisms by which activated macrophages inhibit lymphocyte responses, *Immunology Review* 40: (June 1979), 23-27, ISSN 1550-6606

Ameh, D.A. (1984). Depletion of reduced glutathione and the susceptibility of erythrocytes to oxidative haemolysis in rats infected with *Trypanosoma brucei gambiense*, *Parasitology and Infectious Disease* 12: (March 2008), 130-139, ISSN 1996-0778

Anosa, V.O. (1977). *Studies on the Mechanism of Anaemia and the Pathology of Experimental Trypanosoma vivax (Zieman, 1905) Infection in Sheep and Goats*. PhD Thesis, University of Ibadan, Ibadan, Nigeria

Anosa, V.O. (1988). Haematological and biochemical changes in human and animal trypanosomosis, Parts I & II, *Revue d' Elevage et de Medicine Ve'te'rinaire des pays Tropicaux* 41(2): (June 1988), 65-78, ISSN 151-164

Anosa, V.O. & Isoun, T.T. (1980). Haematological studies on *Trypanosoma vivax* infection of goats and splenectomized sheep, *Journal of Comparative Pathology* 90 (4): (November 1980), 153-168, ISSN 1695-7504

Anosa, V.O. & Isoun, T.T. (1983). Pathology of experimental *Trypanosoma vivax* infection in sheep and goats, *Zentraiblatt fur veterinarmedizin* 30 (1): (November 1983), 685-700, ISSN 0721-1856

Anosa, V.O. & Kaneko, J.J. (1983). Pathogenesis of *Trypanosoma brucei* infection in deer mice (*Peromyscus maniculatus*), Light and electron microscopic studies on erythrocyte pathologic changes and phagocytosis, *American Journal of Veterinary Research* 44 (4): (August 1983) 645-651, ISSN 0002- 9645

Assoku, R.K.G. & Gardiner, P.R. (1992). Detection of antibodies to platelets and erythrocytes during haemorrhagic *Trypanosoma vivax* infection of Ayrshire cattle, *Veterinary Parasitology* 31(2): (April 2009) 199-216, ISSN 1932-6203

Audu, P.A., Esievo, K.A.N., Mohammed, G. & Ajanusi, O.J. (1999). Studies of infectivity and pathogenicity of an isolate of *Trypanosoma evansi* in Yankasa sheep, *Veterinary Parasitology* 86 (4): (October 1999) 185-190, ISSN 0304-4017

Banks, K.L. (1980). Injury induced by *Trypanosoma congolense* adhesions to cell membranes, *Journal of Parasitology* 6(1): (October 1980) 34-37, ISSN 0002-9645

Barret-Connor, E., Ugoretz, J.R. & Braude, A.I. (1973). Disseminated intravascular coagulation in trypanosomiasis, *Archives of Internal Medicine* 131(4): (April 1973) 574-577, ISSN 0003-9926

Bungener, W. & Muller, G. (1976). Adharenz phanomene bei *Trypanosoma congolense* [Adgerence phenomena in *Trypanosoma congolense*], *Tropenmedizin und parasitologie* 27 (2): (September 1976) 370-371, ISSN 0303-4208

Coleman, R.M., Brand, T. & von (1957). Blood pyruvate levels of rats during haematophagus infections, *Journal of Parasitology* 43 (1): (June 1957) 263-270, ISSN 0022-3395

Colley, C.M., Zwaal, R.F.A., Roeofsen, B. & Decssen, L.L.M. van (1973). Lytic and non-lytic degradation of phospholipids in mammalian erythrocytes by pure phospholipase, *Biochimica et Biophsica Acta* 307(1): (April 1973) 74-82, ISSN 0006-3002

Cook, G.M.W., Heard, D.H. & Seaman, G.V.F. (1966). A sialomuscopeptide liberated by trypsin from the human erythrocyte, Nature (*London*) 188 (1): (August 1967) 1011-1012, ISSN 1523-1747

Davies, C.E., Robins, R.S., Weller, R.D. & Broude, A.I. (1974). Thrombocytopenia in experimental trypanosomiasis, *Journal of Clinical Investigation* 53(1): (June 1974) 1359-1367, ISSN 1558-8238

Edwards, E.E., Judd, J.M. & Squire, F.A. (1956). Observations on trypanosomiasis in domestic animals in West Africa II, The effect on erythrocyte sedimentation rate, plasma protein, bilirubin, blood sugar, osmotic fragility, body weight and temperature in goats and sheep infected with *Trypanosoma vivax, T. congolense* and *T. brucei, Annals of Tropical Medicine and Parasitology* 50(2): (December 1957) 242-251, ISSN 0003-4983

Esievo, K.A.N. (1979). *In-vitro* production of neuraminidase (sialidase) by *Trypanosoma vivax, Proceedings of the 16th meeting of the International Scientific Council for Trypanosomiasis. Nairobi, Kenya: Organization of African Unity, Scientific, Technical and Research and Control*, pp. 205-210, ISSN 0372-5480, Yaoundé, Cameroon, August 24-29, 1978

Esievo, K.A.N. (1983). *Trypanosoma vivax*, stock V 953: inhibitory effect of type A influenza virus anti HAV8 serum on *in-vitro* neuraminidase (sialidase) activity, *Journal of Parasitology* 69(1): (December 1983) 491-495, ISSN 0022-3395

Esievo, K.A.N., Saror, D.I., Ilemobade, A.A. & Hallaway, M.H. (1982). Variation in erythrocyte surface and free serum sialic acid concentrations during experimental *Trypanosoma vivax* infection in cattle, *Research in Veterinary Science* 32 (2): (January 1982) 1-5, ISSN 0034-5288

Facer, C.A., Crosskey, J.M., Clarkson, M.J. & Jenkins, G.C. (1982). Immune haemolytic anaemia in bovine trypanosomiasis, *Journal of Comparative Pathology* 92(1): (October 1973) 293-401, ISSN 0721-1856

Goodwin, L.G. & Guy, M.W. (1973). Tissue fluids in rabbits infected with *Trypanosoma (Trypanozoon) brucei, Parasitology* 66 (1): (September, 1973) 499-513, ISSN 0031-1820

Grant, P.T. & Fulton, J.D. (1957). The catabolism of glucose by strains of *Trypanosoma rhodesiense, Biochemical Journal* 66 (2): (October 1957) 242-243, ISSN 0264-6021

Hambry, P.N., Tizard, I.R. & Mellors, A. (1980). Accumulation of phospholipase A1 in tissue fluid of rabbits infected with *Trypanosoma brucei, Tropen medizin und parasitologie* 31(1): (December 1980) 439-443, ISSN 0303-4208

Holmes, P.H. & Jennings, F.W. (1976). *Pathogenicity of parasitic infections*, Academic Press New York, ISBN 0372-5480, New York, USA

Igbokwe, I.O., Obagaiye, I.K., Esievo, K.A.N. & Saror, D.I. (1989). Dyserythropoesis in animal trypanosomiasis, *Revue d'Elavage et de Medicine veterinaire des pays Tropicaux* 42(4): (November 1990) 423-429, ISSN 0035-1865

Igbokwe, I.O. (1994). Mechanisms of cellular injury in African trypanosomiasis, *Veterinary Bulletin* 64(7): (March 1994), 611-620, ISSN 1684-5315

Ikede, B.O. & Losos, G.K. (1972). Pathology of the disease in sheep produced experimentally by *Trypanosoma brucei, Veterinary Pathology* 9(2): (July 1972) 278-289, ISSN 0300-9858

Isoun, T.T. & Esuruoso, G.O. (1972). Pathology of natural infection of *Trypanosoma vivax* in cattle, *Nigerian Veterinary Journal* 1(2): (September 1972), 42-45, ISSN 0721-1856

Jelkmann, W. (1998). Proinflamatory cytokines lowering erythropoietin production, *Journal of Interferon Cytokine Research* 18(2): (March 1998), 555-559, ISSN 0022-3751

Jennings, F.W. (1976). The anaemia of parasitic infections, *Proceedings of the 7th International Conference of the World Association for the Advancement of Veterinary Parasitology*, pp. 41-67, ISBN 0-12655 365- 3, Thessalonica, Greece, October 15-19, 1975

Kaaya, G.P., Valli, V.F., Maxie, M.G. & Losos, G.J. (1979). Inhibition of bovine granulocyte/macrophage colony formation *in-vitro* by serum collected from cattle infected with *Trypanosoma vivax* or *T. congolense, Tropen medizin und parasitologie* 30(2): (June 1979), 230- 235, ISSN 0303-4208

Kaaya, G.P., Tizard, I.R., Maxie, M.G. & Vall, V.O. (1980). Inhibition of leucopoiesis by sera from *Trypanosoma congolense* infected calves, partial characterization of the inhibitory factor, *Tropen medizin und parasitologie* 30(1): (June 1980), 230-235, ISSN 0303-4208

Karle, H. (1974). The pathogenesis of the anaemia of chronic disorders and the role of fever in erythrogenesis, *Scandinavian Journal of Haematology*, 13 (1): (October 1974), 81-86, ISSN 0036- 5534

Kobayashi, A., Tizard, I.R. & Woo, P.T.K. (1976). Studies on the anaemia in experimental African trypanosomiasis II. The pathogenesis of the anaemia in calves infected with *Trypanosoma congolense, American Journal of Tropical Medicine and Hygiene* 25(1): (May 1976), 401-406, ISSN 0002-9637

Liew, F.Y. & Turner, C.M.R. (1999). T. cell responses during *Trypanosoma brucei* infections in mice deficient in inducible nitric oxide synthase, Infection *and Immunology* 67(1): (May 1999), 3334- 3338, ISSN 0022-1767

Lonsdale-Eccles, J.D. & Grab, D.J. (1986). Proteases in African trypanosomes. In: Cytokine proteinases and their inhibitors, V.J. Turk, (Ed.), 189-197, Walter de Grayter, Berlin, Germany

MacLean, L., Odiit, M., & Sternberg, J.M. (2001). Nitric oxide and cytokine synthesis in human African trypanosomiasis, *The Journal of Infectious Disease* 184(4): (July 2001), 1086-1090, ISSN 0022-1899

Mackenzie, P.K.I. & Cruickshank, J.G. (1973). Phagocytosis of erythrocytes and leucocytes in sheep infected with *Trypanosoma congolense* (Broden, 1904), *Research in Veterinary Sciences* 15(1): (February 1973), 256-262, ISSN 0034-5288

Mackenzie, P.K.I., Boyt, W.P., Nesham, V.W. & Pirie, E. (1978). The etiology and significance of the phagocytosis of erythrocytes in sheep infected with *Trypanosoma congolense* (Broden, 1904), *Research in Veterinary Sciences* 24 (1): (April 1978), 4-7, ISSN 0034-5288

Mabbot, N. & Sternberg, J. (1995). Bone marrow nitric oxide production and development of anaemia in *Trypanosoma brucei* infected mice, *Infection and Immunology* 63(4): (June 1995), 1563-1566, ISSN 1098-5522

Magez, S., Radwanaska, M., Beschin, A., Sekikawa, K. & Debaetselier, P. (1999). Tumor necrosis factor alpha is a key mediator in the regulation of experimental *Trypanosoma brucei* infections, *Infection and Immunology* 67(5): (June 1999), 3128-3132, ISSN 1098-5522

Maxie, M.G. & Losos, G.J. (1979). Release of *Trypanosoma vivax* from the microcirculation of cattle by Berenil®, *Veterinary Parasitology* 3: (June 1979), 277-281, ISSN 0019-9867

McCay, P.B. & King, M.M. (1980). Endogenous sources of free radicals, In: Basic and Clinical Nutrition and development of anaemia in *Trypanosoma brucei* infected mice, L.J. Machlin, (Ed.), 269-303, Marcel Decker Inc, New York, USA

Mbaya, A.W., Nwosu, C.O. & Onyeyili, P.A. (2007). Toxicity and anti-trypanosomal effects of ethanolic extract of *Butyrospermum paradoxum* (*Sapotacea*) stem bark in rats infected with *Trypanosoma brucei* and *T. congolence*, *Journal of Ethnopharmacology* 111: (May 2007), 536-530, ISSN 0378-8741

Mbaya, A.W., Aliyu, M.M., Nwosu, C.O., Taiwo, V.O. & Ibrahim, U.I. (2009a). Effects of melarsamine hydrochloride (Cymelarsan®) and diaminazene aceturate (Berenil®) on the pathology of experimental *Trypanosoma brucei* infection in red fronted gazelles (*Gazella rufifrons*), *Veterinary Parasitology*, 163 (1-2): (July 2009), 140-143, ISSN 0304-4071

Mbaya, A.W., Aliyu, M.M., Nwosu, C.O. & Taiwo, V.O. (2009b). An assessment of the efficacy of DFMO in baboons (*Papio anubis*) infected with *Trypanosoma brucei gambiense*, *Global Journal of Pure and Applied Sciences*, 15 (1): (September 2009), 69-78, ISSN 1118-0579

Mbaya, A.W., Aliyu, M.M., Nwosu, C.O. & Ibrahim, U.I. (2009c). Effect of DL-α-difluoromethylornithine on biochemical changes in baboons (*Papio anubis*) experimentally infected with *Trypanosoma brucei gambiense*, *Nigerian Veterinary Journal*, 30(1): (September 2009), 35-44, ISSN 0331-3026

Mbaya, A.W., Aliyu, M.M. & Ibrahim, U.I. (2009d). Clinico-pathology and mechanisms of trypanosomosis in captive and free-living wild animals: A review, *Veterinary Research Communications*, 33: (April 2009), 793 - 809, ISSN 1573-7446

Mbaya, A.W., Aliyu, M.M., Nwosu, C.O. & Egbe-Nwiyi, T.N.C. (2009e). The relationship between parasitaemia and anaemia in a concurrent *Trypanosoma brucei* and *Haemonchus contortus* infection in red fronted gazelles (*Gazella rufifrons*), *Veterenarski Arhiv*, 79 (5): (September 2009), 451-460, ISSN 03720-5480

Mbaya, A.W., Ibrahim, U.I. & Apagu, S. T. (2010). Trypanosomosis of the dromedary camel (*Camelus dromedarius*) and its vectors in the tsetse-free arid zone of northeastern, Nigeria, *Nigerian Veterinary Journal*, 31(3): (September 2010), 195-200, ISSN 0331-3026

Mbaya, A.W. & U.I. Ibrahim (2011). *In-vivo* and *in-vitro* activities of medicinal plants on haemic and humoral trypanosomes: A review, *International Journal of Pharmacology*, 7(1): (January 2011), 1- 11, ISSN 1812-5700

Mbaya, A. W. Nwosu, C. O. & Kumshe, H. A. (2011). Genital lesions in male red fronted gazelles (*Gazella rufifrons*) experimentally infected with *Trypanosoma brucei* and the effect of melarsamine hydrochloride (Cymelarsan®) and diminazene aceturate

(Berenil®) in their treatment. *Theriogenology,* 16: (May 2011) 721-728, ISSN 1879-3231

Morrison, W.I., Max Murray, Sayer, P.D. & Preston, J.M. (1981). The pathogenesis of experimentally induced *Trypanosoma brucei* infection in the dog, Tissue and organ damage, *American Journal of Pathology* 102: (September 1981), 168-181, ISSN 0001-5598

Murray, M. & Dexter, T.M. (1988). Anaemia in bovine African trypanosomiasis: A review, *Acta Tropica* 45: (December 1988), 389-432, ISSN 0001-706X

Murray, M. & Morrison, W.I. (1978). Parasitaemia and host susceptibility in African trypanosomiasis, *Proceedings of a workshop,* pp.71`-81, ISBN 0-088936-214−9, *Nairobi, Kenya,* Nov. 20-23, 1978

Naessens, J., Kitani, H., Yagi, Y., Sekikawa, K., Iraqqi, F. (2005). TNF-a mediates the development of anaemia in a murine *Trypanosoma brucei rhodesiense* infection, but not the anaemia associated with a murine *T. congolense* infection, Clinical and Experimental Immunology 139(3): (March 2005), 403-410, PMID: PMC 180 9320

Nazrul-Islam, A.K.M. & Woo, P.T.K. (1991). Anaemia and its mechanism in goldfish (*Carassius auratus*) infected with *Trypanosoma danilewsky, Disease of Aquatic Organisms* (11): (November 1991), 37- 43, ISSN 0177-5103

Nemeth, E., Rivera, S., Gabayan, V., Keller, C., Taudorf, S., Pedersen, B.K. & Ganz, T. (2004). IL-6 mediates hypoferremia of inflammation by inducing the synthesis of the iron regulatory hormone hepcidin, *Journal of Clinical Investigation* 113: (May 2005), 1271-1276, ISSN 0021- 9738

Newton, B.A. (1978). The metabolism of African trypanosomiasis in relation to pathogenic mechanisms, In: *Pathogenicity of trypanosomes,* G. Losos, A. Chouinard, (Eds.), pp. 17-22, ISBN 0-88936-214-9 Proceedings of a workshop, Nairobi Kenya, November 20-23, 1977

Nwosu, C.O. & Ikeme, M.M. (1992). Parasitaemia and clinical manifestations in *Trypanosoma brucei* infected dogs, *Revue d'Elavage et de Medicine veterinaire des pays Tropicaux* 45(3-4): (September 1992), 273-277, ISSN 0035-1865

Nok, A.J. & Balogun, E.O. (2003). A blood stream *Trypanosoma congolense* sialidase could be involved in anaemia during experimental trypanosomiasis, *The Journal of Biochemistry* 133(6): (June 2003), 725-730, ISSN 1756-2651

Nok, A.J., Esievo, K.A.N., Ukoha, A.I., Ikediobi, C.O., Baba, J., Tekdek, B. & Ndams, I.S. (1992a). Kidney NaK-ATPase: kinetic study of rats during chronic infection with *Trypanosoma congolense, Journal of Clinical Biochemistry and Nutrition* 13: (September 1992), 73-79, ISSN 0912- 0009

Nok, A.J., Esievo, K.A.N., Ajibike, M.O., Achoba, I.I., Tekdek, K., Gimba, C.E., Kagbu, J.A. & Ndams, I.S. (1992b). Modulation of the calcium pump of the kidney and testes of rats infected with *Trypanosoma congolense, Journal of Comparative Pathology,* 107: (July 1992), 119-123, ISSN 0021- 9975

Ogwu, D., Njoku, C.O. & Ogbogu, V.C. (1992). Adrenal and thyroid dysfunction in experimental *Trypanosoma congolense* infection in cattle, *Veterinary Parasitology* 42: (April 1992), 15-26, ISSN 0304-4017

Rabo, J.S. (1995). Toxicity studies and trypanosuppressive effects of stem bark extract of *Butyrospermum paradoxum* in laboratory animals, PhD Thesis, University of Maiduguri, Maiduguri, Nigeria

Rautenberg, P., Schedler, R., Reinwalde, E. & Risse, H.J. (1982). Study on a proteolytic enzyme from *Trypanosoma congolense*, Purification and some biochemical properties, Molecular and some biochemical properties, *Molecular and Cellular Biochemistry* 47: (September 1982), 151-159, ISSN 0300-8177

Rifkin, M.R. & Landsberger, F.R. (1990). Trypanosome variant surface glycoprotein transfer to target membranes: A model for the pathogenesis of trypanosomiasis, *Proceedings of the National Academy of Science,* pp. 801-806, ISSN 0027-8424, May 23-27 USA, 1990

Saror, D.I. (1982). Aspects of the anaemia of acute bovine trypanosomiasis, *Proceedings of the first National Conference on Tsetse and Trypanosomiasis Research*, pp. 12-14, ISSN 0049-4747, August 10-12, Kaduna, Nigeria, 1981

Schauer, R. & Kamerling, J.P. (1997). Chemistry, biochemistry and biology of sialic acid. In: *Glycoptroteins,* J. Montrevil, J. .F. G. Vigenther & H. Shachter (Eds.) 241-400, Elsevier, ISBN 0- 444-80303-3, Amsterdam, The Netherlands

Seed, J.R. and Hall, J.E. (1985). Pathophysiology of African trypanosomiasis. In: *Immunology and pathogenesis of trypanosomiasis,* I.J. Tizard (Ed.), CRC Press, ISBN 0-8493-5640-7, Boca Raton, Florida, USA

Shehu, S.A., Ibrahim, N.D.G., Esievo, K.A.N. & Mohammed, G. (2006). Role of erythrocyte surface sialic acid inducing anaemia in Savannah Brown bucks experimentally infected with *Trypanosoma evansi, Veterenarski Arhiv* 26(6): (October 2006), 521-530, ISSN 0372-5480

Sileghem, M., Flynn, J.N., Logan-Henfrey, L. & Ellis, J. (1994). Tumour necrosis factor production by monocytes from cattle infected with *Trypanosoma* (*Dutonella*) *vivax* and *T.* (*nannomonas*) *congolense*, Possible association with severity of anaemia associated with the disease, *Parasite Immunoassay,* 16(1): (January, 1994), 51-54, ISSN 0141-9838

Slater, T.F. (1984). Free radical mechanism in tissue injury, *Biochemistry Journal* 222: (August 1984), 1-15, ISSN 0264-6021

Solano, P., Dela Roqoes, S. & Duvalet, G. (2003). Biodiversity of trypanosomes pathogenic for cattle and their epidemiological importance, *Annals of Society* 68: 169 - 171.

Soulsby, E.J.L. (1982). *Helminthes, Arthropods and Protozoa parasites of domesticated Animals,* Bailere Tindal, ISBN 0702008206 9780702008207, London

Swallow, B.M. (2000): Impacts of trypanosomosis in African agriculture, Programme against African Trypanosomosis Technical and Scientific series, Food Agriculture Organization (F. A. O.) 2: (April 2000), 45 - 46, ISSN 1020-7163

Tizard, I.R. & Holmes, W.L. (1976). The generation of toxic activity from *Trypanosoma congolense, Experentia* 32: (May 1977), 1533-1534, 0014-4754

Tizard, I.R. & Holmes, W.L. (1977). The release of suitable vasoactive material from *Trypanosoma congolense* intraperitoneal diffusion chambers, *Transactions of the Royal Society of Tropical Medicine and Hygiene,* 71: (June 1977), 52-55, ISSN 0035-9203

Tizard, I.R., Holmes, W.L., Yorke, D.A. & Mellors, A. (1977). The generation and identification of haemolysin of *Trypanosoma congolense, Experintia* 33: (July, 1977), 901-902, ISSN 0014-4754

Tizard, I.R., Holmes, W.L. & Nielsen, K. H. (1978a). Mechanisms of anaemia in trypanosomiasis: Studies on the role of haemolytic fatty acids derived from

*Trypanosoma congolense, Tropen medizin und parasitologie* 29: (March, 1978), 108-114, ISSN 0303-4208

Tizard, I.R., Nielsen, K. H., Mellors, A. & Assoku, R.K.G. (1978b). Biologically active lipids generated by autolysis of *Trypanosoma congolense*. In: *Pathogenecity of Trypanosomes. Proceedings of a workshop*, pp. 103-110, ISBN 0-88936-214-9, Nairobi, Kenya, November 20-23, 1978

Tizard, I.R., Sheppard, J. & Nielsen, K. (1978c). The characterization of a second class of haemolysin from *Trypanosoma brucei, Transactions of the Royal Society of Tropical Mediciene and Hygiene* 72: (July 1978), 198-2000, ISSSN 0035-9203

Umar, I.A., Ogenyi, E., Okodaso, D., Kimeng, E., Stanecheva, G.I., Omage, J.J., Isah, S. & Ibrahim, M.A. (2007). Amelioration of anaemia and organ damage by combined intraperitoneal administration of vitamin A and C to *Trypanosoma brucei brucei* infected rats, *African Journal of Biotechnology* 6(18): (July 2007), 2083-2086, ISSN 0035-9203

Van den Ingh. T.S.G.A.M., Zwart, D., Schotman, A.J.H., Van miert, A.S.J.P.A.M. & Veenaidal, G.H. (1976). The pathology and pathogenesis of *Trypanosoma vivax* infection in the goat, *Research in Veterinary Science* 21: (June 1977), 264-270, ISSN 0034-5288

Varki, A. (1992). Diversity in the sialic acids, *Glycobiology* 2: (February 1992), 25-40, ISSN 0959-6658

Verma, B.B. & Gautam, O.P. (1978). Studies on experimental surra (*T. evansi* infection) in Buffalo and cow calves, *Indian Veterinary Journal* 55: (August 1978), 648-653, ISSN 0019-6479

Vickerman, K. & Tetley, L. (1978). Biology and ultra structure of trypanosomes in relation to pathogenesis. In: *Pathogenecity of trypanosomes*, Proceedings of a workshop, pp. 231-31, ISBN 0- 88936-214-9, Nairobi, Kenya, November 20-23, 1978

Woodruff, A.W., Topley, E., Knight, R. & Downie, C.G.B. (1972). The anaemias of Kalaazar. *British Journal of Haematology* 22: (March 1973), 319-329, ISSN 0007-1048

Wolkmer, P., Shafer da Silva, A., Treasel, C.K., Paim, F.C., Cargncutti., J.F., Pagononcelli, M., Picada, M.E., Monterro, S.G. & Anjus Lopes, S.T. (2009). Lipid peroxidation associated with anaemia in rats experimentally infected with *Trypanosoma evansi, Veterinary Parasitology* 165: (1-2): (October 2009), 41-46, ISSN 1873-2550

Woo P.T.K. & Kobayashi, A. (1975). Studies on the anaemia in experimental African trypanosomiasis, Preliminary communication on the mechanism of the anaemia. *Annals Society Belge Medicine Tropicale* 53(1): (October 1973), 37-45, ISSN 0772-4128

Zwart, D. & Veenendal, G.H. (1978). Pharmacologically active substances in *Trypanosoma vivax* infections. In: *Pathogenecity of trypanosomes*. Proceedings of a workshop, pp. 111-113, ISBN 0-88936-214-9, Nairobi, Kenya, November 20-23, 1978

# 18

# Severe Malaria Anaemia in Children

Ayodotun Olutola and Olugbenga Mokuolu
*University of Maryland/Institute of Human Virology*
*Nigeria*

## 1. Introduction

Severe malaria anaemia is defined as haemoglobin concentration <5g/dl associated with Plasmodium falciparum parasitaemia.(WHO, 1986) Other causes of anaemia have to be excluded as asymptomatic falciparum parasitaemia is common in endemic areas.(Salako et al,1990) Severe anaemia may exist alone or in combination with other complications particularly cerebral malaria and respiratory distress in which it portends worse prognosis.(WHO, 2004)

It is a significant cause of morbidity and mortality in children below five years of age. Children below 3 years are predominantly affected with a mean age of 1.8 years.(Krause,2000) Available data suggests that severe malaria anaemia is the commonest complication of malaria in areas subjected to high inoculation rates throughout the year.(Newton & Krishna, 1998). It accounts for between 26 and 62% of severe malaria admissions in malaria endemic countries (Satpathy et al,2004, Mockenhaupt et al,2004) and up to 29% of total hospital admissions as reported in Ilorin(Ernest,2002) and Kenya.(Lackritz et al,1992). Hospital based data of deaths from anaemia ranges between 11.2% in Sierra Leone and 14% in Kenya for children below 5 years.(Brabin et al,2002). Most deaths occur within 2 days of admission underscoring the importance of adequate blood banking facilities in our primary health care centres. (Newton &Krishna, 1998, Lackritz et al,1992).

## 2. Pathogenesis of severe malaria anaemia

Multiple mechanisms may account for anaemia in children infected with malaria. Host factors, associations with parasitic infections, nutritional deficiencies of iron, Vitamins B12, Vitamin E, and folate, in addition to drug associated causes are important considerations. Children under 5 years are more prone to severe malaria anaemia. The following are some of the key pathogenetic mechanisms:

### 2.1 Host factors

Age: Malaria affects all age groups and congenital malaria is relatively uncommon.(Stephen et al,1996, Falade et al,2007)) There is no sex predilection. It is relatively uncommon in the first few months of life due to the high concentration of haemoglobin F which is not favorable for parasite growth, presence of maternal immunoglobulins (Falade et al,2007) and selective shielding of infants from parasite. Exclusively breastfed infants are also deficient in paraaminobenzoic acid which the parasite thrives upon.(Gilles, 1957)

Immune status: Natural immunity occurs in subjects that are heterozygous for Haemoglobin S, thalassaemia, G6PD deficiency, Human Leucocyte Antigen classes I and II alleles, Band 3, Spectrin, Lewis, Kid Js red cell types.(Luzatto, 1974, Miller et al,1976, Allison 1954, Marsh, 2002) They are believed to be a protective mutation representing a balanced genetic polymorphism that occurred over the years in response to the threat of malaria. Individuals that are duffy negative also lack the receptor for vivax merozoites on their red cells and are resistant to vivax infection. (Miller et al, 1976) Although new evidence is beginning to contradict this age long position and there are increasing reports of P vivax infection in Duffy negative individuals.(Mercereau-Puijalon &Menard, 2010) Acquired immunity which may be passive as in transplacental transfer of maternal IgG to babies(Falade et al, 2007, Marsh,2002) or active immunity following repeated exposure to the parasite determine incidence and severity of infection. IgM and IgG immunoglobulin response to malaria particularly IgG protects against invasion of red cells by merozoites.(Anonymous, 1975) These immunoglobulins also promote phagocytosis of erythrocytes containing maturing schizonts.

Blood group type: Parasite virulence has been found to be reduced in blood group O erythrocytes compared with groups A, B and AB suggesting that Blood group O may confer some resistance to severe falciparum malaria. A matched case-control study of 567 Malian children found that group O was present in only 21% of severe malaria cases compared with 44–45% of uncomplicated malaria controls and healthy controls. Group O was associated with a 66% reduction in the odds of developing severe malaria compared with the non-O blood groups.(Rowe et al, 2007) Others have confirmed that blood group A is a co receptor for plasmodium falciparum rossetting, a mechanism by which the parasite potentiates its virulence causing severe malaria.(Barragan et al, 2000)

Nutritional status: Nutritional status of the host also plays a role as severe malaria has been reported to be uncommon in marasmic and kwarshiokor patients.(Goyal, 1991) Malnutrition is thought to contribute to 53% of under-5 mortality in the developing world.(Caulfield et al, 2004) The global distribution of malnutrition overlaps with that of malaria. However the relationship between malnutrition and malaria is unclear. The pathology of malaria is partly immune mediated requiring both cellular and humoral mechanisms for its evolution.(Jhaveri et al, 1997, Turrini et al, 2003, Sandau,2001) This partly explains why under-nutrition is widely believed to be protective for severe malaria.(Goyal, 1991)

Genetic disorders: Haemoglobinopathies, membranopathies and inherited enzyme deficiencies particularly G6PD all contribute to the anaemia in affected children. In each case multiple mechanisms are at work though one or two mechanisms predominate. (Wickramasinghe & Abdallah,2000) Generally severe malaria anaemia is characterized by a low reticulocyte response and high erythropoietin levels.(Roberts et al, 2005)

### 2.2 Lysis of parasitized erythrocytes

As part of the malaria life cycle, rupture of erythrocytes to release merozoites result in cell lysis. The merozoites destroy the red blood cell by its own protease enzyme. The released merozoites attack other red cells and through the repeated cycles of red cell lysis, anaemia ensues. This is particularly important for falciparum as it has the propensity to invade large cell populations of all age groups.(Miller, 1976) This also partly accounts for the reticulocytopenia as the reticulocytes are not spared of the direct invasion in addition to other mechanisms that suppress regeneration of red cell precursors in the bone marrow (dyserythropoeisis ) In contrast p vivax invades only the young and large cells with less severity of anaemia (Miller et al, 1976) Severe anaemia develops rapidly in children and the rate is directly proportional to the degree of parasitaemia in many cases.(WHO, 2004, Afolabi et al, 2002) However, parasitaemia is not a very reliable indicator of severity as a large number of parasitized red cells may be sequestered in capillaries and venules of vital organs and hence not detected in the peripheral blood film.(Silamut & While, 1993) Prior treatment and continuous immune lysis after parasitic clearance also impair the reliability of parasitaemia as a reliable indicator of severity of anaemia.

### 2.3 Immune mediated lysis

There is evidence for immune mediated lysis of both parasitized and non parasitized red cells as specific antibodies are produced against them. Increased clearance of red blood cells still occur even after parasitic clearance.(Ouma et al, 2008, Edington & Gilles, 1976, Warell et al, 2002, Stouti et al, 2002) This occurs as a result production of antibodies to non parasitized cell, binding of soluble malaria antigens to the red cells, binding of immune complexes to red cell surface with subsequent removal by immune lysis and the erythrophagocytosis. (Warell et al, 2002) The observation of reduced complement particularly C3 during acute attacks, increased destruction of transfused cells in malaria patients also support the possibility of an immune mediated lysis. Complement mediated lysis is increased due to loss of complement regulatory protein CD-55 and CD -59 associated with malaria which protects inadvertent complement mediated lysis. (Stouti et al, 2003) In addition to this the increased production of immune complexes including malaria antigen and drug associated complexes increase complement activation. Non specific polyclonal activation of B cell is a common finding in malaria and may cause production of autoantibodies some of which could conceivably be directed at red cell antigens.(Jhaveri et al, 1997) Transfusion of malaria antigens alone in the absence of infection in animals giving rise to adverse effects on the red cells further strengthen the evidences for immune lysis. (Satpathy et al, 2004)

### 2.4 Removal by the reticuloendothelial system

Removal, particularly in the spleen, of deformed, parasitized red cells and immune sensitized red cells appears to be the most significant mechanism and explains why majority of patients do not present with overt signs of hemolysis such as jaundice and dark colored urine as is commonly found in other causes of intravascular hemolysis. Cytokine dysregulation and increased Tumor Necrosis Factor $\alpha$ (TNF - $\alpha$) can activate macrophages which in a hyperactive stage may even reduce its threshold for amount of antibody coating needed for phagocytosis i.e. minimally sensitized red cells which otherwise would not have been phagocytosed now are actively phagocytosed due to activation of the monocytes and macrophages.(Turrini et al, 2003)

### 2.5 Bone marrow suppression

Anaemia due to malaria is hyporegenerative along with mild to moderate shortening of red cell life span. It is characterized either by normochromic normocytic or hypochromic microcytic features and associated with hypoferinaemia, low total iron binding capacity, transferring, low reticulocyte count and raised levels of inflammatory proteins like fibrinogen.(Abdalla, 1990) These are all features of anaemia of chronic disorder. So long as the insult persists, administration of iron does not correct the anaemia. Interleukins (IL-1 and IL-6) and TNF - α have been found to be significantly elevated in patients with severe anaemia due to malaria and they have an inverse relationship to the degree of anaemia found in such patients.(Issifou et al, 2003, McDevitt et al, 2004) The bone marrow shows a non specific suppression of all cell lines and there is a sequestration of young erythrocytes and reticulocytes.(Edington & Gilles, 1976)

### 2.6 Iron shunting for parasite use

The hypoferrinaemia discussed above can be explained by three mechanisms (Ghosh, 2007)

1. Locking of iron in macrophage stores
2. Synthesis of iron binding proteins with higher affinity for iron than transferrin by inflammatory cells leading to a mop up of available iron
3. Reduction in transferrin synthesis by the hepatocytes

The overall effect is a reduction in iron (a growth promoting nutrient) available to the parasites and the other cells that require iron for their metabolism. This contributes to reduced erythropoiesis. Malaria parasite has an enormous need for iron for its life cycle and extracts iron from host by inserting parasite specific transferring - like receptors on the host red cell membrane. This significantly contributes to the picture of iron deficiency anaemia seen particularly in children with borderline or low iron stores.(Oppenheimer, 1989)

### 2.7 Hypersplenism

Intense stimulation of monocyte macrophage system associated with malaria and hypersplenism persists 4 -6 weeks after parasitic clearance.(Looaressuwan et al, 1997)2 Some non parasitized red blood cells are removed as a result of changes in the membrane and increased osmotic fragility as a result of the changes in the chemical and immunological constituents of plasma.(Ghosh, 2007) Tropical splenomegaly syndrome following repeated or chronic falciparum malaria infection and may contribute to increased red cell removal by the reticulo -endothelial system.

### 2.8 Dyserythropoiesis

High levels of erythropoietin and suppressed marrow response are paradoxically associated with malaria anaemia. The high erythropoietin levels is caused by high levels of hypoxia inducing factor (HIF) induced by a combination of high levels of TNF- α.(Sandau et al 2001) Deficiency of IL -12 and IL - 10 have been found to correlate to the marrow suppression seen in malaria.(Weatherall et al 2002) Erythroid precursors like BFU – E ( Burst forming colonies) and CFU -E (Colony Forming colonies) are inhibited. It is believed that therapeutic application of IL-10 and IL-12 provides prospects for correcting severe malaria anaemia. The inability of young children to maintain IL-10 production in response to inflammatory processes contributes to the anaemia. This cytokine is a growth factor that stimulates the differentiation of haemopoietic progenitor cells in response to anaemia.(Angela O'Donnell et al 2007). Ouma et al investigated the polymorphic variability in innate immune response genes, susceptibility to malaria and circulating inflammatory mediator levels (i.e., IL-10, TNF-alpha, IL-6 and IL-12) in 375 Kenyan children. Results demonstrated that common IL-10 promoter haplotypes modulate susceptibility to severe malaria anaemia and functional changes in circulating IL-10, TNF-alpha, and IL-12 levels in children with falciparum malaria. The expression of these haplotypes have been found to be age dependent and may account for less erythropoeitic response to anaemia in the younger child.

### 2.9 Role of nitric oxide

Acute malaria is associated with increases in Nitric oxide (NO) production.(Clark et al, 1991) High levels of nitric oxide inhibit Na+/K+ ATPase in the red cell membrane and oxidizes the membrane lipids through generation of peroxiynitrate causing poor deformability of red cells. Overactivation of poly-ADP ribose polymerase-1 (PARP-1) by nitric oxide and other proinflammaotry cytokines causes rapid depletion of nicotinamide adenine dinucleotide (NAD) and adenosine triphosphate (ATP) from red cells.(Clark & Cowden,2003) Hence it can inhibit red cell glycolysis. Membrane-damaged red cells are removed by the spleen. Nitric Oxide also suppresses erythropoiesis by mitochondrial damage to erythroid progenitors and early erythroid.(Xie & Wolin, 1996)

### 2.10 Role of haemozoin

Haemozoin, a product of catabolism of haemoglobin by malaria parasite contains iron in the ferrous state which catalyzes the production of free radicals. This leads to increased production of 15-hydroxy-eicosatetraenoic acid (15-HETE) and 4-Hydroxy Nonenal (4HNE) from red cell membrane lipids. These products increase red cell stiffness and shorten red cell life span.(Arese & Schwarzwer, 1997)

### 2.11 Pitting of parasitized red cell

Spherocytes have been found in high prevalence in peripheral blood in malaria endemic areas, and a detailed study of mechanism of whole parasitized red cell removal versus pitting out the parasite from red cell along with some amount of red cell membrane (leading to spherocyte formation) proved that the later mechanism appears to be preferred by the human body.(Anyona et al, 2006) Pitting as one of the major parasite mechanisms is also suggested by high levels of parasite-related antigens on the unaffected spherocytic red cells in malarial infection.(Anyona et al, 2006) Spherocytosis in malarial infection can be caused by several mechanisms. Spherocytes are less compliant than normal red cells and are easily removed by the spleen.

### 2.12 Tropical splenomegaly syndrome (hyperactive malarial splenomegaly)

In some patients with chronic exposure to malaria, P. falciparum leads to chronic and intense stimulation of splenic macrophages leading to gross splenomegaly, low levels of parasitaemia and very high levels of IgM in the serum. These patients have a defect in immunoglobulin class switching and a genetic predisposition to develop this condition. Clonal B cell proliferation in this syndrome has also been recognized.(Bates et al, 1991) Huge spleen and hyperactive reticulo-endothelial system chronically can cause significant anemia by red cell pooling. A small proportion of these patients develop non-Hodgkin lymphoma, which adds to the existent causes of anemia in this infection as a future consequence.

### 2.13 Endothelial injury

Parasitized red cell develops special receptors to stick to endothelial cells. This property is seen particularly with P. falciparum infection. Attachment of these parasites can take place through CD-36 ligand (Gamain et al, 2001) or through interaction with endothelial cell chondroition sulphate-like molecule. Cytokine dysregulation could up regulate endothelial adhesion molecules and converts the anti-coagulant endothelium to a procoagulant surface.

Hence combination of these two mechanisms may cause intense red cell sequestration in deeper capillaries and disseminated intravascular coagulation (DIC) with hemorrhage. Both conditions can contribute to acute anemia in P. falciparum infection. A proportion of patients can also develop microangiopathic hemolysis.

## 3. Clinical features

The features of severe malaria anaemia are those of malaria with or without features of cardio respiratory decompensation. The signs and symptoms of uncomplicated malaria are non specific and there exists a wide range of differential diagnosis for malaria in an endemic region. Many children with malaria parasitemia are asymptomatic particularly in malaria endemic regions. Threshold values of parasitemia based on epidemiological surveys are established for various regions of endemicity to be able to ascribe the clinical features to malaria in the presence of malaria parasitemia.(Salako et al, 1990, Krause, 2000) In malaria endemic regions, a threshold of 5,000 -10,000 parasites/ml is commonly quoted.(Snow et al, 2002) However clinical malaria can occur in the absence of detectable parasite in the blood particularly in falciparum malaria during the process of deep tissue schizogony where the maturing schizonts are sequestered in the capillaries of deep tissues like the muscle and bone marrow.(Taylor & Molyneux, 2002)

Malaria is a febrile illness and majority of patients present with fever.(Ehrhardt et al, 2006) The fever may be of any pattern, the classical intermittent description of fever, within every 48 hours in falciparum, ovale, and vivax and within every 72 hours in malariae is seen if only one brood of parasite causes infection so that the cyclical rupture of erythrocytic schizonts are synchronous with the clinical symptomatology, otherwise fever may be continuous, high or low grade in nature. In cases unmodified by treatment, it starts with malaise, myalgia, anorexia, headache followed by an intense feeling of cold associated with shivering called the cold phase, core temperature is high and tachycardia is common. This lasts for about 15-30 minutes and followed by a rapid rise in temperature to as high as 410C, vomiting, headache, convulsion and delirium may occur while splenomegaly may be detected at this phase. This hot phase lasts 2-4 hours after which is the wet or defervescence where the child sweats profusely and feels better this lasts 2-4 hours. The whole cycle is repeated within 48 hours in falciparum, vivax and ovale malaria and within 72 hours in p. malariae. In the infant and younger child, symptoms are less specific and include irritability, refusal to feed, diarrhea cough and fever of any pattern predominating. (Ehrhardt et al, 2006) Vomiting, diarrhea, cough may occur and confuse the diagnosis with gastroenteritis or an acute upper respiratory tract infection. Anaemia, tachypnea, hepatosplenomegaly and dehydration are common in uncomplicated cases.(Grobusch & Kremsner, 2005) Altered consciousness, repeated convulsions, severe pallor, shock, jaundice, dark or coke colored urine, oliguria, prostration, respiratory distress and hyperpyrexia put patients at a high risk of dying and in addition to laboratory findings of hypoglycemia and hyperparasitemia are classified as forms of severe malaria.(WHO, 2004)

The features of severe malaria anaemia are those enumerated above in addition to symptoms and signs of cardiorespiratory compromise in decompensated children, however many children have severe malarial anaemia with few or no life threatening symptoms (Lackritz et al, 1992, English et al, 2002) and this usually follows when anaemia has developed slowly. Other children with systemic organ diseases particularly cardiac, respiratory, renal diseases

and sepsis may present with signs of decompensation at higher haematocrit levels. If anaemia occurs rapidly or when these compensatory mechanisms are overwhelmed, anaerobic metabolism commences with the generation of acids and development of the signs and symptoms of decompensation. The cardinal signs of decompensation are respiratory distress (tachypnea, chest in-drawing, acidotic breathing)(WHO, 2004, English et al, 1996) tachycardia with or without gallop rhythm and tender hepatomegaly. These signs are also those of congestive cardiac failure.(Afolabi et al, 2002) Others include features of hypovolemic shock, (English et al, 1996a,1996b) cold clammy extremities, weak thready pulses, delayed capillary refill time.(Pamba & Maitland, 2004) An overlap commonly occurs with severe anaemia coexisting with cerebral malaria, respiratory distress and other forms of severe malaria in which it portends worse prognosis.(WHO, 2004)
Pathophysiology of Some Clinical Features of Severe Malaria

| Clinical Features | Pathophysiology |
|---|---|
| Fever | Cytokine mediated |
| Gastrointestinal symptoms (Nausea, Diarrhea) | Mechanism unclear<br>Intestinal dysfunction secondary to hypoxia from parasitic sequestration in splanchnic bed |
| Jaundice and Dark urine | Hemolysis<br>Dehydration |
| Difficulty in breathing | Hypoxia<br>Low pH<br>Lactic acidosis<br>Pyrexia |
| Tachypnea | Hypoxia,<br>Low pH<br>Lactic acidosis<br>Pyrexia |
| Tachycardia | Hypoxia<br>Pyrexia |
| Hepatosplenomegaly | Parasitic sequestration<br>Reticuloendothelial hyperactivity<br>Increased preload from right sided heart failure |
| Loss of consciousness | Cerebral hypoxia and ischaemia,<br>Sludging as a result of parasitic sequestration<br>Micro circulatory obstruction<br>Increased capillary permeability<br>Cerebral oedema |

## 4. Biochemical and laboratory changes

Anaemia is a common finding in malaria and the degree correlates with severity of parasitaemia. (Grobusch & Kremsner, 2005) In severe anaemia, haematocrit is less than 15% or haemoglobin concentration less than 5g/dL. Anaemia is usually haemolytic normochromic and normocytic though macrocytic picture is seen if there is folate deficiency or with marked reticulocytosis. Mean corpuscular volume, however, varies with age in

children and its interpretation has to be related to the expected for age. Leucopenia with a left shift is a common finding though leucocytosis may occur in the early stage of infection or when a concomitant bacterial infection coexists. Monocytosis and malaria pigments in form of granules are found in large monocytes.(Edington & Gilles, 1976, Warrell et al, 2002) Thrombocytopenia (Grobusch & Kremsner, 2005) with some degree of depletion of clotting factors and accumulation of fibrinogen degradation products is seen though disseminated intravascular coagulopathy is very rare.(Warrell et al, 2002) This is as a result of consumption coagulopathy triggered by parasite products, phagocytosis of platelets by the reticuloendothelial system and an inappropriate bone marrow response. The activation of the coagulation cascade is via the intrinsic pathway and has been found to be proportional to disease severity and is least severe in uncomplicated malaria cases.(Clemens et al, 1994)
The peripheral blood film shows parasitized red cells, polychromasia, anisocytosis, poikilocytosis, target cells and in severe cases nucleated red blood cells. The presence of schizont and gametocytes in the peripheral blood film indicates severity of infection. Blood film may show few parasites as a result of deep tissue sequestration or following prior treatment with antimalarial drugs. The bone marrow shows erythroblastic hyperplasia with large eosinophilic normoblastic cells. Erythrocyte sedimentation rate (ESR) is increased in malaria cases and variation due to the intensity of infection can be expected.(Viroj, 2008, Karunaweera et al, 1998) It has been found that an increase in the mass of individual red cell due to inclusion bodies reduce the time for sedimentation.(Viroj, 2008) Malarial parasites act as inclusion bodies thereby increasing red cell mass (weight) and ESR. However ESR is a non specific hematological parameter that cannot be reliably used for diagnosis of malaria or monitoring of response to treatment.
Oxygen delivery is determined by tissue blood flow and the arterial oxygen content.(Moroff & Dend, 1983) While tissue blood flow is dependent on the cardiac output (function of the stroke volume and the heart rate), the arterial oxygen content is a function of haemoglobin concentration and saturation and minimally the amount of oxygen dissolved in plasma. Stroke volume is determined by the preload (venous return), myocardial contractility and the afterload (resistance to flow). All these parameters are delicately regulated by a host of local autoregulatory, hormonal and neural mechanisms to maintain optimal oxygen delivery even in the face of disease. (William, 1997) In anaemic states the arterial partial oxygen pressure (pO2) reduces and pCO2 is elevated. These factors in addition to low pH, fever, lactate, potassium and a host of others are potent stimuli for arteriolar vasodilation increasing tissue blood flow in vital organs like the brain and the heart. (William, 1997b) Autonomic discharges from the sympathetic system results in generalized vasoconstriction and venoconstriction, increase in blood pressure and a reduction in blood pool in the capacitance vessels culminating in an increase in venous return. More importantly in children the sympathetic discharge increases the heart rate by a direct stimulatory effect on the sinoatrial node and a reduction in the vagal inhibitory pulses. Additional effect of the sympathetic discharge on the renal vessels result in increased production of renin by the juxtaglomerular apparatus with subsequent activation of the Renin-Angiotensin-Aldosterone system resulting in water and salt retention further accentuating the preload.( William, 1997b)
Blood viscosity which is a function of the haematocrit drops with a progressive reduction in haematocrit such that resistance to flow further reduces in the blood vessels contributing to the increase in tissue blood flow and the venous return.67 Children in contrast to adults have a greater capacity to increase cardiac output by increasing heart rate than by increasing stroke volume; therefore tachycardia is a more prominent feature in children. Oxygen extraction from

the arterial circulation is enhanced by the higher concentration of 2,3 diphosphoglycerate in children particularly in high oxygen consumption and supply dependent organs which include the brain and the heart(Marsh, 2002) while more is synthesized within 24-36hours of onset of anaemia.(Card & Brain, 1973) This results in a wider arteriovenous oxygen differential across the tissues. Depending on how rapid the anaemia develops in children, these mechanisms are brought to play so that a 50% reduction in oxygen carrying capacity results in less than 25% reduction in tissue oxygen availability.(Moroff & Dend,1983)

## 5. Treatment

Blood transfusion with 10ml/kg of packed cells should be given over 2-4 hours with diuretic therapy to prevent volume overload (Newton et al, 1992) while whole blood transfusion is advocated for patients with proven hypovolemia. There is an increasing tendency towards whole blood transfusion based on evidence that many patients with severe malaria anaemia are actually hypovolemic with hypotension, delayed capillary refill time and low central venous pressures.(Maitland et al, 2003) Based on these findings, this school of thought postulates that cardiac failure does not occur and its features are rather those of a compensated hypovolemic shock,(WHO, 2004) thus they advocate whole blood transfusion or initial volume expansion with colloid to improve tissue perfusion and correct acidosis while awaiting blood transfusion.(Maitland et al, 2003) Severe malaria has been found to be associated with about 6.7% reduction in total body water, a loss slightly more than mild dehydration such that overzealous volume expansion may be detrimental.(Planche et al, 2004)

Blood transfusion is fraught with many risks of immediate and long term complications which must be weighed against their potential benefits. Such risks include transmission of infections including HIV, Hepatitis, Ebstein Barr, cytomegalovirus and other pathogens in screened and unscreened blood. (Halim et al, 1999, Anderson & Weinstein, 1990) Risk of transmitting HIV via transfusion of screened blood in the window period has been estimated to be 1 in 3 x 105 - 2 x 106 while hepatitis is 1 in 1 x 105 transfusions in the USA. (Anderson & Weinstein, 1990) Others include volume overload, electrolyte abnormalities, transfusion reactions, alloimmunization in females and graft vs host disease rarely in immunocompetent hosts. (Anderson & Weinstein, 1990)

Various studies have been done with the aim of increasing the threshold for blood transfusion to limit transfusion to only those at the risk of dying while advocating conservative management for the others with potent anti malarial agents with or without haematinics. (Holzer et al, 1993, Bojang et al, 1997) These studies defined decompensation as respiratory distress or a combination of tachycardia and tachypnea in addition to tender hepatomegaly. Cochrane review of 2 of 42 such studies involving 230 children found no significant tendency towards dying among 2 groups of patients randomized for transfusion and non transfusion. (Meremikwu & Smith, 2004) In one study in Gambia with severe anaemia, those with haematocrit <12 and all those with severe anaemia in association with respiratory distress and cardiac failure were transfused while others were randomized for transfusion and conservative management with antimalarial medication and iron therapy. No stastistical significance in mortality was found and haematologic restoration viz a viz haematocrit at 28 days was better in those treated conservatively.(Bojang et al, 1997) However the need for close monitoring was reduced as well as shortened hospital stay. A study in Tanzania recruited patients with similar criteria and conservative management was with antimalarial alone. They achieved similar result except that haematocrit at 28 days was not significantly different in both groups probably due to the omission of haematinics in their treatment protocol. (Holzer et al, 1993)

Antimalarial drug of choice are Quinine and Artemether. Artemether has a faster parasitic clearance than quinine and the additional advantage of less potential side effects.(Taylor et al, 1998) In comparison to sulphadoxine/pyrimethamine it has both a shorter parasite and fever clearance time but high recrudescence rate.(Salako et al, 1994) Artemisinin based combination therapy is being advocated as a result of this and are now available. However they are expensive, mostly come in oral preparations and may not be easily applicable in emergency situations.(WHO, 2002)

## 6. Findings from a clinical study on severe malaria anaemia in Ilorin, Nigeria

A cross sectional study was carried out in the Emergency Paediatric Unit of the University of Ilorin Teaching Hospital over a ten month period from February to November 2006 to document the clinical profile and haematological indices of children with severe anaemia due to malaria. The study attempted to determine the:

1. Hospital prevalence of severe anaemia in children.
2. Clinical presentation of children with severe anaemia due to malaria
3. Haematological indices (Hb, PCV,MCV,MCH, MCHC), Genotype, and Blood group of children with severe anaemia due to malaria.
4. Factors associated with risk of cardiac decompensation in children with severe anaemia due to malaria

Children between 6 months and 12 years of age with suspected malaria anemia were enrolled into a case control study at the University of Ilorin Teaching Hospital from February to November 2006.

Severe malaria anaemia was defined as haemoglobin concentration <5g/dl associated with Plasmodium falciparum parasitaemia in the absence of other identifiable cause of anaemia. The controls were age and sex matched children with similar characteristics above who had malaria without severe anaemia (Haematocrit >15%).

Detailed history and physical examination were done on all recruited subjects. Venous samples were collected for haematocrit check, haemoglobin electrophoresis, Mean Corpuscular Volume (MCV), Mean Corpuscular Haemoglobin(MCH) and blood film analysis for malaria parasite prior to blood transfusion. Investigations were done using Sysmex 18 auto analyzer and Volkam SAE 2761 electrophoretic tank. Presence of malaria parasitaemia was noted while specie of parasite is detected on the thin film. Parasite count was determined by calculating the number of parasitized red blood cells corresponding to 200 white blood cells multiplied by the total white cell count divided by 200.

All the subjects in the study received blood transfusion. Intravenous fluids and sodium bicarbonate were used as required. Artemether or quinine was administered at the appropriate dose.

Data analysis was done using Epi-info 2004 software package on a microcomputer. For simple proportion, frequency tables were generated. Chi square test and student's 't' test was used to test for significance of the difference between categorical and continuous variable respectively. Yates correction of Chi-square and Fisher's exact were used when appropriate. A p-value of <0.05 was regarded as significant.

## 7. Results

A total of nine hundred and eighty one (981) children were admitted into the Emergency Paediatric Unit from February to November 2006 of which 209 (21.3%) were cases of severe malaria. Among the children admitted with severe malaria, 96 (45.9%) had severe anaemia; thus severe anaemia due to malaria accounted for 9.8% of total admissions in the emergency paediatric unit. One hundred and eighty six children were recruited for the study, 93 each in the subject and control groups. There were 49 males and 44 females in each group with a male to female ratio of 1.1:1. (Table 1) The mean age for the subjects was 24.03 + 14.2 onths (range 6 - 60 onths) compared to 23.97 ± 14.3 onths in the controls and both were comparable (p = 0.91) About a third (32.3%) of the subjects were infants less than 12 months of age while 5.4% were children older than 48 months.

19.4% of the subjects presented to the hospital less within 3 days of onset of illness. A significantly higher proportion of the subjects presented later than 3 days compared to the controls ($\chi2 = 21.24$; $p = 0.001$).

| Parameter | Subjects n | % | Controls n | % | P |
|---|---|---|---|---|---|
| Sex | | | | | |
| Male | 49 | 52.3 | 49 | 52.3 | |
| Female | 44 | 47.7 | 44 | 47.7 | |
| Age in months | | | | | |
| 6 -12months | 30 | 32.3 | 30 | 32.3 | |
| 13-24months | 25 | 26.9 | 27 | 29.0 | |
| 24-36months | 18 | 19.4 | 17 | 18.3 | |
| 37-48months | 15 | 16.1 | 14 | 15.1 | |
| 49-60 months | 5 | 5.4 | 5 | 5.4 | |
| Duration of illness | | | | | |
| <3 days | 18 | 19.4 | 48 | 51.6 | |
| ≥3 days | 75 | 80.6 | 45 | 47.4 | 0.01 |
| Mean age (months) | 24.01 ± 14.2 | | 23.97 ± 14.3 | | |

Table 1. Sex and age distribution of the subjects and controls.

Figure 1 shows that forty five (45%) percent of the subjects were within social class IV-V while thirty two (32%) percent were in social class III using the Oyedeji Social classification Scheme.110 A statistically higher proportion of the subjects were in the lower socio economic classes IV - V compared to the controls. ($\chi2$ - 9.16; $p = 0.002$)

The predominant symptoms in both subjects and controls groups were fever, vomiting and refusal of feeds with comparable proportions as shown in Table 2. Breathlessness and convulsion were significantly prominent among the subjects than controls while easy fatigability, abdominal swelling and loss of consciousness were seen only among the subjects.

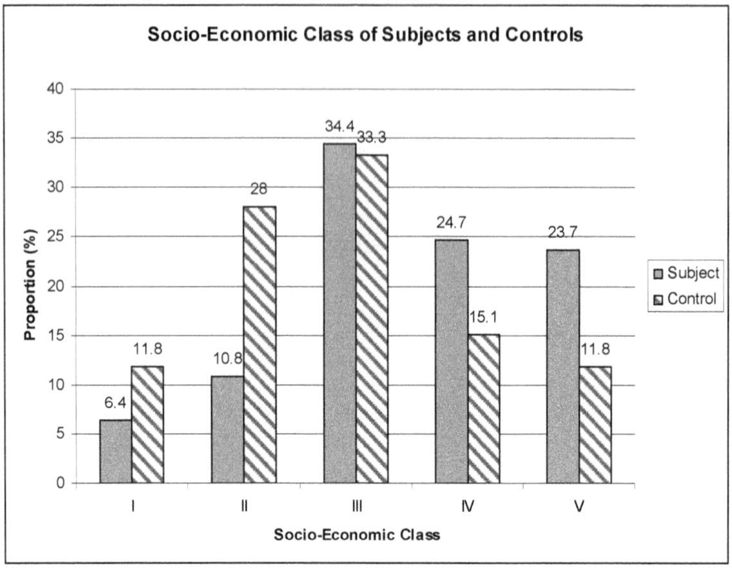


Fig. 1. Socioeconomic class of the subjects and controls.

| Symptom | Subjects | | Controls | | | | |
|---|---|---|---|---|---|---|---|
| | n | % | n | % | $\chi^2$ | p | OR(CI) |
| Fever | 91 | 97.8 | 86 | 92.5 | 2.90 | 0.088 | 1.6(1.1 -2.3) |
| Vomiting | 51 | 54.8 | 43 | 46.2 | 1.38 | 0.241 | 1.18(0.89-1.6) |
| Refusal of feeds | 68 | 73.1 | 56 | 60.2 | 3.48 | 0.062 | 1.32(1.0 -1.8) |
| Diarrhea | 20 | 21.5 | 18 | 19.4 | 0.13 | 0.72 | 1.07(0.74 -1.5) |
| Cough | 22 | 23.7 | 17 | 18.3 | 0.88 | 0.35 | 1.19(0.8 -1.8) |
| Breathlessness | 25 | 26.9 | 4 | 4.3 | 18.0 | 0.001 | 4.1(1.6 -10.3) |
| Convulsion | 26 | 30.0 | 3 | 3.2 | 21.6 | 0.001 | 5.5(1.88 -16.3) |
| Easy fatigability | 3 | 3.2 | 0 | 0 | 3.05 | 0.81 | 0.42(0.42 -0.6) |
| Abdominal swelling | 6 | 6.5 | 0 | 0 | 6.2 | 0.03 | 0.48(0.4 -0.6) |
| Loss of consciousness | 13 | 14.0 | 0 | 0 | 13.9 | 0.01 | 0.46(0.39 -0.5) |

Table 2. Symptoms among subjects and controls.

A combination of tachycardia and tachypnea was found in 33.3% of the subjects and 19.4% of the controls and the difference was statistically significant ($\chi 2 = 4.22$; $p = 0.04$). Among the subjects, 28% had a combination of tachycardia, tachypnea and tender hepatomegaly while 5.4% of the controls demonstrated similar signs and the difference was statistically significant.( $\chi 2 = 17.07$; $p = 0.001$) (Table 3).

| Sign | Subject | | Control | | | | |
|---|---|---|---|---|---|---|---|
| | n | % | n | % | $\chi^2$ | p | OR( CI) |
| Temperature | | | | | | | |
| <37.5⁰C | 19 | 20.4 | 14 | 15.1 | 0.92 | 0.33 | 1.45 (0.64 - 43.31) |
| 37.5-38.5⁰C | 41 | 44.1 | 43 | 46.2 | 0.09 | 0.76 | 0.92 (0.49 - 1.70) |
| >38.5⁰C | 33 | 35.5 | 33 | 38.7 | 0.02 | 0.88 | 1.00 (0.52 - 1.91) |
| Hydration Status | | | | | | | |
| Normal | 62 | 66.7 | 74 | 79.6 | 3.74 | 0.06 | 0.51 (0.25 - 1.05) |
| Mild - Moderate Dehydration | 27 | 29 | 19 | 20.4 | 1.85 | 0.17 | 1.59 (0.77 - 3.30) |
| Severe Dehydration | 4 | 4.3 | 0 | 0 | 4.09 | 0.04 | 2.04 (1.76 - 2.37) |
| Weight(% of expected | | | | | | | |
| <60% | 1 | 1.1 | 0 | 0 | 1.01 | 0.31 | - |
| 60-80% | 27 | 29 | 20 | 21.5 | 1.40 | 0.24 | 1.49 (0.73 - 3.07) |
| >80% | 65 | 69.9 | 73 | 78.5 | 1.80 | 0.18 | 0.64 (0.31 - 1.02) |
| Acidotic breathing | 18 | 19.4 | 7 | 7.5 | 5.6 | 0.01 | 2.95(1.1-8.3) |
| Tachypnea | 33 | 35.5 | 17 | 18.3 | 7.0 | 0.01 | 2.46( 1.2-5.1) |
| Tachycardia | 37 | 39.8 | 30 | 32.3 | 1.14 | 0.28 | 1.39(0.73 -2.65) |
| Gallop rhythm | 15 | 16.1 | 2 | 2.2 | 9.32 | 0.001 | 8.75(1.83 -57.2) |
| Blood pressure for age | | | | | | | |
| Hypotension | 2/31 | 6.5 | 0/42 | 0 | - | | - |
| Normal | 29/31 | 93.5 | 42/42 | 100 | 0.89 | 0.4 | - |
| Hepatomegaly | 87 | 93.5 | 54 | 58.1 | 31.92 | 0.001 | 2.3(1.8 -2.9) |
| Splenomegaly | 58 | 62.4 | 43 | 46.2 | 4.87 | 0.03 | 1.4(1.03-1.1.84) |
| Glasgow Coma Score | | | | | | | |
| ≤ 10 | 5 | 5.4 | 0 | 0 | 3.29 | 0.06 | |
| 11-14 | 8 | 8.7 | 0 | 0 | 6.4 | 0.01 | - |
| 15 | 80 | 85.9 | 93 | 100 | 13.98 | 0.001 | - |
| Tachycardia + Tachypnea | | | | | | | |
| | 31 | 33.3 | 18 | 19.4 | 4.68 | 0.03 | 2.1(1.0- 4.3) |
| Tachycardia+Tachypnea+Tender hepatomegaly | | | | | | | |
| | 26 | 28 | 5 | 5.4 | 17.07 | 0.001 | 3.52(1.56 -7.9) |

Table 3. Physical findings in the subjects and controls at presentation.

Table 4 shows the relationship between selected features and signs of decompensation defined as a combination of tachycardia, tachypnea and tender hepatomegaly among the subjects.

| Parameter | | Compensated n (%) | Decompensated n (%) | $\chi^2$ | p | OR( CI) |
|---|---|---|---|---|---|---|
| Age | <36 months | 48(71.6%) | 19(28.4%) | | | |
| | ≥36months | 19(73.1%) | 7(26.9%) | 0.02 | 0.89 | 1.1(0.50-2.21) |
| Sex | Male | 36(84.7%) | 13(15.3%) | | | |
| | Female | 31(82.9%) | 13(17.1%) | 0.10 | 0.75 | 1.04(0.8-1.34) |
| Social Class | I-II | 13(81.3%) | 3(18.8%) | 0.08 | 0.77 | 1.5(0.35-7.53) |
| | III | 23(71.9%) | 9(28.1%) | 0.3 | 0.58 | 0.76(0.26-2.25) |
| | IV-V | 34(75.6%) | 11(24.4%) | 0.01 | 0.95 | 1.03(0.36-2.93) |
| Duration of illness | ≤3days | 32(71.1%) | 13(28.9%) | | | |
| | >3days | 35(72.9%) | 13(27.1%) | 0.04 | 0.03 | 1.1(0.56-2.0) |
| Weight for age | <80% | 47(72.3%) | 18(27.7%) | | | |
| | ≥80% | 20(71.4%) | 8(28.6%) | 0.01 | 0.93 | 0.97(0.48-2.0) |
| Hydration Status | | | | | | |
| Normal | | 48(75.0%) | 14(25.0%) | 2.09 | 0.14 | 1.93(0.72-5.19) |
| Mild to Moderate dehydration | | 17(65.5%) | 10(34.5%) | 0.44 | 0.51 | 0.73(0.26 -2.05) |
| Severe dehydration | | 1(25.0%) | 3(75.0%) | 1.79 | 0.18 | 0.11(0.1-1.27) |
| Temperature | ≥38.9 | 30(45.5%) | 36(54.5%) | | | |
| | <38.9 | 8(29.6%) | 19(70.4%) | 1.99 | 0.16 | 0.76(0.56-1.1) |
| PCV | ≤ 12% | 41(68.3%) | 19(31.7%) | | | |
| | >12% | 26(78.8%) | 7(21.2%) | 1.16 | 0.28 | 1.5(0.70-3.2) |
| PCV | <15% | 67(72%) | 26(28%) | | | |
| (Controls) | 15 -20% | 26(96.3%) | 1(3.7%) | 2.41 | 0.01 | 0.1(0.00-0.72) |

Table 4. Factors associated with features of decompensation among the subjects.

Cardiac decompensation was not significantly affected by age, sex and social class. However children older than 36 months (OR 1.1(0.5-2.21) and male sex (OR 1.2 (0.5 -2.9) demonstrated an increased risk for decompensation though these were not statistically significant. Though approximately half (49.5%) of the subjects had PCV less than 12%, a higher proportion (31.7%) of the children in this group decompensated compared to 21.2% who decompensated in those with PCV greater than 12%. The difference however was not statistically significant. (p = 0.28 OR 1.5 CI 0.7 -3.2)). A statistically significant relationship was seen between duration of illness and risk of cardiac decompensation.(p = 0.03 OR - 1.1 CI 0.56 - 2.0)

Fifty percent of the subjects had PCV equal or greater than 12% while 36.6% and 12.9% had PCV of 9-11%.and less than 9% respectively. Among the controls, 70.3% had PCV 21-30% while approximately equal proportions had PCV 16-20% and greater than 30%. (Figure 2)

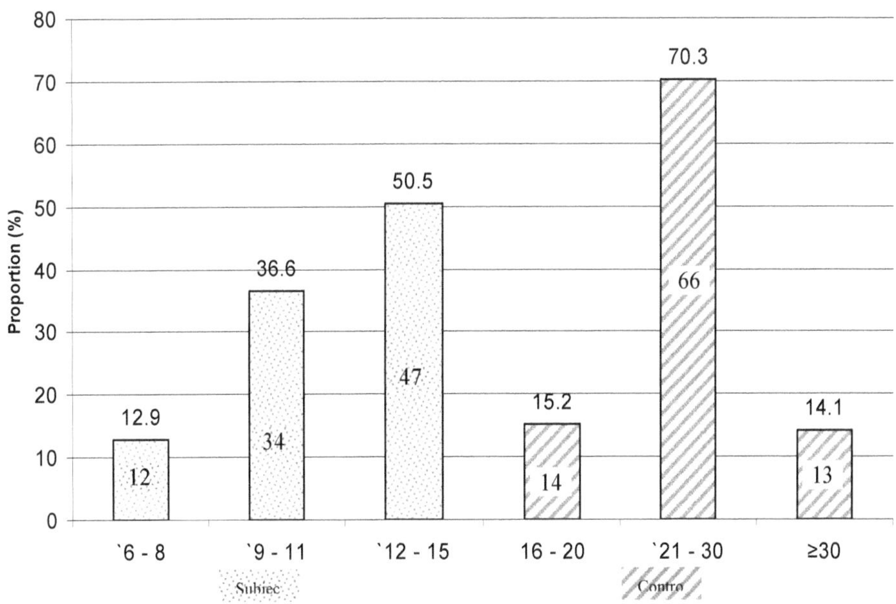


Fig. 2. PCV among subjects and controls.

About a fifth (21.5%) of the patients in both groups had comparable MCV values less than normal for age. However a significantly higher proportion of the subject group had high MCV values for age when compared with those with normal MCV ($\chi 2$ = 5.59; p = 0.02). (Table 5)

A significantly higher proportion of the subjects had low MCH values with 26.8% and 11.8% of subjects and controls respectively demonstrating low MCH values for age. ($\chi 2$ = 7.92; p = 0.004).

Leucocytosis was prominent in 53.7% of the subjects and 41.2% of the controls and a significantly lower proportion of the subjects (4.4%) had WBC less than 4000/mm3 compared to the 17.2% among the controls.($\chi 2$= 8.07;p = 0.01)

Thromobocytopenia was significantly found in 76.4% of the subjects ($\chi 2$ = 6.30; p =0.01).

| Parameter | Subject | Controls | p | $\chi^2$ | t |
|---|---|---|---|---|---|
| MCV | | | | | |
| Low | 20(21.5%) | 18(19.3%) | 0.72 | 0.13 | |
| Normal | 55(59.1%) | 68(73.2%) | 0.04 | 4.06 | |
| Elevated | 18(19.4%) | 7(7.5%) | 0.02 | 5.59 | |
| MCH | | | | | |
| Low | 25(26.8%) | 10(11.8%) | 0.004 | 7.92 | |
| Normal | 66(71%) | 82(88.2%) | 0.003 | 8.47 | |
| Elevated | 2(2.2%) | 1(1.1%) | 0.50 | 0.34 | |
| WBC Count(cells/mm$^3$) | | | | | |
| <4000 | 4(4.4%) | 16(17.2%) | 0.001 | 8.07 | |
| 4-11000 | 39(41.9%) | 35(37.6%) | 0.55 | 0.36 | |
| >11000 | 50(53.7%) | 42(41.2%) | 0.24 | 1.38 | |
| Platelet Count (cells/mm$^3$) | | | | | |
| < 150,000 | 71(76.4%) | 55(59.2%) | 0.01 | 6.30 | |
| 150-450000 | 20(21.5) | 37(38.7%) | 0.006 | 7.31 | |
| >450000 | 2(2.2%) | 1(1.1%) | 1.0 | 0.34 | |
| Blood Group | | | | | |
| A | 28(30.1%) | 33(35.5%) | 0.43 | 0.61 | |
| B | 30(32.3%) | 27(29%) | 0.63 | 0.23 | |
| O | 33(35.5%) | 32(34.4%) | 0.88 | 0.02 | |
| AB | 2(2.2%) | 1(1.1%) | 0.56 | 0.34 | |
| HbGenotype | | | | | |
| AA | 78(83.8%) | 73(78.5%) | 0.35 | 0.88 | |
| AS | 14(15.1%) | 20(21.5%) | 0.26 | 1.30 | |
| AC | 1(1.1%) | 0 | 0.32 | 1.01 | |
| Mean Values | | | | | |
| PCV(%) | 11.2 ± 2.24 | 25.6 ± 5.01 | 0.00 | | 25.0 |
| MCV(μm$^3$) | 79.3 ± 10.28 | 81.5 ± 6 .92 | 0.06 | | 1.9 |
| MCH(pg/cell) | 26.5 ± 4.08 | 28.4 ± 3.64 | 0.001 | | 3.44 |
| MCHC(%Hb/cell) | 31.0 ± 3.68 | 31.4 ± 2.84 | 0.6 | | 0.59 |
| WBC Count (cells/mm$^3$) | 15.1 ±1 2.93 | 10.9 ± 6.94 | 0.03 | | 3.1 |
| Platelet Count(cells/mm$^3$) | 112.8 ± 89.47 | 151.6 ± 86.94 | 0.01 | | 3.5 |

Table 5. Haematological Indices.

Fifty three percent (53%) of the subjeects and 18(19.4%) of the controls had parasite count greater than 250,000. (Figure 3)

The mean parasite count for children in the subject group was 499,450.43 ± 449,018.98 parasites/ml (range 8000 - 3,100,000) while for controls was 283,646 ± 357,224 parasites/ml (range 23000 -730000). Mean parasite count was significantly higher among subjects compared to the controls.($\chi 2 = 2.52$; $p = 0.014$).

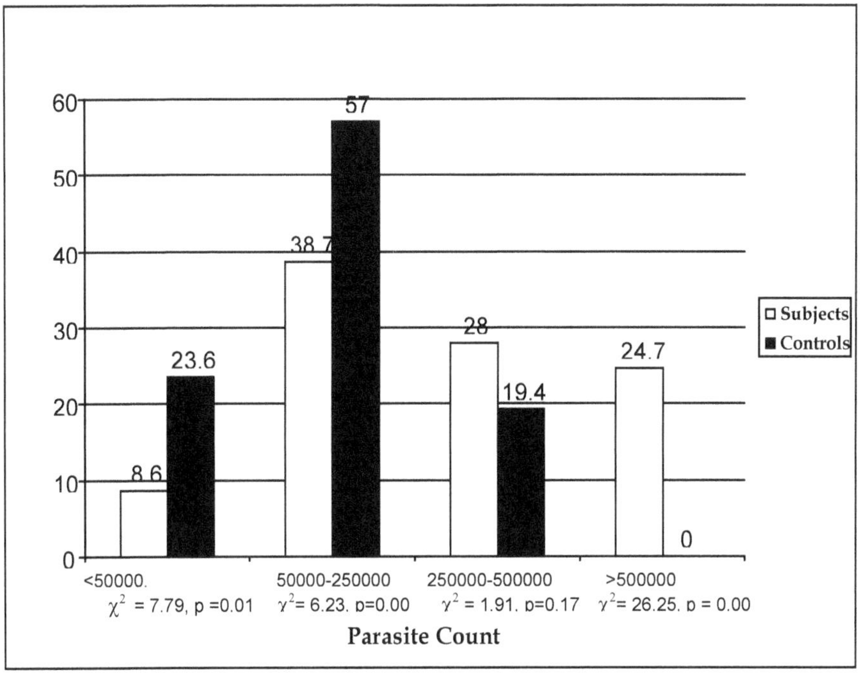


Fig. 3. Parasite Count in the subjects and controls

Table 6 shows the distribution of subjects and controls based on their parasite density across all age bands. Parasite count greater than 250,000 parasites/ml was significantly prominent among children less than 24 months. Sixty percent and forty eight percent of children in age bands 6 -12 months and 12-24 months respectively had parasite density higher than 250,000 parasites/ml ( $p = 0.01$). Among older children the proportions with parasite density higher than 250,000 parasites/ml were comparable with controls.

| Age Range (months) | | Parasite density | | $\chi^2$ | p |
|---|---|---|---|---|---|
| | | <250,000 n(/%) | >250,000 n( %) | | |
| 6-12 | Subjects | 12(40%) | 18(60%) | | |
| | Controls | 22(73%) | 89(27%) | 6.79 | 0.01 |
| 13-24 | Subjects | 13(52%) | 12(48%) | | |
| | Controls | 23(85%) | 4(15%) | 6.71 | 0.01 |
| 25-36 | Subjects | 10(56%) | 8(44%) | | |
| | Controls | 14(82%) | 3(18%) | 2.91 | 0.09 |
| 37-28 | Subjects | 8(53%) | 7(47%) | | |
| | Controls | 13(93%) | 1(7%) | 6.77 | 0.05 |
| 49-61 | Subjects | 3(43%) | 4(57%) | | |
| | Controls | 3(60%) | 2(40%) | 0.00 | 1.00 |

Table 6. Parasite count and age distribution among subjects and controls.

## 8. Discussion

Severe anaemia due to malaria accounted for 9% of all admissions into the Emergency Paediatric Unit (EPU) of the University of Ilorin Teaching Hospital similar to earlier reports of 5.2% in the same facility. (Ernest SK et al) This is comparable to 11.3% reported from Ibadan, Western Nigeria. (Orimadegun et al,2007) and 9.5% from Zambia ( Biemba et al, 2000) Several studies in holoendemic regions have documented severe anaemia as the predominant presentation of severe malaria including this study where it accounted for 45.9% of all cases of severe malaria.( Orimadegun et al,2007, Biemba et al, 2000) This is similar to the WHO report of a multicentre study that attributed a 51.2% contribution of severe anaemia to severe malaria burden in Ibadan.(WHO Report 2002) However Schellenberg et al in Tanzania and Modiano et al in Burkina Faso reported 24 and 21% prevalence of severe anaemia among severe malaria cases respectively. The huge burden of severe malaria and particularly severe malaria anaemia in malaria endemic region may be underestimated as a result of limited access to hospitals in developing countries.

Sixty percent (60%) of the children in the study were less than 24 months of age. This finding supports previous evidence that severe malaria anaemia is seen more frequently below 3 years with a mean age of 1.8 years.(WHO 2004) A reduction in the frequency of severe anaemia beyond 24 months of life with a two fold increase in prevalence of cerebral malaria across same age band had earlier been reported in Ghana and Mali.(Oduro et al, 2007, Ranque et al, 2008) The fact that most cases of severe anaemia are seen in children less than 2years of age is attributable to the smaller red cell mass and the relatively lower immunity to the malaria parasite compared to the older children.(Newton & Krishna, 1998) This study demonstrated a progressive and consistent reduction in proportion of severe malaria anaemia with increasing age supporting the assertion that repeated exposure to malaria with advancing age increased acquired immunity to the parasite with a reduction in severity of malaria presentation. There was a slight male preponderance among children with severe anaemia with a male to female ratio of 1.1:1. This simulates the pattern among general hospital admissions as has been reported in most studies on severe malaria.(Berkley et al, 1999, Chessebrough, 1998) More than half of the children were from the lower socioeconomic classes III-V. Hedberg et al in Kinshasha found low socioeconomic status to be independently associated with anaemia. The children of parents with high socioeconomic status are likely to be relatively shielded from mosquitoes, live in environments with little or no breeding grounds for mosquitoes, have access to malaria prevention methods, early diagnosis and treatment. Poor nutrition, high cost and or unavailability of health services contribute to poor health seeking behaviour in this group of children of parents who belong to low socio economic classes.

Severe malaria anaemia in many cases presents as an acute illness as found in this study with 48% of the patients presenting to the hospital within 3 days after onset of illness. The mean duration of illness of the subjects was 4.3 days. Studies in The Gambia and Burkina Faso reported mean duration of illness of 2 and 3.1 days respectively for children with severe malaria.(Jaff et al, 1997, Modiano et al, 1999) It has been established that severe malaria is rapidly progressive in children with most deaths occurring within 24 hours thus definitive intervention must be undertaken within first 24 -48 hours of the illness if mortality is to be prevented. (Ernest et al, 2002, Greenwood, 1997) Fever was the commonest symptom reported in 97% of patients and pyrexia was documented at presentation in 77.4% of the children with severe malaria anaemia. Vomiting and refusals of feeds were equally prominent symptoms in this study. These are largely nonspecific symptoms and are found in most febrile illnesses in children. In this study, fast breathing and convulsion were more prominent in the patients with severe anaemia than controls. A third of the children in this study were underweight while Kwashiokor and Marasmic Kwashiokor were not common findings. The low weight for age may be related to the socio economic status of the study group and suggests an interplay between nutritional anaemia and malaria amongst them. Several studies have however reported a high incidence of severe anaemia due to malaria among children with low weight for age.(Oduro et al, 2007, Hedberg et al, 1993) The rarity of Marasmus and Marasmic Kwashiokor further confirms earlier findings that severe malaria particularly cerebral malaria is not commonly seen in children with severe malnutrition. Severe malaria anaemia is partly immune mediated requiring both cellular and humoral mechanisms for its evolution.(Turrini et al, 2003, Sandau et al, 2001) Immunosuppression depresses this mechanism and account for the uncommon presentation of severe malaria among children with severe malnutrition. Hepatomegaly, splenomegaly, pyrexia and tachycardia were the most prominent signs. Hepatomegaly and splenomegaly occurred in 94% and 58% of children respectively. A strong correlation between parasitaemia and organ enlargement has been reported.(Hedberg et al, 1993, Mongensen et al, 2006) This is explained by the congestion of parasite infested red cells, hypertrophy and erythrophagocytosis in the reticuloendothelial system particularly the spleen and liver.(Taylor & Molyneux, 2002) The higher preponderance of hepatomegaly over splenomegaly suggests additional mechanism for organ enlargement particularly fluid retention as may occur following anaemic heart failure in decompensated children.

Tachycardia was more prominent among children with severe malaria anaemia (40%) than controls (32%) though this was not found to be statistically significant. The pathophysiology of tachycardia in severe malaria is multifactorial particularly with in the presence of fever, dehydration and anaemia. Therefore tachycardia in isolation may not necessarily imply cardiac decompensation. Slow decline in haematocrit allows for effective adaptation to anaemic states and may reduce the severity of tachycardia seen among the children with severe malaria anaemia who presented late for treatment. (Moroff & Dend, 1983, Card & Brabin, 1973)

Less than a third of the children in both groups had signs of dehydration. Gastrointestinal symptoms (diarrhea, vomiting, anorexia) and late presentation contribute to dehydration. The reduced body water and intravascular space also contribute to tachycardia. In one study, severe malaria was found to be associated with about 6.7% reduction in total body water, a loss, marginally greater than values for mild dehydration such that overzealous volume expansion may be detrimental (Planche et al, 2004) Increased insensible loss from pyrexia, sweating and tachypnea are contributory factors to fluid loss in the study population. Despite the longer duration of illness and prominence of tachypnea, many of the children with severe malaria anaemia showed no or minimal signs of dehydration. We postulate that activation of the renin angiotensin aldosterone system secondary to hypoxia and hypovolemia result in compensatory fluid retention.

Decompensation occurs as a result of a breakdown in maintenance of tissue oxygenation and manifests as signs of cardiorespiratory decompensation or cardiac failure. These signs are tachycardia tachypnea and tender hepatomegaly with or without cardiomegaly. (Orimadegun et al, 2007( A combination of tachycardia, tachypnea and tender hepatomegaly was seen in 28% of the children while the majority of children in the study (72%) were stable. Therefore it may be possible to avoid blood transfusion with its attendant risks among majority of children with SMA if facilities for close observation and early identification of need for transfusion are available. This has been severally reported that many children with severe malaria anaemia remain stable.( Mulenga M et al, 2005, Lackritz et al, 1992, English et al, 2002) The mean PCV of the subjects was 11.2% and half of the children had PCV less than 12%. Signs of cardiac decompensation were demonstrated by similar proportions of subjects with PCV ≤ 12% and those with higher PCV however, among the 26 children who decompensated, seven (27%) had haematocrit levels higher than 12% while 73% had levels ≤ 12%. A study found no difference in mortality among children with a mean of PCV 14.1% randomized for blood transfusion or a more conservative management.(Holzer et al,1993) Mortality was significantly higher in children who had a combination of Hb < 4.7g/dL and clinical findings of respiratory distress. (Lackritz et al, 1992) Similar findings of high mortality in children with PCV < 14% with or without respiratory distress was documented in a study by English et al in 1996. A strict PCV threshold may be insufficient for instituting blood transfusion across board. This study has shown that signs of decompensation become more prominent when PCV declines below 15% compared to higher levels of PCV among controls. However other factors contribute to the risk of decompensation as majority of children remain stable irrespective of haematocrit.

Presentation at a health facility later than 3 days after onset of illness significantly reduced the risk of decompensation ($p = 0.03$). Decompensation occurred within first 72 hours of onset of illness in many cases. This can be attributed to the sudden onset of illness before compensatory mechanisms were well established. Lackritz et al reported that blood transfusion given after a delay of 2 days did not significantly affect mortality suggesting that deaths due to anaemia may be considerably greater in the communities than in hospitals where prompt treatment is administered.(Lacritz et al, 1992) In Ilorin, North Central Nigeria a reduction in mortality in children with severe anaemia who did not receive blood transfusion when they survived longer than 24 hours was found.(Ernest et al, 2002) All these confirm that severe malaria is a rapidly progressing disease and early intervention is required within the first 48hours of illness if mortality is to be limited.(Greenwood, 1997) This also accounts for the relative stability observed in the majority of the study subjects as majority presented later than 72 hours to the facility. Less occurrence of features of decompensation in the children who presented later than 3 days after onset of illness may also be attributed to the possible slower decline in haematocrit during the course of the illness and the gradual deployment of compensatory mechanisms particularly synthesis of 2, 3 diphosphoglycerate which allows for increased oxygen extraction from haemoglobin. (Tuman, 1990)

Age at presentation did not significantly contribute to the risk of decompensation when comparing children younger or older than 36 months. This contrasts with previous works that younger children tolerate anemia better. (Ehrhardt et al, 2006, Tuman,1990) A conclusion however can not be made on the protective value of age as no comparison was made with older children and adults. Dehydration was not significantly associated with decompensation in this study. Ranque et al in Mali reported that SMA was less associated with dehydration than cerebral malaria. (Ranque et al, 1990) Conversely in another study, volume contraction and reduced central venous pressure were found in decompensated children advocating for volume expansion or whole blood transfusion for children presenting with severe anaemia due to malaria.(Marsh et al, 1995) The degree of dehydration is variable and may also be affected by other factors including reduced intake, vomiting and hyperpyrexia. It is therefore difficult to give general recommendations for fluid therapy in severe malaria anaemia cases without individual assessment of hydration status. Other factors that showed no relationship with decompensation include sex, socio economic status and temperature at presentation. High grade pyrexia was seen in 29% of the children, among whom 70.4% were observed to have decompensated compared to 55% that decompensated among children with low grade pyrexia. However this finding was not statistically significant and may be as a result of the small number of children in the category with high grade pyrexia. It does however suggests the contribution of temperature to degree of tachycardia as it is known that heart rate increases by 2.44 beats for every 0.6oC rise above normal temperature.(Mackowaik et al, 1992) The management of pyrexia is therefore of utmost importance not only in prevention of febrile convulsions but also to reduce its contribution to cardiac decompensation.

Hyperparasitaemia was a common laboratory finding in children with severe anaemia in this study as 24.7% and 52.7% of children with severe malaria anaemia had parasite densities greater than 500,000parasites/mL and 250,000parasites/mL respectively. Sowunmi et al in Ibadan, South western Nigeria found age less than 5 years to be an independent risk factor for hyperparasitaemia. (Sowunmi et al, 2004 ) Hyperparasitaemia was significantly prominent in children with severe malaria anaemia who were less than 24 months compared with the controls. This finding can be explained by the waning of maternal antibody protection and increased exposure to the mosquito as the child becomes more ambulant. The prominence of hyperparasitemia in this age range reiterates the need for appropriate chemotherapy for malaria parasitaemia to prevent severe malaria. Leucocytosis was the predominant finding among children with severe anaemia. The possibility of superimposed bacterial sepsis may explain the prominence of leucocytosis in these children as over half of the subjects presented later than 3 days after onset of illness. Researchers have documented 7.8 - 15.6% prevalence of bacteraemia complicating severe malaria particularly in children under 3 years. (Berkley et al, 1999, Enwere et al, 1998) A great overlap exists between severe malaria and the incidence of bacteremia as the two conditions are commoner in younger children.(Newton et al, 1997) Severe malaria potentiates this by reducing splanchnic perfusion and causing intestinal and hepatic hypoxia. This effect is brought about by sequestration of parasites in splanchnic beds and the shunting of blood away from the gastrointestinal tract to essential organs as a compensation for hypoxia associated with severe anaemia. Entry of gram negative organisms and endotoxins from the gut lumen is thus enhanced coupled with the reduction in normal hepatic filtration of these toxins and bacteria.(Usawattanahul et al, 1985) Reduced gastric acidity and immaturity of the gut lymphoid tissue in young children contribute to this.(Miller et al, 1995) Gram negative organisms particularly Non Typhoidal Salmonella sp have been reported in association with severe malaria.(Ayoola et al, 2005) They also found Escherichia coli as the commonest organism isolated in association with malaria parasitaemia. The predisposition to bacteraemia may be related to low socioeconomic status of the study group with associated poor living conditions particularly as enteral organisms have been commonly reported by many studies. WHO recommends that, threshold for administration of broad spectrum antibiotics should be low in severe malaria because of the diagnostic overlap between severe malaria and septicaemia.(WHO Library, 2006) The use of antibiotics for children with severe malaria who demonstrate poor response to potent anti malaria chemotherapy is justified to reduce mortality. Thrombocytopenia was found in 76.4% of the children, however none presented with features of disseminated coagulopathy such as bleeding diathesis. This has been reported to be a feature of falciparum malaria and is more profound in severe forms.(Viroj, 2008) Reasons for thrombocytopenia include reduced platelet survival, bone marrow suppression, destruction by anti platelet antibodies and most significantly sequestration of platelets and removal by the spleen. Disseminated intravascular hemolysis is uncommon and if present suggests an additional pathology in most instances particularly gram negative septicaemia. Normocytic normochromic anaemia with normal MCV and MCH for age was found in majority of the children with severe malaria anaemia. A fifth (21.5%) of the children had microcytic anaemia with low MCV for age. A similar proportion had low MCH values. Isolated SMA presents as normocytic normochromic anaemia however co morbidities like nutritional deficiencies and parasitic infections particularly hook worm infestations may complicate the picture with microcytic or macrocytic features. Iron deficiency anaemia, a common consequence of nutritional deficiency of iron may not be unexpected as a third of children had low weight for age while majority of the children were from low socio economic class. Premji et al reported that majority of children infected with P. falciparum were iron deficient. (Premji et al, 1995) In a randomized study in Tanzania, children given iron supplementation had low incidence of severe anaemia than those who had placebo.( Menendez et al, 1997) These findings support the multifactorial aetiology of severe anaemia and the use of iron supplementation to reduce incidence of severe anaemia in children living in malaria endemic regions. In this study

Children with SMA had a significantly higher incidence of microcytic anaemia than controls with 19.4% presenting with high MCV for age. A co morbid state of megaloblastic anaemia or reticulocytosis following rapid bone marrow response to hemolysis may account for these findings.

AS genotype was found in a smaller proportion (15.1%) of children with severe malaria anaemia compared to controls (22%) though the difference showed no statistical significance. Traditional knowledge AS genotype has been established to protect against the progression to severe forms of malaria. The mechanisms by which mutant haemoglobins protect against severe malaria have not been definitively established and are likely multifactorial. In vitro culture experiments have shown that parasitized AS erythrocytes are more likely to sickle and support reduced parasite growth rates than their non parsitized counterparts under conditions of low oxygen tension.(Pasvol, 1980) The protection is however at the expense of early clearance of parasitized red blood cell by the spleen and contributes to some degree of anemia seen among children with AS genotype in malaria endemic regions. In this study, the lesser proportion of AS genotype found among the children with severe malaria anaemia strengthens the assertion. The ABO blood group also demonstrated no protection against severe malaria anaemia as a similar blood group distribution in the general population was found among children with severe anaemia due to malaria. This is at variance with the findings of other workers who found that parasite virulence is reduced in blood group O erythrocytes compared with groups A, B and AB suggesting that Blood group O may confer resistance to severe falciparum malaria. A matched case-control study of 567 Malian children found that group O was present in only 21% of severe malaria cases compared with 44–45% of uncomplicated malaria controls and healthy controls. Group O was associated with a 66% reduction in the odds of developing severe malaria compared with the non-O blood groups.(Mercereau & Menard, 2010) Others have confirmed that blood group A is a co receptor for plasmodium falciparum rossetting, a mechanism by which the parasite potentiates its virulence causing severe malaria.(Barragan et al, 2000) The sample size may be too small to demonstrate this effect in the study in addition to other findings that suggest the multifactorial aetiology of severe anaemia in children with malaria.

## 9. Conclusion

This study has demonstrated the clinical burden of severe malaria anaemia as a common indication for admission of young children into emergency units particularly children less than 24 months of age. The common clinical and laboratory presentation of this disease were also highlighted.

This study suggests a multifactorial aetiology for SMA and also confirming that majority of affected children are clinically stable without signs of decompensation. Clinical stealth needs to be applied in determining need for transfusion in the current era of blood borne morbidities particularly HIV and hepatitis in malaria prone regions. A larger randomized study with alternative therapies needs to be conducted to prescribe clinical and laboratory guides for transfusion interventions.

But in the interim, a higher threshold has been sensitized particularly in 3 situations;

a. clinical stable children with severe malaria anaemia with PCV >12%,

b. presence of capacity for close monitoring of patient's clinical profile for emergency transfusion while undergoing conservative management
c. availability of potent appropriate anti malaria interventions.

Appropriate preventive strategies should focus on early recognition and prompt treatment of malaria to prevent progression to severe malaria, provision of free or cheap anti malaria medications to reduce progression of malaria to severe forms and improvement in the living conditions particularly appropriate feeding practices to reduce incidence of malaria and anaemia associated with iron deficiency.

## 10. Acknowledgement

We acknowledge the contributions of individuals, paediatricians who have contributed to the body of knowledge on severe malaria and haematological conditions in children. We thank all those whose active or passive participation enriched the process particularly the published works on severe malaria.

## 11. References

Abdalla SH. Hematopoiesis in human malaria. Blood Cells 1990; 16: 401–416.

Afolabi BM, Salako LA, Mafe AG, Ovwigbo UB, Rabiu KA, Sanyaolu NO et al. Malaria in the first six months of life in urban African infants with anaemia. Am J Trop Med Hyg 2002; 65: 822-827.

Allen SJ, O'Donnell A, Alexander ND, Alpers MP, Peto TE, Clegg JB et al. thalassaemia protects children against disease caused by other infections as well as malaria. Proceedings of the National Academy of sciences of the USA. 1997; 94: 14736-14741.

Allison AC. Protection afforded by sickle cell trait against sub tertian malaria infection.Br Med J 1954; 1: 290-294.

Angela O'Donnell, Premawardhena A, Arambepola M, Allen SJ, Peto EA, Fisher CA et al. Age related changes in adaptation to severe anaemia in childhood in developing countries. Proc Natl Acad Sci USA 2007;104:9440-9444.

Anderson KC, Weinstein HS. Transfusion associated graft vs host disease. N Eng J Med 1990; 323: 315-321.

Anonymous: Developments in malaria immunology. WHO Technical Report Series, 1975; 579:1-45.

Anyona SB, Schrier SL, Gichuki CW, Waitumbi JN. Pitting of malaria parasites and spherocytes formation. Malaria Journal 2006; 5: 64-65.

Arese P, Schwarzwer E. Malarial pigment (haemozoin): a very active "inert" substance. Ann Trop Med Parasitol 1997; 91:501–516.

Ayoola OO, Adeyemo AA, Osinusi K. Concurrent bacteraemia and malaria in febrile Nigerian infants. Trop Doct 2005; 35: 34 -36.

Barragan A, Kremsner PG, Wahlgren M, Carlson J. Blood group A antigen is a coreceptor in Plasmodium falciparum rosetting. Infect Immun 2000; 68: 2971-2975.

Bates I, Bedu Addo G, Bevan DH. Use of immunoglobin gene rearrangement to show clonal lymphoproliferative is hypereactive malarial splenomegaly. Lancet 1991; 337:505–507.

Berkley J, Nwarumba S, Bramham K, Lowe B, Marsh K. Bacteraemia complicating severe malaria in children. Trans R Soc Trop Med Hyg 1999; 93: 283-286.

Biemba G, Dolmans D, Thuma PE, Weiss G, Gordeuk VR. Severe anaemia in Zambian children with Plasmodium falciparum malaria. Trop Med Int Health. 2000; 5: 9-16.

Bojang KA, Palmer A, Boelevan Hensbroek M, Banya WA, Greenwood BM.Management of severe malarial anaemia in Gambian children. Trans R Soc Trop Med Hyg 1997; 91: 557-561.

Brabin BJ, Premji Z, Verhoeff F. An analysis of anaemia and child mortality. J Nutr 2002; 131: 636-645.

Card R, Brain M. The "anaemia" of childhood, evidence for physiologic response to hyperphosphatemia. N Eng J Med 1973; 28: 388-392.

Caulfield LE, Richard SA, Black RE: Undernutrition as an underlying cause of malaria morbidity and mortality in children less than five years old. Am J Trop Med Hyg 2004; 71:55-63.

Cheesebrough M. Haematological tests. In Cheesbrough M (eds). District Laboratory Practice in Tropical countries. Cambridge: University Press UK; 1998. pg 320-329..

Clark IA, Cowden WB. The pathophysiology of falciparum malaria. Pharmacol Ther 2003; 99: 221-260.

Clark IA, Rockett KA, Cowden WB. Proposed link between cytokines, nitric acid and human cerebral malaria. Parasitol Today 1991; 7:205-207.

Clemens R, Pramoolsinaap C, Lorenz R, Pukrittayakamee S, Bock HL, white NJ. Activation of the coagulation cascade in severe falciparum malaria through the intrinsic pathway. Bri J Haem 1994; 87:100-105.

Edington GM, Gilles HM. Malaria. In: Pathology in tropics. 2nded. London: Edward Arnold Ltd; 1976. pg 10-34.

Ehrhardt S, Burchard GD, Mantel C, Cramer JP, Kaiser S, Kubo M et al. Malaria, anemia, and malnutrition in african children - defining intervention priorities. J Infect Dis. 2006; 194: 108-114.

English M, Waruiru C, Amukoye E, Murph S, Crawley J, Mwangi I et al. Deep acidotic breathing in children with severe anaemia: Indicator of metabolic acidosis and poor outcome. Am J Trop Med Hyg 1996; 55: 521-524.

English M, Waruiru C, Marsh K. Transfusion for life threatening respiratory distress in severe childhood malaria. Am J Trop Med Hyg 1996; 55: 525-530.

English M, Ahmed M, Ngando C, Berkley J, Ross A. Blood transfusion for severe anaemia in children in a Kenyan hospital. Lancet 2002; 359: 494-5Ernest SK, Anunobi NE, Adeniyi A. Correlates of emergency response and mortality from severe anaemia in childhood. West Afr J Med 2002; 21: 177-179.

Enwere G, Hensbroek MBV, Adegbola R, Palmer A. Bacteraemia in cerebral malaria. Ann Trop Paediatr 1998; 18: 275-278.

Falade C, Mokuolu O, Okafor H, Orogade A, Falade A, Adedoyin O et al. Epidemiology of congenital malaria in Nigeria: a multi-centre study. Trop Med Int Health. 2007; 12 :1279-1287.

Gamain B, Smith JD, Miller LH, Baruch OI. Modification of CD 36 binding domain of P. falciparum variant antigen are responsible for the inability of chondrointin sulphate adherent parasites to bond CD 36. Blood 2001; 97: 3268-3274.

Ghosh K. Pathogenesis of anaemia in malaria, a concise review Parasitol Res. 2007; 101:1463-1469.

Gilles HM. The development of malaria infection in breastfed Gambian infants. Ann Trop Med Parasitol 1957; 51: 58-59.

Grobusch MP, Kremsner PG. Uncomplicated Malaria. Currr Top Microbiol Immunol 2005; 295: 83-104.

Guidelines for red blood cell and plasma transfusion for adults and children. Can Med Ass J 2004; 156: 121-134.

Halim NKD, Offor E, Ajayi OI. Epidemiological study of seroprevalence of Hepatitis B surface antigen and HIV 1 in blood donors. Niger J Clin Pract 1999; 2: 1-34.

Hedberg K, Shaffer N, Davachi F, Hightower A, Lyamba B, Paluku KM et al. Plasmodium falciparum-associated anemia in children at a large urban hospital in Zaire. Am J Trop Med Hyg. 1993; 48: 365-371.

Holzer B, Egger M, Teuscher T. Chidhood anaemia in Africa: To transfuse or not transfuse. Acta Trop 1993; 5: 47-51.

Issifou S, Mavoungou E, Borrmann S, Bouyou-Akotet Mk, Matsiegui PI, Kremsner PG, et al. Severe malarial anaemia associated with increased soluble Fas ligand concentrations in Gabonese children. Eur Cytokine Netw 2003; 14: 238-41.

Jaff S, Hensbroek MBV, Palmer A, Schneider G, Greenwood B. Predictors of a fatal outcome following cerebral malaria. Am J Trop Med Hyg 1997; 57: 20-24.

Jhaveri KN, Ghosh K, Mohanty D, Parmar BD, Surati RR, Camoens HM, Joshi SH et al. Autoantibodies immunoglobulins, complement and circulating immune complexes in acute malaria. Natl Med J India 1997; 54: 23–29.

Karunaweera ND, Carter R, Grau GE, Mendis KN. Demonstration of anti-disease immunity to Plasmodium vivax malaria in Sri Lanka using a quantitative method to assess clinical disease. Am J Trop Med Hyg 1998; 58: 204-210.

Krause PJ. Malaria. In: Behrman RE, Kligman RM, Jenson HB (eds). Nelson textbook of Paediatrics, 18th Ed. Philadelphia: WB Saunders; 2000. pg 1477-1484.

Lackritz EM, Campbell CC, Ruebush TK, Hightower AW, Wakube W, Steketee RW et al. Effect of blood transfusion on survival among children in a Kenyan hospital. Lancet.1992; 340: 524-528.

Looareesuwan S, Ho M, Wattanagoon Y, White NJ, Warrell DA, Bunnaq D et al. Dynamic alterations in splenic function during acute falciparum malaria. N Engl J Med 1997; 317: 678–681.

Luzzattto L. Genetic factors in malaria. Bull WHO 1974; 50: 195-202.

Maitland K, Pamba A, Newton CR, Levin M. Response to volume resuscitation in children with severe anaemia. Paedtr Crit Care Med 2003; 4: 426-431.

Mackowaik PA, Wasseman SS, Levine MM. A critical appraisal of 98.6F, the upper limit of the normal body temperature and other legacies of Carl Reinhold August Wunderlich. JAMA. 1992;268:1578-1580.

Marsh K. Immunology of malaria. In: Warell DA, Gilles HM(ed). Essential Malariology 4th Ed, London: Arnold Publications; 2002. pg 252 – 267.

Marsh K, Forster D, Waruiru C, Mwangi I, Wistanley M, Marsh V et al. Life threatening malaria in African children; clinical spectrum and simplified prognostic criteria. N Eng J Med 1995; 322: 1399-1404.

McDevitt MA, Xie J, Gordeuk V, Bucala R. The anaemia of malaria infection: role of inflammatory cytokines. Curr Haematol Rep 2004; 3: 97-106.

Menendez C, Kahigwa E, Hirt R, Vounatsou P, Aponte JJ, Font F et a. Randomised placebo-controlled trial of iron supplementation and malaria chemoprophylaxis for prevention of severe anaemia and malaria in Tanzanian infants. Lancet. 1997; 350: 844-850.

Mercereau-Puijalon O, Ménard D Plasmodium vivax and the Duffy antigen: a paradigm revisited Transfus Clin Biol. 2010 Sep;17(3):176-83. Epub 2010 Jul 23.

Meremikwu M, Smith HJ. Blood transfusion for treating malarial anaemia. In: The Cochrane Library, 2004; 3:1-76.

Miller SI, Hohmann EL, Pegues DA. Salmonella (including Salmonella typhi ). In: Mandell GL, Bennett JE, Dolin R. (eds). Mandell, Douglas and Bennett's principles and practice of infectious diseases, 4th edn. New York, Churchill Livingstone,1995: 2013

Miller LH, Mason SJ, Clyde DF, McGinniss MH. Innate resistance in malaria. Exp Parasitol 1976; 40: 132-146.

Miller LH, Mason SJ, Clyde DF, McGinniss MH. The resistance factor to plasmodium vivax in blacks. The Duffy-blood-group genotype, Fy Fy. N Engl J Med 1976; 295: 302-304.

Mockenhaupt FP, Eghardt S, Buckhardt J, Bosomtwe SY, Laryea S, Anemana SD, et al. Manifestations and outcome of severe malaria in children in Northern Ghana: Am J Trop Med Hyg 2004; 71: 167-72.

Modiano D, Sirima BS, Sawadogo A, Sanou I,Pare J,Konate A et al. Severe malaria in Burkina Faso: urban and rural environment. Parasitologia 1999; 41: 251-254.

Mongensen CB, Soerensen J, Bjorkman A, Montgomery SM. Algorithm for the diagnosis of anaemia without laboratory facilities among small children in a malaria endemic of rural Tanzania. Acta Trop 2006; 99: 119-125.

Moroff G, Dend D. Characterization of biochemical changes occurring with storage of red cells; comparative studies with CPD and CPDA-1. Transfusion 1983; 23: 484-489.

Mulenga M, Malunga P, Bennett S, Thuma PE, Shulman C, Fielding K et al. Factors associated with severe anaemia in Zambian children admitted with Plasmodium falciparum malarial anaemia. Ann Trop Paediatr 2005; 25: 87-90.

Newton CR, Krishna S. Severe falciparum malaria in children. Current understanding of pathophysiology and supportive treatment. Pharmacol Ther 1998; 79: 1-53.

Newton CR, Marsh K, Peshu N, Mwayi I. Blood transfusion For severe anaemia in African children. Lancet 1992; 340: 917-918.

Newton CR, Warn PA, Winstanley PA, Peshu N, Snow RW, Pasvol G et al. Severe anaemia in children living in a malaria endemic area of Kenya. Trop Med Int Health. 1997; 2: 165-178.

Oduro AR, Koram KA, Rogers W, Atuguba F, Ansah P, Anyorigiya T et al. Severe falciparum malaria in young children of the Kassena-Nankana district of northern Ghana. Malar J. 2007; 6: 96-97.

Okiro EA, Al-Taiar A, Reyburn H, Idro R, Berkley JA, Snow RW. Age patterns of severe paediatric malaria and their relationship to plasmodium falciparum intensity. Malar J. 2009; 8: 4 -5.

Oppenheimer SJ. Iron and malaria. Parasitol Today 1989; 5:77–82.

Orimadegun AE, Fawole O, Okereke JO, Akinbami FO, Sodeinde. Increasing burden of childhood severe malaria in a Nigerian tertiary hospital: implication for control. J Trop Pediatr. 2007; 53: 185-189.WHO Malaria action programme; severe and complicated malaria. Trans R Soc Trop Med & Hyg 1986; 80:1-76.

Ouma C, Davenport GC, Awandare GA, Keller CC, Were T, Otieno MF et al. Polymorphic variability in the interleukin (IL)-1beta promoter conditions susceptibility to severe malaria anaemia and functional changes in IL-1 beta susceptibility. J Infect Dis. 2008;198:1219-1226.

Pamba A, Maitland K. Capillary refill: Prognostic value in Kenyan children. Arch Dis Child 2004; 89: 950-955.

Pasvol G. the interaction between sickle haemoglobin and the malaria parsite. Trans R Soc Trop Med Hyg 1980; 74:701-750.

Planche T, Onanga M, Schwnk A, Dzeing A, Borrman S, Faucher J et al. Assessment of volume depletion in children with malaria. Plos Med 2004; 1:18-20.

Premji Z, Hamisi Y, Shiff C, Minjas J, Lubega P, Makwaya C. Anaemia and Plasmodium falciparum infections among young children in an holoendemic area, Bagamoyo, Tanzania. Acta Trop. 1995; 59: 55-64.

Ranque S, Poudiougou B, Traoré A, Keita M, Oumar AA, Safeukui I et al. Life-threatening malaria in African children: a prospective study in a mesoendemic urban setting: Pediatr Infect Dis J. 2008; 27: 130-135.

Roberts DJ, Casals-Pascul C, Weatherall DJ The clinical and pathophysiological features of malarial anemia. Curr Trop Microbiol Immunol 2005; 295:137–167.

Ronald G. Strauss. Blood and blood component transfusion. In: Behrman RE, Kligman RM, Jenson HB(editors). Nelson textbook of paediatrics 18th Ed. Philadelphia: WB Saunders; 2000. pg 2055 - 2056.

Rowe JA, Handel IG, Thera MA, Deans AM, Lyke KE, Koné A et al. Blood group O protects against severe Plasmodium falciparum malaria through the mechanism of reduced resetting. Proc Natl Acad Sci U S A 2007; 104: 17471-17476

Salako LA, Ajayi FO, Sowunmi A, Walker O. Malaria in Nigeria: a revisit. Ann Trop Med Parasitol 1990; 84: 435-45.

Salako LA, Walker O, Sowunmi A, Omokhodion SJ, Adio R, Oduola AM. Artemether in moderately severe and cerebral malaria in Nigerian children. Trans R Soc Trop Med Hyg 1994; 88: 13-15.

Sandau KB, Zhou J, Kietzmann T, Brune B. Regulation of hypoxia-inducible factoralpha by the inflammatory mediators nitric oxide and tumor necrosis, factor alpha in contrast to desferroxamine and phenylarsine oxide. J Biol Chem 2001; 276: 39805-39811.

Satpathy SK, Mohanby N, Naida P, Samal G. Severe falciparum malaria. Indian J Pediatr 2004; 71: 133-5.

Schellenberg D, Menendez C, Kahigwa E, Font F, Galindo C, Acosta C. African Children with Malaria in Area of Intense Plasmodium Falciparum Transmission : Features on admission to the hospital and risk factors for death. Ann. J Trop Med Hyg 1999; 61: 431-438.

Severe falciparum malaria(WHO).communicable diseases cluster. Trans R Soc Trop Med Hyg 2004; 94:1-90.

Silamut K, White NJ. Relation of the stage of parasite development in the peripheral blood to prognosis in severe falciparum malaria. Trans Roy Soc Trop Med Hyg 1993; 87: 436-443.

Snow RW, Gilles HM. Sinden RE, Gilles HM. The malaria parasite, In: Warell DA, Gilles HM(ed). Essential Malariology 4th Ed. London: Arnold Publications; 2002. pg 85-106.

Sowunmi A, Adedeji AA, Fateye BA, Babalola CP. Plasmodium falciparum hyperparasitaemia in children. Risk factors, treatment outcomes, and gametocytaemia following treatment. Parasite 2004; 11: 317-323.

Stephen CR, Wirima JJ, Steketee RW. Transplacental transmission of p. falciparum in rural Malawi. Am J Trop Med Hyg 1996; 55: 57-60.

Stouti JA, Odindo AO, Owuor BO, Mibei EK, Opollo MO, Waitumbi JN et al. Loss of red blood cell compliment regulatory proteins and susceptibility to severe malarial anemia. J Infect Dis 2003; 187:522–525.

Taylor TE, Molyneux ME. Clinical features of malaria in children. In: Warell DA, Gilles HM(ed). Essential Malariology 4th Ed. London: Arnold Publications; 2002. pg 206-218.

Taylor TE, Willis BA, Courval JK, Molyneux ME. Intramuscular artemether vs intravenous quinine: an open randomized trial in Malawian children with cerebral malaria. Trop Med Int Health 1998; 3: 3-8.

Tuman KJ. Tissue oxygen delivery. The physiology of anaemia\a. Anaesthesiol Clin North Am 1990; 9: 451-469.

Turrini F, Giribaldi G, Carta F, Mannu F, Arese P. Mechanism of band-3 oxidation and clustering in the phagocytosis of Plasmodium falciparum-infected erythrocytes. Rodex Report 2003; 8: 300–303.

Usawattanakulb W, Tharavanij S, Warrell DA, Looareesuwan S, White NJ, Supvej S et al. Factors contributing to the development of cerebral malaria II Endotoxin. Clin Exp Immun 1985; 61:562-568.

Viroj Wiwanitkit. Malarial parasite infection and increase of erythrocyte sedimentation rate. Irn J Med Hypotheses Ideas 2008; 2: 20-23.

Warell DA, Turner GDH, Francis N. Pathology and pathophysiology of human malaria. In: Warell DA, Gilles HM(ed). Essential Malariology 4th Ed. London: Arnold Publications; 2002. pg 236-251.

Weatherall DJ, Miller LH, Barruch DI, Marsh K, Doumbo OK, Casals-Pasual C et al. Malaria and red cell. In "Hematology: ASH education programme book" 2002; 35:1–25.

Wickramasinghe SN, Abdalla SH. Blood and bone marrow changes in malaria. Clin Haematol 2000; 13:277–299.

William F. G.. Cardiovascular regulatory mechanisms. In: Review of medical physiology. 18th ed. Norwalk: Appleton and Lange; 1997. pg 553-566.

William F. G. Endocrine functions of the kidney, heart and pineal gland. . In: Review of medical physiology. 18th ed. Norwalk: Appleton and Lange; 1997. pg 425-434.

World Health Organization. Antimalarial Drug Combination Therapy. Report of a WHO Technical Consultation( document WHO 2002).

WHO Library. WHO guidelines for treatment of malaria. 2006.

WHO Report. Clinical, Behavioral and Socioeconomic factors related to severe malaria. A multicenter study in African Region. 2002.

World Health Organization. Severe falciparum malaria. Trans Roy Soc Trop Med Hyg 2004; 94 : 1-90.

Xie YW, Wolin MS. Role of nitric oxide and its interaction with superoxide in the suppression of cardiac muscle mitochondrial respiration. Involvement in response to hypoxia/ reoxygenation. Circulation 1996; 94: 2580–2586.

# 19

# The Effect of Retinol Supplement on Blood Cytokine Concentrations in Children with Non-Severe Malaria Vivax

Viviana Taylor, Rosa Uscátegui, Adriana Correa, Amanda Maestre and Jaime Carmona
*Universidad de Antioquia/Grupo de Investigación en Alimentación and Nutrición Humana and Grupo Salud y comunidad*
*Colombia*

## 1. Introduction

Malaria, malnutrition, low concentrations of retinol and intestinal parasitism coexist among the habitants of tropical regions of the world (Nacher, 2002). The Turbo municipality is one of the highly endemic malaria regions of Colombia. During 2006, 5.674 cases of malaria were reported in Turbo, corresponding to annual parasite index >10 (number of malaria cases per 1,000 persons per year). From these, 85% were caused by *Plasmodium vivax* (Eventos de interes en salud Pública, 2006). Also, the Urabá region, where Turbo is a major urban area, is one of the regions of Colombia with more cases of malnutrition in children under 15 years; 53.3% of children under 10 years presented chronic malnutrition risk (T/E<-1Unit Z) and 14.9% acute malnutrition (P/T<-1Unit Z), whereas 33.8% of the adolescents had weight deficit according to the Body Mass Index (Alvarez et al., 2005). Furthermore, 85% of children aged 4 to 10 years with malaria had intestinal parasitism (Carmona et al., 2009).

Previous studies in Colombian children with malaria reported low retinol values during the acute phase, which recovered to normal values > 0.7 mmol/l (20 μg/dL) (WHO, 2009) once malaria receded. Within the children with malaria, 85% had anemia, and their haemoglobin values increased after one month of antimalarial treatment, although anemia persisted in 51% of them (Uscátegui & Correa, 2007).

During malaria, TH1 cytokines like interferon gamma (IFN - γ) and tumor necrosis factor alpha (TNF-α), are required to control the primary parasitemia. Nevertheless antinflammatory cytokines or TH2 cytokines, such as interleukin 10 (IL-10) and transforming growth factor beta (TGF-β), that modulate the proinflammatory effect, must be present along with those of the TH1 type, in order to prevent emergence of immune pathology (Schofield et al., 2005). Some in vitro studies revealed that retinol had an effect on the TH1/TH2 balance, as evidenced by reduction of IFN -γ and TNF -α secretion by TH1 cells or by promoting TH2 cells growth and differentiation to produce larger quantities of the IL-10 (Cantorna et al., 1994; Iwata et al., 2003). Vitamin A deficiency has been associated with an increase in TH1 response, intestinal parasitism and malnutrition (Jason et al., 2002; Azevedo et al., 2005). Furthermore, the prevalence of TH1 cytokines in children with malaria has been associated with severe anemia (Kurtzhals et al., 1999).

### 1.1 Anemia and relationship with cytokines TH1 and TH2, in patients with malaria

Ferritin deficiency is defined basically as the reduction of iron in the body and its diagnosis when not associated with anemia is based on quantification of serum ferritin. However, determinations of serum levels of this protein, which are performed systematically to determine the iron status, ferritin acts as a positive acute phase reactant in the presence of inflammatory/infectious disease clinics and subclinics (Aleo et al., 2004) as happens during malaria.

This explains why this protein is not useful tool for evaluating iron stores, and in contrast, constitutes a good indicator of inflammatory status along with the C reactive protein (CRP). CRP is produced by the liver, is also known as a positive acute phase reactant during malaria and main function is to join the organism, acting as an opsonin, with activation of the classical complement pathway, which is responsible for recruitment of inflammatory cells, opsonization and dead direct of the pathogen (Marsh & Kinyanjui, 2006).

Unlike ferritin, hemoglobin is not considered a reactant acute phase and the low concentrations of blood, result in anemia, which is a public health problem in many regions around the world with a high prevalence in economically dependent countries, especially among children and resulting from the interaction between biological, nutritional and cultural factors (Blair et al., 1999). The Anemia is a common complication of malaria and the mechanisms originally involved have not yet been fully defined. The cause is multifactorial and includes aspects related to the increase destruction of parasitized and non-parasitized cells and other factors causing a decreased production of erythrocytes, by alteration in the maturation of erythroid precursors or lack on response of bone marrow to erythropoietin (EPO). Additionally, there are others conditioning agents of anemia related with the characteristics of the parasite and host as resistance to *Plasmodium* or some disease in the host as well as thalassemia or sickle cell anemia, which enhances the severity of anemia, as well as deficiencies of iron and other micronutrients (Llanos et al., 2004).

In adults living in Kenya with acute malaria by *P. falciparum* found that TNF-α, interleukin 1 (IL-1) and IL-6, cytokines produced by monocytes, suppresses the synthesis of erythropoietin (Vedovato et al., 1999). Similar results were seen in children in Ghana (Kurtzhals et al., 1999). In Uganda, children 1 to 10 years who had acute uncomplicated malaria by *P. falciparum*, the authors found that age, high concentrations of erythropoietin, low concentrations of α-1 glycoprotein, and IL-10/TNF-α high proportion were associated with significantly increased hemoglobin concentrations. These data indicate that children younger with malaria do not maintain the production of IL-10 in response to inflammatory process, a mechanism that may contribute to the severity of the anemia (Nussenblatt et al., 2001). A study in Kenya in children with malaria revealed that the TNF-α and IL-10 were significantly higher in those subjects with high parasitemia and anemia, compared with control group, the same age and sex, but without malaria (Othoro et al., 1999). In children Colombians living in El Bagre (Colombia), aged from 4 to 9 years old who had acute uncomplicated malaria, 67% *P. vivax*, 29% *P. falciparum* and 4% mixed infection was found average of IL-10 of 266.18 ± 47.9 pg/ml, highly significant and higher than in children with the same age, but not malaria, which was 8.52 ± 1.17 pg/ml ($P < 0{,}001$); the values of IL-10 in children with malaria correlated with parasitaemia and body temperature. Conversely, TNF-α was only detected in 12% of study subjects, no significant differences between average children malaria and those without the disease. In children with moderate or high parasitemia but not anemia, the proportion was IL-10/TNF-α significantly higher compared with those who did have anemia, indicating that high values of this proportion can prevent

development of anemia with control of excessive inflammatory activity TNF-α (Grencis et al., 1996). The evidence presented shows that high values in the proportion of TH2/TH1 cytokines (IL-10/TNF-α) protect to development severe anemia malaria in children (17). It is proposed that the pathways by which IL-10 exerts its beneficial effects on malaria could be: 1) activating cytotoxic T lymphocytes, with the elimination of cells infected, 2) stimulating the production of antibodies directed against the parasite and 3) inhibiting or blocking the production of cytokines proinflammatory response characteristics TH1 (Blair et al., 1999).
According to the studies presented is clear that, in children with acute malaria, the severity of the anemia is determined by the balance in the production of proinflammatory cytokines such as anti-and IL-10 and TNF-α respectively, which therefore are related to the change in hematological and contribute or not to increase hemoglobin and erythropoietin. Although there is no information linking the paper simultaneously TH1/TH2 response modulator by supplements of vitamin A, with hematological values in children with malaria, there may be this interrelationship, it is clear that supplementation with vitamin A improve hemoglobin levels and erythropoietin and favor mobilization of iron deposits, and also is known its immunomodulatory role, as evidenced by the reduction of proinflammatory cytokines, which are also associated with the severity of anemia, and present during acute malaria. For this reason, further research is required to clarify the relationship between the simultaneous retinol, the immune response and iron metabolism in the population children with acute malaria, especially that produced by *P. vivax* that is more prevalent in Colombia.

## 2. Materials and methods

### 2.1 Study type and sample

A Pilot study balanced, nonblind, with random allocation of the "exposure factor" (retinol supplement) was carried out. Two groups, each of 25 children with nonsevere *P. vivax* malaria were compared according to WHO criteria (Lopez & Schmunis, 1998) and matched according the sex, age and place of residence. One of the group received retinol supplements (200.000 U.I. retinol palmitate, Retiblan®, Procaps laboratories, Colombia), for one year every 3 months, the final dose was administered between one week and six months before the *P. vivax* episode. Te other group did not receive supplement. The "final effect" in each child was the cytokines levels, and nutritional, biochemical and inflammatory indicators.
This project was approved by the committee of ethics of the Centro de Investigaciones Médicas de la Facultad de Medicina, Universidad de Antioquia. A written informed consent was obtained from each patient. The resolution N° 008430 of 1993 of the Ministerio de Salud de Colombia was considered.

### 2.2 Inclusion criteria

It required the following requirements: a) Reside on a regular basis in El Tres, Antioquia, Colombia b) Have not chronic (diabetes) or infectious disease (such as tuberculosis or leprosy) at the time of admission, c) Be free from trauma, accident or poisoning, known and judged as serious by the medical examination; d) A number of 25 children must have participated in research in which they received supplementation with retinol and 25 should not have received such a supplement; e) Have uncomplicated malaria by *P. vivax*; f) Agreeing to participate in the study by signing for his guardian, written informed consent.

### 2.3 Exclusion criteria

Participants were excluded if: a) Occurre done of those events in subparagraphs b) and c) inclusion criteria; b) Withdrawal of informed consent or for any reason of the study.

### 2.4 Diagnosis and treatment of malaria

The parasitological diagnosis of malaria was carried out as recommended by PAHO/WHO (López & Schmunis, 1988) with respect to sampling, processing and reading it. Antimalarial treatment was carried out orally, according to the schemes of the Ministry of Health of Colombia and the Regional Health Direction of Antioquia (drug and dose by age), the drugs are accompanied with water and food as well:

a. Chloroquine: total dose of 25 mg/kg body weight, which is split into three days: day 1 was given 10 mg/kg, days 2 and 3 are supplied 7.5 mg/kg in each.
b. Primaquine at 0.25 mg/kg/day for 14 days, given from day 4 (after completion of chloroquine).

The treatments were obtained in the DSSA-Ministry of Health and were delivered as monitored by the researchers observing the patient during the first half hour, in case of vomiting; the full dose was repeated, with new supervision for 30 minutes. If the patient vomited again, it was excluded from the study and transferred to the municipal hospital.

### 2.5 Anthropometric evaluation

Weight was measured on the children in an standing position, few clothing and without shoes; with an electronic scale of 100 kg capacity and 0.01 kg sensitivity. Height was measured with a flexible estadiometer fixed on the wall, of 2 m capacity and 1 mm sensitivity. Each measurement was evaluated and registered. The mean reading was recorded. The age was calculated as the difference between date of birth and date of evaluation. The height for age index (T/E) was constructed and those who had values <-1 of Z unit were classified as with chronic malnutrition risk and those with equal or greater values to -1 of Z unit as without risk. The population of the National Center of Statistics of Health of the United States (NCHS) was used as reference as accepted by the WHO for international comparisons (WHO, 1995).

Since reference values for weight and height are not available for men higher than 145 cm and children higher than 137 cm, it was not possible to evaluate acute malnutrition with the indicator P/T, hence Body Mass Index (BMI, weight / height $^2$) was used, which is accepted by the WHO for evaluation of children up to 15 years, using as reference values the proposed by the same organization. Those children below percentile 15 (p<15) were classified as low weight.

### 2.6 Laboratory examinations

The procedure followed for each of the laboratory tests was as follows:

#### 2.6.1Testing for malaria

The parasitological diagnosis of malaria to detect the presence of *Plasmodium* parasites by thick film was confirmed in the extended, in the manner provided by the OMS (López & Schmunis, 1988). The spread thin and thick were stained with Field and Giemsa, respectively. The thick smear was observed with 100X magnification and the search for parasites was done in 200 consecutive microscopic fields. The parasitemia was calculated based on 200 leukocytes and a standard of 8,000 cells /mL and expressed in rings/µL. A thick smear was diagnosed as negative when there was no asexually in 200 microscopic fields.

### 2.6.2 Stool

The stool test was conducted on one single sample, once the patient was admitted to the study.
We established the presence of helminths, the eggs were quantified and trophozoites and cysts of protozoa were identified. To do this we proceeded as follows: 3 g of feces was added formaldehyde 10% to cover the sample, which was stored in 4-7days, as was reviewed, consisting of "direct examination "and, if the parasites were not passed to "concentration examination". Treatment with 10% formalin well preserved helminths eggs and protozoan cysts. Direct stool examination with saline-iodine and examination by formalin-ether concentration as Ritchie were made according to the usual procedure only when the second evaluation was negative as declared such to the sample (Botero & Restrepo, 2003). Stool analysis was performed by professional staff of the Laboratory of Intestinal Parasites of the Faculty of Medicine of the University of Antioquia.

### 2.6.3 Determination of biochemical parameters

#### 2.6.3.1 C-reactive protein

Serum was measured by a kit BioSystems (CRP) Latex. C-reactive protein serum causes agglutination of latex particles coated with anti-human C-reactive protein. The agglutination of latex particles is proportional to the concentration of CRP and can be measured by turbidimetry (Rice et al., 1987). Inflammation was considered when the concentration of CRP was 8 mg/L or higher, recommended by the Clinical Laboratory of the IPS at the University of Antioquia, where they processed these samples.

#### 2.6.3.2 Ferritin

The ferritin was measured in serum with Abbott AxSYM kit ® Sistem (reference 7A58-20B7A583 56-4324/R12, Abbott Laboratories, USA). The AxSYM Ferritin assay was based on microparticle enzyme immunoassay technology (MEIA). The determinations were made in Clinical Laboratory of the IPS at the University of Antioquia.

#### 2.6.3.3 Plasma retinol

Chemical analysis was done by affinity high performance liquid chromatography (HPLC) (Talwar et al., 1998), with a team scores Waters, using a manual injection system Reodyne 77251, a solvent delivery system 660E, a UV-VIS detector 400 and a spine C-18 Simetry, using the Millennium software for management. 0.5 mL of plasma were measured and denatured with 0.5 mL of absolute ethanol with BHT (1.0 g/L) as antioxidant and 0.5 mg/mL of ethyl-β-apo-8-carotenoato and 0.5 mg/mL retinol acetate as internal standards.
The mixture was extracted five times with 5 mL of hexane.
The separated hexane was evaporated with N2 and the residue was reconstituted with 200 mL of methanol, an aliquot of 50 mL was injected into the HPLC system, the mobile phase used was methanol, acetonitrile in a proportion 70: 30. There were three chromatograms for each sample to evaluate. It was considered subclinical deficiency of vitamin A, when plasma levels were <20µg/dL. Measurements were made at the Laboratory of the National Institute of Health in Bogotá.

### 2.6.4 Hemoleucogram (cyanmethaemoglobin (g/dL) and Leucogram)

Hemoleucogram became type III-V in automated equipment in the clinical laboratory of hospital Francisco Valderrama of Turbo, Antioquia, Colombia, when it was not possible, was performed manually. The method used was that of the cyanmethaemoglobin recommended by WHO. The reference values for classifying anemia were those recommended by WHO as the concentration of hemoglobin (Hb) as follows: for children 2-4 years <11.0g/dL and the 5 years and older <12 g/dL (WHO, 2001).

Hemoglobin values were not corrected for altitude because Turbo is located less than 200 meters above sea level.

### 2.6.5 Determination of serum cytokines

The cytokines IFNγ, TNFα, IL-10 and TGF-β1 were determined by sandwich ELISA using the Duo Set kit developed by ELISA (R&D systems), the basis and procedure are described below:

#### 2.6.5.1 Fundament

This assay used an ELISA (Enzyme Linked Immuno sorbent Assay) quantitative sandwich, which was based on the detection of cytokines that bind to an immobilized antibody (capture antibody) on a solid phase antibody which directly or indirectly produced a reaction whose product could be measured by spectrophotometry.

#### 2.6.5.2 Reagents and samples required

Were used: a) Polystyrene microplates with 96 wells previously sensitized or attached to a polyclonal antibody capture (From mouse)-specific cytokine (IL-10, IFN-γ, TNF-α and TGF-β1). b) Standard, 1 vial of lyophilized cytokine (IL-10, IFN-γ, TNF-α and TGF-β1) recombinant in a buffered protein base. c) Sample from human serum (approximately alliquotes of 600 mL) and stored in liquid nitrogen or at -70° C. d) 21 mL of concentrated buffer solution mixed with condoms (wash buffer solution). e) Conjugate is 21 mL of polyclonal antibody specific for each cytokine detection coupled with horseradish peroxidase with preservatives. f) Substrate solution de12.5 made mL stabilized hydrogen peroxide (reagent color A) and 12.5 mL of stabilized chromogen (color reagent B). g) 6 mL of 2 N sulfuric acid (stop solution) h) Diluent of standard and diluents of sample RD1-51.

#### 2.6.5.3 Procedure

In the commercial kits used in this procedure microplates were previously coated with a capture antibody polyclonal-specific cytokine (IL-10, IFN-γ, TNF-α and TGF-β1). The standards and samples were added to the wells contained each plate (96 wells per plate) in the amount stated and corresponding cytokine (contained in the standard and samples) are joined to the capture antibody. After the corresponding washes to remove nonspecific binding, was added the respective conjugate (polyclonal antibody specific for each cytokine, together with an enzyme). Subsequently was it washed to remove nonspecific binding to conjugate. Substrate solution was added to the plates, and development color (corresponding to the product) was proportional to the amount of cytokine bound in the initial step of the procedure. After time estimated to measure the color reaction, the development of this stopped with stop solution and the color intensity was measured by a spectrophotometer at the wavelength indicated.

### 2.7 Statistical analysis

For variables exhibiting a normal distribution, the mean values between the groups were compared using the T test for matched groups. For variables lacking a normal distribution, median values were compared using the Mann Whitney test. To explore intragroup relations was applied spearman correlation coefficient. The comparison between the groups of the categorical variables was made using Chi square. The programs Prism, Epi info version 6.4D and SPSS version 15.0 were used and unilateral values of *P<0.05* were set up as significative.

## 3. Results

In total 17 boys and 8 girls in each treatment group were included, they were aged 2.8 -15.7 years old in the supplemented group, and 3.2 - 15.7 years old in the non-supplemented group. The weight, height and parasitemia values were similar in both groups (Table 1).

| Variable | Group with retinol | Group without retinol | p |
|---|---|---|---|
| Weight in kg (X±SD) | 28±10 | 30±13 | 0.621[a] |
| Height in cm (X±SD) | 127±20 | 131±20 | 0.567[a] |
| Parasitemia (P/µl) | 5557±4350 | 5830±3901 | 0.574[a] |
| With chronic under nutrition risk (T/E) (yes/no) | 17/8 | 15/10 | 0.384[b] |
| Low weight for BMI (yes/no) | 6/19 | 4/21 | 0.363[b] |
| Coprologic positive (yes/no) | 19/4 | 20/4 | 0.625[b] |
| Helminths (yes/no) | 10/13 | 17/7 | 0.054[b] |
| Protozoa (yes/no) | 17/6 | 17/7 | 0.536[b] |

X= average, SD= Standard deviation, P/µl= parasites/microlitre, T/E= indicator height for age, BMI= Body Mass Index
a U de Mann-Whitney test p<0.05.
b Chi square p<0.05.

Table 1. Characteristics of the children according to treatment group.

All children were tested for parasitaemia, ferritin, retinol and C reactive protein, 40 of them were tested for cytokines and 47 for haemoglobin and stool tests.

The risk of chronic malnutrition (T/E) in the group with retinol supplement was 68% in contrast to 60% in the non-supplemented group. Prevalence of low weight (IMC) was 24% in the supplemented children versus 16% in the non-supplemented.

Prevalence of intestinal parasites in children was high in both groups; overall 83% of the children had a positive stool test. The group supplemented with retinol exhibited infection in 74% and 43% with protozoa and helminths, respectively; while 71% of the non-supplemented group had protozoa and helminths (Table 1). There was no significant diference in the presence of intestinal parasitism among the groups. With exception of the haemoglobin and retinol, the remaining variables did not exhibit a normal distribution. The cytokines, C reactive protein, ferritin, haemoglobin and retinol, were similar among the groups and only the C reactive protein and haemoglobin values showed significance with the lower concentrations. The TNF- α median values were zero in the non-supplemented group, which means that at least in 50% of the children, this cytokine was not detected (Table 2). For IL-10, the highest concentration for both groups was 677pg/ml, and only 25% of the children from the group supplemented with retinol and 15% of the children from the non-supplemented group reached that value. With the technique used, no TGF-β1 values were detected in any sample tested.

The frequency of inflammation, anemia and subclinic deficiency of vitamin A was similar in both groups (Table 3).

| Variable | With retinol | | | Without retinol | | | p |
|---|---|---|---|---|---|---|---|
| | n | X±SD | Median | n | X±SD | Median | |
| IL-10 (pg/ml) | 20 | 275±283 | 112 | 20 | 233±253 | 125 | 0.989 |
| TNF-α (pg/ml) | 20 | 32.2±66.3 | 5.5 | 20 | 16.2±49.2 | 0.0 | 0.162 |
| IFN-γ (pg/ml) | 20 | 49.1±60.2 | 29.3 | 20 | 68.5±80.3 | 31.1 | 0.473 |
| C reactive protein (mg/l) | 25 | 29±25 | 24 | 25 | 48±39 | 36 | 0.070 |
| Haemoglobin (g/dl) | 23 | 10.5±1.5 | 10.3 | 24 | 11.2±1.8 | 11.1 | 0.054 |
| Ferritin (μg/l) | 25 | 143±191 | 105 | 25 | 154±108 | 113 | 0.160 |
| Retinol (mmol/l) | 25 | 0.59±0.06 | 0.57 | 25 | 0.61±0.08 | 0.59 | 0.786 |

IL-10=interleukyne 10, TNF-α=tumor necrosis factor alpha, IFN-γ=interferon gamma,
SD= Standard desviation.
U de Mann-Whitney test, except haemoglobin and retinol that one became for T pared test $p<0.05$.

Table 2. Comparison of the concentrations of cytokines and nutritional biochemical indicators in children according to treatment group.

| Category | With retinol | Without retinol | p |
|---|---|---|---|
| Inflamation (yes/no) | 21/4 | 23/2 | 0,334 |
| Anemia (yes/no) | 22/1 | 19/5 | 0,104 |
| Subclinic deficiency of vitamin A | 23/2 | 23/2 | 1 |

Inflamation = PCR values ≥ 8 mg/L, Subclinic deficiency of vitamin A = retinol values<20 μg/dL, anemia= haemoglobin in children 2-4 years old <11 g/dL and in children ≥ 5 years old<12 g/dL
Chi square $p<0.05$.

Table 3. Comparison frecuency of Inflamation, anemia and subclinic deficiency of vitamin A according to treatment group

### 3.1 Stratification by nutritional state and presence of intestinal parasitism

Because intestinal parasitosis and malnutrition affect the variables of our interest, results were analyzed according to: 1) absence of malnutrition risk and parasites, 2) at malnutrition risk and without parasites, 3) absence of malnutrition risk and presence of parasites and 4) malnutrition risk and presence of parasites. From these groups, only the group 4 was adequate for statistical analysis and this included, 13 children in the retinol supplemented group and 14 in the group without retinol supplement.

Subjects with T/E <-1 Unit Z o BMI p < 15 were classified as chronic malnutrition risk or with low weight. Since all children who had chronic malnutrition risk simultaneously presented low weight, the number of children with chronic malnutrition risk or low weight, was identical to that of children with chronic malnutrition risk.

In these children, the concentrations of TNF-α, IFN-γ and IL-10 were similar between both groups. Nevertheless, the group that received retinol exhibited a tendency to have lower values of ferritin and C reactive protein (p=0.058 vs 0.089) (Table 4). The parasite blood count was 6.111±3.801 P/μl in the group receiving retinol versus 7.160±4.046 P/μl in the other (p= 0.332).

| Variable | With retinol | | | Without retinol | | | p |
|---|---|---|---|---|---|---|---|
| | n | X±SD | Median | n | X± SD | Median | |
| IL-10 (pg/ml) | 13 | 283±289 | 112 | 8 | 186±219 | 119 | 0.827 |
| TNF-α (pg/ml) | 13 | 43.7±82.7 | 0.0 | 8 | 31.9±74.3 | 0.5 | 0.876 |
| IFN-γ (pg/ml) | 13 | 34.5±25.1 | 24.5 | 8 | 85.4±79.7 | 45.0 | 0.218 |
| C reactive protein (mg/l) | 14 | 30±25 | 25 | 13 | 47±31 | 38 | 0.089 |
| Haemoglobin (g/dl) | 12 | 10.5±1.1 | 10.7 | 13 | 11.6±2.2 | 11.5 | 0.120 |
| Ferritin (μg/l) | 14 | 117±72 | 110 | 13 | 184±127 | 145 | 0.058 |
| Retinol (mmol/l) | 14 | 0.59±0.07 | 0.56 | 13 | 0.61±0.09 | 0.59 | 0.698 |

X= average, SD= Standard desviation, IL-10=interleukyne 10, TNF-α= tumoral necrosis factor alpha, IFN-γ =interferon gamma.
U de Mann-Whitney test p<0.05.

Table 4. Nutritional comparison of the concentrations of cytokines and biochemical indicators in the stratum of children with chronic malnutrition risk and parasites, according to treatment group.

Among children with chronic malnutrition risk and presence of parasites, no differences were observed when the proportions of inflammation, anemia and subclinical deficiency of retinol were compared, regardless of the group (Table 5). Inflammation was detected in 13 out of 14 children from the group administered retinol versus 13 out of 13 children from the group without retinol. Anemia was detected in 11 out of 12 children from the group that receiving retinol and in 9 out of 13 children from the group without retinol. Finally, 12 out of

14 children supplemented with retinol had subclinical deficiency of retinol, while this was evident in 12 out of 13 from the group without retinol.

| Category | With retinol | Without retinol | p |
|---|---|---|---|
| Inflamation (yes/no) | 13/1 | 13/0 | 0,519 |
| Anemia (yes/no) | 11/1 | 9/4 | 0,186 |
| Subclinic deficiency of vitamin A | 12/2 | 12/1 | 0,529 |

Inflamation = values of PCR ≥ 8 mg/L, Subclinic deficiency of vitamin A = values of retinol <20 μg/dL, anemia= haemoglobin in children of 4 years old <11,0 g/dL and children of 5-10 years old <12 g/dL U Mann-Whitney test, except for hemoglobin and retinol was made by paired t test, $p<0.05$.

Table 5. Comparison of intensity of inflammation, anemia and deficiency subclinical vitamin A, in the stratum of chronically malnourished children parasites, according to treatment group.

The immunological and biochemical variables studied, which showed correlation among themselves and with parasitemia in one of the two groups of treatment are shown in Table 6. In the group with retinol it is noted that as the parasitemia increased the values of IL-10 and TNF-α were also increased and this was not observed in children of group without retinol. Similarly, in the group receiving retinol, when ferritin increased so did CRP, IL-10, TNF-α and IFN-γ, variables with ferritin which showed positive correlation behavior was not observed in the group without retinol, in which only one ferritin correlated with parasitemia.

The variables that are similarly associated in both groups were IL-10 and TNF-α, which correlated positively with each other and moreover, were those that showed the highest ratios of all the correlations shown in Table 7, with a Rho = 0.786 in group with retinol and 0.751, which received no retinol. This indicated that as it raised one of the two variables, so did the other with the same strength, regardless of having received or not retinol. This same behavior was observed in the supplemented group, between IL-10 and IFN-γ. In the group without supplement there was no correlation of hemoglobin with IFN-γ, which, though unexpected, was one of the highest in this group (Rho = 0.738) (Table 6).

## 4. Discussion and conclusion

This pilot study answered the need to obtain primary data on the effect of retinol supplements of, on blood concentrations of IL-10, TNF-α, IFN-γ, TGF-β1, C reactive protein, haemoglobin and ferritin, in Colombian children with vivax malaria; as well as the relationships between these variables; aspects rarely addressed .

The prevalence of chronic malnutrition risk (T/E <-1 unit Z) was high (64%), in children with malaria from 6 to 10 years of the same municipality (58.2%) (Uscátegui & Correa, 2007) Similarly, the proportion of children with low weight according to BMI (20%) was higher than in other studies of the region (Alvarez et al., 2005). A common finding within malaria endemic areas is the presence of intestinal parasitism (Nacher, 2002); 83% of our children had a positive stool test, 57.4% with helminths and 73.3% with protozoa, which is similar to previous reports in malaria infected children from the same region (Turbo) (Uscátegui et al., 2008).

| Pairs of variables | Measures (1) | With retinol | Without retinol |
|---|---|---|---|
| Parasitemia (P/μL) -IL-10 (pg/mL) | r | 0,574 | 0,643 |
| | p | 0,040 | 0,086 |
| Parasitemia (P/μL)-TNF-α (pg/mL) | r | 0,693 | 0,621 |
| | p | 0,009 | 0,100 |
| Parasitemia (P/μL)-Ferritin (μg/L) | r | 0, 330 | 0,731 |
| | p | 0, 108 | 0,005 |
| Haemoglobin (g/dL)-IFN- γ (pg/mL) | r | -0, 013 | 0,738 |
| | p | 0,954 | 0,037 |
| Ferritin (μg/L)- CRP (mg/L) | r | 0,574 | 0,330 |
| | p | 0,032 | 0,271 |
| Ferritin (μg/L)-IL-10 (pg/mL) | r | 0,696 | 0,381 |
| | p | 0,008 | 0,108 |
| Ferritin (μg/L)-TNF- α (pg/mL) | r | 0,575 | 0,436 |
| | p | 0,006 | 0,062 |
| Ferritin (μg/L)-IFN- γ (pg/mL) | r | 0,580 | 0,219 |
| | p | 0,006 | 0,367 |
| IL-10 (pg/mL)-TNF- α (pg/mL) | r | 0,751 | 0,786 |
| | p | 0,003 | 0,021 |
| IL-10 (pg/mL)-IFN-γ (pg/mL) | r | 0,569 | 0,068 |
| | p | 0,042 | 0,782 |

(1) r: Rho spearman coefficient, p probability associated with "r".

It is clear that in our study, the small size sample and the great variability in the data are explained partly because we did not found differences between the groups. In our children the age range was wide, 2-16 years. The age might have contributed to variations in the studied parameters. It is known that when children under 5 years are in contact with a pathogen, they produce a very pronounced TH1 cytokine response but as age increases, they shift towards a TH2 response, as a result of the maturation of the immune system (Kovaiou & Grubeck- Loebenstein, 2006).

In spite of the limited scope of our results, we reached some interesting findings. In the supplemented group, C reactive protein values were lower than in the group not supplemented, this was confirmed in children with chronic malnutrition risk and parasitism. In the later group, lower values of ferritin in the group with retinol (117±72 μg/l) versus the group without retinol were also observed (184±127μg/l). Since C reactive protein and ferritin are acute phase reactants increasing during infections (Gruys et al., 2005), our findings suggest that children that received retinol had less intensity on inflammation, which could be of clinical importance, since a exaggerated inflammatory response during malaria, has been associated with development of complications and death (Riley et al., 2006).

Nevertheless, that tendency to present lower intensity of inflammation associated with the retinol supplement was not reflected in the concentrations of cytokines. We expected that in the group with retinol, concentrations of IL-10 would be higher and TNF-α lower, as it has been found *in vitro* murine models of chronic inflammatory processes (Xu & Drew, 2006), but this effect was not seen in our children, which emphasizes the need to be cautious when extrapolating the results of studies from animal models to humans. In addition, it is important to consider that the dose of retinol supplemented to the cultures did not correlate to blood concentrations reached in humans, even after vitamin A administration (Hamzah et al., 2004).

Although no differences were detected in the concentrations of IL-10 neither among the groups with/without retinol in the children of the study, or in the children with chronic under nutrition risk and parasitism, the values of this cytokine were high; 25% of the children with retinol and 15% without retinol, had values exceeding the maximum limit of detection of the kit (677 pg/ml), concentrations very higher than those found in Turkish subjects with *P. vivax* malaria (Yildiz et al., 2006) . These findings led us to think that our subjects had more ability to modulate the immune response, protecting themselves from later complications, since IL-10 is considered very important in the process of malarial immunopathogenesis due to its anti-inflammatory role, and high serum concentrations of this cytokine have been associated with better prognosis of the disease (Shofield et al., 2005).

Haemoglobin concentrations were lower in the group with retinol in comparison to the group without retinol, when the analysis was unstratified. An increase in the destruction of infected red blood cells, which also increases the anemia might be associated to this result as other authors showed that the main receptor that mediates the phagocytosis of the infected erythrocyte by macrophages is CD36 and that the 9-cis-retinoic acid derived from retinol, stimulated the expression of CD36 and increased phagocytosis of erythrocytes infected with *P. falciparum* (Serghides & Kain, 2001).

Nor was there any difference in the prevalence of deficiency subclinical vitamin A, or retinol values between groups. However, we must take into account that concentrations retinol below 20 mg / dL in most children in this study have not really mean deficiency of vitamin A, due to the retinol binding protein is a reactant negative acute phase (Rosales et al., 2000), which decreases their concentrations during malaria and other infections (Ahmed et al., 1993; Rosales et al., 2000).

As for the correlations seen during the malaria episode, in children with and without retinol in the stratified group, most of these corresponded to what was expected. Correlations between parasitemia, CRP, ferritin, proinflammatory cytokines such as TNF-α and IFN-γ and anti-inflammatory such as IL-10, are adjusted as described during the inflammatory process that causes the early phase *Plasmodium* infection as a strategy to control initial parasitemia, limiting the spread of the parasite, with the subsequent removal of circulating forms (Ansar et al., 2006; Torre et al., 2002; Marsh & Kinyanjui, 2006). Additionally, these results allow us to verify has been seen in other previous studies, including: 1) the important role that TNF-α against asexual stages of *Plasmodium* erythrocytic phase early malaria, with a key role in the immune response protective cell, limiting the rate and contributing to death of *Plasmodium* (Maestre et al, 2002), 2) the behavior of ferritin as acute phase protein positive for malaria, which increases their concentrations in the presence of inflammatory/infectious subclinics clinics and, therefore in this research, and similar to observed in other study (Beard et al., 2006) this protein is not considered an adequate indicator of iron stores during

the acute phase infection, and 3) regulation that makes the IL-10 on proinflammatory cytokines, increasing their concentrations simultaneously in to maintain the TH1/TH2 balance, which as mentioned before, important to avoid all the complications associated with immunopathogenesis in malaria (Moormann et al., 2006).
However, an unexpected finding in children in the present study, was the positive correlation between IFN-γ hemoglobin, result which contrasts with other studies that found no association between anemia and iron deficiency in malaria, with high IFN-γ, IL-6, TNF-α and IL-1 (Jason et al., 2002; Kanjaksha et al., 2007; Feelders et al., 1998) situation, although can not be explained, is an interesting finding for further studies.
The undetectable concentrations of TGF-β1 that were found in all subjects might be due to the use of different among the studies (Esmai et al., 2003).
This study is the first one exploring the effect of a supplement of retinol on some immunological parameters in children with *P. vivax* malaria and simultaneous infection with intestinal parasites and at chronic malnutrition risk. Although the results are limited by the small number of the sample and the variability in the data, studies of this type with higher number of subjects and narrower ranges of age, are worthwhile performing to clarify the effect of this supplement on malaria infection. We concluded that: 1) The tendency to have higher values of C reactive protein in the group without retinol and of ferritin in children with chronic malnutrition risk and parasitism of the group without supplement, suggests a possible anti-inflammatory effect of retinol during the acute phase of malaria and 2) A tendency to present lower concentrations of haemoglobin in children of the group that received retinol supplement and 3) The observed positive correlation between IFN-γ and hemoglobin, was a completely unexpected result. These findings could contribute to clarify the issue about the effect of supplemental retinol in children with malaria and relevance of supplementation population, as part of the strategy aimed to control malaria.

## 5. Acknowledgments

To Colombian Institute for the Development of Science and Technology (COLCIENCIAS Cod. 1115-04-16388 Contract 339-2004), Committee for Development of Research of Universidad de Antioquia (CODI), Sectional Direction of Health of Antioquia (DSSA) and Sustainability Strategy 2009-2010 of the Vicerrectory for Research of Universidad de Antioquia, Colombia, by the financial support of the project and publication of manuscript. To the epidemiologist Alejandro Estrada for data analysis.

## 6. References

Aleo, E.; Gil, C., González, F.; Martínez, A. & Valverde, F. (2004). Serum transferring receptor in healthy children: Diagnostic yield in ferropenic and infectious anemia. *An Pediatr.* Vol 60, No. 5, pp. 428-35.

Álvarez, M.; Benjumea, M.; Roldán, P.; Maya, M. & Montoya, E. (2005). Perfil alimentario y nutricional de los hogares de la región del Urabá antioqueño. Medellín: Gobernación de Antioquia, Dirección Seccional de Salud, Programa de mejoramiento alimentario y nutricional de Antioquia, Universidad de Antioquia, Escuela de Nutrición y Dietética.

Ansar, W.; Bandyopadhyay, S.; Chowdhury, S.; Habib, S. & Mandal, C. (2006). Role of C-reactive protein in complement-mediated hemolysis in Malaria. *Glycoconj J.* Vol. 23, No. 3-4, pp. 233-240.

Azevedo, Z.; Victal, L.; Fonseca, K.; Camara, F.; Haeffner-Cavaillon, N.; Cavaillon, J. et al. (2005). Increased production of tumor necrosis factor-α in whole blood cultures from children whit primary malnutrition. *Braz J Med Biol Res.* Vol.38, pp.171-183.

Beard, J.; Rosales, F.; Solomons, N. & Angelilli, M. (2006). Interpretation of serum ferritin concentrations as indicators of total-body iron stores in survey populations: the role of biomarkers for the acute phase response. *Am Clin Nutr.* Vol. 84, pp. 1498- 1505.

Botero, D. & Restrepo M. (2003). *Parasitosis humanas* (4th Edition), Corporación para Investigaciones Biológicas, Medellín, Colombia.

Cantorna, M.; Nashold, F. & Hayes, C. (1994). In vitamin A deficiency multiple mechanisms establish a regulatory T helper cell imbalance with excess TH1 and insufficient TH2 function. *J Immunol.* Vol. 152, No. 4, pp. 1515-1522.

Carmona-Fonseca, J.; Uscátegui, R. & Correa, A. (2009). Parasitosis intestinal en niños de zonas palúdicas de Antioquia (Colombia). *Iatreia.* Vol. 22, pp. 27-49.

Esmai, F.; Ernerudh, J.; Janols, H.; Welin, S.; Ekerfelt, C.; Mining, S. & Fosberg, P. (2003). Cerebral Malaria in children: serum and cerebrospinal fluid TNF-α and TGF-beta levels and their relationship to clinical outcome. *J Trop Pediatr.* Vol. 49, No. 4, pp. 216-223.

Eventos de interés en salud publica, Antioquia. (2006). Available from http://www.dssa.gov.co/dowload/EInteresSP-Ver2007.xls.

Feelders, R.; Vreugdenhil, G.; Eggermont, A.; Kuiper-Kramer, P.; van Eijk, H. & Swaak, A. (1998). Regulation of iron metabolism in the acute-phase response: interferon gamma and tumour necrosis factor alpha induce hypoferraemia, ferritin production and a decrease in circulating transferrin receptors in cancer patients. *Eur J Clin Invest.* Vol 28, No.7, pp. 520-527.

Grencis, R. (1996). T cell and cytokine basis of host variability in response to intestinal nematode infections. *Parasitology.* Vol. 112, pp. 31-37.

Gruys, E.; Toussaint, M.; Niewold, T. & Koopmans, J. (2005). Acute phase reaction and acute phase proteins. *J Zhejiang Univ SCI.* Vol. 6, No. 11, pp. 1045-1056.

Hamzah, J.; Davis, T.; Skinner-Adams, T. & Beilby, J. (2004). Characterization of the effect of retinol on *Plasmodium falciparum* in vitro. *Exp Parasitol.* Vol. 107, No. 7, pp. 136-144.

Iwata, M.; Eshima, Y. & Kagenchika, H. (2003). Retinoic acids exert direct effects on T cells to suppress TH1 development and enhance TH2 development via retinoic acid receptors. *International immunology.* Vol. 15, No. 8, pp. 1017-1025.

Jason, J.; Archibald, L.; Nwanyanwu, OC.; Sowell, AL. & Buchanan, I. (2002). Vitamin A levels and immunity in humans. *Clin Diagn Lab Immuno.* Vol. 9, No. 3, pp. 616-621.

Kanjaksha, G. (2007). Pathogenesis of anemia in malaria: a concise review. *Parasitol Res.* Vol. 101, pp. 1463-1469.

Kovaiou, R. & Grubeck- Loebenstein, B. (2006). Age-associated changes within CD4+ T cells. *Immunology Letters.* Vol. 107, pp. 8-14

Kurtzhals, JA.; Addae, MM. & Akanmori, BD. (1999). Anemia caused by asymptomatic *Plasmodium falciparum* infection in semi-immune African schoolchildren. *Trans R Soc Trop Med Hyg.* Vol. 93, No. 6, pp. 623-627.

Llanos, C.; Flórez, M.; Herrera, M. & Herrera, S. (2004). Mecanismos de generación de anemia en malaria. *Colomb Med.* Vol 35, No.4, pp. 205-214

López, F. & Schmunis, G. (1998). Diagnóstico de malaria. Pub Cient 512. Washington: OPS-OMS.

Marsh, K. & Kinyanjui, S. (2006). Immune effector mechanisms in malaria. *Parasite Immunol.* Vol. 28, No. 1-2, pp. 51-60.

Moormann, A.; John, C.; Sumba, P.; Tisch, D.; Embury, P. & Kazura, J. (2006). Stability of interferon-gamma and interleukin-10 responses to *Plasmodium falciparum* liver stage antigen-1 and thrombospondin-related adhesive protein in residents of a malaria holoendemic area. *Am J Trop Med Hyg.* Vol. 74. No. 4, pp. 585-590.

Nacher, M. (2002). Worms and malaria: noisy nuisances and silent benefits. *Parasite Immunol.* Vol. 24, No. 7, pp. 391-393.

Nussenblatt, V.; Mukasa, G.; Metzger, A.; Ndeezi, G.; Garrett, E. & Semba RD. (2001). Anemia and interleukin-10, tumor necrosis factor alpha, and erythropoietin levels among children with acute, uncomplicated *Plasmodium falciparum* malaria. *Clin Diagn Lab Immunol.* Vol. 8, No. 6, pp. 1164-1170.

Othoro, C.; Lal, A.; Nahlen, B.; Koech, D.; Orago, A. & Udhayakumar V. (1999). A Low Interleukin-10 Tumor Necrosis Factor-α Ratio is associated with Malaria Anemia in Children Residing in a Holoendemic Malaria Region in Western Kenya. *J Infect Dis.* Vol 179, No.1, pp. 279-282.

Rice, C.; Trull, A.; Berry, D. & Gorman, E. (1987). Development and validation of a particle-enhanced turbidimetric immunoassay for C-reactive protein. *J Immunol Methods.* Vol. 99, pp. 205-211.

Riley, E.; Wahl, S.; Perkins, D. & Schofield, L. (2006). Regulating immunity to malaria. *Parasite Immunol.* Vol. 28, No. 1, pp. 35-49.

Schofield, L. & Grau, G. (2005). Immunological processes in malaria pathogenesis. *Nature reviews immunology.* Vol. 5, pp. 722-734.

Serghides, L. & Kain, K. (2001). Peroxisome proliferator-activated receptor gamma-retinoid X receptor agonists increase CD36-dependent phagocytosis of *Plasmodium falciparum*-parasitized erythrocytes and decrease malaria-induced TNF-alpha secretion by monocytes/macrophages. *J Immunol.* Vol. 166, No. 11, pp. 6742-6748.

Talwar, D.; Ha, T.; Cooney, J.; Brownlee, C. & O'Reilly, D. (1998). A routine method for the simultaneous measurement of retinol, alpha-tocopherol and five carotenoids in human plasma by reverse phase HPLC. *Clin Chim Acta.* Vol. 270, No. 2, pp. 85-100.

Torre, D.; Speranza, F. & Martegani, R. (2002). Role of proinflammatory and anti-inflammatory cytokines in the immune response to *Plasmodium falciparum* malaria. *Lancet Infect Dis,* Vol. 2, No. 12, pp. 719-720.

Uscátegui, R.; Correa, A. & Carmona, J. (2008). Efecto de los suplementos de retinol y antiparasitarios intestinales, sobre valores sanguíneos de retinol, hemoglobina, proteína C reactiva y ferritina en niños maláricos y su relación con estado nutricional e inflamación. Memorias quinto premio fundación éxito por la nutrición infantil. Bogotá: Fundación Éxito.

Vedovato, M.; De Paoli Vitali, E.; Dapporto, M. & Salvatorelli, G. (1999). Defective erythropoietin production in the anaemia of malaria. *Nephrol Dial Transplant.* Vol. 14, No. 4, pp. 1043-1044.

WHO/NHD/01.3 I. (2001). Iron deficiency anemia, assessment, prevention, and control a guide for programme managers. United Nations Children's Fund United Nations University, World Health Organization, pp 10.

World Health Organization. (1995). El estado físico: uso e interpretación de la antropometría. Ginebra: OMS. Serie Informes Técnicos: 854

World Health Organization. (2009). Global prevalence of vitamin A deficiency in populations at risk 1995-2005. WHO Global Database on Vitamin A Deficiency. Geneva, World Health Organization. Available from http://whqlibdoc.who.int/publications/2009/9789241598019_eng.pdf

Xu, J. & Drew, P. (2006). 9-Cis-retinoic acid suppresses inflammatory responses of microglia and astrocytes. *J Neuroimmunol*. Vol. 171, No. 1, pp. 135-144.

Yildiz, F.; Kurcer, M.; Zeyrek, D. & Simsek, Z. (2006). Parasite density and serum cytokine levels in *Plasmodium vivax* malaria in Turkey. *Parasite immunology*. Vol. 28, pp. 201-207

# 20

# Elevated System Energy Expenditure in Sickle Cell Anemia

Chidi G. Osuagwu
*Department of Biomedical Technology*
*Federal University of Technology, Owerri, Imo State*
*Nigeria*

## 1. Introduction

*In Sickle-cell Anemia (SCA), anergy (lack of metabolic energy) and elevated resting energy expenditure (REE) are commonly observed phenomena. The many systemic changes in Sickle-cell anemia are, therefore, associated with measurable changes in patterns of energy uptake, utilization and efficiency. Understanding the scientific basis of these structural and energy changes suggest mechanisms of possible amelioration.The structural and energy changes in sickle-cell anemia can be viewed at different levels: at the level of the whole person, as reflected in anergy and elevated resting energy expenditure. At the level of the whole blood tissue, as shown in lowered blood pH (high hydrogen ion, $H^+$, concentration). This is also associated with structural changes in polyhedral charge-packing of hydrogen and hydroxyl ions (octahedral charge-packing, which is the ideal is not achieved). At the specific organ level, this is shown in the elevated energy cost of kidney proton-dialysis. Because of this kidney disease is a major cause of death among sickle cell sufferers. The cellular level shows the disruption of the erythrocyte membrane itself. The anti-turbulence biconcave 'erythrocytoid' shape is changed to the sickle-shape, resulting to increased blood flow-turbulence. This overworks the heart; causing high heart disease rates among patients. At the molecular level, this results to, for example, the inability to metabolize the key energy-source molecule glucose. This results to, as well as inability to extract energy from glucose, glycation of hemoglobin. Glycated hemoglobin has poor oxygen-carrying power, compounding the problem of the little hemoglobin available. Also there are shifts in redox equilibriums, enzyme and metabolite concentrations and activities, and so on. All these result to extra-energy costs to try to restore system optimal state of efficiency and stability. All these, together, explain elevated resting energy expenditure in sickle cell disease.*

Different researchers have, over the years, discovered that sufferers from sickle cell anemia (SCA) expend more energy maintaining the same mass of their bodies than normal people (Kopp-Hollihan *et al*, 1999; Borrel *et al*, 1998). Some have worked to establish more efficient measurements of the observed differences from normal (Buchowski *et al*, 2002). Others have worked on theories and experiments towards remediation (Bourre, 2006; Enwonwu, 1988). On the internet, there are sites actively publicizing high-energy foods they consider ideal for sickle cell sufferers (Sherry, 2011). In folk medicine in the African communities, where sickle anemia is common, easy to digest high-energy foods are usually recommended for sickle cell patients.

To appreciate why a sick body, such as that of the sufferers of sickle-cell anemia, would cost more energy to maintain, as reflected in the higher resting energy expenditure (REE), than normal people's, we have to, first, appreciate some simple rules, with respect to energy economy; that nature employs in the design of natural systems. The living system, including the human body, is the ideal natural energy-using system. The living system is energy-conservative; efficient, compared to any other known system, in nature.

The rule is that for a given system in nature there is a functionally ideal arrangement. This ideal or optimal (not perfect, but best possible) arrangement is most energy efficient. It offers the best stability (*stay-ability*) to the system. The human body is designed to operate at optimal conditions; where it is most bio-energetically efficient and stable. Stability in human terms means good health, less stress and pain, and long life. Sickness, generally, is a state of body-system displacement from the optimal conditions of function and is, therefore, energy costly. The fever (abnormally high body temperature) commonly associated with sick people results from the decrease in efficiency of body energy use.We recall that entropy, disorderly flow of system energy, increases with temperature. Such elevated basal body temperature (high metabolic entropy) is commonly found in sickle-cell anemia sufferers, particularly during crisis.

The following statement by the researcher Zora Rogers (2011) "Fever is a common presenting symptom in many manifestations of sickle cell disease" summarizes the situation. Heat loss (fever) is sign of wasting energy. That is why the sufferer, inspite of higher *Resting Metabolic Energy* (RME) utilization, suffers from anergy (a state of lack of energy). Much of the energy and nutrients, including ascorbic acid, the reducing metabolite glutathione, etc, consumed or produced by patients of this disease are wasted (Fakhri *et al*, 1991; Kiessling *et al*, 2000; Reid *et al*, 2006). They go into the dissipative chaos of entropy, instead of being organized as parts of stable system structures such as fat, healthy nerves and muscles, which SCA sufferers lack. In this sense sickle cell anemia is, literally, a wasting disease. Energy and structures are dissipated.

## 2. Some contributing factors to energy wastage in sickle cell anemia (SCA)

There are so many factors that contribute to systemic energy wastage in sickle cell anemia. Because of its dramatic manifestations as anemia, particularly during crisis, sickle cell disease is seen, primarily as an anemia. The catastrophic fall in red blood cell concentration; and the accompanying yellow eyes, caused by excess bilirubin (a by-product of hemoglobin breakdown) would easily identify the disease as of blood origin. This assumption is sustained by the direct link between hemoglobin and blood oxygen concentration on the one hand and body energy generation on the other. Anemia can, therefore, be thought of, equally, as low energy metabolism syndrome; and more so for a chronic condition like sickle cell anemia. The first major factor that leads to anergy in sickle cell anemia is inefficient glucose metabolism.

### 2.1 Inefficient glucose metabolism in sickle cell anemia

Glucose is the main fuel molecule of the human body. Some key body cells depend mostly or solely on glucose for energy metabolism. Two of these glucose-dependent body cells include the red blood cell (rbc) and nerve cells, including brain cells. It is clear that anybody in whose body system glucose metabolism is compromised is in trouble with the vital tissues and organs associated with these cells; blood system and nervous system. This happens to be the case in sickle cell anemia. In SCA hexose metabolism is deranged

(Osuagwu and Mbeyi, 2007). Table 1 below shows the consistent rise in blood glucose level from the normal genotype (HbAA), through the one-gene (HbAS) and double gene-dose (HbSS) to the crisis (HbSS-crisis) state. The diminishing capacity to utilize glucose is seen to be, inadequately, compensated by the consistently enhanced utilization of extra fructose, from one state to the other.The differences are statistically significant between the states (Osuagwu and Mbeyi, 2007). This implies that the issue of capacity to utilize glucose should, by itself, be considered seriously, in handling anemia cases. Part of the explanation for this is that glucose is activated with the high energy molecule adenosine-triphosphate (ATP) by phosphorylation, before it can go into a cell. In a person with anergy (lack of metabolic energy), such as SCA patients, there is a shortage of the ATP to phosphorylate glucose. Fructose that gets into cells by passive transport or facilitated diffusion is consumed, in partial compensation. Exhaustive depletion of fructose in SCA should, by itself, be of primary concern. This is because the basic metabolism of cells that depend mainly on fructose, such as spermatozoa, would be compromised in the sickle cell disease state. This could be a major explanation for the poor spermatozoa health; and infertility observed in sickle cell males. The number, motility and other indices of spermatozoa vitality are all poor in men with SCA (Osegbe et al, 1981).
Any measure to promote glucose uptake into the cell would be of much help to SCA sufferers. Administration of insulin to facilitate glucose uptake for sickle cell sufferers in crisis is a management measure that logically suggests itself.This should be systematically investigated. By facilitating trans-membrane glucose transport, this measure will also result to better fructose conservation; and better sperm health and fertility. This should help sickle cell males live better lives; and bear healthier children.

| Sickle Cell State | Number of Subjects In Group | Plasma Glucose Level, mg/dl | Plasma Fructose Level, mg/dl |
|---|---|---|---|
| **HbAA** | 35 | 70.10 ± 7.50 | 1.32 ± 0.08 |
| **HbAS** | 32 | 74.75 ± 6.20 | 1.25 ± 0.05 |
| **HbSS** | 34 | 78.59 ± 4.20 | 1.09 ± 0.05 |
| **HbSSc** | 33 | 84.80 ± 4.10 | 0.99 0.04 |

Table 1. Plasma Glucose and Fructose Levels in Sickle Cell States.

### 2.2 Deranged pyruvate metabolism

Another major cause of poor glucose metabolism in sickle cell anemia is the non-efficient utilization of the end product of glycolysis; pyruvate. Table 2 summarizes this condition. The critical step in the generation of most energy (ATP) and reducing power (NADH) for the whole system fails in sickle cell disease; See Fig 1. Fig1, Fig 2 and Table 2 help to explain both anergy and acidosis in sickle cell anemia.

| **Sickle Cell State** | HbAA | HbAS | HbSS | HbSS-crisis |
|---|---|---|---|---|
| Lactate Level, mM-L$^{-1}$ | 0.74 ± 0.19 | 0.75 ± 0.23 | 27.60 ± 1.39 | 31.40 ± 2.56 |
| Lactate ratio | 1.00 | 1.01 | 37.30 | 42.43 |
| Pyruvate Level, mM-L$^{-1}$ | 0.11 ± 0.02 | 0.11 ± 0.03 | 2.03 ± 0.05 | 2.08 ± 0.11 |
| Pyruvate ratio | 1.00 | 1.00 | 18.45 | 18.91 |
| Lactate/pyruvate | 7.01 | 7.02 | 13.60 | 15.07 |

Table 2. Lactate and pyruvate levels in different sickle cell states.

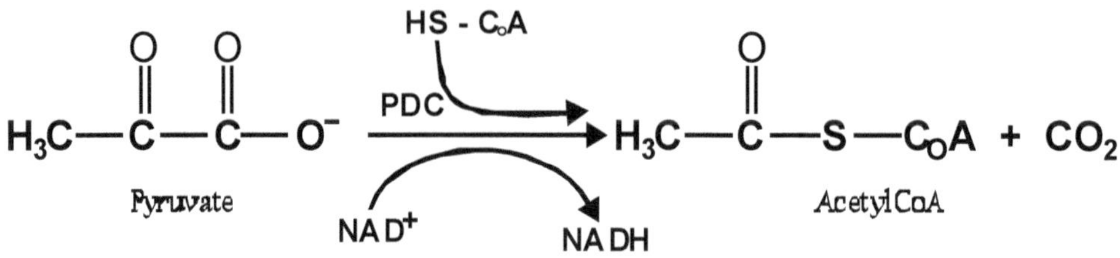


Fig. 1. Pyruvate dehydrogenase complex (PDC) links glycolysis to tissue respiration.

Pyruvate is the end-product of glycolysis and feedstock material for the production of Acetyl-CoA for the TCA cycle. If acetyl-CoA, the gate-substrate of the tricarboxylic acid (TCA) cycle is not generated, by successful pyruvate conversion, then most of the free energy stored in glucose cannot be extracted. This would, and does, result to anergy.

If reduced nicotinamide adenine dinucleotide (NADH) is not generated, there would be insufficient reducing power for the body system, down the electron transport chain; hyper-oxidation, excess free radicals, etc., will result. There is indeed observed hyper-oxidation and excess free radicals found in the body system of sickle cell patients, as theory indicated.

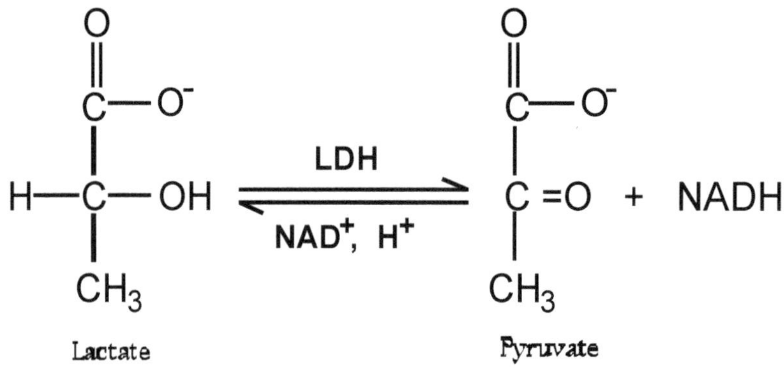


Fig. 2. Reversible oxidation of lactate to pyruvate.

If pyruvate accumulates, the equilibrium of Fig 2, which naturally favours the generation of lactate from pyruvate (Murray et al, 2006), will result to what is displayed in Table 2; a higher and higher ratio of lactate to pyruvate. Lactate acidosis will be the end result as observed in sickle cell patients. See Table 3. The data of Table 2 also best explains the dramatically different existential outcomes for single gene carriers (HbAS) as compared to double dose carriers (HbSS). The expression of the Sickle cell gene in relation to the pyruvate dehydrogenase complex is sigmoid (Osuagwu, 2009). Both the HbAA and HbAS values fall around the same point; which is why the HbAS, trait-carrier group, do not manifest the proportionate impact of the disease, as expected from theory. This suggests that the system-equilibrium mechanism of the HbAS is much better preserved than theory would suggest. But there is still an energy cost. The HbAS are not a hundred percent free of the pathological manifestation of the gene, as the popular notion suggests. They pay a smaller than expected energy price.

## 2.3 Energy cost of acidosis in SCA

A look at Fig 3 tells a simple story; the human body was designed by nature to be, overall, alkaline. The human body is by design an electron-rich system (alkaline). Food is a neutral substance that the human body can absorb, extract electrons (mostly as H· attached $NAD^+$; NADH, etc) from. It then safely excretes the associated positive charges, particularly hydrogen ion, $H^+$. As Fig 3 shows all the major body fluids are alkaline (electron-rich); all the excretory body fluids are acidic (hydrogen-ion rich).Part of the reason for this alkaline design is body energy economics. It is more efficient to extract energy from energy-rich molecules in an alkaline medium.

Consider the hydrolysis reaction that extracts energy from the key energy currency of the body adenosine triphosphate, ATP:

$$ATP^{4-} + H_2O \rightleftharpoons ADP^{3-} + HPO_4^{2-} + H^+ + \text{Energy}$$

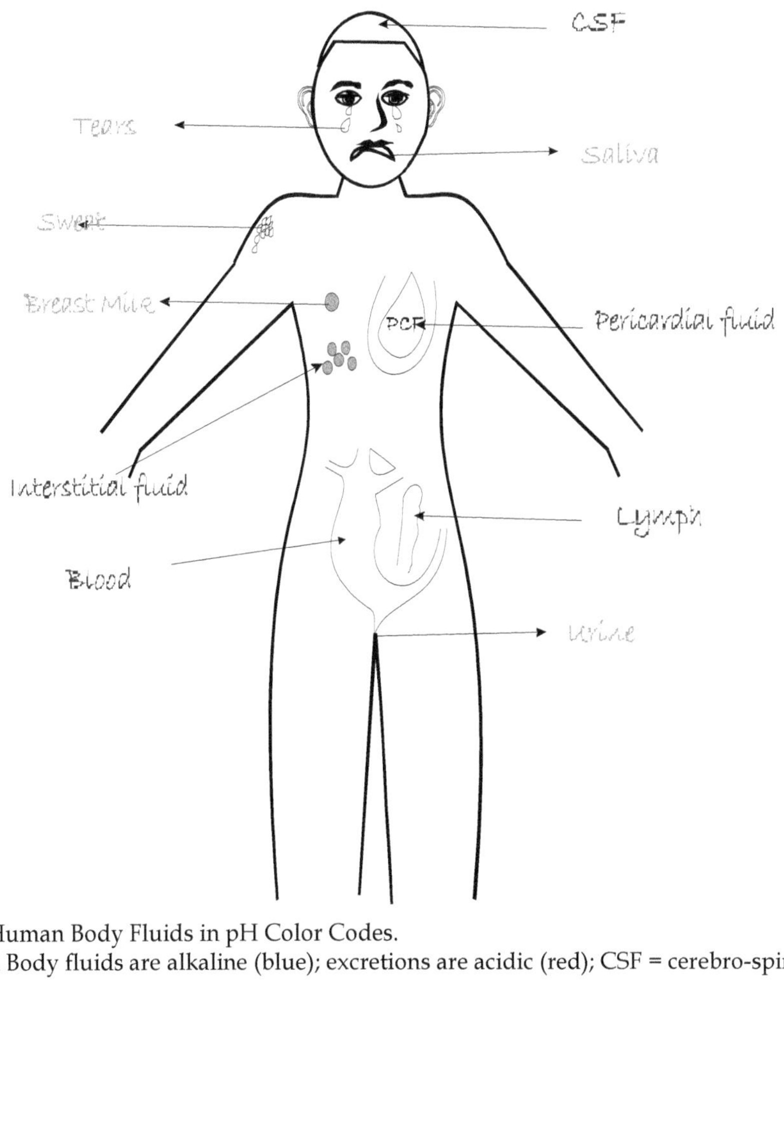


Fig. 3. Human Body Fluids in pH Color Codes.
Internal Body fluids are alkaline (blue); excretions are acidic (red); CSF = cerebro-spinal fluid.

A product of this reaction is the hydrogen ion, $H^+$, which gives acids their character. Le Chatellier's principle, on the self-restoring tendency of displaced equilibrium systems, teaches that ATP hydrolysis in acid medium would be resisted, because one of the products is an acid, $H^+$. To push ATP hydrolysis under such condition would in itself cost energy. In addition, the efficiency of the ATP hydrolyzing enzyme, ATPase, decreases with increasing acidity (Bronk, 1973). We know enzymes are denatured by acids, outside normal range of function. This implies extra energy cost and waste. On the other hand ATP hydrolysis would proceed rapidly in a more alkaline medium that would consume the produced $H^+$. The more alkaline the better; within physiological range. ATP hydrolysis is more efficient, yields more energy, in more alkaline medium (Manchester, 1980).

In recent times, there have been groups or movements, particularly via the internet, promoting the '*Alkaline Body*' as the ideal body. Their arguments are based on some of the points noted here. The problem with their position is they don't seem to realize that excess alkalinity of the body (alkalosis) is in itself a disease. The body is designed on the optimality principle. And human survival at beyond pH 7.65 is difficult.

### 2.4 Low blood pH in SCA

Table 3 shows clear tendency towards more acid body fluid, as the sickle-gene dose/state increases.Therefore the sickle cell sufferer's body consumes more ATP to do the same amount of, say, muscular work. The energy cost of extracting the same amounts of hydrogen ion, $H^+$, from blood into urine illustrates this point well. This data agrees with the theory outlined above.The more energy exerted to do the same amount of work, the more stress would be associated with it.

| S/No | Genotype/State | n | Blood pH, | Urine pH, |
|---|---|---|---|---|
| 1 | HbAA = 0 | 42 | $7.39 \pm 0.07$ | $6.54 \pm 0.15$ |
| 2 | HbAS = 1 | 42 | $7.35 \pm 0.09$ | $6.44 \pm 3.15$ |
| 3 | HbSS = 2 | 42 | $7.32 \pm 0.08$ | $5.89 \pm 0.39$ |
| 4 | HbSS-crisis = 3 | 42 | $7.15 \pm 0.12$ | $4.75 \pm 0.46$ |

Table 3. Sickle State, Blood and Urine pH.

#### 2.4.1 Energy cost of kidney hydrogen ion dialysis in SCA

From the data of Table 3, the estimated enthalpies of dialysis, $\Delta H_d$, for each of the four states are: HbAA = 1.96RT; HbAS = 2.10RT; HBSS = 3.29RT; HbSS-crisis = 5.53RT. The estimated entropies of dialysis $T\Delta S_d$, compared to the normal HbAA state are: HbAA = 0.00RT; HbAS = 0.14RT; HbSS = 1.34RT and HbSS-crisis = 3.57RT (R = 8.31Jmol$^{-1}$ K$^{-1}$ and T = 303K). This offers a bio-energetic explanation of why the kidney of the sickle cell disease sufferer, on average, fails at an early age; and is the top source of morbidity (Saborio and Scheinman, 1999; Osuagwu, 2007). The kidney hydrogen, $H^+$, dialysis energy expenditure gap between SCA sufferers and normal is so wide that it is somewhat surprising.

| S/No | Genotype/State | n | $\Delta H_d$ | $T\Delta S_d$ |
|---|---|---|---|---|
| 1 | HbAA = 0 | 42 | 1.96RT | 0.00RT |
| 2 | HbAS = 1 | 42 | 2.10RT | 0.14RT |
| 3 | HbSS = 2 | 42 | 3.29RT | 1.34RT |
| 4 | HbSS-crisis = 3 | 42 | 5.53RT | 3.57RT |

Table 4. Indices of Energy Cost of KidneyHydrogen Ion DialysisIn SCA.

This data confirms that the stress, in this specific case of kidney proton dialysis, suffered by the HbAS individuals (7% more) compared HbSS-steady-state (68% more) and HbSS-crisis (182% more) for doing the same amount of system work compared to the HbAA, non-carrier individuals are high. In the specific case of HbSS-crisis, three times normal. This, among others, explains why resting energy expenditure of the SCA sufferer is high. This phenomenon, of disproportionate severity of gene expression in genotypic disease conditions, is likely to be observed in varying amounts in other genetic diseases. The explanation is likely due to interaction with other genes, which help buffer the effect of the defective gene. Also noteworthy is the general fact that a complex system under stress tends to self-conserve; and does so better the closer it is to ideal state, as HbAS is compared to HbSS. Any SCA anemia management measure that reduces hydrogen ion accumulation, or that can provide an alternative route for its excretion would be of major relief to the patient.

### 2.5 Energy cost of change in blood system charge-parking arrangement

Nature, always, prefers the optimal structure and associated energy expenditure in designs of system. One of these choices for optimality is in the packing of charges in living things (Osuagwu, 2010). The pH values we are familiar with represent ratios of hydrogen ions, $H^+$, and hydroxyl ions, $OH^-$, that can be packed together, with optimal stability.

Comparing the concentrations of hydroxyl and hydrogen ions in the bloods of normal (HbAA) and sickle sufferers at their measured pHs from Table 3 above reveals the data of Table 5. Similar charges repel and opposite charges attract each other. The most efficient way to arrange six hydroxyl ions to one hydrogen ion in the normal, HbAA, blood (pH = 7.39) would be as octahedron; the most efficient way to arrange four to one in HbSS blood (pH = 7.32) would be as tetrahedron (Fuller, 1975). The octahedral arrangement is the optimal considering, jointly, energy efficiency and stability. Any shift from this ideal is less efficient; and energy costly. This is one other way sickle cell sufferers pay a higher energy cost to try to maintain their body system. The stress wears their system down with time, faster than for normal people.

It has been noted that, generally, any shift from the ideal charge-packing arrangement would result to sickness (Osuagwu, 2007). Larger hydroxyl to hydrogen ratios, such as found in alkalosis is also troublesome; and disease-causing. The pH 7.65, which affords a hydroxyl to hydrogen ion ratio of 20: 1, is consistent with packing on the twenty vertices of the dodecahedron with the lone hydrogen ion at the centre of the structure, held in place by weak coordinate bonds to the surrounding hydroxyl ions. 20: 1 is the largest ratio consistent with life. Beyond that, death occurs.

| GENOTYPE | HbAA | HbSS |
|---|---|---|
| **PARAMETER** | | |
| pH | 7.39 | 7.32 |
| $[H^+]$, mol-$L^{-1}$ | $10^{-7.39}$ | $10^{-7.32}$ |
| pOH | 6.61 | 6.68 |
| $[OH^-]$, mol-$L^{-1}$ | $10^{-6.61}$ | $10^{-6.68}$ |
| $[OH^-]/[H^+]$ | $6.03 \approx 6$ | $4.37 \approx 4$ |
| Efficient -packing Structure | Octahedron | Tetrahedron |

Table 5. Hydroxyl to Hydrogen ion Concentrations and Ratios Represented by Measured pH.

### 2.6 Energy cost of stresses on the erythrocyte

The red blood cell, erythrocyte, whose structural and physical collapse, sickling, has given the name to SCA is of special interest in accounting for the high energy expenditure in the disease state. Sickling, erythrocyte structural collapse, occurs because the cell is overwhelmed by stresses. Two such stresses are:

#### 2.6.1 Erythrocyte and failure of glucose metabolism in SCA

What happens to a cell that depends solely on glucose if its metabolism fails? From significant data, some presented here, and published work (Osuagwu and Mbeyi, 2007), glucose metabolism is subnormal in SCA. But the erythrocyte, like the nerve cell, depends mostly on glucose for energy. SCA erythrocyte lacks the energy to maintain the integrity of its cell membrane (Osuagwu et al, 2008). This is a significant reason for SCA erythrocyte instability.

#### 2.6.2 Excessive oxidative stress

An acidic medium is an oxidizing medium. The proton, $H^+$, is nature's unit oxidant. The acidic sickle cell sufferer's body-fluid, such as blood is, therefore, inherently oxidizing. Red blood cell that is embedded in this oxidizing medium, in this case the blood stream, becomes a victim. Its lipid, electron-rich membrane is oxidized; becomes rigid and breaks down.

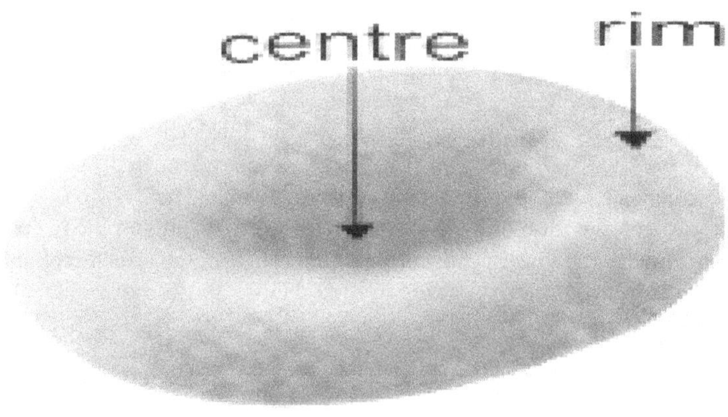


Fig. 4. Dimensions of the erythrocyte; ratios are powers of pi (3.14...).

The dimensions of the erythrocyte (Centre thickness: rim thickness: diameter: circumference) are fractal, sequential, powers of pi ($\pi$ = 3.14...). This is the origin of the pi-discoid shape of the erythrocyte (Osuagwu, 2007).This pi-biconcave shape locates the greater part of the mass of the cell at the rim. This results to a very large moment of inertia; low angular momentum and great resistance to turbulence (Uzoigwe, 2006). This 'erthrocytoid' shape is the best to minimize frictional breakdown of the erythrocyte in the very viscid blood stream, through which it is propelled at great blood pressure, and speed, by the heart.Oxidative damage, by contributing to sickling, destroys this energy efficient pi-biconcave structure; increasing energy cost of blood-stream transport; and energy cost of forming new cells, with a rapid bone-marrow turnover. This is why sickle cell anemia also involves cardiovascular problems (Serjeant, 1974). Studies show that movement across the cell membrane is deranged; and the ion pumps that help maintain the trans-membrane concentration gradients consistent with life are compromised (see Table 6). It is observed that the concentration gradients of these cations deviate from the normal as the sickle condition intensifies.

| Measure | HbAA | HbAS | HbSS | HbSS-c |
|---|---|---|---|---|
| No. of Subjects | 62 | 62 | 62 | 62 |
| $Na^+$, out, mmol/L | 139.59 ± 2.89 | 139.05 ± 2.73 | 133.74 ± 2.44 | 109.02 ± 1.93 |
| $Na^+$, in, mmol/L | 15.42 ± 2.48 | 19.03 ± 3.25 | 20.64 ± 2.51 | 28.20 ± 1.69 |
| $K_{eq}$-$Na^+$(out/in) | 9.0525 | 7.3069 | 6.4797 | 3.8660 |
| $K^+$, out, mmol/L | 3.51 ± 0.33 | 4.05 ± 0.39 | 4.72 ± 0.42 | 5.52 ± 0.48 |
| $K^+$, in, mmol/L | 103.35 ± 4.49 | 97.91 ± 3.86 | 88.08 ± 3.80 | 83.94 ± 3.56 |
| $K_{eq}$-$K^+$(in/out) | 29.4444 | 24.1753 | 18.6610 | 15.2065 |
| $Ca^{2+}$, out, mmol/L | 8.48 ± 0.42 | 8.04 ± 0.11 | 7.90 ± 0.21 | 5.06 ± 0.32 |
| $Ca^{2+}$ , in, mmol/L | 0.46 ± 0.09 | 0.58 ± 0.08 | 0.60 ± 0.70 | 2.30 ± 0.32 |
| $K_{eq}$-$Ca^+$(out/in) | 18.4348 | 13.8621 | 13.1667 | 2.2000 |

Table 6. Trans-membrane Cation Concentrations and Gradients, Keq, in Different Sickle cell States.

If the concentration of the potassium ions, $K^+$, which is more representative of the potential across the membrane, is looked at; it is observed that the energy to maintain the cell membrane integrity decreases as the sickle cell gene dosage increases. There is consistent drop in system-maintaining energy; as shown across the cell membrane.

| Measure | HbAA | HbAS | HbSS | HbSS-c |
|---|---|---|---|---|
| No. subjects | 62 | 62 | 62 | 62 |
| Keq | 29.44 | 24.18 | 18.66 | 15.21 |
| $\Delta H_p$, $K^+$; J | 8362.55±35.00 | 7988.33±253.66 | 7274.03±229.12 | 6952.29±211.49 |
| Ratio | 1.00 | 0.96 | 0.87 | 0.83 |

Table 7. Energy Decrease Across Cell Membrane as Sickle Cell Intensity Increases.

Because of this extra need for energy, the need for extra nutrients by the sickle cell sufferer has been known for a long time (Reed *et al*, 1987).

## 3. System energy wastage and sickle cell anemia management

The different points of energy wastage (high entropy) in sickle cell anemia, outlined above, have helped to explain the anergy (system lack of energy), instability and other symptoms of the disease. They also offer clues as to points and modes of possible intervention for disease management. They also offer the possibility of rationalizing existing interventions that appear effective. Inability to extract reducing power/hyper-oxidation from nutrients; the build-up of glucose, acidosis, the viscid blood and erythrocyte lysis, etc., are all issues that can be dealt with by rational intervention.

Diet or nutritional management is already well-established as a method of sickle cell disease management. But from the facts outlined here, one can see that intervention to improve glucose metabolism would be very helpful to the SCA patients. Also would dietary supplements that promote pyruvate metabolism; such as lipoic acid. Alkalinizing nutrients would be of overall good. But acid-forming nutrients would need to be taken with care; as are agents that support free-radical generation and propagation.

Special care would have to be taken in relation to the impact of any management strategy on the kidney. As observed the organ is under severe energy stress in the sickle cell patients' system.We learn from Fig 3 that sweat-inducing exercises would do some good to the SCA patients, as part of the excess acidity will be excreted that way; taken care not to over-do it and induce crisis.

Overall, the observed elevation in resting energy expenditure (REE) by the sickle cell disease sufferer can be understood in terms of known energy-related physiological, anatomical and biochemical processes. They can, therefore, be managed, for amelioration, from the careful consideration of these.

## 4. Summary

The observed elevation of basal energy expenditure in sickle cell anemia has been explained, in this work, in terms of established principles' of nature and bioenergetics. The genetic programme that results to sickle cell anemia appears to involve more than the genes coding for hemoglobin formation; and bone marrow metabolism. Energy metabolism is, critically, involved. And the derangements along the energy pathways have consequences that affect different levels of system function and integrity. It is shown that management of sickle cell anemia by intervention along the body's energy metabolism pathways can be helpful, in relieving the anergy (lack of energy) experienced by the sufferers of the disease. This can come about, for instance, by stabilizing erythrocyte cell membrane; minimizing blood turbulence, cell lysis and enhancing oxygen carrying capacity. The consumption of foods or supplements that supply reducing power, in the form of say ascorbic acid, glutathione or alkalinizing nutrients would be of help to the sickle cell sufferer in this regard. They would do this by free-radical-scavenging, reduction of acidity and the enhancement of ATP hydrolysis efficiency.

Enhancing glucose and pyruvate metabolism and hydrogen ion excretion, perhaps more than anything, would enhance the energy efficiency of the SCA blood system; lowering the resting energy expenditure. Achieving this would improve the energy status and general well-being of the sickle cell sufferer.

## 5. References

[1] Borel, MJ; Buchowski, MS; Turner, EA; Peeler, BB; Goldstein, RE and Flakoll, PJ. Alteration in Basal Nutrient Metabolism Increase Resting Energy Expenditure in Sickle Cell Disease. American Journal of Physiology: Endocrinology and Metabolism; Feb 1998; 274(2): 257-264.

[2] Bourre, JM; Effects of Nutrients (in Foods) on Structure and Function of the Nervous System: Update on the Dietary Requirement for Brain; Part I: Micronutrients. Journal of Nutrition in Health and Aging; 2006, Sept-Oct, 10 (5):377-85.

[3] Bronk, JR (1973). Chemical Biology, An Introduction to Biochemistry; The MacMillan Company, NY. p. 247.

[4] Buchowski, MS; Chen KW; Bryne D and Wang, WC. Equation to Estimate Resting Energy Expenditure in Adolescents with Sickle Cell Anemia. The American Journal of Clinical Nuitrition; Dec. 2002; 76(6):1335-1344.

[5] Enwonwu, CO 1988; Nutritional Support in Sickle Cell Anemia: Theoretical Considerations. Journal of National Medical Association; 1988, Feb; 80(2):139-44.

[6] Fakhri, ME; Aggarwal, SK; Gayoum, A and Sherrif, DS. Reduced Plasma Ascorbic Acid and Red Cell Glutathione Contents in Sickle Cell Disease- A Preliminary Report. Indian Journal of Biochemistry; 6(1): 47-50, 1991.

[7] Fuller, RB (1975). Synergetics. Macmillan Publishers, NY; p. 321.

[8] Kiessling, K; Roberts, N; Gibson, JS and Ellroy, JC. A Comparison in Normal Individuals and Sickle Cell Patients of Reduced Glutathione Precursors and their Transport between Plasma and Red Cells. Hematological Journal, 2000; 1(4): 243-249.

[9] Kopp-Hollihan, LE; van Loan, MD; Mentzer, WC and Heyman, MD; Elevated Resting Energy metabolism in Adolescents with Sickle Cell Anemia; Journal of American Dietetics Association; 1999, Feb 99(22):195-9.

[10] Manchester, KL; Free Energy, ATP Hydrolysis and Phosphorylation Potential. Biochemical Education; 8(3), 1980.

[11] Murray, R; Cramer, D; Mayes, P and Rodwell, V (2006). Glycolysis and the Oxidation of pyruvate. Harper Illustrated Biochemistry (27thedn). McGraw-Hill, NY.

[12] Osegbe, DN; Akinyanju, O and Amaku,EO; Fertility in males with sickle cell disease. Lancet; 318 (8241- 2): 275-276; August 1981.

[13] Osuagwu, CG and Mbeyi CU; Altered Plasma Hexose Sugar Metabolism in Sickle Cell Anemia. African Journal of Biotechnology; 1(3): pp 037-40; August, 2007.

[14] Osuagwu, CG. The Energy Cost of Kidney Proton Dialysis in Sickle Cell Anemia. African Journal of Biotechnology, 2007; 6 (2): 128-130.

[15] Osuagwu, CG. Polyhedral Charge-packing Model of Blood pH Changes in the Disease State. African Journal of Biotechnology, 2007; 6 (9): 1128-1131.

[16] Osuagwu, CG; Nwanjo, HU and Ajaegbu, VU. Decreased Erythrocyte Resting Membrane Potential in Sickle Cell Anaemia. Nigerian Journal of Biochemistry and molecular Biology, 2008; 24(2): 51.54.

[17] Osuagwu, CG. Turbulence: Erythrocyte Structure and Fluid-dynamic Pi (π) Designs. Journal of Medical Research and Technology, December 2007; 4 (2).

[18] Osuagwu, CG; Primary Pyruvate Acidosis in Sickle Cell Anaemia. Nigerian Journal of Biochemistry and Molecular Biology, 2009; 24 (2): 48-51

[19] Osuagwu, CG. Physiochemical Logics of Natural Selection of Biostructural Elements. Nigerian Journal of Biochemistry and Molecular biology, 2010; 25 (1): 73-76.

[20] Reed, OJ; Redding-Lallinger, R and Orringer, EP. Nutrition and Sickle Cell Disease. American Journal of Hematology, 1987; 24(4): 441-455.

[21] Reid, M; Badaloo, A; Forrester, T and Jahoor, F. In Vivo Rates of Erythrocytes Synthesis in Adults with Sickle Cell Disease. American Journal of Physiology, Endocrinology and Metabolism; 291: E73-E79; 2006.

[22] Rogers, ZR. Management of Fever in Sickle Cell Disease. *UptoDate*, June 10, 2011. UptoDate, Inc. www.uptodate.com.

[23] Saborio P and Scheinman, JI. Sickle Cell Nephropathy; Journal of the American Society of Nephrology, 1999; 10: 187-192.

[24] Serjeant, GR (1974). The Clinical Features of Sickle Cell Disease. North Holland Publishing Co, Amsterdam.

[25] Sherry, E. Foods High in Energy for Sickle Cell Anemia Patients. Livestrong.com; Demand Media Inc. (2011).

[26] Uzoigwe, C. The Human Erythrocyte Has Developed the Biconcave Shape to Optimize the Flow Property of Blood. Medical hypothesis, 2006; 7 (5):1159-1163.

# 21

# Molecular Basis of Thalassemia

Michela Grosso, Raffaele Sessa, Stella Puzone,
Maria Rosaria Storino and Paola Izzo
*Dipartimento di Biochimica e Biotecnologie Mediche,*
*University of Naples Federico II*
*Italy*

## 1. Introduction

Hemoglobinopathies are a heterogeneous group of monogenic disorders widespread overall. They are commonly subdivided into three partially overlapping subgroups: structural variants which comprise the sickle cell anemia syndrome; thalassemias, characterized by a reduced rate of synthesis of one or more globin chains of hemoglobin; conditions of high persistence of fetal hemoglobin in adulthood (HPFH) (Weatherall & Clegg, 2001).

As a group, they are the commonest monogenic disorders in the world population. It is thought that the high prevalence of these defects could be due to selective advantage of the carrier state to malaria infection. However, in spite of epidemiological evidences supporting this hypothesis as well as of extensive hematological studies, the mechanisms underlying this protection still remain unknown. It is, however, evident that as a consequence of this positive selection, these diseases are mostly common in geographic areas extending from the Mediterranean region through tropical countries including Sub-Saharian Africa, the Middle East, India, Southeast Asia and Indonesia, where malaria was or still is endemic (Weatherall & Clegg, 2001). In many of these areas the estimated frequencies of these disorders range from 3 to 10 percent, even though in some specific areas the carrier frequencies may be higher, reaching 80-90% in some tribal populations in India (Harteveld & Higgs, 2010). Because of their high frequencies, different hemoglobin defects may be co-inherited, giving rise to an extremely complex series of genotypes and clinical phenotypes. In fact, in many regions thalassemic defects coexist with structural Hb variants; it is also quite common for individuals from areas at high frequency of thalassemic defects to inherit genes for more than one type of thalassemia. Furthermore, some Hb variants are synthesized at reduced rate or are highly instable, leading both to functional and structural deficiency of the affected globin chain, thus resulting in a thalassemic condition, generally showing dominant inheritance. These complex interactions contribute to generate a wide range of clinical disorders that, taken together, constitute the thalassemic syndromes (Weatherall, 2001).

The complex and heterogeneous spectrum of molecular defects underlying these inherited conditions is regionally specific and in most cases the geographic and ethnic distributions have been determined, providing support for prevention programs based on screening, genetic counselling and prenatal diagnosis in couples at risk.

On the other hand, as the result of mass migration of populations from areas at high risk, hemoglobinopathies are being seen with increasing frequency even in regions where they were rather uncommon.

In Italy eight point mutations represent about 90% of β-thalassemia defects (Rosatelli et al., 1992) with the remaining 10% being represented by a wide array of molecular defects, some of which very rare. Furthermore, recent intensive immigration flows moving from countries with high incidence of hemoglobinopathies (Middle East, Southeast Asia and Northern Africa) with their own specific pattern of mutations as well, has rapidly increased the molecular heterogeneity of hemoglobinopathies in our region. This condition requires additional efforts to allow rapid and feasible carrier and prenatal screening programs.

## 2. Organization and structure of human globin genes

Hemoglobin tetramer is composed by two α-like and two β-like globin chains which are encoded by genes localized in two clusters where they are arranged in a sequential mode in the 5'→3' direction, according to their order of activation and expression during ontogenesis (Weatherall & Clegg, 2001). The α-like gene cluster is located in a region of about 30 kb in the telomeric region on the short arm of chromosome 16 (Fig. 1). It includes in the 5'→3' order an embryonal gene (ζ2), three pseudogenes, (Ψζ1, Ψα2, Ψα1), the α2 and α1 genes and the pseudogene θ. The β-like gene cluster is located in a region of DNA of about 60 kb on the short arm of chromosome 11 (Fig. 2). It includes in the 5'→3' order the genes ε, $^{G}\gamma$, $^{A}\gamma$, the pseudogene Ψβ followed by the δ and β genes (Weatherall & Clegg, 2001). All globin genes share a similar structure which includes three coding exons separated by two introns. Conserved sequences critical for gene expression are found in the proximal promoter regions, at the exon-intron boundaries and in the 5′ and 3′ untranslated (UTR) regions. The fetal globin chains are encoded by two genes, $^{G}\gamma$ and $^{A}\gamma$ which share the same sequence, except in the proximal promoter region and at codon 136, where a glicine residue ($^{G}\gamma$) is replaced by alanine ($^{A}\gamma$). Besides typical promoter and enhancer elements, each globin gene cluster has an upstream regulatory region which plays a crucial role to promote erythroid-specific gene expression and to coordinate the developmental regulation of each gene. In the β-gene cluster this region is known as Locus Control Region (LCR), a relatively large element, encompassing ~20 Kb. It is located approximately 25 Kb upstream of the most proximal ε-globin gene and contains five DNase I hypersensitive (HS) erythroid specific sites (HS-1 HS-2 HS-3 HS-4 HS-5). These sites define sub-regions of open chromatin that are bound by multi-protein complexes (Fig. 2). Similarly a regulatory region, known as HS-40, is located in the α-gene cluster, upstream of the embryonal α-like globin gene (Fig. 1) (Cao & Moi, 2002; Ho & Thein, 2000; Weatherall & Clegg, 2001).

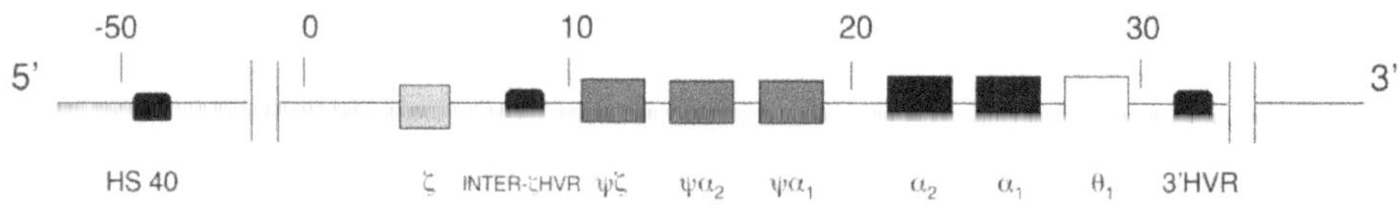


Fig. 1. **Structure of the α-gene cluster on chromosome 16.** The genes are arranged spatially in the order of their expression during ontogeny.

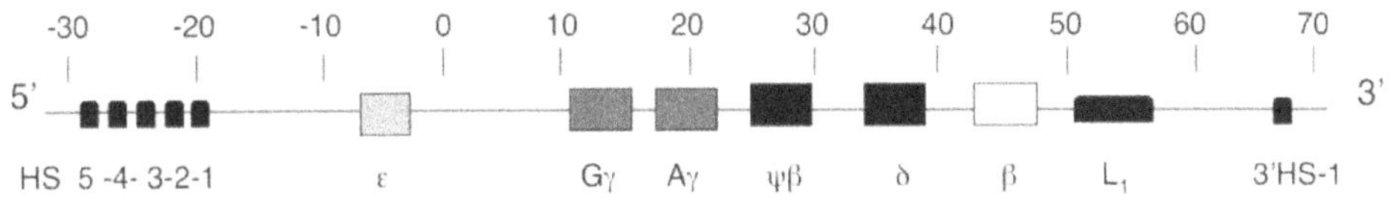


Fig. 2. **Structure of the β-gene cluster on chromosome 11**. The genes are arranged spatially in the order of their expression during ontogeny.

## 3. Regulation of globin gene expression

The expression of human globin genes is regulated throughout ontogeny by fine and complex mechanisms involving transcriptional, post-transcriptional and post-translational processes. The function of such a tight control is to assure that, at any stage of development, the production of α-like globin chains equals that of β-like globin chains (α/non-α ratio = 1) for the correct hemoglobin assembling (Cao & Moi, 2000). However, this mechanism of control is not able to detect whether a gene which is to be activated is functional or not. Therefore if a mutation that impairs gene expression occurs in any globin gene, it will give rise to an imbalanced globin chain production. When synthesis of α-globin genes is defective, β-like globin chains will be in excess, thus leading to α-thalassemia, whereas impaired β-globin chain output will lead to excess of α-globin chains and β-thalassemia conditions.

Transcriptional control of each globin gene expression requires distant upstream regulatory regions as well as proximal promoter regions. All proximal regulatory elements are located within the first 500 base pairs (bp), 5′ to the transcriptional start (Cap) site. The promoters of all the globin genes share high homology but they also show unique sequences that may be responsible for their developmental stage-specific regulation. Three major regulatory elements with minor sequence variations are common to all globin promoter regions: the TATA, CCAAT and CACCC boxes. In the β-globin gene promoter the TATA box is located at positions -28 to -31, the CCAAT box at positions -72 to -76 and the duplicated CACCC sequences at positions -86 to -90 (proximal element) and at position -101 to -105 (distal element), respectively. It is noteworthy that, with respect to the β-globin gene promoter, the γ-globin gene shows a single CACCC element and a duplication of the CAAT box, which may have implications in the different developmental regulation of these genes. All promoter regions also contain binding sites for specific erythroid transacting factors (Cao & Moi, 2002; Ho & Thein, 2000).

All these elements, through direct interactions with the LCR and transcriptional factors, act as positive regulators and are required for optimal transcription. In fact, mutations in these sequences lead to impaired globin gene expression levels.

Several other positive regulatory elements known as enhancers have been identified within gene sequences or in intergenic regions which increase transcriptional activity of certain promoters. In the β-globin gene, enhancers are found in intron 2 and 3′ to the gene, 600 to 900 bp downstream of the polyadenylation site. Silencer elements which repress gene expression play a role in the developmental control of globin gene expression, in the switch from embryonal to fetal to adult hemoglobin production. Indeed, these elements

are found in the distal promoter region of the ε-globin gene and in the γ-globin genes (Oneal et al., 2006).
The primary role of the LCR in the β-globin cluster is to confer a tissue specific state of open chromatin at the globin gene loci and also to allow interaction of transacting factors with specific globin gene promoters in a developmental stage-specific manner. Specific binding site for EKLF, GATA-1 and NF-E2, three erythroid-specific transcriptional factors that play critical roles in activation of the β-globin genes, have been described both in the LCR and in the promoters of the globin genes, thus allowing speculations on the complex function of the LCR on globin gene expression. Therefore, the stage-specific expression of globin genes could depend on the location of the genes in the cluster as well as on the availability of stage-specific transcription factors (Cao & Moi, 2002; Ho & Thein, 2000).

## 4. Switching of globin gene expression

During ontogenesis, physiological changes in oxygen requirements are accompanied by the switching of globin gene expression (Stamatoyannopoulos G. & Gronsveld F., 2001). This process represents one of the most intriguing and studied regulatory mechanisms of gene expression which leads to progressive and sequential changes in the expression of embryonic, fetal and adult globin genes and thus allows to synthesize different types of hemoglobin tetramers. However, the detailed mechanisms that control this process are still not fully understood (Pi et al., 2010; Ross et al., 2009).
Human hemoglobin synthesis requires two switches: from embryonic to fetal hemoglobin at 6 week of gestation and from fetal to adult production at birth (Fig. 3). The first genes to be expressed are those of the ζ-chain (α-like) and ε-chain (β-like), synthesized in the embryonic yolk sac until 4-5 weeks of gestation, which lead to the formation of Hb Gowers I (ζ2ε2). Then, with the change of the liver as the main erythropoietic compartment, synthesis of α and γ chains is activated. At this stage the embryonic Hb Gowers II (α2ε2) and Hb Portland (ζ2γ2) are progressively and completely substituted by the fetal hemoglobin Hb F (α2γ2). Around birth, when the bone marrow becomes the main erythropoietic site, β-globin gene expression is activated to synthesize the adult Hb A (α2β2), which at birth is about 20% of total hemoglobin. The switch from fetal to adult hemoglobin is completed within the first two years of life and leads to the pattern in which adult globin expression HbA (α2β2) comprises about 97%, HbA2 (α2δ2) 2-3% and HbF (α2γ2) less than 1% of total hemoglobin, respectively (Stamatoyannopoulos G. & Gronsveld F., 2001).
The control of tissue and developmental expression of specific globin genes is exerted by physical interactions between the different globin gene promoters and the LCR through binding of both ubiquitous and erythroid-specific transacting factors. The sequential expression of different globin genes requires coordinated mechanisms of gene silencing and gene competition for the LCR sequences, as well as chromatin remodelling and complex chromosomal looping and tracking processes (Pi et al., 2010; Ross et al., 2009).
The switching of the expression of β-globin genes is not only a fascinating and complex model used for studying regulation mechanisms of gene expression in space and time, but its full understanding could also have important therapeutic implications in the treatment of sickle cell anemia and β-thalassemia. Indeed, the clinical picture of these conditions can improve in the presence of sufficiently high levels of HbF: in β-thalassemia syndromes, in

fact, hereditary persistence or drug-mediated reactivation of γ-globin chain output may result in a reduction of the α/non α globin chain imbalance which represents the main pathogenetic factor influencing the severity of these conditions, whereas in sickle cell anemia an increase in HbF contributes to ameliorate the severity of disease by inhibiting the polymerization of sickle hemoglobin and its related pathophysiological effects (Fathallah & Atweh, 2006).

Persistent expression of fetal hemoglobin may be associated with specific genotypes (as described below in detail) or induced by appropriate drug treatments. In fact, fetal globin genes can be reactivated by demethylation of regulatory sequences generated by hydroxyurea or 5-azacytidine or by histone deacetylation induced by treatment with short-chain fatty acids (Fathallah & Atweh, 2006). However, besides toxic side effects of these drugs, response to treatment is transient and highly variable. Thus, a better understanding of the switching processes and regulatory mechanisms of fetal globin genes may indicate new therapeutic approaches in the treatment of thalassemia and sickle cell anemia by means of a permanent reactivation of the γ-globin genes.

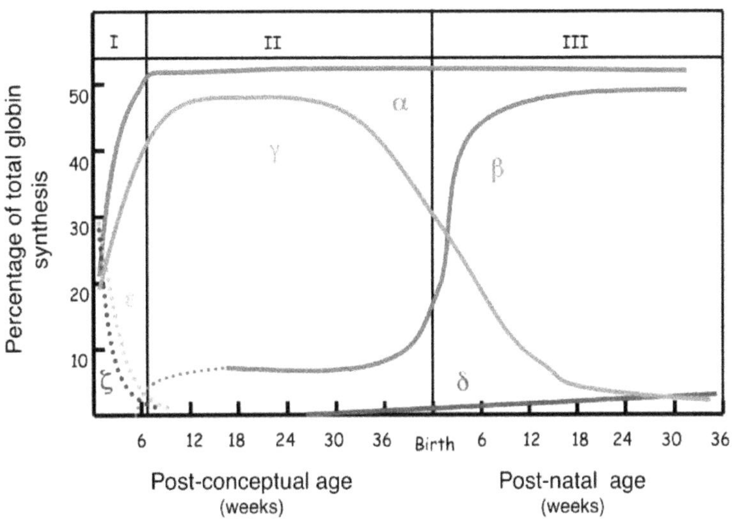


Fig. 3. **Changes in globin gene expression profile during ontogeny.** The x-axis represents the age of the fetus in weeks. The y-axis corresponds to the expression of each globin gene as a percentage of total globin gene expression. Time of birth is denoted with a vertical line. The embryonic genes are expressed during the first six weeks of gestation. The first switch from ε- to γ-globin occurs within 6 weeks after conception, and the second switch from γ- to β-globin occurs shortly after birth.

## 5. Molecular basis of hemoglobinopathies

With few exceptions, molecular defects affecting the globin genes are transmitted in an autosomal recessive manner and can result in:

1. Structural variants, characterized by the production of abnormal globin chains;
2. Thalassemias due to a quantitative defect in the synthesis of one or more globin chains;
3. Hereditary persistence of fetal haemoglobin (HPFH), a heterogeneous group of defects in the switch from fetal to adult globin gene expression which leads to persistent fetal hemoglobin synthesis in adult life. This condition, without any clinical relevance, is of great interest because it represents a useful model for studying the regulation of globin gene switching during development and because of its potential therapeutic role, since high HbF levels can ameliorate the severity of clinical phenotypes associated with some structural hemoglobin variants or thalassemias.

### 5.1 The structural variants

Over 900 hemoglobin variants have been identified so far (Weatherall & Clegg, 2001). Although their frequencies vary greatly in different ethnic groups, only three of them occur at high frequency in different populations: the Hb S, responsible of the sickle cell anemia which is distributed in the sub-Saharan region, in the Mediterranean area, in Middle East and in some Indian regions; the Hb C which is present in West Africa and certain parts of the Mediterranean area; the Hb E which occurs at very high frequency in Indian and Southern Asian populations.
The majority of human Hb variants result from single amino acid substitutions in one of the globin chains. Some rarer variants are instead characterized by elongated or shortened globin chains. Another type of structural variant is due to unequal crossing-over events with the formation of hybrid or fusion globin chains, as in the case of the Hb Lepore which involves the δ- and β-globin genes. All variants have the $\alpha_2\beta_2$ tetrameric structure, with the exception of the non-functional Hb Bart's and HbH, which are $\gamma_4$ and $\beta_4$ homotetramers, respectively.

### 5.2 The thalassemias

The thalassemias are a heterogeneous group of inherited disorders of hemoglobin synthesis, all characterized by the absent or reduced output of one or more globin chains. They are classified into α-, β-, δβ-, γδβ- and εγδβ-thalassemias, according to the particular globin chain(s) which is ineffectively synthesized. However, since the prevalent hemoglobin tetramer in adulthood is composed by α- and β-globin chains ($\alpha_2\beta_2$), the most relevant clinical forms are thus α- and β-thalassemias, respectively. In recent years, the molecular basis of the thalassemia syndromes have been described in detail, revealing the wide range of mutations encountered in each type of thalassemia (Galanello & Ortiga, 2010).

#### 5.2.1 The β-thalassemias

The β-thalassemias are subdivided into the $\beta^0$-, $\beta^+$ and $\beta^{++}$ groups, to designate a complete, severe or mild defect in β-globin chain synthesis, respectively (Weatherall & Clegg, 2001). This results in excess of α-globin chains and, consequently, various degrees of imbalanced α/non α chain output, which is the main determinant of the typical hematological phenotypes and the clinical severity of these conditions (Cao & Moi, 2000; Weatherall, 2001).

Molecular basis of β-thalassemia are extremely heterogeneous. So far, more than 200 different β-thalassemic mutations have been described. Most of them are point mutations (single base changes, small deletions or insertions), whereas only a minority are due to large deletions encompassing the β-globin cluster (a comprehensive database of thalassemia and other globin gene defects is available at http://globin.cse.psu.edu/).

These mutations may occur in exon or intron sequences, as well as in the promoter or the 5′ and 3′ flanking UTR sequences (Fig. 4). As a consequence of the type and the position in which these defects fall, they have been reported to affect expression of the β-globin gene at the following stages:

- transcription efficiency, for mutations occurring in the promoter region, i.e., recognition sequences for proteins involved in transcriptional or post-transcriptional mechanisms such as the conserved TATA, CCAAT and CACCC boxes. Generally, such mutations are of $\beta^+$ or $\beta^{++}$ types, thus resulting in mild forms of β-thalassemia;
- maturation of pre-mRNA, if they fall into splicing or polyadenylation sites. RNA-splicing mutations are fairly common and represent a large portion of all β-thalassemic mutations. These mutations affect the splicing process at variable degree, depending on the position in which the mutation occurs. Mutations that affect either of the invariant dinucleotide at the intron-exon junction (the GT motif at the 5' or donor site and the AG motif at the 3' or acceptor site) completely abolish normal splicing and result in $\beta^0$-thalassemia. Mutations occurring in the splicing consensus sequences are instead of $\beta^+$ type, resulting in variable degrees of defective splicing and causing milder types of β-thalassemia. Other mutations occurring in exon or intron sequences may activate a cryptic splicing site, thus leading to abnormal mRNA processing. Even in these cases defective splicing occurs at variable degrees, resulting in phenotypes that range from mild to severe;
- RNA stability, if they occur in the 5′ UTR, Cap site, 3′ UTR or the polyadenylation site. These mutations are generally associated with mild β-thalassemia phenotypes. In particular, mutations occurring in the 5′ UTR are so mild that they act as silent β-thalassemic alleles which generally show normal hematological phenotypes in heterozygotes.
- mRNA translation, if they generate premature nonsense codons. Premature termination of globin chain synthesis generally leads to the production of short, nonviable β-chains or to nonsense mediated decay (NMD) of abnormal mRNA. In all these cases mutations are of $\beta^0$-type and result in severe thalassemia;
- protein instability, if they give rise to truncated or elongated globin chains which tend to form insoluble tetrameters.

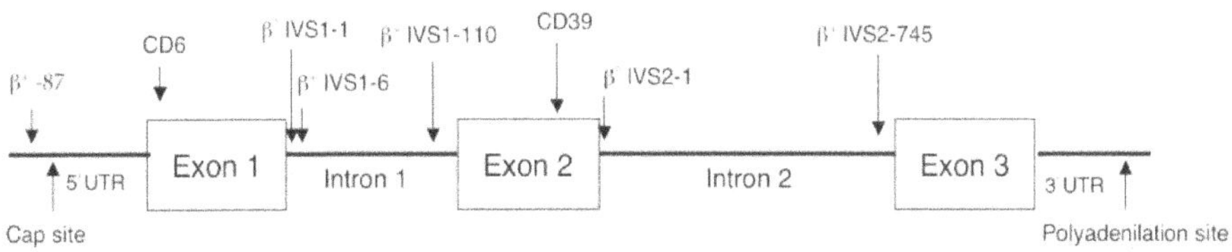


Fig. 4. **Schematic representation of the β-globin gene.** The arrows show the positions of the most frequent β-thalassemic mutations in the Mediterranean area (Rosatelli et al., 1992).

### 5.2.2 The α-thalassemias

Alpha thalassemias are characterized by absent ($\alpha^0$-thalassemia) or reduced ($\alpha^+$-thalassemia) output of α-globin chains, thus resulting in globin chain imbalance. As a consequence, there is a relative excess of γ-and β-globin chains which aggregate to form the homotetramers Hb Bart's and HbH, respectively, and are responsible of a severe hemolytic anemia. The two main groups of α-thalassemia can be further subdivided into deletional and non-deletional forms, according to the specific type of the underlying molecular defect. In fact, the majority of the α-thalassemia defects result from deletions involving one or both α-globin genes on the same chromosome whereas point mutations affecting the functional expression of one of the two α-globin genes ($\alpha_2$ or $\alpha_1$ globin gene) are less common (Harteveld & Higgs, 2010; Higgs & Gibbons, 2010). The cause of the increased susceptibility to such deletional defects for the α-globin cluster with respect to the β-globin cluster is due to the presence of highly homologous regions scattered within this cluster which predispose to events of unequal recombination. Normal individuals have four α-globin genes since each chromosome 16 carries two α-globin genes (Fig. 1); therefore, normal genotypes can be written as αα/αα. Deletions so far reported result in loss of one (-α) or both (--α) of the duplicated α-globin genes from the same chromosome (Kattamis et al., 1996). The clinical picture of α-thalassemia is determined by the number of the remaining functional genes. The deletional loss of the $\alpha_2$ or $\alpha_1$ gene (namely, the $-\alpha^{4.2}$ and $-\alpha^{3.7}$ deletion, respectively) are the most common molecular defects responsible for α-thalassemia. These two mutations have been found, even with different frequencies, in all populations in which thalassemia defects are common. The unequal crossing-over events responsible for their origin give also rise to the corresponding triplicated or quadruplicated α-gene arrangements which are referred to as $\alpha\alpha\alpha^{anti3.7}$ and $\alpha\alpha\alpha^{anti4.2}$ or $\alpha\alpha\alpha\alpha^{anti3.7}$ and $\alpha\alpha\alpha\alpha^{anti4.2}$, respectively. In $\alpha^0$-thalassemias large deletions almost entirely remove the α-globin cluster region. The two most common $\alpha^0$-thalassemias, the $--^{SEA}$ and $-^{MED}$ occur in Southeast Asia and Mediterranean area, respectively (Sessa et al., 2010; Harteveld & Higgs, 2010; Kattamis et al., 1996; Mesbah-Amroun et al., 2008) (Fig. 5).

Non-deletional α-thalassemias (indicated at the heterozygous state as $\alpha\alpha^T/\alpha\alpha$) are due to point mutations that, similarly to the mutations responsible for β-thalassemia, occur in genomic regions critical for normal expression of the α-genes. Furthermore, as for the β-thalassemia defects, they may be classified according to the level of gene expression that is affected and also their distribution is population-specific. However, point mutations affecting the $\alpha_2$ gene are able to impair more greatly α-globin gene expression since in normal conditions the $\alpha_2$ globin gene expression is about three times greater than that of the $\alpha_1$ gene. Therefore, such mutations have more relevant effects on phenotype and it is expected that they could provide a greater selective advantage with respect to malaria infection. It is thus evident that they are more common than those occurring in the $\alpha_1$ gene. On the other hand, non deletional α-thalassemia mutations have also a greater effect on phenotype than -α deletions. In fact, the $-\alpha^{4.2}$ deletional form of α-thalassemia which involves the $\alpha_2$-globin gene results in a compensatory increase in the remaining intact $\alpha_1$ gene, whereas no increased expression in the remaining functional gene is detected when the $\alpha_2$ globin gene is inactivated by a point mutation.

Alpha thalassemia point mutations so far detected may have effects either on RNA processing, as in the case of $\alpha^{Hph}$ mutation, or on RNA translation, as for the $\alpha^{Nco}$ defect, or on protein instability, as for the Hb Suan Dok or the Hb Evanston. Some point mutations affecting the termination codon give rise to elongated α-globin chains, as in the case of Hb Constant Spring which is found with relatively high frequency in Southeast Asia (Harteveld & Higgs, 2010; Weatherall, 2001).

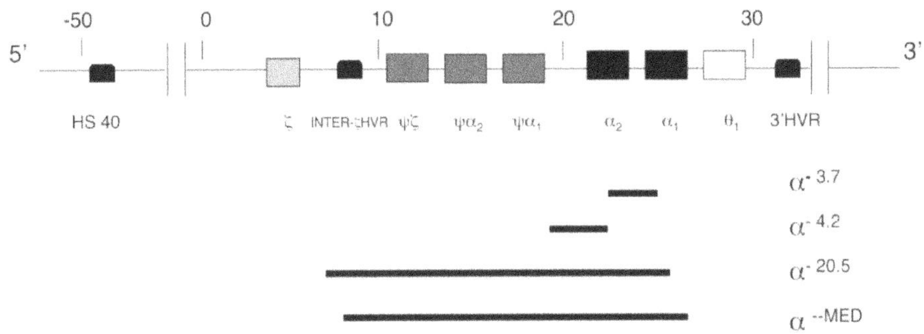


Fig. 5. Schematic representation of the α-globin cluster showing the regions removed by the most frequent α-thalassemic deletions in the Mediterranean area (Harteveld & Higgs, 2010).

### 5.3 High persistence of fetal hemoglobin (HPFH)

Generally, fetal hemoglobin production declines rapidly within few months after birth and in adult life it is detected only in traces (<1% of total hemogobin). This production is normally confined to a particular small subpopulation of red cells, called F cells (fetal cells), in which the fetal profile of globin gene expression is still active. Persistent expression of fetal hemoglobin in adulthood represents a group of conditions which are referred to as HPFH (high persistence of fetal hemoglobin). The mechanisms and the molecular basis underlying these conditions are very heterogeneous. In conditions of hematopoietic stress, such as β-thalassemia, an increased number of F cells may be detected along with higher HbF levels. In these cases the γ-chains have an ameliorative effect on the thalassemic phenotype, since they reduce the excess of α-globin chains. Consequently, the erythroid precursors which produce high γ-chain levels undergo positive selection, thus increasing the number of circulating F cells.

However, because the number of F cells is largely under genetic control, the HbF levels vary considerably in these patients and this contributes to the remarkable diversity in the severity of these diseases (see also the 6.1 paragraph, for further discussion). HbF levels vary considerably not only in thalassemic patients but also in healthy adults, where it represents a benign and clinically silent condition (Thein et al., 2009; Weatherall, 2001).

Besides epigenetic factors such as gender and age (Chang et al., 1995), the molecular basis of this variation largely depends on genetic determinants which may be linked or unlinked to the β-globin cluster. Forms of HPFH may be caused by large deletions within the β-globin cluster or point mutations in the proximal or distant promoter regions of the fetal globin genes (Cao & Moi, 2000). These rare forms, in which all red blood cells show increased levels of HbF, are referred to as pancellular HPFH and are transmitted in a simple Mendelian manner. Large deletions involving intergenic γ-δ sequences, the structural δ- and β-globin genes as well as regulatory regions at the 3′ end of the β-globin cluster (Thein et al., 2009) are associated with reactivation of fetal globin gene expression. These types of rearrangements may indeed cause a loss of regulatory regions involved in globin gene switching or may result in enhancer regions brought in apposition to the γ genes as well. Examples of HPFH deletions in the β-globin cluster are the Sicilian $\delta\beta^0$ deletion (Esposito G. et al., 1994) and the Corfù deletion (Bank A. et al., 2005). A similar but less marked effect on HbF increase is found in the Hb Lepore, a δβ hybrid hemoglobin variant caused by a deletion originated from a mechanism of non homologous recombination between the δ- and β-globin genes. It is thought that this deletion also removes putative elements involved in globin gene switching located between these two genes, thus leading to persistent expression of fetal hemoglobin (Weaterall & Clegg, 2001).

Point mutations responsible for this form of HPFH are thought to modify the binding of transacting factors involved either in the mechanisms of globin gene switching or in γ-globin gene silencing. Among these defects, the most common mutations are those occurring in the proximal promoter region of the $^{G}\gamma$ gene at position -202 (C→G) and –175 (T→C) or in the proximal promoter of the $^{A}\gamma$ gene at position -196 (C→T), -175 (T→C) and -117 (G→A) (Olave et al., 2007). A relatively common C→T polymorphism at position -158 in the $^{G}\gamma$-globin gene, altering a Xmn I recognition site, is associated with increased HbF levels in conditions of hematopoietic stress whereas it has no or little effects in normal individuals. Its presence has also been associated with a delayed decline of γ-globin gene expression in infant age (Grosso et al., 2007).

In heterocellular HPFH, a more common set of conditions, the HbF is distributed in an uneven fashion among F cells. Heterocellular HPFH forms are generally characterized by a structurally intact β-globin cluster and are inherited as a quantitative genetic trait (Thein et al., 2009). Extensive linkage studies have so far identified three major quantitative trait loci (QTLs) involved in the heterocellular HPFH phenotype: the Xmn I-158 $^{G}\gamma$ polymorphism, the HBS1L-MYB intergenic region on chromosome 6q23 and the BCL11A on chromosome 2p16 (Craig et al., 1996; Manzel et al., 2007). The role for one of these QTLs has been recently described. It had been found that the BCL11A locus codifies for a transfactor acting as repressor of fetal globin genes (Xu et al., 2011). Recently, another repressor of fetal globin genes, the Cold Shock Domain Protein A or CSDA, has been identified and characterized (Petruzzelli et al., 2010). Therefore, both these two factors may be directly involved in the switching of globin gene expression through silencing of the transcriptional activity of γ-globin genes in adult life, although additional studies are required in order to define better their role in the regulation of this complex mechanism of gene expression.

## 6. Clinical phenotypes

### 6.1 β-thalassemias

The hallmark of β-thalassemias is the quantitative defect in the production of β-globin chains which leads to imbalanced α-/non α-globin chain ratio and an excess of α-chains. This condition is the main determinant in the pathophysiology of β-thalassemia. Alpha-globin chains in excess precipitate in red-cell precursors, causing oxidative membrane damage, abnormal cell maturation and erythroid premature destruction in the bone marrow with consequent ineffective erythropoiesis. These abnormalities are responsible for the subsequent erythroid marrow expansion and characteristic skeletal deformities. Marrow expansion leads ultimately to increased iron absorption and progressive deposition of iron in tissues (Weatherall & Clegg, 2001). Severity of clinical conditions is thus clearly related to the degree of globin chain imbalance which gives rise to a wide array of extremely diverse hematological phenotypes. The most severe forms are represented by β-thalassemia major, a set of conditions characterized by severe anemia requiring regular blood transfusion treatments for survival since early childhood. These forms most often result from homozygosity or compound heterozygosity for β-globin gene mutations and, in rarer cases, from heterozygosity for dominant mutations. In some cases, however, the same genotypes may lead to milder conditions, referred to as thalassemia intermedia. These intermediate forms show very heterogeneous clinical pictures that range in severity from the asymptomatic condition to transfusion-dependent anemia, generally only slightly less severe than thalassemia major. Since, as above discussed, severity of disease is related to the degree of globin chain imbalance, the milder clinical phenotype of these conditions can be explained by coinheritance of genetic factors that are able to reduce the excess of α-globin chains, such as α-thalassemia that reduce the α-globin chain production, or genetic determinants that lead to persistent expression of γ-globin chains in adulthood, thus increasing the β-like globin chain production. Alternatively, these attenuated phenotypes may also be due to homozygosity for mild mutations or compound heterozygosity for a mild or silent mutation and a more severe defect in the β-globin genes. On the other hand, triplication or quadruplication rearrangements of α-globin genes may produce a more marked imbalance in globin chain production thus leading to a clinical picture of thalassemia intermedia even in simple heterozygotes for β-thalassemia, who are otherwise generally clinically silent (Cao & Moi, 2002; Thein, 2005; Weatherall, 2001; Wong et al., 2004). This latter condition, also referred to as β-thalassemia minor, is characterized by mild anemia and morphological changes of the red blood cells, which are tipically hypochromic and microcitic. Other typical features are represented by increased $HbA_2$ levels and slight increase of HbF (Steinberg & Adams J.G. III, Weatherall & Clegg, 2001). Finally, a rarer form of β-thalassemia trait is characterized by normal $HbA_2$ and thalassemia-like red cell indices (Moi et al., 1988). This condition may represent co-inheritance of mutations, associated or not on the same chromosome and decreasing both β- and δ-globin gene function. Increased HbF levels are usually detected in δβ-thalassemia characterized by deletions involving both δ- and β-globin genes.

### 6.2 α-thalassemias

The clinical phenotypes of α-thalassemia are classified in four types that range from mild to severe conditions, depending on the degree of defective α-globin gene output. The wide heterogeneity in clinical and hematological pictures is largely related on the wide spectrum of molecular defects which may lead to a great variety of genotypes characterized by loss of one, two, three or all four α-globin genes. In general, the loss of only one α-gene leads to very mild clinical conditions, with the $-\alpha^{3.7}$ producing milder phenotypes respect to the $-\alpha^{4.2}$. Non deletional mutants involving the $\alpha_2$ gene are responsible of a more pronounced phenotype, as already discussed, whereas deletional loss of both α genes leads to more severe conditions (Higgs & Gibbons, 2010; Weatherall, 2010).

Deletion of one α gene (-α/αα) is associated to the milder clinical forms of α-thalassemia, referred to as silent carrier state, which are characterized by slight imbalanced α/non-α globin chain production, normal values of $HbA_2$ and mild microcytosis, with or without anemia. The α-thalassemia trait is instead characterized by mild or moderate microcytic and hypochromic anemia, which is clinically asymptomatic and is generally diagnosed during regular health checks or prenatal screening. This condition is commonly generated by loss of two α genes (-α/-α or --/αα genotypes). On the other hand, the homozygous condition of the non deletional form of α-thalassemia responsible for the synthesis of Hb Constant Spring ($\alpha\alpha^{CS}/\alpha\alpha^{CS}$) causes a more severe phenotype respect to the α-thalassemia trait. This condition is characterized by severe anemia, typical thalassemic changes in hematological indices, moderate jaundice and a variable degree of hepatosplenomegaly, a clinical picture more similar to the HbH disease than to the mild thalassemic trait. The HbH disease is most frequently the result of compound heterozygosity for $\alpha^+$ and $\alpha^0$ mutations (--/-α) and is therefore predominantly found in Southeast Asia and in the Mediterranean region, where these defects are more common. HbH disease forms produced by non deletional defects are more severe than those caused by the more common deletional α-thalassemic types. The clinical conditions resemble those of β-thalassemia intermedia. Similarly to these intermediate conditions, the HbH disease is characterized by considerable variation in the severity of hematological conditions. The predominant features are variable degrees of anemia, with hemoglobin levels ranging from 2.6 to 12.4 g/dl, and amounts of HbH from 2 to 40% of total hemoglobin. Hb Bart's is occasionally detected in the peripheral blood. HbH patients usually have hepatosplenomegaly, jaundice in variable degrees, gall stones and acute hemolytic episodes induced by infections or drug treatments. In fact, with respect to the β-thalassemia conditions characterized by ineffective erythropoiesis, in α-thalassemia the main mechanism of anemia is due to hemolysis. The most severe deficiencies in α-globin chain production lead to Hb Bart's hydrops fetalis syndrome, which is commonly the result of inheritance of two $\alpha^0$ determinants, although it may also result from compound heterozygosity for a severe non deletional determinant with a deletional $\alpha^0$ mutant allele. In this syndrome most of the circulating hemoglobin is constituted by the non functional homotetramers γ4 and β4, with also variable amounts of the embryonic Hb Portland, the only functional type of hemoglobin in these patients. The severity of anemia conditions and cardiac failure, along with the other prominent features of this syndrome, often leads to death *in utero* (23-38 weeks of pregnancy) or soon after birth (Weatherall & Clegg, 2001).

## 7. Unusual forms of thalassemia

Over the last two decades, our group has been involved in a prevention program for hemoglobinopathies based on screening and molecular characterization of carriers and on prenatal diagnosis in couples at-risk. In the course of this activity we have defined the molecular basis of several atypical thalassemic phenotypes which have been found to be associated with complex and unusual interactions of mutations affecting the expression of one or more globin genes. Our study provides further indications on the complexity and heterogeneity of molecular basis of thalassemia in our region. Our experience also highlights the potential pitfalls in genetic counselling in areas where globin gene disorders are most common. Some of the most intriguing cases are now being discussed in detail.

### 7.1 A δβ thalassemia phenotype associated with a complex interaction of mutations in the γ-, δ- and β-globin genes

In this case the propositus was a 2 year-old girl of Italian descent showing a mild hypochromic microcytic anemia (Fig. 6) (Grosso M al., 2007). The peripheral blood film showed anisopoikilocytosis and marked microcytosis; she had normal serum iron values and increased osmotic fragility; the hemoglobin analysis, carried out by cation exchange HPLC, revealed normal Hb $A_2$ (2.5%) and increased Hb F (6.4%) levels. This condition was consistent with a δβ-thalassemia trait. To confirm this hypothesis, hematological studies were extended to all family members. Unexpectedly, the father was found to be a typical β-thalassemia carrier with a mild increase of Hb $A_2$ (3.5%) and no Hb F, while the mother showed normal red blood cell indices and iron balance with a low Hb $A_2$ level (1.5%) and no HbF. Her two siblings, a 4 year old brother and a 13 month old sister, had both normal red blood cell indices and iron balance with $HbA_2$=2.1% , HbF=1% and $HbA_2$ 0.8%, HbF 6%, respectively.

Molecular analysis was performed for all family members on genomic DNA. The propositus and her father were heterozygotes for the $\beta^+$IVS I-6 (C→T) mutation. The propositus, her mother and the younger sister were all carriers of the δ+27 (G→T), the Mediterranean most common δ-thalassemia defect (Pirastu et al., 1983) and the -158 $^G\gamma$ gene polymorphism (C→T) (Fig. 6). The molecular study thus showed that in the propositus co-inheritance of the $\beta^+$IVS I-6 with the $\delta^+$27 mutation was responsible for the normalization of the $HbA_2$ level, whereas the HbF increase was associated with the -158 $^G\gamma$-globin gene polymorphism. The δ- and γ-globin gene defects had been co-inherited *in cis* on the maternal chromosome. However, the mother had normal HbF values. In fact, carriers for the -158 $^G\gamma$- gene polymorphism have increased HbF levels only in conditions of erythropoietic stress, which may be caused by a β-thalassemic trait, as found in the propositus and not in her mother. This case also allowed us to detect a novel *in cis* association of the -158 $^G\gamma$ polymorphism with a δ-thalassemic defect, thus providing further evidence of the complex effects on the hematological phenotype when different thalassemic defects are co-inherited.

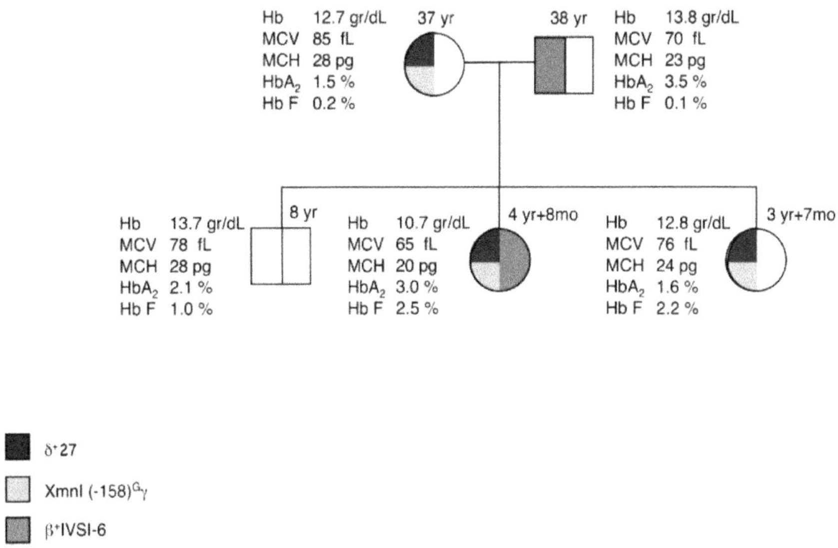


Fig. 6. **Complex interaction of mutations in the γ-, δ- and β-globin genes.** Pedigree with hematological data of the propositus and her family. The propositus had inherited the β-thalassemic defect from her father and the maternal chromosome bearing both the $\delta^+$27 mutation, which is responsible for the normalization of the $HbA_2$ level, and the -158 (C→T) $^G\gamma$-globin gene polymorphism associated with increased HbF levels.

### 7.2 An unusual δβ-thalassemia phenotype associated with a complex interaction of mutations in the δ- and β-globin genes

We investigated the molecular basis of a mild hypochromic microcytic anemia in a 5-year-old boy from Naples, Italy (Grosso et al., 2001). The patient had normal $HbA_2$ (2.5%) and no HbF. Osmotic resistance, serum iron and transferrin concentrations were within normal values. His father had normal red blood indices and iron balance, low $HbA_2$ (1.5%) and normal HbF (0.3%) levels. His mother had mildly hypochromic microcytic red blood indices, normal $HbA_2$ (2.7%) and HbF (0.6%). This phenotype could have been explained by either double heterozygosity for δ- and β-thalassemia or heterozygosity for α-thalassemia. Globin chain synthesis analysis allowed to exclude the α-thalassemia carrier status since the α/non-α globin chain ratio was 2.27 for the patient, and 1.66 and 0.96 for his mother and father, respectively. Reverse phase HPLC performed in the course of globin chain synthesis analysis revealed in the patient and his mother an anomalous β-globin peak that showed features comparable to those of Hb Neapolis (beta 126 (H4) Val→Gly). Hb Neapolis is a rare unstable hemoglobin variant undetectable by conventional hematological HPLC screening methods and showing mild thalassemic features. Subjects heterozygous for this variant are characterized by mild microcytosis and slightly increased Hb $A_2$ levels (Pagano et al., 1991; Pagano et al., 1997). DNA sequence analysis confirmed the presence of the mutation causing the synthesis of Hb Neapolis in the propositus and his mother.

Our study also revealed the $\delta^{+}27$ (G→T) mutation in the heterozygote state, in the patient and his father.

These results indicated that the atypical δβ-thalassemia phenotype was determined in this patient by coinheritance *in trans* of $\delta^{+}27$ (G→T) and β-globin codon 126 (T→G) mutations. The δ-thalassemic trait completely normalized $HbA_2$ concentration, thus almost completely silencing the mild β-thalassemic phenotype produced by Hb Neapolis (Fig. 7).

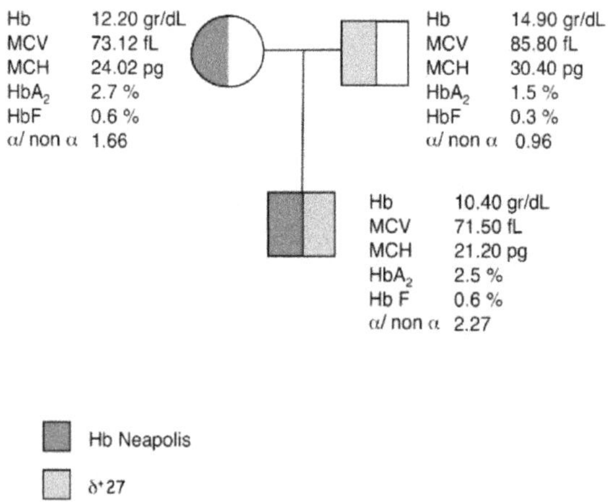


Fig. 7. **An unusual δβ-thalassemia phenotype associated with a complex interaction of mutations in the δ- and β-globin genes.** Pedigree with hematological data of the propositus and his family. The propositus was found to be a compound heterozygous for two rare mutations: a rare hemoglobin variant, the Hb Neapolis, associated with a mild thalassemic phenotype, inherited from his mother, and a δ-thalassemic defect ($\delta^{+}27$) of paternal origin, which was responsible for the normalization of the HbA2 level (2.5%).

It is noteworthy that the $HbA_2$ level detected in the mother is lower comparable to that expected for carriers of the Hb Neapolis variant. In this case the slightly increased $HbA_2$ level reported for this mutation was reduced to normal values by coexistence of iron deficiency (Moi et al., 1988). This condition might have masked the underlying mild β-thalassemia carrier status, thus strengthening the importance of accurate evaluation of hematological features in families at-risk for hemoglobinopathies.

### 7.3 Interaction of α- and β-globin gene mutations in a couple at risk for thalassemia

A couple at risk for hemoglobinophaties, originated from Nigeria, was referred to our Prenatal Centre for genetic counselling. The woman showed slight microcytic indices with normal iron and ferritin serum values. Cation exchange HPLC analysis of hemoglobin showed mild increase of Hb F and normal HbA2 level, along with an abnormal peak consistent with the presence of the HbS variant at the heterozygous state. The Hb S is characterized by the replacement of the glutamic acid residue at position 6 with a valine residue in the β-globin chain. At the DNA level a point mutation (A→T) at codon 6 modifies the codon GAG (glutamic acid) into GTG (valine) (Weatherall & Clegg, 2001). Molecular analysis confirmed the presence of this mutation and excluded other β-globin gene defects.

Her partner showed a slight microcytic anemia, normal HbA2 values (2.9%) with both serum iron and ferritin low levels (Fig. 8).

We hypothesized that the hematological phenotype in both cases could be explained by the presence of α-thalassemia defects. Indeed, both partners were found to be heterozygous for the $-\alpha^{3.7}$ deletion, one of the most common *thalassemic* defects in their country of origin along with the hemoglobin variant HbS (Galanello & Origa, 2010). Transmission of both these defects does not represent a factor of risk for hemoglobinopathy since when combined with α-thalassemic determinants, the HbS defect remains in a carrier state (Cao & Moi, 2000).

However, it is known that iron deficiency contributes to slightly reduce HbA2 levels. Therefore, we could not exclude that the normal HbA2 value detected in the male could have been the result of a complex combination of both genetic and epigenetic factors. We thus performed extensive β-globin gene sequence analysis also in this subject, in order to verify the hypothesis that the α-thalassemic defect associated with iron deficiency could have masked a mild β-thalassemic trait. Indeed, if this was the case, co-inheritance of the paternal β-thalassemic allele with the maternal HbS defect, which also occurs within the β-globin gene, would affect the production of functional hemoglobin with varying degree of severity and cause a disease known as HbS-β thalassemia (Weatherhall & Clegg, 2001).

This analysis showed the presence at the heterozygous state of a single nucleotide substitution at the position 108 in the first intron of the β-globin gene (IVS1-108), a defect reported to be associated with a mild β-thalassemic trait phenotype in a Cuban patient of European origin (Muñiz et al., 2000). It has been hypothesized that this point mutation may activate an intronic cryptic branch site, resulting in defective β-globin gene splicing efficiency.

Our study thus allowed us to define the risk of this couple having a child with HbS-β thalassemia disease which, on the basis of the mild β-thalassemic defect, we might expect would present with mild or moderate symptoms.

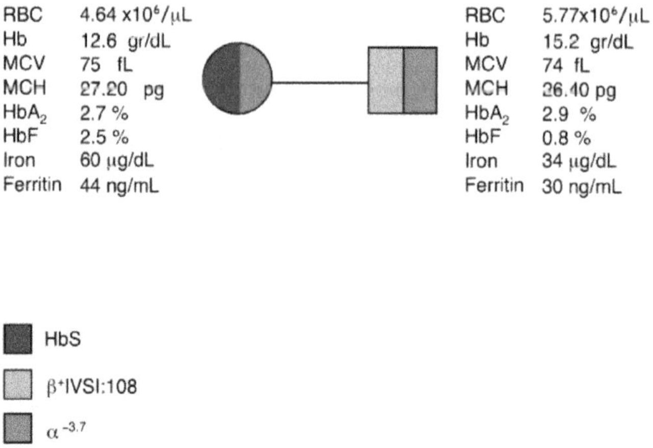


Fig. 8. **Interaction of α- and β-globin gene mutations in a couple at risk for thalassemia.** Genotypes and hematological phenotypes of the couple at-risk for hemoglobinopathy. Serum iron and ferritin values are also reported, showing a mild hyposideremic condition in the male partner.

### 7.4 Rare α-thalassemic genotypes detected in a family at-risk for thalassemia.

A couple of Italian descend at risk for thalassemia was referred to our Prenatal Centre for genetic counselling and further investigations. The woman who was at the 8th week of pregnancy showed slight microcythemia (MCV=78.40 fl) with normal values of $HbA_2$ and Hb F. This phenotype was consistent with a typical α-thalassemia carrier state. However, the proband was found negative for the most common deletional forms of α-thalassemia. Since her partner was a typical carrier of β-thalassemic trait, extensive molecular studies were performed in the woman to exclude the presence of any silent or mild β-thalassemia defect.
Furthermore, to investigate the molecular basis of this very mild phenotype, we extended our study to her parents.
We found that whereas her mother had normal hematological indices, her father showed a more relevant reduction of both MCV and $HbA_2$ values with respect to her daughter (Fig. 9). In this subject, analysis of α-thalassemic deletions revealed the heterozygous condition for the thalassemic $-\alpha^{-3.7}$ defect. Sequencing analysis performed on the α-globin genes revealed in both the propositus and her father the heterozygous state for a deletion of five nucleotides in the 5′ donor site of the first intron (-TGAGG) of the α2-globin gene that abolishes a restriction site for the Hph I restriction enzyme. This mutation, like other non deletional α-thalassemic determinants, has a more severe effect on the hematological phenotype with respect to deletions of single α-globin genes. Our study thus allowed us to define the complex α-globin gene genotypes in this family: the propositus was a carrier of a non deletional defect ($\alpha\alpha^T/\alpha\alpha$) whereas her father had a more complex genotype ($\alpha\alpha^T/-\alpha$), consistent with his more prominent α-thalassemic phenotype.
These investigations also allowed us to exclude the risk for thalassemia and the requirement for prenatal diagnosis in this couple since, as already discussed, co-inheritance of α-thalassemia trait has ameliorative effects on the β-thalassemic phenotype.

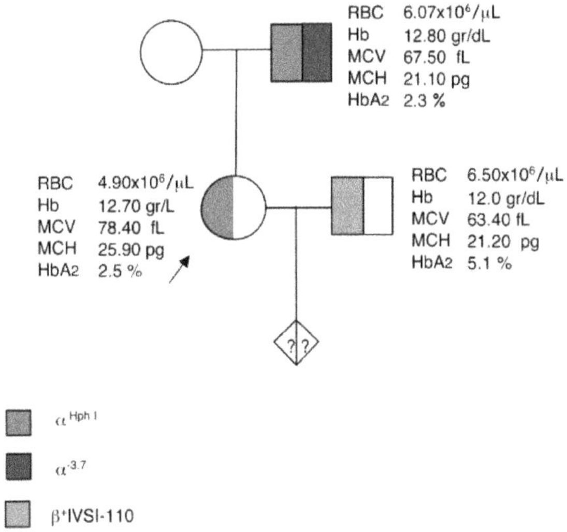


Fig. 9. **Rare α-thalassemic genotypes detected in a family at-risk for thalassemia.** Pedigree with hematological data of the propositus and her family. The arrow shows the proband who was found to be a carrier of a rare point mutation in the α-globin gene ($\alpha^{Hph\,I}$), inherited from her father who instead is a compound heterozygous for a common deletional defect ($-\alpha^{-3.7}$) and the rarer non deletional $\alpha^{Hph\,I}$ mutation.

## 8. Conclusions

The thalassemias, together with sickle cell anemia, are the most common group of inherited monogenic disorders in the world. Their high incidence is related to selective advantage of the carrier state to malaria infection. As a result, these diseases are mostly common in geographic areas extending from the Mediterranean region through tropical countries including Sub-Saharian Africa, the Middle East, India, Southeast Asia and Indonesia, where malaria was or still is endemic. Their clinical severity varies greatly, from asymptomatic hypochromia and microcytosis conditions to life-threatening ineffective erythropoiesis and hemolytic anemia. The more severe conditions require intensive medical treatments throughout life, even though, as a result of advances in transfusion, iron chelation and bone marrow transplantation therapies, expectancy as well as quality of life have increased very considerably in the last years.

Among the first diseases to be studied at the molecular level, the thalassemias still remain a paradigm for understanding the pathogenetic basis of inherited disorders, as well as the molecular mechanisms involved in the regulation of gene expression. In fact, since late 70's when DNA recombinant technologies emerged as a powerful tool for the identification of the molecular defects of the human inherited diseases, the experimental strategies and the methods firstly developed to study hemoglobinopathies were subsequently applied to define the molecular basis of other genetic diseases. These studies have also contributed to define the complex pathophysiological mechanisms underlying these syndromes and have made possible prevention programs based on large-scale screening and prenatal diagnosis in populations at high risk for hemoglobinopathies.

Molecular and clinical investigations have also provided powerful insights into the relationships between the molecular basis of thalassemias and their clinical diversity and have contributed to clarify the effects of the interactions among different genetic determinants on the thalassemic phenotypes, providing in the meantime the basis for accurate genetic counselling and preventive medicine services.

More recently, many efforts have been made toward the definition of the molecular basis of globin gene switching which represents a fascinating and unique model to study the mechanisms of gene expression regulation in space and time. Furthermore, these studies are also expected to provide novel therapeutic targets in the treatment of sickle cell anemia and β-thalassemia, as conditions of high persistence of fetal hemoglobin (HPFH) or drug-mediated reactivation of fetal globin gene expression have considerable ameliorating effects on the severity of these conditions.

A vast body of knowledge has been gained so far and great progress has been made in the understanding of these mechanisms. It is expected that these advances will rapidly lead to novel molecular approaches to the treatment of hemoglobinopathies, before definitive gene therapy strategies will enter clinical practice.

## 9. References


Bank A., O'Neill D., Lopez L., Pulte D., Ward M., Mantha S. & Richardson C. (2005). Role of intergenic human γ-δ globin sequences in human hemoglobin switching and reactivation of fetal hemoglobin in adult erythroid cells. *Annals of the New York Academy of Science*, 1054, pp. 48-54

Cao A. & Moi P. (2000). Genetic modifying factors in beta-thalassemia. *Clinical Chemistry and Laboratory Medicine*, 38, pp. 123-132

Cao A. & Moi P. (2002). Regulation of the globin genes. *Pediatric Research*, 51, 4, pp. 415-421

Chang Y.C., Smith K.D., Moore R.D., Serjeant G.R. & Dover G.J. (1995). An analysis of fetal hemoglobin variation in sickle cell disease: the relative contribution of the X-linked factor, β-globin haplotypes, α-globin gene number, gender and age. *Blood*, 8, pp.1111-1117

Craig J.E., Rochette J., Fisher C.A., Weatherall D.J., Marc S., Lathrop G.M., Demenais F. & Thein S.L. (1996). Dissecting the loci controlling fetal haemoglobin production on chromosomes 11p and 6p by the regressive approach. *Nature Genetics*, 12, pp. 58-64.

Esposito G., Grosso M., Gottardi E., Izzo P., Camaschella C. & Salvatore F. (1994). A unique origin for the Sicilian (δβ)°-thalassemia in 33 unrelated families and its rapid diagnostic characterization by PCR analysis. *Human Genetics*, 93, pp. 691-693.

Fathallah H. & Atweh G.F. (2006). Induction of fetal hemoglobin in the treatment of Sickle Cell Disease. *Hematology American Society of Hematological Education Program*, pp. 58-62

Galanello R. & Origa R. (2010). β-thalassemia. *Orphanet Journal of Rare Diseases*, 5: 11

Grosso M., Rescigno G., Zevino C., Matarazzo M., Poggi V. & Izzo P. (2001). A rare case of compound heterozygosity for δ+27 and Hb Neapolis (Dhonburi) associated to an atypical β-thalassemia phenotype. *Haematologica*, 86, pp. 985-986

Grosso M., Amendolara M., Rescigno G., Danise P., Todisco N., Izzo P. & Amendola G. (2008). Delayed decline of γ-globin expression in infant age associated with the presence of $^{G}\gamma$-158 (C→T) polymorphism. *International Journal of Laboratory Hematology*, 31, pp. 359-363.

Harteveld C.L. & Higgs D.R. (2010). α-thalassaemia. *Orphanet Journal of Rare Diseases*, 5: 13

Higgs D.R. & Gibbons R.J. (2010). The molecular basis of α-thalassemia: a model for understanding human molecular genetics. *Hematology/Oncology Clinics of North America*, 24, 6, pp. 1033-1054

Ho P.J. & Thein S.L. (2000). Gene regulation and deregulation: a β globin perspective. *Blood reviews*, 14, pp. 78-93

Kattamis A.C., Camaschella C., Sivera P., Surrey S. & Fortina P. (1996). Human α-thalassemia syndromes: Detection of molecular defects. *American Journal of Hematology*, 53, pp. 81-91

Mesbah-Amroun H., Rouabhi F., Ducrocq R. & Elion J. (2008). Molecular basis of alpha-thalassemia in Algeria. *Hemoglobin*, 32, 3, pp. 273-278

Menzel S., Garner C., Gut I., Matsuda F., Yamaguchi M., Health S., Foglio M., Zelenika D., Boland A., Rooks H., Best S., Spector T.D., Farrall M., Lathrop M. & Thein S.L. (2007). A QTL influencing F cell production maps to a gene encoding a zinc-finger protein on chromosome 2p15. *Nature Genetics*, 39, 10, pp. 1197-1199

Moi P., Paglietti E., Sanna A., Brancati C., Tagarelli A., Galanello R., Cao A. & Pirastu M. (1988). Delineation of the molecular basis of delta- and normal $HbA_2$ β-thalassemia. *Blood*, 72, pp. 530-533

Muñiz A., Martinez G., Lavinha J. & Pacheco P. (2000).Beta-thassaemia in Cubans: novel allele increases the genetic diversity at the HBB locus in the Caribbean. *American Journal of Hematology*, 64, 1, pp. 7-14

Olave I.A., Doneanu C., Fang X., Stamatoyannopoulos G. & Li Q. (2007). Purification and identification of proteins that bind the Hereditary Persistence of fetal Hemoglobin -198 mutation in the γ-globin gene promoter. *The Journal of Biological Chemistry*, 282, 2, pp. 853-862

Oneal P., Gantt N.M., Schwartz J.D., Bhanu N.V., Lee Y.T., Moroney J.W., Reed C.H., Schechter A., Ludan N.L. & Miller J.L. (2006). Fetal hemoglobin silencing in human. *Blood*, 108, pp. 2081-2086

Pagano L., Lacerra G., Camardella L., De Angioletti M., Fioretti G., Maglione G., de Bonis C., Guarino E., Viola A. & Cutolo R. (1991). Hemoglobin Neapolis, beta 126 (H4) Val → Gly: a novel beta-chain variant associated with a mild beta-thalassemia phenotype and displaying anomalous stability features. *Blood*, 78, pp. 3070-3075

Pagano L., Carbone V., Fioretti G., Viola A., Buffardi S., Rametta V., Desicato S., Pucci P. & De Rosa C. (1997). Compound heterozygosity for Hb Lepore-Boston and Hb Neapolis (Dhonburi) (beta 126 (H4) Val→Gly) in a patient from Naples, Italy. *Hemoglobin*, 21, pp. 1-15

Petruzzelli R., Gaudino S., Amendola G., Sessa R., Puzone S., Di Concilio R., d'Urzo G., Amendolara M., Izzo P. & Grosso M. (2010). Role of the Cold Shock Domain Protein A in the transcriptional regulation of HBG expression. *British Journal of Haematology*, 150, 6, pp. 689-699

Pi W., Zhu X., Wu M., Sessa R., Whang Y., Fulzele S., Eroglu A., Ling J. & Tuan D. (2010). Long-range function of the intergenic retrotransposon. *Proceedings of the National Academy of Sciences, USA*, 150, 6, pp. 689-699

Pirastu M., Galanello R., Melis M.A., Brancati C., Tagarelli A., Cao A. & Kan Y.W. (1983). Delta (+)-thalassemia in Sardinia. *Blood*, 62, pp. 341-345

Rosatelli M.C., Tuveri T., Scalas M.T., Leono G.B., Sardu R., Faà V., Meloni A., Pischedda M.A. & Monni G. (1992). Molecular screening and fetal diagnosis of β-thalassemia in the Italian population. *Human Genetics*, 89, pp. 585-589

Ross J., Bottardi S., Bourgoin V., Wollenschlaeger A., Drobetsky E., Trudel M. & Milot E. (2009). Differential requirement of distal regulatory region for pre-initiation complex formation at globin gene promoters. *Nucleic Acids Research*, 37, 16, pp. 5295-5308

Sessa R., Puzone S., Ammirabile M., Piscopo C., Pagano L., Colucci S., Izzo P. & Grosso M. (2010). Identification and molecular characterization of the --CAMPANIA deletion, a novel alpha (0)-thalassemic defect, in two unrelated Italian families. *American Journal of Hematology*, 85, pp.143-144

Stamatoyannopoulos G. & Gronsveld F. (2001). Hemoglobin switching, In: *The Molecular Basis of Blood Diseases*, G. Stamatoyannopoulos G., Majerus P.W., Perlmutter R.M. & Varmus H. Eds., pp. 135-182, Saunders, ISBN-10: 0721676715, Philadelphia, PA, USA

Steinberg M.H. and Adams J.G. III (1991). Hemoglobin $A_2$: origin, evolution and aftermath. *Blood*, 78, pp. 2165-2177

Thein S.L. (2005). Genetic modifiers of beta-thalassemia. *Human Molecular Genetics*, 18, 90, 5, pp. 649-660

Thein S.L., Menzel S., Lathrop M. & Garner C. (2009). Control of fetal hemoglobin: new insights emerging from genomics and clinical implications. *Human Molecular Genetics*, 18, pp. 216-223

Weatherall D.J. (2001). Phenotype-genotype relationships in monogenic disease: lessons from the thalassaemias. *Nature Reviews*, 2, pp. 245-255

Weatherall D.J. & Clegg J.B. (2001). *The thalassaemia syndrome* (Fourth edition), *Blackwell Science, ISBN*-10: 0865426643, *Oxford, UK*

Wong W.S., Chan A.Y., Yip S.F., Ma E.S. (2004). Thalassemia intermedia due to co-inheritance of beta0/beta(+)-thalassemia and (--SEA) alpha-thalassemia/Hb Westmead [alpha122 (H5) His→Gln (alpha2)] in a Chinese family. *Hemoglobin*, 28, 2, pp. 151-156

Xu J., Sankaran V.G., Ni M., Menne T.F., Puram R.V., Kim W. & Orkin S.H. (2011). Transcriptional silencing of γ-globin by BCL11A involves long-range interactions and cooperation with SOX6. *Genes & Development*, 24, pp. 783-798

# 22

# Paroxysmal Nocturnal Hemoglobinuria

Antonio M. Risitano
*Head of Bone Marrow Transplant Clinical Unit*
*Department of Biochemistry and Medical Biotechnologies*
*Federico II University of Naples, Naples*
*Italy*

## 1. Introduction

Paroxysmal nocturnal hemoglobinuria (PNH) is a complex hematological disorder resulting in a quite unique clinical syndrome. In fact, the typical clinical presentation encompasses three distinct hematological manifestations, i.e., hemolytic anemia, bone marrow failure and thrombophilia (Dunn et al 2000; Parker & Ware 2003; Notaro & Luzzatto 2003). Thus, the term PNH covers only one feature of the disease - the one that is the most evident to patients, even if it does not reveal the actual clinical and pathophysiological complexity of the disease. The first extensive description of PNH was made by Dr. Strübing in 1882, although some cases could be identified even in older reports (maybe the first one dates back to 1678 by Dr. Schmidt from Gdanks). Remarkably, Dr. Strübing recognized the uniqueness of the clinical syndrome (hemolytic anemia with possible thrombosis), anticipating some of the pathophysiological implications that were unraveled decades later. In fact, he hypothesized that hemoglobinuria was due to "*red blood cells which dissolve into the vessels*" (corresponding to intravascular hemolysis in current terminology), possibly secondary to a "*disordered blood production*" of erythrocytes which are "*abnormally sensitive*" to acidification (namely, the production of blood cells with the aberrant PNH phenotype, that makes them susceptible to complement-mediated lysis) (Crosby 1951). However, it was with Marchiafava and Nazari (Marchiafava & Nazari 1911) in 1911 that the disease was recognized as a distinct medical entity, characterized by "*chronic hemolytic anemia with perpetual hemosiderinuria*", subsequently known as the *Marchiafava-Micheli syndrome* (Micheli 1928); the current name "*paroxysmal nocturnal hemoglobinuria*" was eventually coined by Dr. Enneking in 1928 (Enneking 1928). In the last century, a number of reports on PNH were subsequently published because the puzzling nature of the disease has intrigued generations of investigators; however, PNH remained a mystery until the 1980s, when most of its pathophysiology was progressively elucidated, first with the description of the molecular defect of PNH cells, and then with the identification of the underlying genetic defect. By that time it was already known that PNH erythrocytes are exquisitely sensitive to lysis upon complement activation, both *in vivo* and *in vitro*. Thus, the observation that PNH cells lack from their surface some complement regulators, all included in a specific class of membrane-bound proteins (the so-called glycosyl phosphatidyl-inositol (GPI)-anchored proteins [GPI-APs]), clearly explained the reason for such sensitivity. Thereafter, the biochemical pathway accounting for GPI-AP surface expression was described, as well as its impairment in PNH cells. Finally, the genetic lesion leading to the aberrant phenotype was identified in distinct mutations in the *phosphatidyl-inositol glycan class A (PIG-A)* gene. This formally demonstrated that PNH is a clonal hematological disorder characterized by the expansion of abnormal (GPI-AP deficient, *PIG-A* mutated) hematopoietic stem cells (HSCs) carrying an intrinsic defect, that accounts for the clinical phenoptype of the disease. Nowadays most pathophysiological events occurring in PNH patients have been extensively described, even if definitive explanations for some disease manifestations (i.e., thromboembolic events) are still elusive. In the last few years, insights into the field pertain to the new treatment strategies that have drastically changed the management and clinical outcome of PNH patients. In fact, the availability of an inhibitor of the complement cascade - the actual effector mechanism of hemolysis in PNH - has led to the first etiological treatment for PNH, which seems to have a superb impact on the natural history of the disease.

## 2. Epidemiology

PNH is a rare acquired disease, with a worldwide prevalence estimated in the range of 1-5 cases per million (Rosse 1996; Orphanet 2004) regardless of the ethnicity; however, given the rarity of the disease and possible reporting biases, its incidence and prevalence remain largely unknown. Indeed, most reports deal with retrospective data, but formal epidemiological studies are lacking. A recent analysis from a well-defined geographical area (Hill et al 2006c) suggests that the actual incidence could be higher than previously reported, in the range of about 1.3/1,000,000/year, leading to a prevalence of about 15 cases per million in a 15 year observation period; however, these data may suffer from biases due to referral center, as well as to inclusion criteria (Parker et al 2005; De Latour et al 2008) In fact, a higher incidence might reflect the inclusion of patients with subclinical PNH, who have not been included in previous studies. In additional, geographical variations in PNH incidence should be considered; for instance, an increased prevalence is reported in some regions which also harbor higher incidence of aplastic anemia (e.g., Thailand and some other Asian countries) (Pramoonjago et al 1999). A multi-national prospective PNH registry is currently ongoing, and possibly will provide more definitive data on the actual incidence and prevalence of PNH in different geographical areas (Muus et al 2010). The incidence of PNH is similar in both genders, and most patients are diagnosed in their middle age (third or fourth decades), although cases have been reported in adolescents, children and even the elderly (De Latour et al 2008; Ware et al 1991).

## 3. Genetic basis

### 3.1 The GPI anchor and the *PIG-A* gene

The hallmark of PNH is hemolytic anemia secondary to the intrinsic susceptibility of affected red cells to complement activation (Ham & Dingle 1939; Rosse & Dacie 1966); thus, the presence of intrinsically abnormal blood cells is the cause of the disease phenotype. However, in PNH patients not all blood cells are affected, as they in fact present a mosaicism of normal and abnormal blood cells; therefore, a putative genetic cause was unlikely to be inherited or transmitted to the progeny. The clonal origin of PNH hematopoiesis was first demonstrated in 1970 by Dr. Luzzatto's group, who showed that, in patients heterozygous for the glucose-6-phosphate-dehydrogenase (G6PD), affected red blood cells (RBCs) all share the same G6PD allele (which, on the other hand, is not involved in pathophysiology of the disease *per se*) (Oni et al 1970). Subsequently, the biochemical defect of PNH cells was identified in a specific molecular abnormality, consisting in the bizarre lack of several proteins from the cell surface. This peculiar defect was first described in the 1980s (Kunstling & Rosse 1969; Nicholson-Weller et al 1983; Selvaraj et al 1988), and rapidly became the hallmark of PNH, although its relationship with the pathophysiology of the disease remained obscure at that time. Notably, this abnormal phenotype pertained not only to erythrocytes, rather it included myeloid and megakaryocytic lineages too, suggesting that it derived from either multi-potent hematopoietic progenitors or even hematopoietic stem cells (Kinoshita et al 1985). Focusing on the underlying intrinsic abnormality rather than on the consequences of individual protein deficiency (which accounts for the susceptibility to hemolysis, as discussed later on), it became clear that all the proteins missing from the PNH cell surface shared a common mechanism responsible for their attachment to the cell membrane (Medof et al 1987). This is a specific glycolipid structure named glycosyl-phosphatidyl inositol (GPI) anchor (Mahoney et al 1992). The functional implications of the GPI-anchoring of proteins are not completely understood; they include ease of assemblage and shedding, lateral mobility, capping, involvement in endo-, exo-, and potocytosis (a clathrin-independent form of endocytosis and recycling). The strongest evidence that this type of membrane anchoring is important in cell biology is its high conservation among eukaryotic cells; indeed, it is found even in yeast and trypanosome. In 1993, using complementation of GPI-anchored protein deficient cell lines and expression cloning, Kinoshita and colleagues first isolated the cDNA of the *PIG-A* gene (Takeda et al 1993; Miyata et al 1993). *PIG-A* is a housekeeping gene located on the short arm of the X chromosome (Xp22.1); the organization of the genomic gene was described in 1994 (Bessler et al 1994). The *PIG-A* gene, in combination with at least two other proteins, encodes an enzyme essential to transfer N-acetyl glucosamine to phosphatidyl inositol; this is the very first step of the GPI-anchor biosynthesis (Armostrong et al 1992; Hirose et al 1992; Takahashi et al 1993). GPI-deficient cell lines showing defects in any of the various metabolic steps have been produced by experimental mutagenesis (Kinoshita et al 1995); however, the study of PNH has shown, at the very beginning surprisingly, that the same early step is impaired in all patients, and all patients have a mutation in the *PIG-A* gene (Takeda et al 1993, Luzzatto et al 1997, Nafa et al 1995). The present explanation for this finding is that among the various genes involved in the GPI-anchor synthesis, *PIG-A* may be the only one that is X-linked (Almeida et al 2009). As a consequence, a single mutation in that gene will produce an abnormal cell in either sex: males have only one allele and females have only one functional allele (as result of X-chromosome inactivation). Although females have two *PIG-A* alleles, only half of the mutation will occur in the functional X; thus, the risk of having the disease is the same in both genders. Since a defect causing a metabolic block is generally recessive, it is very unlikely (although not impossible) that a double mutation targeting both alleles of an autosomal gene in the same cell may occur in vivo. In keeping with this assumption, quite recently two kindreds harboring a mutation in the *PIG-M* gene were described (hence, with the genetic lesion inherited, not acquired). Indeed, all affected members did not develop PNH, but presented a quite distinct clinical syndrome characterized by a partial GPI deficiency associated with a propensity to thrombosis and seizures, in the absence of significant hemolysis (Almeida et al 2006).

### 3.2 *PIG-A* mutations in PNH

Direct sequencing of the *PIG-A* gene has demonstrated distinct mutations in all PNH patients (Luzzatto et al 2000; Nishimura et al 1999); in most cases, each patient has a single mutation (even if distinct *PIG-A* mutated clones may co-exist in some patients) and mutations are unique to each patient (private mutations). These mutations can be found in all blood lineages, consistent with a genetic lesion occurring in hematopoietic stem cell(s) (Takeda et al 1993; Endo et al 1995). All types of mutations have been observed (Nafa et al 1995; Nafa et al 1998): small deletions or insertions producing frameshift (the most frequent), nucleotide substitutions resulting in stop codon, large deletions, missense mutations causing amino acids substitutions or new sites for alternative splicing. No particular clustering of mutations has emerged, even if most of the mutations occur in exon 2, probably because it is the largest. If we compare the type of mutations found in PNH with those found in G6PD deficiency -- another (this time inherited) X-linked disorder of a housekeeping gene -- a clear discrepancy is evident. In PNH, a vast majority of mutations have extremely severe functional consequences, (i.e., production of truncated proteins, leading to a complete GPI deficiency - the PNH type III phenotype), whereas missense mutations are rare (usually resulting in the PNH type II phenotype); in G6PD deficiency almost all mutations are missense, leading to single amino acid substitutions with conserved (although possibly altered) function. Two considerations may be relevant to this discrepancy: i. in inherited disorders, mutations in a housekeeping gene may be lethal, and thus have been selected to allow residual functional activity; by contrast, null mutations can be seen if they are somatically acquired, because they do not affect organ development and pertains only to a small fraction of somatic cells, which may survive albeit with some functional abnormality; ii. if missense mutations in PNH are rare, it means that the gene must be seriously damaged for leading to a clonal expansion. Indeed, the rare missense mutations found in PNH patients are associated with a marked reduction of GPI-linked proteins, indicating that they usually have affected either mRNA stability or protein function, or both. Remarkably, different types of mutations may account for different cell phenotypes in PNH patients, especially when the erythrocytes are considered. In fact, RBCs harboring a mutation leading to the complete inactivation of the *PIG-A* gene product will unequivocally show a complete deficiency of all GPI-APs from their surface (the so-called PNH type III phenotype). In contrast, mutations leading to partial inactivation of the *PIG-A* gene (for instance missence mutations) may lead to a partial deficiency of GPI-APs, known as the PNH type II phenotype. Of note, this biochemical finding has direct functional consequences; in fact, as discussed later on, type II and type III erythrocytes have a quite distinct susceptibility to complement-mediated lysis (Rosse & Dacie 1966). Quite surprisingly, some PNH patients may harbor at the same time type II and type III cells, suggesting that distinct *PIG-A* mutated HSCs may expand concomitantly (Endo et al 1995; Nafa et al 1998). Indeed, even phenotypically identical PNH cells may carry distinct *PIG-A* genotypes (Endo et al 1995, Nishimura et al 1997), suggesting that the functional phenotype rather than the specific genetic defect may play a major role in the development of the disease (Luzzatto et al 1997), as discussed below.

## 4. Pathophysiology

### 4.1 The dual pathophysiology theory

PNH develops through a somatic mutation in the *PIG-A* gene occurring in HSC(s), which originate progeny mature blood cells uniquely lacking of all GPI-APs from their surface.

PNH is therefore an acquired genetic blood disorder, that cannot be transmitted to the progeny; however, the *PIG-A* mutation is likely insufficient to cause the disease and additional events are thought to be involved (Rotoli & Luzzatto 1989).

#### 4.1.1 The *PIG-A* mutation is not sufficient for the development of clinical PNH

A number of observations support the idea that the *PIG-A* mutation itself is necessary, but not sufficient to cause PNH. In fact, the expansion of PNH cells over normal hematopoiesis remains a key step to develop the disease phenotype. These observations include both findings from tentative animal models of PNH, as well as findings from human individuals, with or without PNH.

*Murine models of PNH.* In order to explore experimentally the causal relationship between the *PIG*-A mutation and the development of PNH, murine models have been generated in the last few years to recapitulate human PNH (Rosti 2002). Initially, a complete knockout animal has been attempted, but it could not be produced due to fetal loss, demonstrating that *pig-a* is necessary for embryogenesis (Kawagoe et al 1996). Thus, a different strategy was devised, aiming to inactivate the mouse *pig-a* gene directly in embryonic stem (ES) cells, using the conventional knock-out gene targeting technique. Preliminary *in vitro* studies demonstrated that *pig-a* deficient ES cells were able to differentiate into mature cells of various hematopoietic lineages, thus showing that *pig-a* is not necessary for the differentiation and maturation of hematopoietic progenitors (Rosti et al 1997). However, when this approach was challenged *in vivo*, using chimeras obtained by inserting *pig-a* knocked out ES cells in early embryonic development, only a few chimeras survived (pointing out, once again, the pivotal role of the GPI-anchor for embryonic development), showing a low proportion of GPI-deficient blood cells at birth, which subsequently decreased with aging (Tremml et al 1999). These data support the theory that there was no absolute growth advantage for *pig-a* mutated cells as compared to normal cells coexisting in the same organism. Notably, the generation of a mouse model showing *in vivo* expansion of *pig-a* mutated hematopoiesis, thus better mimicking the human PNH disease, required a more sophisticated experimental approach (Keller et al 2001; Jasinski et al 2001). This included a conditional inactivation of the murine *pig-a* gene implemented using Cre recombinase and its specific recombination sites loxP; when the Cre/loxP system was targeted to the hematopoietic stem cells or the erythroid/megakaryocytic lineage using tissue-specific c-FES and GATA-1 regulatory sequences, respectively, the generation of mice having almost 100% of red cells with the PNH phenotype was obtained. However, even these mice do not really mimic the disease phenotype seen in humans, because PNH hematopoiesis tends to decrease over time (Jasinski et al 2001). Indeed, the conclusion from murine models is that the *pig-a* mutation is not sufficient itself to sustain the expansion of PNH-like hematopoiesis over time, suggesting the presence of additional causal factors.

*PIG-A mutations in human individuals. PIG-A* mutation may be identified in affected cells from all PNH patients, demonstrating a clear etiological role in the development of PNH. However, it is not true that all individuals who undergo inactivating mutations in the *PIG-A* gene develop clinical PNH. In fact, it has been shown that a few blood cells harboring the PNH phenotype (namely, a complete or partial deficiency in all GPI-APs) may be detected even in normal individuals, at a frequency of 10 to 50 cells per million (Araten et al 1999). This was possible thanks to an ultra-sensitive flow cytometry analysis (see above, diagnosis of PNH) of large numbers of circulating granulocytes or erythrocytes obtained from healthy subjects. When these phenotypically abnormal cells were selected and studied at the genetic level, they revealed themselves to be clonal, and to carry specific *PIG-A* mutations (as demonstrated by a nested PCR technique) undistinguishable from those identified in PNH patients (Araten et al 1999). This clearly demonstrated that, *in vivo*, a *PIG-A* mutation was not sufficient to cause the disease, for at least two different reasons. First, to sustain clonal expansion, such mutations have to occur in multipotent HSC, while in most cases they statistically could pertain to cells without self-renewal capability, such as differentiated blood cells or committed hematopoietic progenitors. Second, a *PIG-A* mutation, even when occurring in a HSC, could simply confers a biological phenotype (the GPI deficiency) that requires additional, *PIG-A*-independent, conditions for further clonal expansion leading to the disease. The latter view is also supported by the observation that, at least in some patients, PNH hematopoiesis may include more than one abnormal clone. This was initially postulated based on the differential susceptibility of erythrocyte population to complement lysis (Rosse & Dacie 1966; Rotoli et al 1984), as subsequently demonstrated by flow cytometry (van der Schoot et al 1990), and finally confirmed by *PIG-A* sequencing (Endo et al 1996; Nishimura et al 1997)). In keeping, the expansion of distinct clones carrying the same, albeit molecularly heterogeneous, functional defect seems to suggest an expansion based on non-stochastic processes, such as selection, rather than a random process. This is also supported by the observation that relapse of PNH may be sustained by clones harboring *PIG-A* mutations different from those identified at diagnosis (Nafa et al 1998).

#### 4.1.2 Clonal expansion of the *PIG-A* mutated clone(s) and development of clinical PNH

This background raised the hypothesis of a dual pathophysiology for PNH: the *PIG-A* mutation is not sufficient to cause the disease, and requires a second, independent event (Rotoli & Luzzatto 1989). This theory is also known as the "relative advantage" (Luzzatto et al 1997) or "escape" theory (Young & Maciejewski 2000). According to this view, a mutation in the *PIG-A* gene might be a fairly common phenomenon, with no major biological consequences, because in physiological conditions the mutated cell has no reason for expanding in the presence of a vast majority of normal cells. In fact, no intrinsic proliferative advantage has been demonstrated in PNH hematopoietic progenitors in comparison to normal ones (Araten et al 2002). However, additional factors may alter this equilibrium, creating the conditions for the expansion of PNH clone(s), and possibly leading to the occurrence of a single *PIG-A* mutated stem cell sustaining hematopoiesis even for the rest of the patient's life (Nishimura et al 2002; Nishimura et al 2004). The nature of such second event(s) can be of various origin, and distinct pathways -- not necessarily mutually exclusive -- have been postulated.

*An immune-mediated damage of hematopoiesis sparing PNH cells.* The well-accepted theory of PNH pathophysiology claims that such second event is a change in the microenvironment of hematopoiesis, leading to the selective expansion of the *PIG-A* mutated cells. It is quite accepted that such external factor, which does not affect the intrinsic features of the *PIG-A* mutated cells, is an (auto)-immune attack against hematopoiesis. Several clinical and experimental observations support the presence of such auto-immune attack in PNH; they include the well-known clinical overlap between PNH and aplastic anemia (AA, which is in most cases immune-mediated) (Lewis & Dacie 1967), as well as the direct demonstration of immune abnormalities in PNH patients. All these observations are discussed later on in this chapter. Indeed, normal and PNH cells are not different in terms of growth or survival, but PNH cells could be spared by immune-mediated damage, finally resulting in a progressive consumption of normal hematopoiesis, with relative expansion of PNH hematopoiesis (Rotoli & Luzzatto 1989; Luzzatto et al 1997; Young & Maciejewski 2000). This was confirmed by gene expression profiling performed in normal and PNH HSCs: when CD34+ cells from PNH patients were separated according to the presence or absence of GPI-APs on their surface, distinct patterns of gene expression were identified. In fact, phenotypically normal (GPI-AP positive) CD34+ cells harbored diffuse abnormalities of their transcriptome, with over-expression of genes involved in apoptosis and immune activity, paralleling the findings seen in CD34+ cells of AA patients. By contrast, phenotypically abnormal PNH CD34+ (GPI-AP negative) showed a gene expression profiling closer to that obtained in CD34+ cells from healthy individuals (Chen et al 2005). Notably, normal and PNH CD34+ cells did not show any difference in the genes involved in growth or proliferation, rather suggesting the presence of sublethal extrinsic damage in phenotypically normal HSCs but not in their *PIG-A* mutated counterpart. Indeed, PNH cells ultimately expand as a result of a selective pressure that acts negatively on normal hematopoiesis; however, the molecular reasons underlying the "escape" still remain elusive. Contradictory data have been produced on a putative differential sensitivity to inhibitory stimuli between normal and PNH cells; susceptibility to apoptosis has been reported to be increased, normal or decreased in different models. It has been shown that human cell lines carrying the *PIG-A* mutation are less susceptible to NK-mediated killing compared to their normal counterpart (Nagakura et al 2002). In a more sophisticated model, GPI-deficient cells were not able to induce primary and secondary stimulation of both antigen-specific and alloreactive T cells, providing experimental support to the hypothesis that the PNH clone could inefficiently interact with the immune system (Murakami et al 2002). Indeed, the actual mechanisms causing the escape may include the absence of specific GPI-APs directly targeted by effector immune cells, or a protection due to the absence of important molecules involved in cell-cell interaction (e.g., accessory molecules). Alternatively, a broader impaired sensitivity to common effector mechanisms may be hypothesized, possibly due to the lack of GPI-APs or to non specific structural changes of the raft structure in the outer surface. Remarkably, the observation that patients with a B-cell lymphoproliferative disorder treated by alemtuzumab may develop expansion of GPI-deficient (PNH-like) T cells indirectly confirms the escape theory. Alemtuzumab is a monoclonal antibody that kills lymphocytes targeting the GPI-linked protein CD52; after treatment, CD52-negative lymphocytes may be found, which also lack all other GPI-APs. Once such lymphocytes are cloned, mutations in the *PIG-A* gene can be demonstrated; interestingly, the same mutation can be found also in a few cells from pre-treatment blood samples. In most cases these expansions are self-limiting and transient, and GPI-deficient T-cells gradually disappear after alemtuzumab discontinuation. Thus, this model elucidates most features of the PNH pathogenesis: the pre-existence of *PIG-A* mutated cells, their expansion only in the presence of a selective pressure negatively acting on normal cells (mutated cells are intrinsically resistant to alemtuzumab due to the absence of CD52), and the gradual disappearance of the mutated clone once the selective mechanism has been removed (Hertestein et al 2005). It has to be remarked that none of these alemtuzumab-treated patients developed PNH, because the expansion of GPI-AP deficient clones includes only mature lymphocytes and not multipotent HSCs (alemtuzumab does not kill HSC or hematopoietic progenitors, because CD52 expression is restricted to the lymphoid cells).

*Additional mutations conferring growing advantage.* The selective advantage of the *PIG-A* mutated clone could also be explained by a second (or a pre-existing) mutation of the aberrant clone, which confers an absolute growth advantage. The most striking evidence supporting this theory is the observation that a few PNH patients may harbor, in the *PIG-A* mutated clone, an additional concomitant genetic lesion in the chromosome 12. This lesion was identified in a mutation in the 3′ of the *HMGA2* gene, which leads to HMGA2 over-expression and subsequent proliferative advantage (Inoue et al 2006). However, this mutation has not been found in larger series of PNH patients, making the pathogenic role of this lesion questionable. Clonal dominance of the PNH clone may also be due to other, still unknown, additional mutation(s) of the *PIG-A* mutated cells, possibly secondary to an intrinsic genetic instability of the abnormal clone. However, recent data exclude that *PIG-A* mutated cells have any increase in genetic instability. In fact, using the *PIG-A* itself as sentinel gene, the intrinsic rate of somatic mutation in PNH cells did not differ from that of normal cells, and it was remarkable less than that of cells with known genetic instability (i.e., Fanconi Anemia cells) (Araten et al 2007). Thus, these data argue against the possibility that PNH can be due to either a pre-existing genetic instability favoring the *PIG-A* mutation, or to a genetic instability secondary to the *PIG-A* mutation itself, which could predispose to additional genetic events necessary for PNH development. This is also supported, *in vivo*, by the clinical observation that malignant evolution in PNH patients is extremely rare, even if possible (Krause 1983; Devine et al 1987a); karyotypic abnormalities can been found in a few PNH patients, but in most cases they are transient and do not lead to leukemic transformation (Araten et al 2001). Remarkably, both MDS and truly leukemic cells not necessarily come from the *PIG-A* mutated clone; in fact, even more frequently they arise from the non-PNH, normal, residual hematopoiesis (van Kamp et al 1994; Araten et al 2001). Thus, the malignant evolution seems not related to any intrinsic feature secondary to the *PIG-A* mutation, but rather to the underlying bone marrow disorder, possibly including even clonal dominance itself.

*The neutral evolution theory*. More recently, a third possibility has been postulated, that even the expansion of the *PIG-A* mutated HSC could be a simple stochastic phenomenon, not requiring any additional event; this theory has been described as the "neutral evolution" hypothesis. According to the mathematic model provided by Dingli (Dingli et al 2008), given the stochastic nature of hematopoiesis (Notaro & Luzzatto et al 2010), a *PIG-A* mutation may randomly occur within the active HSCs pool, which in adults comprises about 400 cells, each replicating, on average, once per year. Subsequently, the expansion of the mutant clone may simply reflect the stochastic dominance of a few HSC, regardless of any functional feature (either absolute or conditional growth advantage), which may lead to a PNH clone size large enough to cause the disease. According to the authors, this model would fit the actual (expected) incidence of PNH (Hill et al 2006c). The chances that a single clone (even carrying a neutral mutation like the *PIG-A*) overcomes residual hematopoiesis increases with oligoclonal hematopoiesis, reconciling the model with the observation that clinical PNH mostly develop in patients with an underlying bone marrow failure.

### 4.2 Hematopoiesis in PNH patients

#### 4.2.1 Marrow failure and PNH

As discussed later on, anemia is a typical presentation of PNH; however, cytopenias involving other blood lineages are also common in PNH patients. Cytopenia in these patients is mainly due to impaired production by the bone marrow, as confirmed by the reduction in hematopoietic progenitors assessed by culture assays. In fact, it has been demonstrated that bone marrow from PNH patients show a significant reduction in all lineage-committed progenitors (CFU-E, BFU-E, CFU-GM, CFU-GEMM) (Rotoli et al 1984; Maciejewski et al 1997) , as well as in stem cells/multi-potent progenitors (LTC-IC) (Maciejewski et al 1997). This was demonstrated in all PNH patients, regardless of their clinical presentation (see disease classification) (Parker et al 2005); namely, a subclinical marrow failure can be detected even in patients with hypercellular bone marrow. The functional impairment of the bone marrow may become clinically evident in a fraction of patients (at least one third), leading to mild cytopenia up to clinically significant bone marrow failure, seen as aplastic anemia (AA) (Lewis & Dacie 1967). In fact, many PNH patients may sooner or later develop frank aplastic anemia during the course of their disease (Hillmen et al 1995; Sociè et al 1996; De Latour et al 2008); conversely, AA patients may also develop PNH. Indeed, a substantial fraction of AA patients (up to 40%) may have detectable PNH clone (Nissen et al 1999; Mukhina et al 2001; Sugimori et al 2006; Scheinberg et al 2010), in most cases not large enough to cause evident hemolysis; however, the size of the PNH clone may vary over time, possibly leading to clinical PNH. Thus, PNH and AA are closely embedded (Dameshek 1967), and should be considered as different presentations of the same disorder rather than independent conditions. Furthermore, regardless of its clinical presentation, PNH must be considered by definition a bone marrow disorder because of its impairment of hematopoiesis, which is both quantitative (clinical or subclinical) and qualitative (the aberrant phenotype stems from the *PIG-A* mutated HSC). To some extent, PNH could be considered an attempt of the body to prevent the development of AA by rescuing hematopoiesis with PNH cells (Rotoli & Luzzatto 1989); in fact, the PNH clone ensures some mature blood cells, even if it leads to specific consequences secondary to the abnormality of the PNH cells (i.e., hemolysis and thrombophilia).

### 4.2.2 Immune derangement in PNH patients

Given the clinical overlap between PNH and AA, it is reasonable to hypothesize that pathogenic mechanisms involved in AA may also play a pivotal role in PNH, representing the additional factor required for developing clinical PNH once a *PIG-A* mutation has occurred (without any specific chronologic order). The immunological mechanisms in idiopathic AA play a pivotal role in damaging the hematopoietic compartment, leading to HSC pool consumption or to functional impairment and subsequent pancytopenia (Young & Maciejewski 2000; Young et al 2006). A number of experimental observations supports the presence of an anti-hematopoiesis immune attack, although the target antigens are still undefined, as are the mechanisms leading to the breach in immune tolerance. Unknown triggers of autoimmunity induce a cellular immune response resulting in a preferential expansion of specific T cell clones that may damage the hematopoietic progenitors, directly or through indirect mechanisms, such as the production of inhibitory cytokines. Stem cell damage can be mediated by cytokine-transduced inhibition (mostly type I cytokines, such as interferon-γ and tumor necrosis factor-α), or by direct cell-mediated killing due to cytotoxic lymphocytes (CTLs) (reviewed in Young et al 2006). Such mechanisms, which may attack innocent bystander cells in addition to the primary target cells, ultimately result in apoptosis, the main key mechanism of HSC damage. Circulating and marrow CTLs have been demonstrated in vivo in AA patients, and their inhibitory effect on hematopoiesis has been documented in vitro (reviewed in Young et al 2006); this cellular immune response has been dissected at the molecular level through the identification of in vivo-dominant T cell clonotypes, which are evidence of a pathogenic antigen-driven immune response (Risitano et al 2004). Since in PNH a similar antigen-driven immune response targeting marrow tissue may be postulated, investigators have evaluated the same pathways of the immune system for possible abnormalities. As for AA, evidence of immune derangement in PNH has been produced, mostly pointing out the pivotal role of cell-mediated immunity. In fact, oligoclonality of the T cell pool has been reported (Karadimitris et al 2000), and immunodominant pathogenic CTL clones may be detected in most PNH patients (Risitano et al 2004; Plasilova et al 2004). Notably, immunodominant T-cell clones identified in PNH patients may share highly homologous T-cell receptor beta (TCR-beta) sequences, and additional closely related sub-dominant T-cell clones may be identified, consistent with an antigen-driven public immune response (Gargiulo et al 2007). The observation that recurrent or highly homologous TCR-beta sequences may be identified regardless of the individual patient's HLA background (in contrast with what is seen in AA) (Risitano et al 2004), may also suggest that a non-peptidic triggering antigen may be involved, possibly related to the GPI-anchor itself (Gargiulo et al 2007). Functionally, these pathogenic T cells harbor an effector, cytotoxic phenotype, characterized by expression of CD8 and CD57. These effector lymphocytes also show an imbalance in the expression of the activating and inhibitory surface receptors; in fact, they tend to over-express the activating isoforms of inhibiting superfamily receptors, which elicit a powerful cytolytic activity (Poggi et al 2005). Notably, in some PNH patients these CTL clonal populations may expand to represent a subclinical (Risitano et al 2005) or even clinically meaningful LGL proliferations (Karadimitris et al 2001).

### 4.3 Hemolysis in PNH patients

#### 4.3.1 The complement system

The complement system is a key component of innate immunity, that has evolved to recognize both exogenous pathogenic microorganisms as well as injured self tissues, and to amplify adaptive immunity (Müller-Eberhard 1988; Holers 2008). The complement system encompasses distinct functional pathways with unique mechanisms of activation, which then all merge into a common final effector mechanism -- the cytolytic membrane attack complex (MAC). Thus, initiation of complement activation may occur along three different pathways - classical, alternative or lectin - which independently lead to activation of C3 and C5 convertases. While the classical and the lectin pathways require specific triggers to be activated, usually infectious agents, it has been known for decades that the complement alternative pathway (CAP) exhibits low-grade continuous activation due to spontaneous hydrolysis of C3 (the so-called tick-over phenomenon) (Pangburn et al 1981; Pangburn & Müller-Eberhard 1983). In addition, some components of the CAP constitute an amplification mechanism (the so called CAP amplification loop), which amplifies complement activation regardless of the specific pathway that initially generates the first C3b molecule. Fine mechanisms have evolved to control the complement system, including membrane bound proteins (complement receptor 1 [CR1], membrane cofactor protein [MCP], and the membrane proteins CD55 and CD59) as well as fluid-phase components, including complement factor I (FI) and factor H (FH). Among these, CD55 and CD59 are of pivotal importance in PNH, given that they are normally expressed on blood cells through the GPI-anchor (Medof et al 1986).

#### 4.3.2 Complement regulatory proteins and PNH erythrocytes

CD55, also known as Decay Accelerating Factor (DAF), is a 70-kd protein first isolated in 1969 (Hoffman 1969) and subsequently purified in 1982 (Nicholson-Weller et al 1982) which inhibits the formation and the stability of C3 convertase (both C3bBb and C4b2a) (Nicholson-Weller 1992). Historically, CD55 was the first complement regulator reported to be absent on PNH erythrocytes (Pangburn et al 1983(a); Pangburn et al 1983(b); Nicholson-Weller et al 1983) possibly accounting for the increased susceptibility of PNH erythrocytes to complement mediated lysis. However, further studies suggested that factors other than CD55 should also be involved, possibly acting downstream on the complement cascade (Medof et al 1987; Shin et al 1986). Subsequently, CD59 (also known as Membrane Inhibitor of Reactive Lysis , MIRL) was identified as an additional complement inhibitor expressed on normal erythrocytes, while PNH erythrocytes were demonstrated deficient in CD59 (Holguin et al 1989(a)). CD59 interferes with the terminal effector complement, blocking the incorporation of C9 onto the C5b-C8 complex, forming the membrane attack complex (MAC) (Meri et al 1990). Thus, independently from CD59 the lack of CD50 may explain complement-mediated hemolysis of PNH erythrocytes (Holguin et al 1989(b)). The hierarchical contribution of CD55 and CD59 to hemolysis suggests that CD59 is the key molecule which, if absent, leads to lysis (Wilcox et al 1991); in contrast, redundant mechanisms (including CD59 itself) usually overcome the isolated deficiency of CD55 (Holguin et al 1992). This is also confirmed by clinical observations: in fact, patients carrying the so-called Inab phenotype (an isolated CD55 deficiency, with normal CD59 expression) do not suffer from hemolysis (Telen & Green 1989; Merry et al 1992) whereas anecdotic cases of CD59 deficiency lead to a clinical phenotype undistinguishable from PNH (Yamashina et al 1990; Motoyama et al 1992).

#### 4.3.3 Increased susceptibility of PNH erythrocytes to complement-mediated lysis in vitro and in vivo

It is intelligible that the deficiency of the complement regulatory proteins CD55 and CD59 renders PNH erythrocytes susceptible to uncontrolled complement activation and subsequent lysis.

*In vitro*. The very initial studies on PNH performed by Dr. Ham associated the hemolysis observed in PNH patients with an intrinsic susceptibility of red cells to complement activation *in vitro* (Ham 1937; Ham & Dingle 1939). In fact, the acidified serum assay (also known as the Ham test) - where the acidification activates the complement through the alternative pathway - became the standard technique for the diagnosis of PNH. The abnormality resulted intrinsic to patient erythrocytes, given that hemolysis occurs regardless of the origin of serum, while sera from patients do not result into the lysis of erythrocytes from normal individuals. This assumption was also confirmed in cross-transfusion studies (Rosse 1971). Since these initial studies it was evident that not all the erythrocytes drawn from a patient had the same susceptibility to complement-mediated lysis, making the point that all patients presented a mosaicism of normal and affected erythrocytes. Rosse and Dacie clearly elucidated that in erythrocytes obtained from PNH patients three different phenotypes could be identified, differing in their sensitivity to complement-mediated lysis *in vitro* (Rosse & Dacie 1966; Rosse 1973) . The first phenotype had a normal (equal to that of erythrocytes from healthy individuals) sensitivity to complement, while abnormal cells could have a dramatic hypersensitivity to complement-mediated lysis (15-25 times the normal one), or just a moderate hypersentivity (3-5 times normal). These phenotypes are referred as PNH type I, type III and type II, respectively (Rosse & Dacie 1966; Rosse 1973); now we know that they correspond to a normal expression of GPI-APs (type I), or to a complete (type III) or partial (type II) deficiency of GPI-APs, as documented by flow cytometry (van der Schoot et al 1990). Notably, PNH patients may have either PNH type II or type III only, or may harbor a combination of both phenotypes. As anticipated, the proportion of the specific phenotype shapes the clinical manifestations of an individual patients (especially the extent of hemolysis), and may vary greatly not only among patients, but even in the same patient during the course of the disease.

*In vivo*. The *in vivo* consequence of the hypersensitivity of PNH erythrocyte to complement activation accounts for the most obvious manifestation of PNH, namely intravascular hemolysis and subsequent hemoglobinuria. Indeed, it is well known that PNH erythrocytes chronically undergo intravascular hemolysis in PNH patients *in vivo*, with a lifespan reduced to 10% compared to normal RBCs. This chronic hemolysis likely results from steady-state complement activation, due to the low-grade spontaneous C3 tick-over leads to chronic CAP activation on the PNH erythrocyte surface (Pangburn et al 1981; Pangburh & Müller-Eberhard 1983). It should be reiterated that both the initial complement activation and the down-stream effector mechanisms are uncontrolled on PNH erythrocytes. Specifically, the lack of CD55 impairs the regulation of C3 convertases (regardless the triggering pathway - classical or alternative) (Mold et al 1990), leading to increased C3 activation and further progression along the subsequent steps of the complement cascade. Thus on PNH erythrocytes -- due to the lack of CD55 -- the complement cascade activated by the CAP continues through to MAC assembly, finally coming to lysis for the lack of CD59. In this view, PNH can be considered mostly a CAP-mediated disease (Holers 2008); in real life, this physiological low-level complement activation is greatly amplified during inflammatory or infectious diseases. Indeed, overt hemolysis and paroxysms of PNH patients likely results from a specific triggering action on the complement cascade, which may occur along each of the three distinct complement pathways. There are no data demonstrating which is the complement pathway activated in specific conditions *in vivo* (i.e. infections); however one may speculate that all the three pathways may co-operate, with a possible hierarchical dominance of the CAP, given its capability to amplify any complement activation regardless the initial triggering pathway.

### 4.4 Thrombophilia and PNH

In addition to hemolytic anemia and bone marrow failure, thrombophilia is the third typical manifestation of PNH; however, in contrast to the other two, much less is known about its pathophysiology. A number of possible mechanisms have been hypothesized, and some pieces of evidence have been provided, although the final mechanism remains speculative, possibly because it can be multifactorial. The clinical observation that thrombotic complications are more common in patients with larger PNH clones (Hall et al 2003; Grünewald et al 2003; Moyo et al 2004) and greater hemolysis may suggest that the pathogenic mechanism could be in some way embedded with complement activation (Markiewski et al 2007) and hemolysis itself. At least four distinct (but not mutually exclusive) mechanisms can be hypothesized. First, uncontrolled complement regulation on platelet surface might lead to platelet activation and aggregation, enhancing clot formation (Gralnick et al 1995; Louwes et al 2001). Second, thrombophilia may directly results from hemolysis, due to the build-up of cell-free plasma hemoglobin released by the erythrocytes. This may occur through the ability of free hemoglobin to scavenge nitric oxide from plasma, blocking its inhibitory action on platelet aggregation and adhesion to endothelium, as well as its regulatory effect on vessel wall tone (Schafer et al 2004; Rother et al 2005). An other mechanism by which hemolysis might lead to thrombophilia includes the generation of procoagulant particles. In fact, microvesicles are known to be released in PNH patients upon hemolysis and complement activation from RBCs (Hugel et al 1999), WBCs (monocytes) and platelets, (Wiedmer et al 1993; Simak et al 2004) and even from the endothelium. However, even if their procoagulant action is commonly accepted (van Beers et al 2009), their specific role in the pathophysiology of thromboembolisms in PNH is not yet proven. The fourth possible mechanism of thrombophilia in PNH might be an impairment of the fibrinolytic system, due to the lack of membrane-bound urokinase-type plasminogen activator receptor (uPAR) -- which is GPI-linked, and to the excess of its soluble form (Ninomiya et al 1997; Sloand et al 2006).

## 5. Clinical features

PNH is characterized by a unique triad of clinical features: intravascular hemolysis, thromboembolic events and cytopenia (Dunn et al 2000; Parker & Ware 2003; Notaro & Luzzatto 2003). However, not all three manifestations are presents in all the patients, and the individual presentation of each patient may greatly vary according to the most dominant signs and symptoms. Thus, many investigators have tried to classify PNH according to the most typical clinical presentations; however, distinct categories are hard to define for a disease with such an unpredictable presentation and evolution.

### 5.1 Classification

The most adopted classification of PNH was proposed by the International PNH Interest Group in 2005 (Parker et al 2005), whereby PNH patients are grouped according to the presence of hemolysys and of an underlying bone marrow disorder. Accordingly, three distinct subtypes are identified: i. classic PNH, characterized by hemolysis without other marrow disorder (i.e., hemolytic PNH patients without relevant cytopenia); ii. PNH in the setting of another bone marrow disorder, characterized by hemolysis associated with an underlying marrow disorder, usually AA or MDS (i.e., hemolytic PNH patients with cytopenia; AA or MDS may be concomitant or have preceded PNH); iii. subclinical PNH, characterized by the presence of PNH cells in the absence of any clinical or laboratory sign of hemolysis, in the setting of other hematological disorders (i.e., AA or MDS patients with GPI-AP deficient cells, but not clinical PNH). This classification does not completely take into account that, by definition, PNH carries an underlying bone marrow disorder, and as a result most PNH patients have cytopenia or some signs of marrow failure. In fact, a recent registry study (de Latour et al 2008) made the point that many PNH patients do not fit either one of the two major categories, and a fourth subgroup has been included (intermediate PNH, characterized by hemolysis and mild cytopenia not qualifying for the diagnosis of AA). However, even this classification seems to fail the goal of identifying patient subgroups with distinct clinical outcome (de Latour et al 2008). Some other groups have used in the past a different classification (Notaro & Luzzatto 2003), where the category of AA/PNH patients is restricted to those with concomitant severe AA and clinically meaningful hemolysis, who require more intensive care and are supposed to have a worse prognosis. According to this classification, classic PNH patients are further grouped into hyperplastic and hypoplastic (based on peripheral counts and bone marrow analysis), AA/PNH patients are only those with severe marrow failure and concomitant clinically relevant hemolysis, whereas subclinical PNH patients are characterized by small PNH clone(s) (even with minimal signs of hemolysis) associated with either AA or thromboembolic disease (the latter are very rare cases with a clinical PNH that does not include relevant hemolysis).

### 5.2 Hemolysis

Hemolysis is the most typical manifestation of PNH, which by definition affects all patients with clinical PNH. However, the extent of hemolysis varies among patients, according to size of the PNH clone(s), type of PNH erythrocytes (type II versus type III), and possibly the level of complement activation (which may vary according to specific medical conditions or patient-specific features). Typically, hemolysis is chronic (secondary to the low-level spontaneous complement activation), with possible exacerbations (the paroxysms) consequent to a massive complement activation, often in association with infections or other triggering events. Hemolysis of PNH erythrocytes occurs in the vessels (intravascular hemolysis), and leads to a number of clinical consequences. The most evident sign to the patient is the hemoglobinuria, with the emission of dark urine, whose aspect is commonly defined as "*marsala wine*" or coke-like, according to the Country of origin of the observer and/or the time of the report (Parker 2002) . The color of urine is not constant over time, with the most typical dark urine often seen in the morning (hence the name "*paroxysmal nocturnal hemoglobinuria*"); however, the patient's urine mostly range from dark yellow to orange and dark red, with very rapid variations during the day. Even if nocturnal $CO_2$ retention has been hypothesized as possible cause of plasma pH fall and subsequent complement activation (Ham 1937), the reasons underlying nocturnal exacerbation of hemolysis are not yet fully understood (unless first-morning hyperconcentrated urine is not by itself an explanation for evident hemoglobinuria). The typical biochemical marker of hemolysis is the increase in lactate dehydrogenase (LDH), which may be as high as tenfold the upper normal value; additional intra-erythrocytary components may also increase, such as aminotransferases (especially the alanine one). As in other hemolytic disorders, unconjugated bilirubin levels may increase, even up to frank jaundice; compensatory erythropoiesis is usually demonstrated by very high reticulocyte counts, even if the latter value greatly depends upon the underlying marrow function (patients with hyperproliferative PNH may show even 300000-400000 cell x $10^9$/L, while those with AA/PNH usually have less than 60000 cell x $10^9$/L). Secondary iron deficiency may appear as a consequence of perpetual iron loss through urine. Clinically, the main consequence of continuous hemolysis is the development of anemia, and possibly other related symptoms such as asthenia and weakness. The extent of anemia is very heterogeneous among patients, also depending on other factors such as compensatory erythropoiesis (which may be impaired in patients with more severe marrow failure) or even iron/vitamin deficiency. As a result, anemia may be severe in some patients and requiring frequent transfusions, or well-compensated in other cases, even with normal-like hemoglobin levels. Furthermore, anemia may greatly vary even in the clinical course of an individual patients, with sudden worsening or unexpected improvements in the absence of any known reason; anecdotic cases showing spontaneous remission of the disease have also been reported (Hillmen et al 1995; Sociè et al 1996; de Latour et al 2008). In addition to anemia, it is now accepted that hemolysis may induce by itself specific disabling symptoms. This is usually seen in concomitance with the typical "paroxysms" of PNH, which are massive hemolytic crises often triggered by specific conditions (e.g., infections, surgery). These disabling symptoms include malaise and fatigue, with possible painful crises; the latter are quite typical, and mostly involve the abdomen, mimicking an acute abdomen. Some patients also report lumbar or sub-sternal pain, headache, dysphagia (both painful and difficult swallowing) and erectile dysfunction (Rother et al 2005). PNH paroxysms are irregular and unpredictable in individual patients, although most show a quite regular recurrence in the long run period. However, some of these hemolysis-related symptoms (especially malaise and fatigue exceeding those expected based on the low hemoglobin level) can be also seen as a consequence of chronic hemolysis. All these symptoms, which significantly impact patient well-being , are thought to be due to smooth muscle dystonia secondary to local nitric oxide (NO) consumption by plasma free-hemoglobin (Rosse 2000, Moyo et al 2004, Rother et al 2005).

### 5.3 Bone marrow failure

The second key clinical feature of PNH is cytopenia; in contrast to erythrocytes, PNH granulocytes and paltelets have anormal lifespan *in vivo* (Brubaker et al 1977; Devine et al 1987b); as discussed above, an underlying marrow disorder is embedded in the dual pathophysiology of the disease and with PNH clone expansion (Rotoli & Luzzatto 1989). Thus, some degree of marrow failure is common or even expected in PNH patients, ranging from mild cytopenias to severe aplastic anemia (Dunn et al 2000; Parker & Ware 2003; Notaro and Luzzatto 2003), and it may qualify for distinct disease categories (Parker et al 2005). Remarkably, the specific picture of each individual patient may change during the course of the disease, with patients initially presenting with normal marrow function and subsequently developing more severe marrow failure, as well as patients initially diagnosed with aplastic anemia subsequently developing frank hemolytic PNH (Tichelli et al 1992; Scheinberg et al 2010). Bone marrow failure usually becomes evident because of neutropenia and thrombocytopenia; however, it has to be remarked that marrow failure may also contribute to anemia in PNH patients. In fact, many PNH patients have a reticulocyte count that is inadequate to the hemoglobin level (iron deficiency may also contribute to that). The proportion of PNH patients with marrow failure ranges from 30 to 70% in different series, possibly because of heterogeneous definitions of bone marrow failure itself. The most homogeneous data from the French registry indicate that over 430 PNH patients 26% presented with normal counts (neutrophils > 1.5 x $10^9$/L, platelets > 120 x $10^9$/L) at diagnosis, 52% were classified as AA/PNH (with at least two of the following: Hb < 10gr/dL, neutrophils < 1.0 x $10^9$/L, platelets > 80 x $10^9$/L) and the remaining 22% as intermediate PNH (de Latour et al 2008).

### 5.4 Thrombophilia

The third typical manifestation of PNH is thrombophilia, with thrombosis developing in about 40% of all patients; accordingly, PNH is the medical condition with the higher risk of thrombosis. Unfortunately, as the underlying pathogenic mechanisms are not fully understood, thromboses are largely unpredictable in PNH patients, even if according to most series they generally develop in patients with large clones and massive hemolysis (Hall et al 2003; Moyo et al 2004). The thrombotic risk is peculiar to each patient, possibly as a result of additional independent (environmental or genetic) risk factors that may shape the individual predisposition to thrombosis. For instance, inherited polymorphisms such as Factor V Leiden mutation and the 677 C>T methylenetetrahydrofolate reductase gene variant (as well as other polymorphisms leading to hyperhomocysteinemia) may have a relevant role, although this has not been proven so far (Nafa et al 1996). However, this concept has in someway been confirmed by the observation that the thrombotic risk is different in PNH patients with specific ethnicity; in fact, Asian patients have a lower incidence of thrombosis (Nishimura et al 2004), while Afro-Americans and Latin-Americans seem to have an increased incidence (Araten et al 2005). Thrombosis of PNH is quite unique, because it mostly occurs at venous sites which are unusual for other non-PNH-related thrombosis. Intra-abdominal veins are the most frequent sites, followed by cerebral and limb veins; other possible sites include dermal veins, the lungs - with pulmonary embolus - and the artheries - leading to arterial thrombosis. Thrombotic disease may be life-threatening and is the main cause of death for PNH patients (Hillmen et al 1995; Socie et al 1996; de Latour et al 2008). Typical severe presentations of thrombotic PNH include hepatic venous (Budd-Chiari syndrome) (Hoekstra et al 2009), portal, mesenteric, and renal vein thrombosis. Usually patients are asymptomatic, until clinical manifestations appear, especially pain; other signs and symptoms are specific according to the vessel involved (e.g., ascites, varices and splenomegaly in hepatic/portal thrombosis, or stroke in cerebral vein thrombosis). Unfortunately, pain is not a useful symptom by itself, because it may also be due to vessel wall dystonia or to a transient ischemic attack (especially of the intestine) rather than to true thrombosis. However, a thrombotic episode has to be suspected in all PNH patients with obscure pain, even when it may mimic acute abdomen; ultra sound scan and magnetic resonance imaging (especially angiography) are useful to rule out these dangerous complications. Recurrence after the first episode and/or development of chronic thrombotic disease is typical of PNH (Hillmen et al 1995; Socie et al 1996; de Latour et al 2008; Audebert et al 2005; Moyo et al 2004); this is especially common in the setting of the Budd-Chiari syndrome, when the thrombotic process initially affects small veins, and then progressively involves large hepatic veins, with the development of life-threatening manifestations like variceal bleeding, jaundice, ascitis and liver failure. At this stage, liver regenerative nodules may also appear, which may erroneously suggest the presence of hepatocellular carcinoma. Thrombosis of other splancnic vein may usually lead to secondary ischemia and infarction, possibly leading to gangrene of the peripheral organ. Even if thromboses in PNH are unpredictable, recent data suggest that some biochemical parameters may work as surrogate markers of overt thrombophilia in PNH. They include D-dimers and other plasma markers of coagulation pathway activation, reactive fibrinolysis and endothelial cell activation (Helley et al 2010). However, their use has not been validated yet.

### 5.5 Other clinical manifestations

*Renal failure.* Both acute and chronic renal failure have been described in PNH patients (Nair et al 2008). Acute renal insufficiency is usually seen in concomitance with hemolytic crisis, as a result of massive hemoglobinuria. This condition is usually self-limiting and tends to

recover spontaneously in a few days after the resolution of the crisis, although specific interventions (even dialysis) may be needed in the acute phase. Chronic kidney disease (CKD) has also been reported; in a recent paper the incidence of clinically relevant CKD was estimated in the range of 20% (Hillmen et al 2010), but these data have not been confirmed by other groups (nor in previous large retrospective studies) (Hillmen et al 1995; Socie et al 1996; de Latour et al 2008). Pathophysiologically, CKD might be related to microthrombi of the renal vessels, as well as to renal cortex siderosis, which can be easily demonstrated in PNH patients by magnetic resonance imaging.
*Infections.* Infectious complications are common in PNH patients; they mostly pertain to cases with concomitant marrow failure, as a direct consequence of neutropenia. However, they could also be related to some functional impairment of PNH neuthrophils and monocytes, and especially of their oxidative response - which is necessary for microorganism destruction - as documented by some *in vitro* data (Cacciapuoti et al 2007).
*Pulmonary hypertension.* Pulmonary hypertension (PH) has also been reported as possible complication of PNH by a single group (Hill et al 2006b); however, the clinical relevance of this observation remains to be confirmed in larger studies.

### 5.6 Pregnancy

Pregnancy is a specific issue which deserves an appropriate discussion in the setting of PNH. In fact, pregnancy in PNH certainly carries a high risk of complications for both mother and fetus. The main cause of complications is thrombophilia, which obviously worsen during pregnancy, and may lead to any of the thrombotic presentations described above. Additional risks may be related to suboptimal hemoglobin levels that hamper normal fetal development, as well as to cytopenia secondary to marrow failure, which may lead to infectious and hemorrhagic complications. It has to be remarked that, as for AA, pregnancy rarely causes worsening or recurrence of underlying bone marrow failure. A recent review (Fieni et al 2006) collecting 43 patients reported between 1965 and 2005 estimated the range of maternal and fetal mortality to 11.6% and 7.2%, respectively, which is quite lower than what previously thought. All the deaths were due to thrombotic complications, including fetal loss secondary to placental vein thrombosis; no case of fetal malformation was reported. Other major maternal complications included hemorrhage and infections; the most common fetal complication was pre-term delivery due to maternal complications (including placental vein thrombosis). On the other hand, pregnancies with successful outcome in the absence of any complication have lso been described. Thus, caution should be advised in counseling PNH women about a possible pregnancy, for both maternal and fetal risk. Regardless of the absolute contraindication to pregnancy (which could be re-discussed in the era of new treatment strategies), pregnancy in PNH remains a high-risk medical condition which requires an experienced caring team.

## 6. Natural history

The natural history of PNH is quite unpredictable, given the very heterogeneous disease presentation and evolution. In fact, some patients may live with the disease for decades, without major complications, whereas some others present with life-threatening medical complications, which in any case may develop at any moment during the course of the disease. Thus, the evolution and outcome of an individual patient is largely unpredictable.

Despite the rarity of the disease, some information from large series is available, although it might suffer from possible selection biases (e.g., exclusion of patients with early death due to dramatic presentation, such as lethal thrombosis) (Hillmen et al 1995; Socie et al 1996; de Latour et al 2008). Median survival was estimated above 10 years in the past decade in two independent series, with one fourth of patients surviving longer than 25 years (Hillmen et al 1995; Sociè et al 1996); more recently, the update of the French registry has revealed a median survival of about 22 years from diagnosis (de Latour et al 2008). Notably, these changes in median survival refer to the years before the introduction of the anti-complement therapy, and survival improvement was time-dependent (10-year survival was 63%, 76% and 92% according to diagnosis before 1995, 1995-2005 and after 2005, respectively), suggesting a relevant improvement in supportive care. Survival does not differ according to disease category: in fact, 10-year overall survival was 75%, 82% and 74% in classic PNH, intermediate PNH and AA/PNH, respectively. The main causes of death were thrombosis (cerebral thrombosis 25%, Budd-Chiari 23% - expressed as percentage of all deaths) and infectious complications (25%); they were both major causes of morbidity too. Even if PNH is not a malignant disease, progression to myelodysplastic syndrome and acute leukemia was observed with a 10-year cumulative incidence of 3.8%, which is similar to previous series (Hillmen et al 1995; Sociè et al 1996; Fujioka & Asai 1989) and to that reported for AA patients. Thrombosis developed in about 50% of classic PNH and 30% of intermediate PNH or AA/PNH patients; marrow failure developed in about 25% of classic and intermediate PNH patients. In the whole series, thrombosis was the main negative prognostic factor, followed by development of by- or pan-cytopenia, lower hemoglobin levels and previous diagnosis. Thrombosis affected long-term survival in all disease categories, including AA/PNH; risk factors for the development of thrombosis included thrombosis at diagnosis, old age, transfusion and lack of immunosuppressive treatment, and PNH clone size. Recurrent infections affected up to 40% of patients, representing the second main clinical complications of PNH; hemorrhage was an other relevant complication, especially in thrombocytopenic patients. Thus, even if most PNH patients may have a quite long life expectancy, the course of their disease may be stormy, with frequent hospitalizations, possible comorbidities and subsequent impaired quality of life. On the other hand, some patients may experience an indolent course, without major complications; a few PNH patients may also undergo spontaneous clinical remission of their disease, which can be estimated in about 5% (de Latour et al 2008) (even if an older study reported up to 15%, possibly due to definition bias) (Hillmen et al 1995). It has to be underlined that these data on the natural history of the disease might significantly change in the current era of effective anti-PNH treatment, mainly eculizumab or even bone marrow transplantation.

## 7. Diagnosis

PNH has to be suspected in patients showing mild to severe anemia with moderate reticulocytosis, elevated serum LDH and possibly mild jaundice, with negative Coombs test; all these clues suggest a non-immune hemolytic anemia. The occurrence of dark urine and urinary hemosiderin, both evidence of intravascular hemolysis, strongly support the suspect of PNH; haptoglobin is usually very low or undetectable. Additional signs to be considered are the presence of mild to severe leuko-thrombocytopenia and/or a history of thromboembolic events of unknown origin, including cerebrovascular accidents. In specific conditions, PNH may be considered even in the absence of clinically evident hemolytic anemia, such as in patients with AA or those showing recurrent thromboembolic events in the absence of documented risk factors; all these patients may deserve a careful screening for PNH. Diagnostic tests for PNH have much changed in the past three decades: the Ham test, which was the diagnostic test until the 1980s, has been completely replaced by flow cytometry.

**The Ham test**

Historically, the Ham test, also known as acidified serum assay, was since its identification in the 1930s the best test to diagnose PNH. Indeed, even the pathophysiological definition of PNH is based on the increased susceptibility of affected erythrocytes to complement mediated lysis (Rosse & Dacie 1966; Rosse 1991). The Ham test is an *in vitro* assay which employs this unique feature of PNH erythrocytes, testing the lysis in sera where the complement cascade (and specifically the complement alternative pathway) has been activated by pH lowering (by the addition of HCl). In these conditions, erythrocytes from PNH patients show a substantial lysis, which may vary according to the proportion of affected (*PIG-A* mutated) cells and to the type of mutation (type II versus type II PNH). Hemolysis occurs in both autologous and ABO-matched sera; as a control, lysis does not occur if the serum has been inactivated at 56° C (which inactivates some complement components), or when erythrocytes from healthy individuals are tested. In experienced hands, the test is relatively simple, and quite specific; however, its sensitivity is limited, with a threshold of about 5-10% PNH erythrocytes required for a definitive diagnosis. Other lysis assays exist, such as the sucrose lysis (or sugar water test); they exploit reduced ionic strength rather than acidification-based complement activation. However, their sensitivity and specificity for PNH are worse than those of the Ham test, and false positive may be common in other inherited hemolytic conditions. Obviously, all these lysis assays may only detect the presence of PNH erythrocytes, but cannot be utilized to detect cells with a PNH phenotype within any other blood lineage.

**Flow cytometry**

At present the diagnosis of PNH is based on flow cytometry analysis of blood cells (Parker et al 2005; Richards et al 2002); the high sensitivity and specificity of this analysis has made the Ham and similar tests obsolete. In fact, fluorochrome-conjugated monoclonal antibodies specific to several GPI-APs expressed on the various blood cell lineages are available for routine testing; thus, simultaneous multi-parameter analysis allows accurate detection of GPI-AP deficient cell populations, measuring their extent within each blood lineage (erythrocytes, granulocytes, monocytes and lymphocytes). By this technique, one or two erythrocyte populations with abnormal expression of GPI-APs may be found in PNH patients: one completely lacking GPI-AP expression (type III PNH cells), and another characterized by GPI-AP faint (dim) expression (type II PNH cells). These findings match the observation initially made by Dr. Rosse, demonstrating the presence of distinct subpopulations of erythrocytes with different sensitivity to complement-mediated lysis (Rosse & Dacie 1966); as discussed above, this may also imply that different populations may be genetically different. The demonstration of GPI-AP deficient populations is easy for all cell lineage, even if discrimination between type II and type III PNH cells is more difficult for white blood cells; antibodies specific for GPI-APs selectively expressed by specific cell lineage may render the test more sensitive and specific. Different panels of monoclonal antibodies have been proposed by different groups (Richards et al 2000;

Borowitz et al 2010); they usually include CD55 and CD59 for erythrocytes, CD66b, CD66c and CD24 for granulocytes, CD14 or CD48 for monocytes, CD48 or CD59 for lymphocytes. A counter-staining for gating strategies on specific blood cell populations may be included; in fact, a complete testing for PNH includes the analysis of erythrocytes, granulocytes, monocytes, and possibly lymphocytes (even if they are usually minimally affected, because most of them are long-living cells sustained by peripheral homeostasis). Platelets are usually not tested for PNH phenotype, due to the difficulty to separate normal platelets from PNHs (Maciejewski et al 1996; Vu et al 1996). The simultaneous absence of different GPI-linked proteins on the same cells validates the specificity of the test; as far as the sensitivity is concerned, flow cytometry analysis in experienced hands may detect even very small PNH clones (below 1% in routine testing, (Borowitz et al 2010) up to 0.01% in ultra-sensitive analysis for research purpose) (Araten et al 1999; Sugimori et al 2006). More recently, the novel fluorescent reagent aerolysin (FLAER), which specifically binds to the GPI anchor, showed even greater sensitivity for the detection of small PNH cell population, up to 0.01% as a single marker (Brodsky et al 2000; Sutherland et al 2007). FLAER can be easily combined with other monoclonal antibodies for a comprehensive and simultaneous study of all blood leukocytes. However, given that FLAER requires to be processed by proteolytic enzymes expressed on leucocyte surface, it cannot be utilized detect PNH erythrocytes or platelets.

**Molecular studies**

Molecular studies on DNA or mRNA, aimed to identify the specific causative mutation within the *PIG-A* gene, are usually considered superfluous rather than confirmatory. In fact, they do not add any clinically informative data and can even be somewhat misleading. Indeed, a false negative result may occur, especially when mononuclear cells are used as nucleid acid source (proportion of PNH lymphocytes are minimal in the majority of patients), or in case of some intronic mutations; on the other hand, false positive results may also occur due to the intrinsic sensitivity of the technique. Notably, molecular studies do not deliver the most relevant information as flow cytometry-based assay, which is the exact proportion of affected GPI-deficient (thus *PIG-A* mutated) cells. Thus, molecular testing is not recommended for the diagnosis of PNH.

**Blood**

The blood film is usually not very informative in PNH patients. Red blood cells are usually macrocytic due to reticulocytosis (which can be demonstrated by vital dyes), but cell size may greatly vary. Polychromatophilic or even nucleated erythrocytes may be present as a result of compensatory erythropoiesis. Microcytic hypocromic erythrocytes may also be present, because of the secondary iron deficiency; red cell fragments may be observed, especially in concomitance with thrombotic complications. Leukocytes do not show any abnormality, even if neutropenia is commonly seen in patients with AA/PNH; thrombocytopenia is also quite frequent.

**Coombs test**

The differential diagnosis of PNH includes all other hemolytic conditions, thus, the Coombs test should be performed as initial assay. By definition, the Coombs test is negative in PNH, as it is a non-immune hemolytic anemia. However, it has to be remarked that a positive Coombs test may result from allo-immunization secondary to transfusion. More recently, it has been shown that a C3-only positive Coombs test may develop in most PNH patients on eculizumab treatment (Risitano et al 2009a); this finding is not due to any antibody, but rather it derives from mechanistic reasons that will be discussed later on.

**Bone marrow**

The bone marrow pattern may be significantly different according to the presentation of the disease. In fact, patients with classic PNH may present with hyperproliferative bone marrow, and markedly increased erythropoiesis; however, due to the underlying bone marrow disorder, they may also present normal or even reduced marrow cellularity. The latter pattern is typical in AA/PNH patients, where cellularity is below 30%, as assessed by threphine biopsy. Commonly, morphological abnormalities may be observed, sometimes leading to the misdiagnosis of MDS; it has to be underlined that in most cases such abnormalities are not specific and simply reflect the stressed erythropoiesis. Additional tests can be performed on bone marrow specimens. Cytogenetic studies may occasionally reveal karyotypic abnormalities, which may occur in either PNH or normal cells; however, they do not necessarily carry a bad prognosis as for MDS (Araten et al 2001). Flow cytometry may be used to rule out leukemic transformation; given that surface expression of most GPI-APs undergoes changes during differentiation and maturation, bone marrow flow cytometry is not recommended for the diagnosis of PNH.

**Urine**

Even a macroscopic observation of urine may be a useful tool for the diagnosis of PNH; in fact, eye-evident hemoglobinuria may be one of the clinical presentations. Plasma free hemoglobin secondary to intravascular hemolysis depletes haptoglobin; as a result, free hemoglobin is continuously present in the glomerular filtrate. The excess hemoglobin is partially reabsorbed in the proximal tubule, and the iron stored as intracellular ferritin granules easily detected in the urine cast by appropriate iron (Perl's) staining - as hemosiderin granules. Hemosiderinuria is constantly present in all hemolytic PNH patients (even in the absence of hemoglobinuria, which fluctuates according to the concomitant hemolysis), thus it still represents an easy test to support the initial suspect of PNH.

**Other instrumental studies**

The management of PNH patients may require many other laboratory and instrumental studies useful to investigate the evolution of the disease and its possible complications. They especially include all the techniques useful to assess the presence of possible thrombosis; according to the specific sites, the most useful are computed tomography or magnetic resonance based, (for the cerebral and sometimes the hepatic districts), or ultra-sound based (for the abdomen and limbs). Specific angiographic studies are always helpful, especially once a thrombotic episode has been demonstrated (and always for the assessment of the cerebral district), to better assess the extent of the clot and its evolution. All these studies should be performed without delay, at diagnosis and/or in the presence of specific symptoms.

## 8. Treatment

The treatment of PNH is driven by the specific disease presentations (Brodsky 2009; Luzzatto et al 2011); however, in most cases treatment is essentially supportive, aiming at living with the disease with the least clinical burden. Thus, the main goals of PNH treatment includes the control of anemia and possibly of hemolysis; in patients with either marrow failure or thrombosis additional specific treatments are needed. Given the chronic course of PNH, an other major goal is the prevention of possible complications, mainly thrombosis and infections, to ensure long-term survival. More recently, etiological treatments for PNH have become available with the introduction of the first anti-complement agent, the anti-complement component 5 (C5) eculizumab. Finally, the only curative option for PNH is allogeneic stem cell transplantation.

### 8.1 Supportive therapies

The supportive treatment of PNH aims to control the main clinical manifestations of the disease; thus, it can be split according to specific manifestation - hemolysis and subsequent anemia, bone marrow failure and thrombocytopenia.

#### 8.1.1 Management of hemolysis and anemia

Hemolysis and subsequent anemia are the hallmarks of PNH, affect most PNH patients and often require specific treatment. Unfortunately, until the new millennium there was no specific option for controlling hemolysis. Steroids were broadly used as chronic administration or for acute hemolytic crises, without any proof of efficacy. Indeed, some investigators claimed that steroids are useful in controlling chronic complement-mediated hemolysis (Issaragrisil et al 1987; Bourantas 1994) and, even more, paroxysmal crises likely interfering with complement activation and/or the underlying conditions (i.e., inflammation) triggering the complement cascade; however, so far no mechanism of action has been provided. It has been suggested that steroids might ameliorate patient well-being even in the absence of any direct control of hemolysis (Parker et al 2005); in particular, they may be effective in improving the symptoms associated with paroxysmal crises, such as dysphagia and abdominal pain, although this effect in most cases may result from the self-limiting behavior of the paroxysms. However, a continuous use of steroids is discouraged in PNH patients, given the long-term toxicity of chronic steroidal therapy; a short-term use in presence of the paroxysms is not harmful but likely useless. Androgens have been utilized as well, with limited benefit (Harrington et al 1997); however, given their potential utility in stimulating erythropoiesis and especially megakaryocytopoiesis (Katayama et al 2001), they are primarily indicated in the presence of marrow impairment rather than to control hemolysis (see below). Once again, a risk-to-benefit evaluation should be specifically made for all individual cases, given that liver toxicity, virilizing action and other side effects have to be considered; in addition, some concerns about a potential increase in the Budd-Chiari syndrome have been raised by some physicians (Parker et al 2005). Regardless of the possibility to block hemolysis, in many patients anemia leads to clinically relevant symptoms requiring specific interventions. As remarked in the pathophysiology section, anemia of PNH patients is someway multi-factorial; thus, if the main contributor (hemolysis) cannot be affected, one may try to interfere with the additional mechanisms to improve hemoglobin levels. Besides hemolysis, the main factor affecting hemoglobin level is the bone marrow function, especially its capability to adequately compensate the ongoing hemolysis. By definition, erythropoiesis is usually impaired in patients with AA/PNH syndrome, who may require specific treatments (see below); however, ineffective erythropoiesis is commonly seen even in classic PNH patients. Given the perpetual hemosiderinuria, iron deficiency is common in PNH patients (Luzzatto et al 2011), and simple iron supplementation may increase hemoglobin levels in many patients. Similarly, vitamin B12 and folate supplementation are usually indicated to sustain the compensatory erythropoiesis secondary to hemolysis (Luzzatto et al 2011). Erythroid stimulating agents, essentially recombinant erythropoietin, may also help enhance erythropoiesis (Stebler et al 1990; Bourantas et 1994), especially in cases showing inadequate production of endogenous erythropoietin (McMullin et al 1996). Paradoxically, all these strategies may be of limited clinical benefit, because of the increased hemolysis (and hemolysis-related symptoms) resulting from the production of PNH erythrocytes susceptible to complement-mediated lysis. Notwithstanding these interventions, moderate to severe anemia may develop in a substantial proportion of PNH patients, for whom transfusions are the main strategy to control anemia. RBC transfusions are given to PNH patients according to their hemoglobin level; as for other chronic anemic patients, transfusions should be administered to maintain hemoglobin levels above 8 gr/dL. Transfusions transiently improve anemia-related symptoms, as well as hemolysis-related symptoms (the production of PNH erythrocytes temporarily decreases by effect of the higher hemoglobin levels). Remarkably, in contrast to other transfusion-dependent patients, iron overload is usually not a transfusion-related complication in PNH, given the massive iron loss through urine; this may change in PNH patients receiving transfusions during eculizumab treatment (Risitano et al, 2009b). However, as in other transfusion-dependent patients, refractoriness to transfusion may develop, mostly due to allo-sensitization. Refractoriness to transfusions was considered a severe complication requiring alternative treatment – even stem cell transplantation; however, nowadays it is not necessarily a severe complication, given the availability of the anti-complement treatment by eculizumab. Eculizumab has also dramatically changed the management of hemolysis for all PNH patients with meaningful hemolysis, as discussed later on.

### 8.1.2 Management of marrow failure

The management of marrow failure in PNH patients is the same as for AA patients, and represents the main challenge for physicians dealing with the treatment of this condition (Risitano 2011). Indeed, in addition to supportive strategies such as anti-infectious, anti-thrombotic and anti-hemorrhagic prophylaxis and/or treatment, etiologic therapies can also be attempted. According to the pathogenic mechanisms and the dual hypothesis described above, an immune-mediated inhibition of hematopoiesis is postulated in PNH, similar to that demonstrated in AA. Thus, immunosuppressive strategies have been reasonably utilized in PNH patients, even if large prospective studies are lacking. Cyclosporine A has led some improvement in a few series (Schubert et al 1997; Stoppa et al 1996; van Kamp et al 1995). More intensive regimens (as those recommended in severe AA) using the anti-thymocyte globulin associated with high dose prednisone and cyclosporin A have also been exploited; however, the available results are quite heterogeneous (Tichelli et al 1992; Sanchez-Valle et al 1993). Alternative immunosuppressive agents such as cyclophosphamide (Brodsky et al 2010) or the anti-CD52 monoclonal antibody alemtuzumab (Risitano et al 2010a) may be an alternative option (as salvage treatment); in the setting of alemtuzumab-based treatment, there is no concern over the potential selection risk for PNH hematopoiesis, given that the GPI-linked CD52 is not expressed on HSCs. Regardless of the specific immunosuppressive regimen, when this etiological treatment leads to an improvement of the underlying bone marrow impairment, usually normal (non-

PNH) hematopoiesis may be restored, possibly resulting in a progressive dilution (or even extinction) of the PNH clone. However, some patients may continue to have remarkable hemolysis due to the persistence of the PNH clone(s). In addition to the immunosuppressive therapy, it has to be pointed out that marrow failure represents the main indication to allogeneic stem cell transplantation for PNH patients; in fact, all young PNH patients with bone marrow failure should be considered for transplantation if they have a HLA-matched donor (Luzzatto et al 2011), or even if they have an unrelated donor (later in their disease course). Indeed, marrow failure of PNH patients has to be treated as aplastic anemia by either immunosuppression or allogeneic stem cell transplantation, regardless of the presence of the PNH clone(s) (Risitano 2011).

### 8.1.3 Management of thrombophilia

The management of the propensity to develop thrombosis is the hottest issue in PNH, since this complication represents the first cause of death. Unfortunately, there are no controlled prospective clinical trials concerning either primary and secondary thrombosis prophylaxis, or acute treatment of the event. The issue of primary prophylaxis is controversial, and no consensus exists; some physicians advocate the use of warfarin for all newly diagnosed PNH patients, while others do not use any prophylaxis. Both approaches are reasonable, given the unpredictability of thromboembolic events and the lack of evidence supporting any of these strategies; possible benefits are counterbalanced by the risk of hemorrhage from warfarin therapy, which may be considerable in PNH patients with low platelet count. Given that up to two thirds of PNH patients may never develop any thrombosis during the course of their disease, some physicians consider unacceptable to risk hemorrhagic complications (especially in those who are thrombocytopenic); this perception is strengthened by the fact that current primary prophylaxis is not necessarily protective in all patients (de Latour et al 2008; Luzzatto et al 2011). A reasonable compromise may be the adoption of primary prophylaxis for patients at higher risk of thrombosis, which can be identified by the presence of additional inherited (e.g., ethnicity, factor V Leiden) or acquired (e.g., lupus anti-coagulant, pregnancy) risk factors for thrombosis. A single group reported that prophylaxis by warfarin in patients with WBC PNH clones larger than 50% resulted in a very low incidence of thromboembolic events compared to historical controls (Hall et al 2003); however, hemorrhagic complications (even fatal) were also observed, and these date need to be confirmed in larger, possibly prospective studies. To data, there is no experience with newer and possibly more manageable agents, such as thrombin inhibitors, which might play a major role in the future. In contrast, as far as secondary prophylaxis is concerned, there is general agreement that all PNH patients experiencing any thromboembolic event should remain life-long on anticoagulants; however, even in this setting, no consensus exists about the best strategy. Low-molecular-weight heparin, as well as warfarin at different therapeutic ranges, are both utilized, with some physicians even considering the addition of anti-platelet agents; most physicians start with heparin, and subsequently shift to warfarin. However, despite the extended prophylaxis, recurrence of thrombosis (either as new events or progression of the existing ones) is frequent and affects the survival of PNH patients (Audebert et al 2005; de Latour et al 2008). Moreover, life-threatening hemorrhagic events are quite frequent in this cohort of patients, mostly when concomitant thrombocytopenia is present (Hall et al 2003, Moyo et al 2004). Finally, the management of an acute thromboembolic disease may require an intensive therapy similar to that for myocardial infarct; in addition to anti-coagulants at therapeutical doses, fibrinolytic therapies using tissue plasminogen activator have been exploited, showing efficient clearance of the thrombus in individual cases (McCullin et al 1994; Hauser et al 2003; Sholar & Bell 1985; Araten et al 2010). As for hemolytic anemia, the management of thrombophilia has substantially changed with the introduction of eculizumab.

### 8.2 Anti-complement treatment

#### 8.2.1 Eculizumab: A humanized anti-complement component 5 monoclonal antibody

Eculizumab (h5G1.1-mAb, Soliris®, Alexion Pharmaceuticals) is a humanized monoclonal antibody (mAb) (Rother et al 2007) derived from the murine anti-human C5 mAb; it specifically binds the terminal complement component 5, thereby inhibiting its cleavage to C5a and C5b (Matis & Rollins 1995). Thus, eculizumab blocks the formation of MAC, the terminal effector mechanism leading to intravascular hemolysis of PNH erythcocytes. The blockade of the complement cascade at the level of C5 does not affect early complement components, preserving pivotal functions such as clearance of immune complexes and microorganisms (Matis and Rollins 1995). Eculizumab was initially investigated in patients suffering from other complement-mediated disorders; however, PNH appeared the best candidate disease to benefit from eculizumab treatment. In fact, eculizumab may compensate for the absence of CD59 on PNH erythrocytes, preventing their lysis upon complement activation (which is also uncontrolled given the absence of CD55). Eculizumab is administered intravenously, thus its bioavailability is 100%; its estimated half-life is 271 hours. Eculizumab therapy was designed to rapidly reach pharmacodynamic levels using an induction regimen, followed by a maintenance dosage schedule aiming to avoid concentration drops below the plasma level of 35 μg/mL (Hillmen et al 2006), which is the threshold level for pharmacodymanic effectiveness (based on *in vitro* data). In all PNH studies eculizumab has been administered intravenously as 4 weekly doses of 600 mg (induction regimen), followed by 900 mg doses every other week (maintenance regimen), starting 1 week after induction (week 5); this is the standard schedule, approved by the FDA for the treatment of hemolysis in PNH patients.

#### 8.2.2 Safety and efficacy of eculizumab

*Eculizumab and intravascular hemolysis: efficacy from the registration studies.* The management of hemolysis of PNH, which was palliative until 2000, has dramatically changed with the availability of eculizumab (Brodsky 2009; Luzzatto et al 2011). In the last few years eculizumab has been extensively investigated for the treatment of hemolysis in patients with transfusion-dependent PNH. Safety and efficacy of eculizumab were initially established in a phase II pilot study (Hillmen et al 2004) as well as in two phase III clinical studies (TRIUMPH and SHEPHERD) (Hillmen et al 2006; Brodsky et al 2008), and subsequently were confirmed in a common open-label Extension study (Hillmen et al 2007). All patients receiving eculizumab were vaccinated against *Neisseria Meningiditis* at least two weeks before starting treatment. After the initial pilot study, which provided the proof-of-principle of effective blockade of intravascular hemolysis in eleven heavily transfused PNH patients (Hillmen et al 2004), eculizumab was tested in a double-blind, placebo-controlled, multinational randomized trial which enrolled 86 patients (Hillmen et al 2006). The eligibility criteria included at least 4 red cell transfusions in the previous 12 months, a PNH type III erythrocyte population ≥10%, platelets ≥100 x $10^9$/L, and lactate dehydrogenase (LDH) ≥1.5 times the upper limit of normal (Hillmen et al 2006). Treatment with eculizumab resulted in a dramatic reduction of intravascular hemolysis, as measured by LDH, leading to hemoglobin stabilization and transfusion independence in about half the patients. Control of intravascular hemolysis was achieved in all patients, and even cases who still required transfusions showed a reduction of their transfusional needs. The effects of eculizumab on hemolysis were evident after the first administration, and lasted for the whole study period. Compared to placebo, eculizumab significantly improved fatigue and quality of life, as measured by validated questionnaires (Hillmen et al 2006). These data were confirmed in the open-label phase III study SHEPHERD, which included a broader PNH population (minimum pretreatment transfusion requirement was one, and minimum platelet count requirement was 30 x $10^9$/L) (Brodsky et al 2008). In the 96 patients enrolled in the study, treatment with eculizumab resulted in an almost complete control of intravascular hemolysis, regardless of the pretreatment transfusion requirement, with transfusion independence achieved in half the patients, and significant improvement in fatigue and quality of life (Brodsky et al 2008). The subsequent open-label Extension study enrolled a total of 187 patients who had previously completed one of the parent clinical trials (Hillmen et al 2007). The Extension study confirmed the efficacy and safety of eculizumab with a longer follow up, confirming that the effects of eculizumab treatment on intravascular hemolysis were retained over time (Hillmen et al 2007).

*Eculizumab and thrombophilia.* The Extension study included as a secondary endpoint the assessment of thrombotic risk in PNH patients chronically receiving eculizumab treatment, by looking to the incidence of thromboembolic events in the pretreatment and treatment periods in the same patients (Hillmen et al 2007). The rate of thromboembolism decreased from 7.37 to 1.07 events/100 patient-years after eculizumab treatment, with a 85% relative reduction. This reduction was preserved even in patients on anticoagulants, suggesting that eculizumab may be the most effective agent to prevent thromboembolisms in PNH patients (Hillmen et al 2007). Whether eculizumab exerts its effect on thrombophilia of PNH directly, or through the blockade of intravascular hemolysis (e.g., by reduction of NO consumption or reduced release of procoagulant microvesicles), it is still unknown. Recently, it has been reported that eculizumab treatment results in a significant decrease in the plasma markers of coagulation pathway activation, reactive fibrinolysis and endothelial cell activation (Helley et al 2010). This finding suggests that the pathophysiology of thrombosis in PNH may involve multiple pathways, and that the triggering events possibly affected by eculizumab have not been yet identified. However, if the protective effect of eculizumab on the thromboembolic risk are confirmed in a long-term period, it is reasonable to anticipate that eculizumab may result in an improvement of survival of PNH patients. Such effect on survival has been recently shown in a limited cohort of patients (Kelly et al 2011).

*Eculizumab and PNH: any additional benefit?* More recently, it has been reported that eculizumab may lead to additional beneficial effects for PNH patients. As stated before, by inhibiting intravascular hemolysis eculizumab controls all hemolysis-related symptoms, including painful crisis, dysphagia and erectile dysfunction (Hill et al 2005). In addition, by counteracting NO consumption, eculizumab might reduce the risk of pulmonary hypertension (PH) (Hill et al 2010b). This conclusion was mainly derived from the 50% reduction of N-terminal pro-brain natriuretic peptide (NT-proBNP), which was elevated at baseline in about 50% of PNH patients. Unfortunately this study does not include a direct estimation of pulmonary artery pressure by doppler echocardiography, making it uncertain as to whether these PNH patients exhibited clinically relevant PH. However, even if NT-proBNP can be considered a non-invasive marker for PH, possibly reflecting increased pulmonary vascular resistance and right ventricular dysfunction, it is usually utilized as prognostic marker in patients with proven diagnosis of PH. In another study, eculizumab appeared to improve renal function of PNH patients, as measured by estimated glomerular filtration rate (eGFR), preventing possible CKD (Hillmen et al 2010). The authors report that before treatment a fraction of PNH patients may have decreased eGFR, qualifying for stage 3-5 CKD (about 20%); eculizumab treatment resulted in an improvement of eGFR, and reduced the risk of major clinical kidney events. Nevertheless, PH and CKD are not commonly described in PNH patients (de Latour et al 2008); therefore, the real clinical impact of these finding has to be assessed in appropriate studies.

*Eculizumab and pregnancy.* Most hematologists try to dissuade PNH women from pursuing pregnancy, due to both maternal and fetal risk of complications, mainly secondary to thrombosis. Since eculizumab has became available, three pregnancies have been reported in women on this agent all through the gestation period; all of them had healthy newborns, without any maternal complication (Kelly et al 2010; Marasca et al 2010). Thus, even if eculizumab is formally not indicated in PNH pregnant women, and indeed the label for eculizumab classifies it as a pregnancy class C drug, common sense suggests that eculizumab be not automatically withdrawn in the case of pregnancy, giving careful consideration to the need to control the major causes of both maternal and fetal morbidity (intravascular hemolysis and subsequent anemia, and thrombophilia). It is still a matter of debate whether these data are sufficient to change our current counseling, allowing highly motivated PNH women to start pregnancy during eculizumab treatment.

*Safety and tolerability of eculizumab treatment.* The safety profile of eculizumab was assessed in the six studies involving PNH patients (Hillmen et al 2006; Brodsky et al 2008; Hillmen et al 2007), as well as on eleven studies utilizing eculizumab for different indications; the cumulative exposure was 147.44 and 492.20 patient-years in the two populations, respectively. Three deaths were reported in the PNH studies, all related to the underlying disease in two cases (one cerebral vascular accident and one progression to chronic myelomonocytic leukemia) and to an unrelated accident in the third (cerebral herniation). The main concern was a putative increased risk of infections, mostly by encapsulated bacteria, namely *Neisseria Spp.* Given the occurrence of a single case of meningitis by *Neisseria meningitidis* in the initial non-PNH cohort, all patients exposed to eculizumab were vaccinated against *Neisseria meningitidis* using a polyvalent vaccine. In addition, all patients received a warning on meningitis and infectious symptoms, as well as a rescue antibiotic prescription. No case of meningitis has been documented among the 195 PNH patients receiving eculizumab in the clinical trials; however, three patients developed a *Neisseria meningitidis* infection (possibly from *N. meningitidis* groups not covered by the prescribed vaccine), with sepsis in two cases. None of these patients developed meningitis or other complications, and all recovered promptly as a result of early diagnosis and treatment. The incidence of serious adverse events was similar in eculizumab-treated patients and in those receiving the placebo within the TRIUMPH trial; furthermore, none of the serious adverse events was considered as possibly, probably or definitely related to eculizumab. The overall rate of infectious events did not increase compared to the placebo group; however, herpes simplex and some other site-specific infections (nasopharyngitis, upper respiratory tract infection, urinary tract infection and sinusitis) appeared to be more frequent within the eculizumab-treated population. However, in all cases the intensity was mild and the clinical resolution prompt. The occurrence of immunogenity was assessed, and was demonstrated to be very infrequent, if at all present, and without consequence on drug efficacy. In summary, the treatment with eculizumab is safe and well-tolerated for the treatment of PNH, with negligible side effects (Hillmen et al 2006). Long-term treatment has not shown any deviation from this safety profile, as confirmed by post-marketing experience; however, anti-meningococcal vaccination and warning for symptoms of meningitis remains mandatory.

### 8.2.3 Emerging observations during treatment with eculizumab

*C3-mediated extravascular hemolysis during eculizumab treatment.* Since the introduction of eculizumab in 2005, growing evidence suggests that its effect on MAC inhibition may unmask a biologically relevant and potentially pathogenic role for the early phases of the complement cascade. We have recently documented that a novel, clinically significant finding may appear in PNH patients receiving eculizumab, accounting for some portion of residual anemia and heterogeneous hematological benefit from treatment (Risitano et al 2009a). In fact, while basically all patients achieve normal or almost normal LDH levels (pointing out an adequate control of intravascular hemolysis), only about a third reach a hemoglobin value above 11 gr/dL). In contrast, the remaining patients on eculizumab continue to exhibit moderate to severe (transfusion-dependent) anemia, in about equal proportions. In our initial series of 56 PNH patients, we have demonstrated by flow cytometry that all the 41 PNH patients on eculizumab harbored C3 fragments bound to a substantial portion of their PNH erythrocytes (while none of the untreated patients did) (Risitano et al 2009a). Our data were confirmed in an independent series by an other group that exploited a direct antiglobulin test using C3d-specific anti-sera (Hill et al 2010a). We concluded that membrane-bound C3 fragments work as opsonins on PNH erythrocytes, resulting in their entrapment by reticuloendothelial cells through specific C3 receptors and subsequent extravascular hemolysis (Risitano et al 2009a; Luzzatto et al 2010). This mechanism is supported by persistent reticulocytosis, hyperbilirubinemia and anemia in patients on eculizumab, and was also confirmed by an *in vivo* erythrocyte survival study by $^{51}$Cr labeling (which showed reduced survival and hepatosplenic $^{51}$Cr uptake) (Risitano et al 2009a).

*The complement cascade regulation during eculizumab treatment.* Pathophysiologically, it is clear that such a mechanism becomes evident only when eculizumab prevents MAC-mediated hemolysis, allowing longer survival of PNH erythrocytes, which continue to suffer from uncontrolled C3 convertase activation and C3 fragment deposition due to CD55 deficiency (Luzzatto et al 2010; Risitano et al 2011). Indeed, CAP is physiologically in a state of continuous activation because spontaneous (low-grade) hydrolysis of an internal thioester bond of C3 generates a C3b-like molecule, C3($H_2O$); nascent C3($H_2O$) is able to recruit factor B in forming (in the fluid phase) an unstable pro-C3 convertase. Once cleaved by factor D (generating C3($H_2O$)Bb), this complex will in turn cleave additional C3 molecules to generate C3b, which binds predominantly to glycophorin A and activate (now in a membrane-bound phase) the CAP amplification loop (Parker et al 1982; Pangburn et al 1983c; Müller-Eberhard 1988; Risitano et al 2011). On PNH erythrocytes, the lack of CD55 will allow this process (which is self-limiting on normal cells) to continue, leading to progressive CAP-mediated amplification, even in the presence of eculizumab (which acts downstream). The reasons why only a fraction of PNH erythrocytes has membrane-bound C3, and why the proportion varies among patients, are not fully understood. Nevertheless, *in vitro* data support the concept that PNH erythrocytes are all susceptible to C3 deposition once exposed to conditions causing complement activation (Sica et al 2010). We have hypothesized that inter-individual differences in other physiological inhibitors (such as CR1 , complement FH and complement FI) may modulate the complement activation in a patient-specific fashion, leading to distinct patterns of C3 deposition. In addition, even more complex factors may drive the subsequent fate of C3-bound PNH erythrocytes; in fact, some patients may harbor large proportion of C3-bound PNH erythrocytes, without showing a clinically relevant extravascular hemolysis (Risitano et al 2010b). At the moment, there is yet no ability to predict before starting eculizumab which patients will develop C3-mediated extravascular hemolysis.

*Current strategies to overcome C3-mediated extravascular hemolysis.* C3 opsonization of PNH erythrocytes is a common phenomenon for PNH patients treated with eculizumab, even if the subsequent extravascular hemolysis may remain limited or well-compensated in most cases (Luzzatto et al 2010). However, additional therapeutic strategies are needed for patients developing a clinically relevant C3-mediated extravascular hemolysis, because they may continue to require frequent red cell transfusions, possibly developing subsequent iron overload (Risitano et al 2009a). We reported a patient managed by splenectomy (Risitano et al 2008), who achieved a substantial improvement of hemoglobin level without any medical complication; however, many physicians raise the concern that this approach may carry an increased life-long risk of infections (Brodsky 2009). In addition, the risk of intra- or peri-operatory complications (especially thrombosis, or hemorrhage in thrombocytopenic patients) might also argue against this therapeutic option. Very recently a group reported a single case where steroids were beneficial in controlling C3-mediated extravascular hemolysis (Berzuini et al 2010). To best of our knowledge, this observation has not been confirmed in a larger series, and the well known side effects of long-term steroid use should advise against the use of steroids in PNH patients on eculizumab (Risitano et al 2010b). In some patients, the use of recombinant erythropoietin has proven beneficial by increasing compensatory erythropoiesis (Hill et al 2007).

*A look into the future of complement inhibition.* The emergence of experimental and clinical evidence for CAP-initiated and C3 fragment-mediated extravascular hemolysis suggests that new treatment strategies appropriately targeting the early phases of the complement cascade should be assessed. The ideal agent should prevent the early phase of complement activation on PNH cells and defuse the amplification mechanisms (e.g., the CAP amplification loop). A systemic blockade of C3 activation through all pathways by monoclonal antibodies (similar to the anti-C5 eculizumab) could be considered (e.g., by anti-C3 monoclonal antobiiodies) (Lindorfer et al 2010); however this approach may carry the risk of infectious and autoimmune complications secondary to a complete switching off of the complement system at this point. A novel candidate agent has been designed by creating a recombinant fusion protein between two endogenous complement-related proteins, complement factor H (FH) and complement receptor 2 (CR2). FH is a physiological complement inhibitor that modulates the initial CAP activation in the fluid phase by preventing C3 convertase activity and by promoting C3b inactivation into iC3b (Whaley et al 1976). Indeed, FH defuses the CAP amplification loop, and it has been demonstrated protective from lysis for PNH erythrocytes *in vitro* (Ferreira & Pangburn 2007). In the aim to deliver FH activity locally at the site of complement activation, FH was fused with the iC3b/C3d-binding domain of CR2. The resulting CR2-FH fusion protein has shown a dramatic inhibition of hemolysis of PNH erythrocytes *in vitro* (Risitano et al 2009c), and further investigations are currently under way. A phase I clinical trial has just started to enroll PNH patients (Alexion Pharmaceuticals, personal communication). Once these or other next generation complement inhibitors proceed to clinical development, then we can determine whether such targeted inhibition should be additional or alternative to eculizumab. Indeed, the adequate control of C3, or both C3 and C5 activation on PNH red cells might make the downstream blockade by eculizumab redundant.

### 8.3 Hematopoietic stem cell transplantation

Cell therapy (insertion of molecules on the outer surface of blood cells) (Hill et al 2006a) and gene therapy (insertion of a functional *PIG-A* gene in early hematopoietic progenitors) have been hypothesized in the past as a curative approach for PNH. However, they seem unfeasible or even inappropriate; in fact, if the escape theory is correct, the gene therapy approach may not result in clinical benefit in PNH, since a repair of the damaged cell should result in cell destruction, as is believed to occur for normal hematopoiesis in PNH patients. The only curative strategy for PNH is allogeneic hematopoietic stem cell transplantation (SCT); SCT has been exploited since the late '80, and has proven effective in eradicating the abnormal PNH clone possibly leading to definitive cure of PNH, even if morbidity and mortality remain a major limitation. Most reports in the literature refer to single cases or small series from single-institutions (Bemba et al 1999, Raiola et al 2000; Saso et al 1999), while large prospective studies are lacking. In an overview, Parker et al (Parker et al 2005) collected data from 67 patients transplanted from different types of donors (syngeneic, sibling or HLA-identical unrelated) and using different types of conditioning (myeloablative or reduced-intensity). The results from the entire group showed a 75% long-term survival, which is quite higher than that reported in individual series (55-100%), likely as a result of a reporting bias. Data from two large registry studies are also available. The International Bone Marrow Transplant Registry reported 57 consecutive SCT performed for PNH (16 AA/PNH) between 1978 and 1995 (Matos-Fernandez et al 2009), showing a 2-year survival of 56% in 48 HLA-identical sibling transplants (the median follow-up was 44 months). The incidence of grade II or more severe acute GvHD was 34%, and that of chronic GvHD of 33%; graft failure (n=7) and infections (n=3) were the most common causes of treatment failure. An other retrospective study from the Italian Transplant Group (GITMO) on 26 PNH patients (4 AA/PNH) transplanted between 1998 and 2006 showed a 57& survival rate at 10 years. Acute and chronic GvHD were 42% (grade III-IV 12%) and 50% (extensive 16%), respectively (Santarone et al 2010). Given these results, guidelines for SCT in PNH are hard to define; the most difficult task today is to identify PNH patients who could benefit from HSCT (Brodsly 2010). At the moment, the main indication for SCT in PNH patients is an underlying bone marrow failure; as for AA patients, SCT may be performed as first-line therapy in the presence of an HLA-identical sibling donor, or in case of treatment failure in patients with an HLA-matched unrelated donor (Risitano 2011). The patient's age largely drives the choice of treatment, given that transplant-related mortality and morbidity increase with age. Refractoriness to transfusions and life-threatening thrombosis were also indications to SCT in the past, but nowadays they rather represent indications to anti-complement treatment, with the exception of Countries where eculizumab is not available (yet). However, SCT remains a worthy second-line therapy for the few patients not achieving a good response to eculizumab. As for AA, SCT (regardless of the type of donor, sibling or unrelated donor) is the treatment of choice for PNH patients developing a clonal evolution to MDS or even AML. The Working Party for Severe Aplastic Anemia of the European Bone Marrow Transplantation Group, together with the French PNH Registry, are currently running a retrospective studies comparing the outcome of all BMT performed in Europe with the natural history of PNH (in the pre-eculizumab era). Likely the results from this study will guide future treatment strategies for PNH patients, according to specific disease presentation and complications. A number of questions remain open in the setting of SCT for PNH, to improve the clinical outcome: the most relevant is the choice of the conditioning regimen. Based on available data, AA/PNH patients should be treated as non-PNH AA patients; thus, the conditioning should be cyclophosphamide/ATG for sibling transplants, and fludarabine-based RIC for unrelated transplants (to be performed as in case of failure of IST) (Bacigalupo et al 2010). In contrast, classic, non-hypoplastic, PNH patients receiving SCT should benefit from myeloablative conditioning (e.g., busulphan-based) (Raiola et al 2000); however, RIC regimens (fludarabine-based) (Takahashi et al 2004) may be appropriate for patients who are older or who present with relevant comorbidities.

## 9. Conclusion

PNH has attracted the efforts of several generations of investigators in the last three decades for its biological and clinical uniqueness. While the '80s unraveled the GPI-anchor and the functional defect of the PNH clone, and the '90s revealed the *PIG-A* gene and its role in the pathophysiology of the disease, this new century brought forth innovative therapeutic approaches. Thanks to current treatment options, we are finally able to change the natural history of PNH, possibly giving back to PNH patients a normal-like life expectancy, in addition to a significant reduction of disease manifestations and improvement in their quality of life. As often occurs in medicine, thanks to these novel treatments we are also improving our biological knowledge of the disease and of current treatments. Thus, the scientific community has already accepted the next challenge: utilize these recent insights to develop novel targeted treatment strategies, for further improvement of current management of PNH patients.

## 10. Acknowledgments

I am grateful to Professor Bruno Rotoli who handed down to myself his devotion to PNH patients and PNH science; this chapter mostly stems from his long-lasting thoughtful teachings. I also thank Dr. Rosario Notaro, Professor Lucio Luzzatto, Dr. Jaroslaw Maciejewski and Dr. Neal Young for their contribution to my knowledge of PNH.

## 11. References

[1] Almeida AM, Murakami Y, Layton DM, et al. Hypomorphic promoter mutation in PIGM causes inherited glycosylphosphatidylinositol deficiency. Nat Med. 2006; 12:846-51.

[2] Almeida A, Layton M & Karadimitris A. Inherited glycosylphosphatidyl inositol deficiency: a treatable CDG. Biochim Biophys Acta. 2009; 1792:874-80.
[3] Araten DJ, Nafa K, Pakdeesuwan K, et al. Clonal populations of hematopoietic cells with paroxysmal nocturnal hemoglobinuria genotype and phenotype are present in normal individuals. Proc Natl Acad Sci U S A. 1999; 96:5209-5214.
[4] Araten DJ, Swirsky D, Karadimitris A, et al. Cytogenetic and morphological abnormalities in paroxysmal nocturnal haemoglobinuria. Br J Haematol. 2001; 115:360-8.
[5] Araten DJ, Bessler M, McKenzie S, et al. Dynamics of hematopoiesis in paroxysmal nocturnal hemoglobinuria (PNH): no evidence for intrinsic growth advantage of PNH clones. Leukemia. 2002; 16:2243-8.
[6] Araten DJ, Thaler HT & Luzzatto L. High incidence of thrombosis in African-American and Latin-American patients with Paroxysmal Nocturnal Haemoglobinuria. Thromb Haemost. 2005; 93:88-91.
[7] Araten DJ & Luzzatto L. The mutation rate in PIG-A is normal in patients with paroxysmal nocturnal hemoglobinuria (PNH). Blood. 2006; 108:734-6.
[8] Araten DJ, Notaro R, Thaler H, et al. Thrombolytic therapy for reversal of thrombosis in paroxysmal nocturnal hemoglobinuria. Blood. 2010; 116:1721(a).
[9] Armstrong C, Schubert J, Ueda E, et al. Affected paroxysmal nocturnal hemoglobinuria T lymphocytes harbor a common defect in assembly of N-acetyl-D-glucosamine inositol phospholipid corresponding to that in class A Thy-1- murine lymphoma mutants. J Biol Chem. 1999; 267:25347-51.
[10] Audebert HJ, Planck J, Eisenburg M, et al. Cerebral ischemic infarction in paroxysmal nocturnal hemoglobinuria report of 2 cases and updated review of 7 previously published patients. J Neurol. 2005; 252:1379-86.
[11] Bacigalupo A, Socie' G, Lanino E, et al; Severe Aplastic Anemia Working Party of the European Group for Blood and Marrow Transplantation. Fludarabine, cyclophosphamide, antithymocyte globulin, with or without low dose total body irradiation, for alternative donor transplants, in acquired severe aplastic anemia: a retrospective study from the EBMT-SAA working party. Haematologica. 2010; 95: 976-82.
[12] Bemba M, Guardiola P, Gardret L et al. Bone marrow transplantation for paroxysmal nocturnal haemoglobinuria. Br J Haematol. 1999; 105 :366-368.
[13] Berzuini A, Montanelli F & Prati D. Hemolytic anemia after eculizumab in paroxysmal nocturnal hemoglobinuria. N Engl J Med. 2010; 363:993-4.
[14] Bessler M, Hillmen P, Longo L, et al. Genomic organization of the X-linked gene (PIG-A) that is mutated in paroxysmal nocturnal haemoglobinuria and of a related autosomal pseudogene mapped to 12q21. Hum Mol Genet. 1994; 3:751-7.
[15] Borowitz MJ, Craig FE, Digiuseppe JA, et al; Clinical Cytometry Society. Guidelines for the diagnosis and monitoring of paroxysmal nocturnal hemoglobinuria and related disorders by flow cytometry. Cytometry B Clin Cytom. 2010; 78:211-30.
[16] Bourantas K. High-dose recombinant erythropoietin and low-dose corticosteroids for treatment of anemia in paroxysmal nocturnal hemoglobinuria. Acta Haematol 1994; 91-62-5.
[17] Brodsky RA, Mukhina GL, Li S, et al. Improved detection and characterization of paroxysmal nocturnal hemoglobinuria using fluorescent aerolysin. Am J Clin Pathol. 2000; 114:459-66.

[18] Brodsky RA, Young NS, Antonioli E, et al. Multicenter phase III study of the complement inhibitor eculizumab for the treatment of patients with paroxysmal nocturnal hemoglobinuria. Blood. 2008; 114:1840-47.
[19] Brodsky RA. How I treat paroxysmal nocturnal hemoglobinuria. Blood. 2009; 113:6522-7.
[20] Brodsky RA, Chen AR, Dorr D, et al. High-dose cyclophosphamide for severe aplastic anemia: long-term follow-up. Blood. 2010; 115:2136-41.
[21] Brodsky RA. Stem cell transplantation for paroxysmal nocturnal hemoglobinuria. Haematologica. 2010; 95:855-6.
[22] Brubaker LH, Essig LJ & Mengel CE. Neutrophil life span in paroxysmal nocturnal hemoglobinuria. Blood. 1977; 50:657-62.
[23] Cacciapuoti C, Terrazzano G, Barone L, et al. Glycosyl-phosphatidyl-inositol-defective granulocytes from paroxysmal nocturnal haemoglobinuria patients show increased bacterial ingestion but reduced respiratory burst induction. Am J Hematol. 2007; 82:98-107.
[24] Chen G, Zeng W, Maciejewski JP, et al. Differential gene expression in hematopoietic progenitors from paroxysmal nocturnal hemoglobinuria patients reveals an apoptosis/immune response in 'normal' phenotype cells. Leukemia. 2005; 19:862-8.
[25] Crosby WH. Paroxysmal nocturnal hemoglobinuria; a classic description by Paul Strübling in 1882, and a bibliography of the disease. Blood. 1951; 63:270-84.
[26] Dameshek W. Riddle: what do aplastic anemia, paroxysmal nocturnal hemoglobinuria (PNH) and "hypoplastic" leukemia have in common? Blood. 1967; 30:251-254.
[27] de Latour RP, Mary JY, Salanoubat C, et al; French Association of Young Hematologists. Paroxysmal nocturnal hemoglobinuria: natural history of disease subcategories. Blood. 2008; 112:3099-106.
[28] Devine DV, Siegel RS & Rosse WF. Interactions of the platelets in paroxysmal nocturnal hemoglobinuria with complement. Relationship to defects in the regulation of complement and to platelet survival in vivo. J Clin Invest. 1987a; 79:131-7.
[29] Devine DV, Gluck WL, Rosse WF, et al. Acute myeloblastic leukemia in paroxysmal nocturnal hemoglobinuria. Evidence of evolution from the abnormal paroxysmal nocturnal hemoglobinuria clone. J Clin Invest. 1987b; 79:314-7.
[30] Dingli D, Luzzatto L & Pacheco JM. Neutral evolution in paroxysmal nocturnal hemoglobinuria. Proc Natl Acad Sci U S A. 2008; 105:18496-500.
[31] Dunn DE, Liu JM & Young NS. 2000. Paroxysmal nocturnal hemoglobinuria. In: Young NS (ed). Bone Marrow Failure Syndromes. Philadelphia: W.B. Saunders Company. p 99-121.
[32] Endo M, Ware RE, Vreeke TM, et al. Molecular basis of the heterogeneity of expression of glycosyl phosphatidylinositol anchored proteins in paroxysmal nocturnal hemoglobinuria. Blood. 1996; 87:2546-57.
[33] Enneking J. Eine neue form intermittierender Haemoglobinurie (Haemoglobinuria paroxysmalis nocturna). Klin. Wehnschr. 1928. 7: 2045.
[34] Ferreira VP & Pangburn MK. Factor H mediated cell surface protection from complement is critical for the survival of PNH erythrocytes. Blood. 2007; 15;110:1290-2.
[35] Fieni S, Bonfanti L, Gramellini D, et al. Clinical management of paroxysmal nocturnal hemoglobinuria in pregnancy: a case report and updated review. Obstet Gynecol Surv. 2006; 61:593-601.

[36] Fujioka S & Asai T. Prognostic features of paroxysmal nocturnal hemoglobinuria in Japan. Nihon Ketsueki Gakkai Zasshi. 1989; 52:1386-94.

[37] Gargiulo L, Lastraioli S, Cerruti G, et al. Highly homologous T-cell receptor beta sequences support a common target for autoreactive T cells in most patients with paroxysmal nocturnal hemoglobinuria. Blood.2007; 109:5036-42.

[38] Gralnick HR, Vail M, McKeown LP, et al. Activated platelets in paroxysmal nocturnal haemoglobinuria. Br J Haematol. 1995; 91:697-702.

[39] Grünewald M, Siegemund A, Grünewald A, et al. Plasmatic coagulation and fibrinolytic system alterations in PNH: relation to clone size. Blood Coagul Fibrinolysis. 2003; 14:685-95.

[40] Ham TH. Chronic hemolytic anemia with paroxysmal nocturnal hemoglobinuria. A study of mechanism of hemolysis to acid-base equilibrium. N Engl J Med. 1937; 217:915-917.

[41] Ham TH & Dingle JH. Studies on the destruction of red blood cells. II. Chronic hemolytic anemia with paroxysmal nocturnal hemoglobinuria: certain immunological aspects of the hemolytic mechanism with special reference to serum complement. J Clin Invest. 1939; 18:657-672.

[42] Hall C, Richards S & Hillmen P. Primary prophylaxis with warfarin prevents thrombosis in paroxysmal nocturnal hemoglobinuria (PNH). Blood. 2003; 102:3587-91.

[43] Harrington WJ Sr, Kolodny R, Horstmann LL et al. Danazol for paroxysmal nocturnal hemoglobinuria. Am J Hematol. 1997; 54:149-54.

[44] Hauser AC, Brichta A, Pabinger-Fasching I, et al. Fibrinolytic therapy with rt-PA in a patient with paroxysmal nocturnal hemoglobinuria and Budd-Chiari syndrome. Ann Hematol. 2003; 82:299-302.

[45] Helley D, de Latour RP, Porcher R, et al; French Society of Hematology. Evaluation of hemostasis and endothelial function in patients with paroxysmal nocturnal hemoglobinuria receiving eculizumab. Haematologica. 2010; 95:574-81.

[46] Hertenstein B, Wagner B, Bunjes D, et al. Emergence of CD52-, phosphatidylinositolglycan-anchor-deficient T lymphocytes after in vivo application of Campath-1H for refractory B-cell non-Hodgkin lymphoma. Blood. 1995; 86:1487-1492.

[47] Hill A, Rother RP & Hillmen P. Improvement in the symptoms of smooth muscle dystonia during eculizumab therapy in paroxysmal nocturnal hemoglobinuria. Haematologica. 2005; 90:ECR40.

[48] Hill A, Ridley SH, Esser D, et al. Protection of erythrocytes from human complement-mediated lysis by membrane-targeted recombinant soluble CD59: a new approach to PNH therapy. Blood. 2006a; 107:2131-7.

[49] Hill A, Wang X, Sapsford RJ, et al. Nitric oxide consumption and pulmonary hypertension in patients with paroxysmal nocturnal hemoglobinuria. Blood. 2006b; 108:305a.

[50] Hill A et al. The incidence and prevalence of Paroxysmal Nocturnal Hemoglobinuria (PNH) and survival of patients in Yorkshire. Blood 2006c; 108:985a.

[51] Hill A, Richards SJ, Rother RP, et al. Erythopoietin treatment during complement inhibition with eculizumab in a patient with paroxysmal nocturnal hemoglobinuria. Haematologica. 2007; 92:ECR14.

[52] Hill A, Rother RP, Arnold L, et al. Eculizumab prevents intravascular hemolysis in patients with paroxysmal nocturnal hemoglobinuria and unmasks low-level extravascular hemolysis occurring through C3 opsonization. Haematologica. 2010a; 95,567-573.

[53] Hill A, Rother RP, Wang X, et al. Effect of eculizumab on haemolysis-associated nitric oxide depletion, dyspnoea, and measures of pulmonary hypertension in patients with paroxysmal nocturnal haemoglobinuria. Br J Haematol. 2010b; 149:414-25.

[54] Hillmen P, Lewis SM, Bessler M, et al. Natural history of paroxysmal nocturnal hemoglobinuria. N Engl J Med. 1995; 333:1253-1258.

[55] Hillmen P, Hall C, Marsh JC, et al. Effect of eculizumab on hemolysis and transfusion requirements in patients with paroxysmal nocturnal hemoglobinuria. N Engl J Med. 2004; 350:552-559.

[56] Hillmen P, Young NS, Schubert J, et al. The complement inhibitor eculizumab in paroxysmal nocturnal hemoglobinuria. N Engl J Med. 2006; 355:1233-43.

[57] Hillmen P, Muus P, Duhrsen U, et al. Effect of the complement inhibitor eculizumab on thromboembolism in patients with paroxysmal nocturnal hemoglobinuria. Blood. 2007; 110:4123-8.

[58] Hillmen P, Elebute M, Kelly R, et al. Long-term effect of the complement inhibitor eculizumab on kidney function in patients with paroxysmal nocturnal hemoglobinuria. Am J Hematol. 2010; 85:553-9.

[59] Hirose S, Ravi L, Prince GM, et al. Synthesis of mannosylglucosaminylinositol phospholipids in normal but not paroxysmal nocturnal hemoglobinuria cells. Proc Natl Acad Sci U S A. 1992; 89:6025-9.

[60] Hoekstra J, Leebeek FW, Plessier A, et al. Paroxysmal nocturnal hemoglobinuria in Budd-Chiari Syndrome: findings from a cohort study. Journal of hepatology. 2009; 51:696-706.

[61] Hoffman EM. Inhibition of complement by a substance isolated from human erythrocytes. I. Extraction from human erythrocyte stromata. Immunochemistry. 1969; 6:391-403.

[62] Holers VM. The spectrum of complement alternative pathway-mediated diseases. Immunol Rev. 2008; 223:300-16.

[63] Holguin MH, Fredrick LR, Bernshaw NJ, et al. Isolation and characterization of a membrane protein from normal human erythrocytes that inhibits reactive lysis of the erythrocytes of paroxysmal nocturnal hemoglobinuria. J Clin Invest. 1989; 84:7-17.

[64] Holguin MH, Wilcox LA, Bernshaw NJ, et al. Relationship between the membrane inhibitor of reactive lysis and the erythrocyte phenotypes of paroxysmal nocturnal hemoglobinuria. J Clin Invest. 1989; 84:1387-94.

[65] Holguin MH, Wilcox LA, Bernshaw NJ, et al. Erythrocyte membrane inhibitor of reactive lysis: effects of phosphatidylinositol-specific phospholipase C on the isolated and cell-associated protein. Blood. 1990; 75:284-9.

[66] Holguin MH, Martin CB, Bernshaw NJ, et al. Analysis of the effects of activation of the alternative pathway of complement on erythrocytes with an isolated deficiency of decay accelerating factor. J Immunol. 1992; 148:498-502.

[67] Hugel B, Socié G, Vu T, et al. Elevated levels of circulating procoagulant microparticles in patients with paroxysmal nocturnal hemoglobinuria and aplastic anemia. Blood. 1999; 93:3451-6.

[68] Inoue N, Izui-Sarumaru T, Murakami Y, et al. Molecular basis of clonal expansion of hematopoiesis in 2 patients with paroxysmal nocturnal hemoglobinuria (PNH). Blood. 2006; 108:4232-6.

[69] Issaragrisil S, Piankijagum A & Tang.Naitrisorana Y. Corticosteroid therapy in paroxysmal nocturnal hemoglobinuria. Am J Hemato. 1987; 25:77-83.

[70] Jasinski M, Keller P, Fujiwara Y, et al. GATA1-Cre mediates Piga gene inactivation in the erythroid/megakaryocytic lineage and leads to circulating red cells with a partial deficiency in glycosyl phosphatidylinositol-linked proteins (paroxysmal nocturnal hemoglobinuria type II cells). Blood. 2001 ; 98:2248-2255.

[71] Karadimitris A, Manavalan JS, Thaler HT, et al. Abnormal T-cell repertoire is consistent with immune process underlying the pathogenesis of paroxysmal nocturnal hemoglobinuria. Blood. 2001; 96:2613-262.

[72] Karadimitris A, Li K, Notaro R, et al. Association of clonal T-cell large granular lymphocyte disease and paroxysmal nocturnal haemoglobinuria (PNH): further evidence for a pathogenetic link between T cells, aplastic anaemia and PNH. Br J Haematol. 2001; 115:1010-4.

[73] Katayama Y, Hiramatsu Y & Kohriyama H. Monitoring of Cd59 expression in paroxysmal nocturnal hemoglobinuria treated with danazol. Am J Hematol. 2001; 68:280-3.

[74] Kawagoe K, Kitamura D, Okabe M, et al. Glycosylphosphatidylinositol-anchor-deficient mice: implications for clonal dominance of mutant cells in paroxysmal nocturnal hemoglobinuria. Blood. 1996; 87:3600-6.

[75] Keller P, Payne JL, Tremml G, et al. FES-Cre targets phosphatidylinositol glycan class A (PIGA) inactivation to hematopoietic stem cells in the bone marrow. J Exp Med. 2001; 194:581-589.

[76] Kelly RJ, Hill A, Arnold LM, et al. Long-term treatment with eculizumab in paroxysmal nocturnal hemoglobinuria: sustained efficacy and improved survival. Blood. 2011;117:6786-92.

[77] Kelly R, Arnold L, Richards S, et al. The management of pregnancy in paroxysmal nocturnal haemoglobinuria on long term eculizumab. Br J Haematol. 2010; 149:446-450.

[78] Krause JR. Paroxysmal nocturnal hemoglobinuria and acute non-lymphocytic leukemia. A report of three cases exhibiting different cytologic types. Cancer. 1983; 51:2078-82.

[79] Kinoshita T, Medof ME, Silber R, et al. Distribution of decay-accelerating factor in the peripheral blood of normal individuals and patients with paroxysmal nocturnal hemoglobinuria. J Exp Med. 1985; 162:75-92.

[80] Kunstling TR & Rosse WF. Erythrocyte acetylcholinesterase deficiency in paroxysmal nocturnal hemoglobinuria (PNH). A comparison of the complement-sensitive and insensitive populations. Blood. 1969; 33:607-16.

[81] Lewis SM & Dacie JV. The aplastic anaemia--paroxysmal nocturnal haemoglobinuria syndrome. Br J Haematol. 1967; 13:236-51.

[82] Lindorfer MA, Pawluczkowycz AW, Peek EM, et al. A novel approach to preventing the hemolysis of paroxysmal nocturnal hemoglobinuria: both complement-mediated cytolysis and C3 deposition are blocked by a monoclonal antibody specific for the alternative pathway of complement. Blood. 2010; 115:2283-91.

[83] Louwes H, Vellenga E & de Wolf JT. Abnormal platelet adhesion on abdominal vessels in asymptomatic patients with paroxysmal nocturnal hemoglobinuria. Ann Hematol. 2001; 80:573-6.
[84] Luzzatto L, Bessler M & Rotoli B. Somatic mutations in paroxysmal nocturnal hemoglobinuria: a blessing in disguise? Cell. 1997; 88:1-4.
[85] Luzzatto L & Nafa G. Genetics of PNH. 2000. In: Young NS, Moss J (ed). Paroxysmal nocturnal hemoglobinuria and the glycosylphosphatidylinositol-linked proteins. Sa Diego: Academic Press. p 21-47.
[86] Luzzatto L & Notaro R. 2003. Paroxysmal nocturnal hemoglobinuria. In Handin RI, Lux SE, Stossel TP (eds): Blood, principles and practice of hematology (2nd ed.). Philadelphia, PA (USA), Lippincot Williams & Wilkins; p 319-34.
[87] Luzzatto L, Risitano AM & Notaro R. Paroxysmal nocturnal hemoglobinuria and eculizumab. Haematologica. 2010; 95:523-6.
[88] Luzzatto L, Gianfaldoni G & Notaro R. Management of paroxysmal nocturnal haemoglobinuria: a personal view. Br J Haematol. 2011; 153:709-20.
[89] Luzzatto L & Notaro R. Biological basis of paroxysmal nocturnal hemoglobinuria. Hematology education: the educational program for the annual congress of European Hematology Association. 2010;222-227.
[90] Maciejewski JP, Sloand EM, Sato T, et al. Impaired hematopoiesis in paroxysmal nocturnal hemoglobinuria/aplastic anemia is not associated with a selective proliferative defect in the glycosylphosphatidylinositol-anchored protein-deficient clone. Blood. 1997; 89:1173-81.
[91] Maciejewski JP, Young NS, Yu M, et al. Analysis of the expression of glycosylphosphatidylinositol anchored proteins on platelets from patients with paroxysmal nocturnal hemoglobinuria. Thromb Res. 1996; 83:433-47.
[92] Mahoney JF, Urakaze M, Hall S, et al. Defective glycosylphosphatidylinositol anchor synthesis in paroxysmal nocturnal hemoglobinuria granulocytes. Blood. 1992; 79:1400-3.
[93] Marasca R, Coluccio V, Santachiara R, et al. Pregnancy in PNH: another eculizumab baby. Br J Haematol. 2010; 150:707-708.
[94] Marchiafava E & Nazari A. Nuovo contributo allo studio degli itteri emolotici cronici. Policlinico, (sez. med.). 1911. 18: 241.
[95] Markiewski MM, Nilsson B, Ekdahl KN, et al. Complement and coagulation: strangers or partners in crime? Trends in immunology. 2007; 28:184-92.
[96] Matis LA & Rollins SA. Complement-specific antibodies: designing novel anti-inflammatories. Nat Med. 1995; 1:839-42.
[97] Matos-Fernandez NA, Abou Mourad YR, Caceres W, et al. Current status of allogeneic hematopoietic stem cell transplantation for paroxysmal nocturnal hemoglobinuria. Biol Blood Marrow Transplant. 2009; 15:656-61.
[98] McMullin MF, Hillmen P, Elder GE, et al. Serum erythropoietin level in paroxysmal nocturnal hemoglobinuria: implications for therapy. Br J Haematol. 1996; 92:815-7.
[99] McMullin MF, Hillmen P, Jackson J, et al. Tissue plasminogen activator for hepatic vein thrombosis in paroxysmal nocturnal haemoglobinuria. J Intern Med. 1994; 235:85-9.
[100] Medof ME, Walter EI, Roberts WL, et al. Decay accelerating factor of complement is anchored to cells by a C-terminal glycolipid. Biochemistry. 1986; 25:6740-7.
[101] Medof ME, Gottlieb A, Kinoshita T, et al. Relationship between decay accelerating factor deficiency, diminished acetylcholinesterase activity, and defective terminal

complement pathway restriction in paroxysmal nocturnal hemoglobinuria erythrocytes. J Clin Invest. 1987; 80:165-74.

[102] Meri S, Morgan BP, Davies A, et al. Human protectin (CD59), an 18,000-20,000 MW complement lysis restricting factor, inhibits C5b-8 catalysed insertion of C9 into lipid bilayers. Immunology. 1990; 71:1-9.

[103] Merry AH, Rawlinson VI, Uchikawa M, et al. Studies on the sensitivity to complement-mediated lysis of erythrocytes (Inab phenotype) with a deficiency of DAF (decay accelerating factor). Br J Haematol. 1989; 73:248-53.

[104] Micheli N. Anemia emolitica cronica con emosiderinuria perpetua. Policlinico, (sez. prat.). 1928; 35:2574.

[105] Miyata T, Takeda J, Iida Y, et al. The cloning of PIG-A, a component in the early step of GPI-anchor biosynthesis. Science. 1993; 259:1318-1320.

[106] Motoyama N, Okada N, Yamashina M, et al. Paroxysmal nocturnal hemoglobinuria due to hereditary nucleotide deletion in the HRF20 (CD59) gene. Eur J Immunol. 1992; 22:2669-73.

[107] Mold C, Walter EI, Medof ME. The influence of membrane components on regulation of alternative pathway activation by decay-accelerating factor. J Immunol. 1990; 145:3836-41.

[108] Moyo VM, Mukhina GL, Garrett ES, et al. Natural history of paroxysmal nocturnal haemoglobinuria using modern diagnostic assays. Br J Haematol. 2004; 126:133-8.

[109] Mukhina GL, Buckley JT, Barber JP, et al. Multilineage glycosylphosphatidylinositol anchor-deficient haematopoiesis in untreated aplastic anaemia. Br J Haematol. 2001; 115:476-82.

[110] Müller-Eberhard HJ. Molecular organization and function of the complement system. Annu Rev Biochem. 1988; 57:321-47.

[111] Murakami Y, Kosaka H, Maeda Y, et al. Inefficient response of T lymphocytes to glycosylphosphatidylinositol anchor-negative cells: implications for paroxysmal nocturnal hemoglobinuria. Blood. 2002; 100:4116-4122.

[112] Muus P, Szer J, Schrezenmeier H, et al. Evaluation of Paroxysmal Nocturnal Hemoglobinuria Disease Burden: The Patient's Perspective. A Report From the International PNH Registry. Blood. 2010; 116:1525a.

[113] Nagakura S, Ishihara S, Dunn DE, et al. Decreased susceptibility of leukemic cells with PIG-A mutation to natural killer cells in vitro. Blood. 2002; 100:1031-1037.

[114] Nafa K, Mason PJ, Hillmen P, et al. Mutations in the PIG-A gene causing paroxysmal nocturnal hemoglobinuria are mainly of the frameshift type. Blood. 1995; 86:4650-5.

[115] Nafa K, Bessler M, Castro-Malaspina H, et al. The spectrum of somatic mutations in the PIG-A gene in paroxysmal nocturnal hemoglobinuria includes large deletions and small duplications. Blood Cells Mol Dis. 1998a; 24:370-84.

[116] Nafa K, Bessler M, Deeg HJ, et al. New somatic mutation in the PIG-A gene emerges at relapse of paroxysmal nocturnal hemoglobinuria. Blood.1998b; 92:3422-7.

[117] Nafa K, Bessler M, Mason P, et al. Factor V Leiden mutation investigated by amplification created restriction enzyme site (ACRES) in PNH patients with and without thrombosis. Haematologica. 1996; 81:540-2.

[118] Nakakuma H, Nagakura S, Iwamoto N, et al. Paroxysmal nocturnal hemoglobinuria clone in bone marrow of patients with pancytopenia. Blood. 1995; 85:1371-6.

[119] Nair RK, Khaira A, Sharma A, et al. Spectrum of renal involvement in paroxysmal nocturnal hemoglobinuria: report of three cases and a brief review of the literature. Int Urol Nephrol. 2008; 40:471-5.

[120] Nicholson-Weller A, Burge J, Fearon DT, et al. Isolation of a human erythrocyte membrane glycoprotein with decay-accelerating activity for C3 convertases of the complement system. J Immunol. 1982; 129:184-9.

[121] Nicholson-Weller A, March JP, Rosenfeld SI, et al. Affected erythrocytes of patients with paroxysmal nocturnal hemoglobinuria are deficient in the complement regulatory protein, decay accelerating factor. Proc Natl Acad Sci U S A. 1983; 80:5066-70.

[122] Nicholson-Weller A. Decay accelerating factor (CD55). Curr Top Microbiol Immunol. 1992; 178:7-30.

[123] Ninomiya H, Hasegawa Y, Nagasawa T, et al. Excess soluble urokinase-type plasminogen activator receptor in the plasma of patients with paroxysmal nocturnal hemoglobinuria inhibits cell-associated fibrinolytic activity. Int J Hematol. 1997; 65:285-91.

[124] Nishimura J, Inoue N, Wada H, et al. A patient with paroxysmal nocturnal hemoglobinuria bearing four independent PIG-A mutant clones. Blood. 1997; 89:3470-6.

[125] Nishimura J, Murakami Y, Kinoshita T. Paroxysmal nocturnal hemoglobinuria: An acquired genetic disease. Am J Hematol. 1999; 62:175-82.

[126] Nishimura Ji J, Hirota T, Kanakura Y, et al. Long-term support of hematopoiesis by a single stem cell clone in patients with paroxysmal nocturnal hemoglobinuria. Blood. 2002; 99:2748-2751.

[127] Nishimura J, Kanakura Y, Ware RE, et al. Clinical course and flow cytometric analysis of paroxysmal nocturnal hemoglobinuria in the United States and Japan. Medicine (Baltimore). 2004; 83:193-207.

[128] Nissen C, Tichelli A, Gratwohl A, et al. High incidence of transiently appearing complement-sensitive bone marrow precursor cells in patients with severe aplastic anemia--A possible role of high endogenous IL-2 in their suppression. Acta Haematol. 1999; 101:165-72.

[129] Oni BS, Osunkoya BO & Luzzatto L. Paroxysmal nocturnal hemoglobinuria: evidence for monoclonal origin of abnormal red cells. Blood. 1970; 36:145-152.

[130] Orphanet. Paroxysmal Nocturnal Hemoglobinuria. 1-12-2004. Ref Type: Internet Communication

[131] Pangburn MK, Schreiber RD & Müller-Eberhard HJ. Formation of the initial C3 convertase of the alternative complement pathway. Acquisition of C3b-like activities by spontaneous hydrolysis of the putative thioester in native C3. J Exp Med. 1981; 154:856–67.

[132] Pangburn MK, Schreiber RD, Trombold JS, et al. Paroxysmal nocturnal hemoglobinuria: deficiency in factor H-like functions of the abnormal erythrocytes. J Exp Med. 1983a; 157:1971-80.

[133] Pangburn MK & Müller-Eberhard HJ. Initiation of the alternative complement pathway due to spontaneous hydrolysis of the thioester of C3. Ann N Y Acad Sci. 1983; 421:291–8.

[134] Pangburn MK, Schreiber RD & Müller-Eberhard HJ. Deficiency of an erythrocyte membrane protein with complement regulatory activity in paroxysmal nocturnal hemoglobinuria. Proc Natl Acad Sci U S A. 1983b; 80:5430-4.

[135] Pangburn MK, Schreiber RD & Müller-Eberhard HJ. C3b deposition during activation of the alternative complement pathway and the effect of deposition on the activating surface. J Immunol. 1983c; 131:1930-5.

[136] Parker CJ, Baker PJ & Rosse WF. Increased enzymatic activity of the alternative pathway convertase when bound to the erythrocytes of paroxysmal nocturnal hemoglobinuria. J Clin Invest. 1982; 69:337-46.

[137] Parker CJ. Historical aspects of paroxysmal nocturnal hemoglobinuria; "defining the disease". Br J Haematol. 2002; 117:3-22.

[138] Parker CJ & Ware RE. 2003. Paroxysmal nocturnal hemoglobinuria. In: Greer J et al (ed). Wintrobe's clinical hematology - 11th ed. Philadelphia: Lippincott Williams & Wilkins. p 1203-1221.

[139] Parker C, Omine M, Richards S, et al; International PNH Interest Group. Diagnosis and management of paroxysmal nocturnal hemoglobinuria. Blood. 2005; 106:3699-709.

[140] Parker C. Eculizumab for paroxysmal nocturnal haemoglobinuria. Lancet. 2009; 373:759-67.

[141] Plasilova M, Risitano AM, O'Keefe CL, et al. Shared and individual specificities of immunodominant cytotoxic T cell clones in Paroxysmal Nocturnal Hemoglobinuria as determined by molecular analysis. Exp Hematol. 2004; 32:261-269.

[142] Poggi A, Negrini S, Zocchi MR, et al. Patients with paroxysmal nocturnal hemoglobinuria have a high frequency of peripheral-blood T cells expressing activating isoforms of inhibiting superfamily receptors. Blood. 2005; 106:2399-408.

[143] Pramoonjago P, Pakdeesuwan K, Siripanyaphinyo U, et al. Genotypic, immunophenotypic and clinical features of Thai patients with paroxysmal nocturnal haemoglobinuria. Br J Haematol.1999; 105:497-504.

[144] Raiola AM, Van Lint MT, Lamparelli T, et al. Bone marrow transplantation for paroxysmal nocturnal hemoglobinuria. Haematologica. 2000; 85:59-62.

[145] Richards SJ, Rawstron AC, Hillmen P. Application of flow cytometry to the diagnosis of paroxysmal nocturnal hemoglobinuria. Cytometry. 2000; 42:223-33.

[146] Risitano AM, Maciejewski JP, Green S, et al. In vivo dominant immune responses in aplastic anemia patients: molecular tracking of putatively pathogenic T cells by TCRβ-CDR3 sequencing. Lancet. 2004 ; 364:353-363.

[147] Risitano AM, Maciejewski JP, Muranski P, et al. Large granular lymphocyte (LGL)-like clonal expansions in paroxysmal nocturnal hemoglobinuria (PNH) patients. Leukemia. 2005; 19:217-22.

[148] Risitano AM, Marando L, Seneca E, et al. Hemoglobin normalization after splenectomy in a paroxysmal nocturnal hemoglobinuria patient treated by eculizumab. Blood. 2008; 112:449-51.

[149] Risitano AM, Notaro R, Marando L, et al. Complement fraction 3 binding on erythrocytes as additional mechanism of disease in paroxysmal nocturnal hemoglobinuria patients treated by eculizumab. Blood. 2009a; 113:4094-100.

[150] Risitano AM, Seneca E, Marando L, et al. From Renal Siderosis Due to Perpetual Hemosiderinuria to Possible Liver Overload Due to Extravascular Hemolysis: Changes in Iron Metabolism in Paroxysmal Nocturnal Hemoglobinuria (PNH) Patients on Eculizumab. Blood. 2009b; 114:4031a.

[151] Risitano AM, Holers VM & Rotoli B. TT30, a Novel Regulator of the Complement Alternative Pathway (CAP), Inhibits Hemolysis of Paroxysmal Nocturnal Hemoglobinuria (PNH) Erythrocytes and Prevents Upstream C3 Binding On Their Surface in An in Vitro Model. Blood. 2009c; 114:158a.

[152] Risitano AM, Selleri C, Serio B, et al; Working Party Severe Aplastic Anaemia (WPSAA) of the European Group for Blood and Marrow Transplantation (EBMT). Alemtuzumab is safe and effective as immunosuppressive treatment for aplastic anaemia and single-lineage marrow failure: a pilot study and a survey from the EBMT WPSAA. British Journal of Haematology. 2010a; 148, 791-6.

[153] Risitano AM, Notaro R, Luzzatto L, et al. Paroxysmal Nocturnal Hemoglobinuria: Hemolysis Before and After Eculizumab. New Engl J Med. 2010b; 363:2270-2.

[154] Risitano AM. Immunosuppressive therapies in the management of immune-mediated marrow failures in adults: where we stand and where we are going. Br J Haematol. 2011; 152:127-40.

[155] Risitano AM, Perna F & Selleri C. Achievements and limitations of complement inhibition by eculizumab in paroxysmal nocturnal hemoglobinuria: the role of complement component 3. Mini Rev Med Chem. 2011; 11:528-35.

[156] Rosse WF & Dacie JV. Immune lysis of normal human and paroxysmal nocturnal hemoglobinuria (PNH) red blood cells. I. The sensitivity of PNH red cells to lysis by complement and specific antibody. J Clin Invest. 1966; 45:736-748.

[157] Rosse WF. The life-span of complement-sensitive and –insensitive red cells in paroxysmal nocturnal hemoglobinuria. Blood. 1971; 37:556-562.

[158] Rosse WF. Variations in the red cells in paroxysmal nocturnal haemoglobinuria. Br J Haematol. 1973; 24:327-342.

[159] Rosse WF. Dr Ham's test revisited. Blood. 1991; 78:547-550.

[160] Rosse WF. Epidemiology of PNH. Lancet 1996; 348:560.

[161] Rosti V, Tremml G, Soares V, et al. Murine embryonic stem cells without pig-a gene activity are competent for hematopoiesis with the PNH phenotype but not for clonal expansion. J Clin Invest. 1997; 100:1028-1036.

[162] Rosti V. Murine models of paroxysmal nocturnal hemoglobinuria. Ann N Y Acad Sci. 2002; 963:290-6.

[163] Rother RP, Bell L, Hillmen P, et al. The clinical sequelae of intravascular hemolysis and extracellular plasma hemoglobin: a novel mechanism of human disease. JAMA. 2005; 293:1653-62.

[164] Rother RP, Rollins SA, Mojcik CF, et al. Discovery and development of the complement inhibitor eculizumab for the treatment of paroxysmal nocturnal hemoglobinuria. Nat Biotechnol. 2007; 25:1256-64.

[165] Rotoli B, Robledo R & Luzzatto L. Decreased number of circulating BFU-Es in paroxysmal nocturnal hemoglobinuria. Blood. 1982; 60:157-9.

[166] Rotoli B, Robledo R, Scarpato N, et al. Two populations of erythroid cell progenitors in paroxysmal nocturnal hemoglobinuria. Blood. 1984; 64:847-851.

[167] Rotoli B & Luzzatto L. Paroxysmal nocturnal haemoglobinuria. Baillieres Clin Haematol 1989; 2:113-138.

[168] Sanchez-Valle E, Morales-Polanco MR, Gomez-Morales E, et al. Treatment of paroxysmal nocturnal hemoglobinuria with antilymphocyte globulin. Rev Invest Clin. 1993; 45:457-461.

[169] Santarone S, Bacigalupo A, Risitano AM, et al. Hematopoietic stem cell transplantation for paroxysmal nocturnal hemoglobinuria: long-term results of a retrospective study on behalf of the Gruppo Italiano Trapianto Midollo Osseo (GITMO). Haematologica. 2010; 95:983-8.
[170] Saso R, Marsh J, Cevreska L, et al. Bone marrow transplants for paroxysmal nocturnal haemoglobinuria. Br J Haematol. 1999; 104:392-396.
[171] Schafer A, Wiesmann F, Neubauer S, et al. Rapid regulation of platelet activation in vivo by nitric oxide. Circulation. 2004; 109:1819-22.
[172] Scheinberg P, Marte M, Nunez O, et al. Paroxysmal nocturnal hemoglobinuria clones in severe aplastic anemia patients treated with horse anti-thymocyte globulin plus cyclosporine. Haematologica. 2010; 95:1075-80.
[173] Schubert J, Scholz C, Geissler RG, et al. G-CSF and cyclosporin induce an increase of normal cells in hypoplastic paroxysmal nocturnal hemoglobinuria. Ann Hematol. 1997; 74:225-30.
[174] Selvaraj P, Rosse WF, Silber R, et al. The major Fc receptor in blood has a phosphatidylinositol anchor and is deficient in paroxysmal nocturnal haemoglobinuria. Nature. 1988; 333:565-7.
[175] Shin ML, Hänsch G, Hu VW, et al. Membrane factors responsible for homologous species restriction of complement-mediated lysis: evidence for a factor other than DAF operating at the stage of C8 and C9. J Immunol. 1986; 136:1777-82.
[176] Sholar PW & Bell WR. Thrombolytic therapy for inferior vena cava thrombosis in paroxysmal nocturnal hemoglobinuria. Ann Intern Med. 1985; 103:539-41.
[177] Sica M, Pascariello C, Rondelli T, et al. In vitro complement protein 5 (C5) blockade recapitulates the Complement protein 3 (C3) binding to GPI-negative erythrocytes observed in Paroxysmal Nocturnal Hemoglobinuria (PNH) patients on e.culizumab. Haematologica. 2010; 95(s2):196(a).
[178] Simak J, Holada K, Risitano AM, et al. Elevated counts of circulating endothelial membrane microparticles in paroxysmal nocturnal hemoglobinuria indicate inflammatory status and ongoing stimulation of vascular endothelium. Br J Hemat. 2004; 125:804-813.
[179] Sloand EM, Pfannes L, Scheinberg P, et al. Increased soluble urokinase plasminogen activator receptor (suPAR) is associated with thrombosis and inhibition of plasmin generation in paroxysmal nocturnal hemoglobinuria (PNH) patients. Exp Hematol. 2008; 36:1616-24.
[180] Socie G, Mary JY, de Gramont A, et al. Paroxysmal nocturnal haemoglobinuria: long-term follow-up and prognostic factors. French Society of Haematology. Lancet. 1996; 348:573-7.
[181] Stebler C, Tichelli A, Dazzi H, et al. High-dose recombinant human erythropoietin for treatment of anemia in myelodysplastic syndromes and paroxysmal nocturnal hemoglobinuria: a pilot study. Exp Hematol. 1990; 18:1204-8.
[182] Stoppa AM, Vey N, Sainty D, et al. Correction of aplastic anaemia complicating paroxysmal nocturnal haemoglobinuria: absence of eradication of the PNH clone and dependence of response on cyclosporin A administration. Br J Haematol. 1996; 93:42-4.
[183] Sugimori C, Chuhjo T, Feng X, et al. Minor population of CD55-CD59- blood cells predicts response to immunosuppressive therapy and prognosis in patients with aplastic anemia. Blood. 2006; 107:1308-14.

[184] Sutherland DR, Kuek N, Davidson J, et al. Diagnosing PNH with FLAER and multiparameter flow cytometry. Cytometry B Clin Cytom. 2007; 72:167-77.
[185] Takahashi M, Takeda J, Hirose S, et al. Deficient biosynthesis of N-acetylglucosaminyl-phosphatidylinositol, the first intermediate of glycosyl phosphatidylinositol anchor biosynthesis, in cell lines established from patients with paroxysmal nocturnal hemoglobinuria. J Exp Med. 1993; 177:517-21.
[186] Takahashi Y, McCoy JP Jr., Carvallo C, et al. In vitro and in vivo evidence of PNH cell sensitivity to immune attack after nonmyeloablative allogeneic hematopoietic cell transplantation. Blood. 2004; 103:1383-1390.
[187] Takeda J, Miyata T, Kawagoe K, et al. Deficiency of the GPI anchor caused by a somatic mutation of the PIG-A gene in paroxysmal nocturnal hemoglobinuria. Cell. 1993; 73:703-11.
[188] Takeda J & Kinoshita T. GPI-anchor biosynthesis. Trends Biochem Sci. 1995; 20:367-71.
[189] Telen MJ & Green AM. The Inab phenotype: characterization of the membrane protein and complement regulatory defect. Blood. 1989; 74:437-41.
[190] Tichelli A, Gratwohl A, Nissen C, et al. Morphology in patients with severe aplastic anemia treated with antilymphocyte globulin. Blood. 1992; 80:337-45.
[191] Tremml G, Dominguez C, Rosti V, et al. Increased sensitivity to complement and a decreased red blood cell life span in mice mosaic for a nonfunctional Piga gene. Blood. 1999; 94:2945-54.
[192] van Beers EJ, Schaap MC, Berckmans RJ, et al; CURAMA study group. Circulating erythrocyte-derived microparticles are associated with coagulation activation in sickle cell disease. Haematologica. 2009; 94:1513-9.
[193] van der Schoot CE, Huizinga TW, van 't Veer-Korthof ET, et al. Deficiency of glycosyl-phosphatidylinositol-linked membrane glycoproteins of leukocytes in paroxysmal nocturnal hemoglobinuria, description of a new diagnostic cytofluorometric assay. Blood. 1990; 76:1853-1859.
[194] van Kamp H, Smit JW, van den Berg E, et al. Myelodysplasia following paroxysmal nocturnal haemoglobinuria: evidence for the emergence of a separate clone. Br J Haematol. 1994; 87:399-400.
[195] van Kamp H, van Imhoff GW, de Wolf JT, et al. The effect of cyclosporine on haematological parameters in patients with paroxysmal nocturnal haemoglobinuria. Br J Haematol. 1995; 89:79-82.
[196] Vu T, Griscelli-Bennaceur A, Gluckman E, et al. Aplastic anaemia and paroxysmal nocturnal haemoglobinuria: a study of the GPI-anchored proteins on human platelets. Br J Haematol. 1996; 93:586-9.
[197] Ware RE, Hall SE & Rosse WF. Paroxysmal nocturnal hemoglobinuria with onset in childhood and adolescence. N Engl J Med. 1991; 325:991-996.
[198] Whaley K & Ruddy S. Modulation of the alternative complement pathway by β1H globulin. J Exp Med. 1976; 144:1147-63
[199] Wiedmer T, Hall SE, Ortel TL, et al. Complement-induced vesiculation and exposure of membrane prothrombinase sites in platelets of paroxysmal nocturnal hemoglobinuria. Blood. 1993; 82:1192-6.
[200] Wilcox LA, Ezzell JL, Bernshaw NJ, et al. Molecular basis of the enhanced susceptibility of the erythrocytes of paroxysmal nocturnal hemoglobinuria to hemolysis in acidified serum. Blood. 1991; 78:820-9.

[201] Yamashina M, Ueda E, Kinoshita T, et al. Inherited complete deficiency of 20-kilodalton homologous restriction factor (CD59) as a cause of paroxysmal nocturnal hemoglobinuria. N Engl J Med. 1990; 323:1184-9.

[202] Young NS & Maciejewski JP. Genetic and environmental effects in paroxysmal nocturnal hemoglobinuria: this little PIG-A goes "Why? Why? Why?". J Clin Invest. 2000; 106:637-641.

[203] Young NS, Calado RT & Scheinberg P. Current concepts in the pathophysiology and treatment of aplastic anemia. Blood. 2006; 108, 2509-19.

# 23

# Anemia in Chronic Obstructive Pulmonary Disease

Karina Portillo Carroz and Josep Morera
*Department of Pneumology Hospital Germans Trias i Pujol. Universitat Autónoma de Barcelona Spain*

## 1. Introduction

Chronic obstructive pulmonary disease (COPD) is the fourth leading cause of death worldwide, and it is projected to be the third by 2020 or earlier. Patients with COPD frequently have other chronic diseases and systemic effects that worsen their clinical status and prognosis. The best recognized manifestations include the presence of concomitant cardiovascular disease, skeletal muscle wasting, osteoporosis and lung cancer. Although COPD is "traditionally" associated with polycythemia there is a growing body of literature on the relationship between anemia and COPD. Recent studies described that anemia in patients with COPD is more frequent than expected, with a prevalence ranging from 8 to 33%. Systemic inflammation may be an important pathogenic factor, but anemia in COPD can also be the result of a number of factors, such as nutritional and endocrine disorders, treatment with certain drugs (theophylline or angiotensin-converting enzyme inhibitors), acute exacerbations and oxygen therapy.

The level of hemoglobin in COPD patients is strongly associated with increased functional dyspnea, decreased exercise capacity as well as a poor quality of life. Moreover, some studies have showed that anemia is an independent predictor of mortality. Despite the possible clinical benefit of successfully treating anemia in these patients, evidence supporting the importance of its effect on the prognosis of COPD is limited.

## 2. Prevalence of anemia in COPD

The prevalence of anemia in COPD remains unclear and varies widely. This variability depends on the population under study (stable COPD or patients hospitalized for acute exacerbation), the tools to identifying anemic subjects, and the definitions used for anemia. Contrary to common thinking, recent studies have shown that anemia is a frequent comorbid associated disease in COPD, ranging from nearly 10 to 30% of patients, particularly in patients with severe disease, whereas polycythemia (erythrocytosis) is relatively rare (Barnes & Celli, 2009).The World Health Organization defines anemia in the general population as hemoglobin concentration of less than 13.0 g/dL in men and less than 12.0 g/dL in women (WHO 1968). However, when determining anemia using hemoglobin, it is important to account for the following aspects: firstly, the prevalence of anemia in the general population increases with age and COPD is a chronic disease that affects an aging population; secondly, appropriate hemoglobin threshold for anemia definition in older post-menopausal females remains controversial (Cote et al, 2007) and finally, COPD patients could have a "relative anemia"—a term used to describe cases in which apparently normal hemoglobin values do not correlate with level of hypoxemia.

John et al., reported for first time anemia prevalence in a stable COPD population. They found that among 101 severe COPD patients (forced expiratory volume in one second [$FEV_1$]37 ±2% predicted) 13 were anemic, which means a prevalence of 13%. (John et al, 2005) The data extracted from large national database in France maintained by the Association Nationale pour le Traitement à Domicile de l'Insuffisance Respiratoire (ANTADIR study) showed a similar prevalence in a cohort of 2524 COPD individuals under long-term oxygen therapy (LTOT) (12.6% in males and 8.2% in females) (Chambellan et al, 2005). Cote and colleagues estimated a prevalence of anemia of 17% in contrast with 6% of polycythemia among 683 COPD outpatients. (Cote et al, 2007). In hospitalized patients, described prevalence in anemia rises up to 33%.John and colleagues compared the prevalence of anemia between hospital-admitted COPD and other chronic diseases (asthma, chronic heart failure, chronic renal insufficiency, and cancer).They found in a sample of 7,337 patients an overall prevalence of anemia in COPD of 23%. This was comparable to that in patients with heart failure, higher than in asthmatic individuals, but lower than that in the groups with cancer or chronic renal insufficiency (John et al, 2006). In another study, based on 177 COPD admitted patients due to acute exacerbation (AECOPD) the prevalence reported was 31%. The normocytic normochromic anemia was the most common morphological pattern in 32 cases (58%) and anemia of chronic disease (ACD)or anemia of inflammation was also the more frequent etiology founded. Ultimately, only 8 (4.5%) had polycytemia. (Portillo et al, 2007).

It is worthwhile saying that studying the prevalence of anemia in patients with acute syndromes may overestimate the real number of cases, however, the frequency of anemia during AECOPD is also a relevant issue, since it represents a state of augmented systemic inflammation which also could affect hemoglobin levels in COPD, as described later.

Two recent reports have provided data in large series of patients, obtained from ICD-9/10 code of the discharge diagnoses in order to analyze mortality and healthcare resource variables. In a study performed on US Medicare population, anemia was diagnosed in 21% of COPD patients (Halpern et al, 2006); whereas Shorr and co-workers identified 788 cases in a population of 2404 COPD patients (33%). Anemic patients were older, more likely to be male and non-caucasian, and had a greater co-morbidity burden than non-anemic individuals. (Shorr et al, 2008)

In summary, anemia seems to be common entity among COPD patients, but current available data about its frequency are provided from retrospective analysis or single-center studies, therefore, are subject to the general biases inherent in such designs. Efforts to determine the true prevalence of anemia as comorbid disease in COPD are needed.

## 3. Mechanisms of anemia in COPD

Increasing evidence indicates that COPD is a complex disease involving more than airflow obstruction (Barnes & Celli 2009).In many patients the disease is associated with several extra pulmonary manifestations that could be the expression of systemic inflammatory state of COPD. In the light of this and together with presence of normocytic anemia in some reported series, it has considered that COPD is another disease likely to be associated with anemia of chronic disease or anemia of inflammation (ACD) (Similowski et al, 2006). In any case, besides the possible role that inflammation may play in the etiology of anemia in COPD, it should not forget that the aging process itself increases the prevalence of anemia as mentioned above and the hemoglobin concentration in COPD can also be influenced by intervention of other mechanisms (Fig. 1). There is a growing interest in the literature about this issue, but the evidence is still scarce. We briefly review the most cited pathophysiologic aspects of this association.

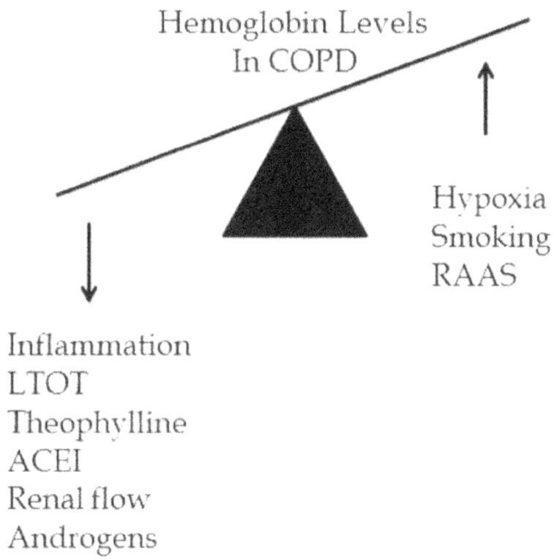


Fig. 1. Possible factors related to hemoglobin levels in COPD. ACEI indicates angiotensin-converting enzyme inhibitors; LTOT, long-term oxygen therapy; and RAAS, renin-angiotensin-aldosterone system.

### 3.1 Anemia of chronic disease

ACD is an immune disorder that has been reported in numerous diseases with an inflammatory component. Inflammatory cytokines exert various effects on pathogenesis of this form of anemia and ultimately interfere with the normal process of erythropoiesis. The underlying mechanisms are complex, including dysregulation in iron homeostasis and erythropoietin production, impaired proliferation of erythroid progenitor cells and reduced life span of red blood cells. (Weiss 2005). In addition, activation of these inflammatory mediators may stimulate the production of hepcidin, a polypeptide that is the principal regulator of extracellular iron homeostasis and is thought to play a key role of development of ACD.

ACD is usually normocytic, normochromic anemia, but it can become microcytic and hypochromic as the disease progresses. Characteristic changes in systemic iron distribution develop such that the serum iron concentration and transferrin saturation are low, while macrophage iron stores remain replete (Roy, 2010).

COPD is a disorder that could be related with ACD, due the existence of systemic inflammation documented in some patients with COPD. A wide variety of inflamatory markers are isolated in both peripheral blood and sputum in these patients and are higher than controls (Gan et al, 2004). The most important mediators that have been identified are: C-reactive protein (CRP), fibrinogen, circulating leukocytes, and several interleukines (IL) such as IL- 6, IL-8 and tumor necrosis factor alfa (TNF-α) (Fig. 2). Increased of oxidative stress also have been demonstrated in COPD, especially during exacerbations. (McNee 2005).

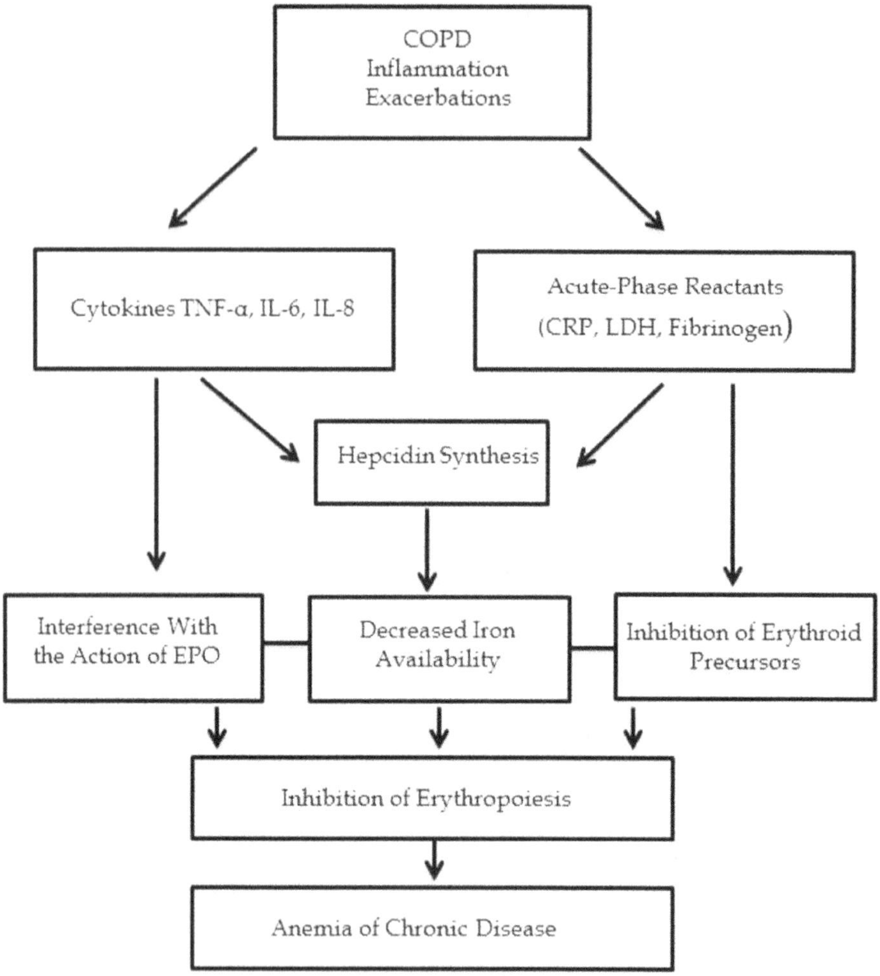


Fig. 2. Possible mechanisms of anemia of inflammation, or anemia of chronic disease, in chronic obstructive pulmonary disease (COPD). EPO indicates erythropoietin; IL, interleukin; LDH, lactate dehydrogenase; CRP, C-reactive protein; and TNF-α, tumor necrosis factor α. (Taken from Portillo, 2007)

One of the first studies that linked the ACD in patients with COPD was made by Tassiopoulos and co-workers, in 2001. Their initial objective was to evaluate the characteristics of anemia and compare the compensatory erythropoietic response in clinically stable patients with idiopathic pulmonary fibrosis and COPD individuals in respiratory failure. The assumption was that the hematologic mechanism would function differently in these two diseases and that the phenomenon of secondary erythrocytosis would be retained in COPD hypoxemic patients. However, they found that the expected response (an increase in red cell mass) was inconsistent in a subgroup of patients with COPD. These individuals had normal or below normal hemoglobin values in spite of higher than normal concentrations of erythropoietin (EPO) in plasma, a suggestion that inflammation was probably the cause of the inconsistent response (Tassiopoulus et al, 2001). These observations were confirmed later by the previously mentioned study performed by John and colleagues. In these patients, the serum levels of CRP and IL-6 were significantly higher than in a group of control subjects. CRP was significantly higher in the anemic subgroup than in non anemic patients as well the level of serum EPO. Moreover, an inverse correlation was showed between hemoglobin and EPO levels, an indication of the existence of a certain resistance to the action of this hormone. These results, together with the lack of any correlation between anemia with nutritional abnormalities present in these patients (weight loss and cachexia), led to the conclusion that the development of anemia in some patients with COPD may fulfilled the criteria for ACD. (John et al, 2005).

### 3.2 Exacerbations

One of the inherent characteristics of COPD is the occurrence of exacerbations, (AECOPD) which succeed in the curse of the natural history of disease. During AECOPD typically occurs an amplification inflammatory response, both locally and systemically. It has been postulated that the existence of this increased systemic inflammation may worsen some of extrapulmonary manifestations of COPD including anemia. (Portillo 2007; Soler- Cataluña et al, 2010)

Two recent reports assessed the role of inflammatory mechanisms over hemoglobin levels during AEPOC with dissimilar results regarding EPO response. Sala et al., compared the plasma levels of EPO and CRP in patients hospitalized because of AECOPD (n = 26; $FEV_1$: 48 ±15% predicted), patients with clinically stable COPD (n = 31; $FEV_1$ :49 ± 17% predicted), smokers with normal lung function (n = 9), and healthy never smokers (n = 9). The main findings were: 1) EPO plasma levels were significantly lower during AECOPD and 2) in COPD group EPO was significantly related to CRP ($r = -0.55$, $p < 0.0001$) and with circulating neutrophils ($r = -0.48$, $p <0.0001$). Finally, in a subset of 8 COPD patients who could be studied both during AECOPD and clinical stability, EPO levels were significantly higher in stability compared to those recorded during the AECOPD ($p < 0.0001$). These observations suggest that EPO is downregulated during AECOPD related to the burst of systemic inflammation. (Sala et al, 2010)

In the other study, hemoglobin, EPO and serum biomarkers of systemic inflammation (CRP, TNF-α, fibrinogen and IL-6]) were measured at three time points (admission, resolution and stable phases) in a selected cohort of 93 COPD patients. Hemoglobin levels were significantly lower on admission compared to resolution and stable phases ($p=0.002$), whereas EPO was significantly higher on admission compared to resolution and stable phases. EPO and hemoglobin were negatively associated during AECOPD. This association was related to increased IL-6 levels, indicating a possible EPO resistance through the mechanism of increased systemic inflammatory process (Markoulaki et al, 2011).

### 3.3 Macrocytosis

An increase in mean corpuscular volume (MCV) has been reported in patients with COPD, although the cause is still poorly understood. Tsantes et al., investigated this phenomenon among 32 hypoxemic COPD patients and 34 healthy volunteers. They evaluated the following parameters: complete blood count, percentage of F-cells (erythrocytes containing fetal hemoglobin), arterial blood gases, and EPO levels. Red cell macrocytosis (defined as MCV>94 fL) was found in almost half of the patients with COPD (43.75%), and 37% of this group had erythrocytosis. The EPO response was not associated with the degree of hypoxemia, erythrocytosis, or macrocytosis, and in some cases the phenomenon occurred independently. The F-cell percentage was significantly higher in the patients with COPD, and this parameter correlated with MCV values. Based on their findings, the authors hypothesized that erythropoietic stress occurs repeatedly in COPD as a result of exacerbations and nocturnal or exercise-related desaturation. This may triggers a compensatory mechanism, as the release of immature cell forms in the bone marrow to optimize oxygen carrying capacity. Even when they are within the normal range, hemoglobin concentrations can be suboptimal in these patients given the severity of their baseline hypoxemia (Tsantes et al, 2004). Garcia-Pachón et al., also reported macrocytosis in COPD patients but without respiratory insufficiency. It was present in 17 of the 58 stable COPD patients (29%). The most interesting finding, was a significant correlation between macrocytosis, dyspnea, and $FEV_1$ in a subgroup of 9 COPD (36%), that presumably reflects a correlation between macrocytosis and a deterioration in the clinical situation (García-Pachón & Padilla-Navas 2007).

### 3.4 Renin-angiotensin-aldosterone system

There are some clinical and experimental studies demonstrating that COPD causes neurohumoral activation, which presumably contributes to a self- maintaining pathogenic cycle that may be related to the systemic effects of the disease (Andreas et al, 2005). An increase in EPO secretion has been observed in experimental animals after administration of renin or angiotensin II. Thus, administration of angiotensin converting enzyme inhibitors is accompanied by a reduction in EPO and hematocrit values. Vlahakos et al., analyzed the degree to which activation of renin-angiotensin system (RAS) was associated with the development of compensatory erythrocytosis in hypoxemic COPD individuals. Renin and aldosterone levels were 3 times higher in the patients with erythrocytosis than in the control group of hypoxemic COPD patients who did not have erythrocytosis. Therefore, it has been contemplated that the alteration in the activation could, partially, help to explain the differences found in the values of hemoglobin in patients with COPD with the same degree of hypoxemia (Vlahakos et al, 1999).

### 3.5 Renal flow

As EPO is synthesized primarily in the kidney, any impairment of renal hemodynamics—a comorbidity also reported in COPD as a consequence of decreased renal blood flow—causes an imbalance in the supply and demand of oxygen that affects the production of this hormone possibly as a result of an effect on the oxygen sensor (Pham et al, 2001).

### 3.6 Androgens

Androgens can also stimulate erythropoiesis directly by stimulation of erythroid progenitors or indirectly by activating the renin-angiotensin-aldosterone system; in fact, anemia is a common finding in men who have hypogonadism or are receiving antiandrogenic treatment. Furthermore, testosterone levels decline with age. There is evidence that testosterone concentrations are low in men with COPD (Casaburi et al, 2004).Various predisposing factors for these low values have been proposed, including hypoxia, corticosteroid treatment, and the chronic nature of the disease. A published study of a sample of 905 patients over 65 years of age concluded that low testosterone levels are associated with a higher risk of developing anemia (Ferrucci et al, 2003).

### 3.7 Other factors

It has been observed that, like the angiotensin-converting enzyme inhibitors, which reduce hematocrit values, theophylline also gives rise to a reduction in the production of red blood cells. The suppression mechanism is complex and in principle may be the result of direct inhibition of erythropoiesis through apoptosis induced by this drug rather than any effect on EPO (Tsantes et al, 2003).

Oxygen therapy can theoretically blunt hypoxia-driven erythropoyiesis, (Similowski et al, 2005) while smoking habit might exert negative effect on folate status and oxygen carrying capacity through tendency to increase red blood cell mass.

## 4. The effects of anemia in COPD

The relationship between anemia and adverse clinical outcomes is wide recognized in other chronic disease states. The hemoglobin is the principal oxygen transport molecule. Any decrease in hemoglobin levels results in a corresponding reduction in the oxygen-carrying capacity of the blood. Thus, while arterial oxygen pressure may remain normal, the absolute amount of oxygen transported per unit blood volume declines. Impairment of this mechanism exerts a negative impact on clinical status. Although there are few related studies, those published so far it appears that anemia plays an important role in various domains and outcomes of disease including mortality.

### 4.1 Symptoms, exercise tolerance

It is well known that anemia is a cause per se of dyspnea and that it contributes to functional limitation in the anemic individual. Fatigue is also a common finding among COPD and is the primary symptom of anemia. In fact, anemia is one of the most treatable causes of fatigue in general. Cote and colleagues demonstrated that anemia was independently associated with increased dyspnea, by means modified Medical Research Council dyspnea scale (MRC) and reduced exercise capacity measured by 6- min walk distance in a cohort of stable COPD patients (Cote et al, 2007). Recently, another study was aimed to investigated specifically the impact of ACD on dyspnea and exercise capacity utilizing cardiopulmonary exercise testing (CPET) in a group of 283 COPD patients. The results of these report also showed a negative effect of low hemoglobin on breathlessness. COPD patients whom fulfilled criteria of ACD had higher MRC dyspnea score compared to controls and lower exercise capacity (lower peak oxygen uptake[VO2], peak work rate, peak VO2/heart rate, as well a trend for lower anaerobic threshold) (Boutou et al, 2010).

There is only restrospective study that analyzed the relationship between anemia in COPD and health related quality of life (HRQL) based on general population (n=2704). Among patients with COPD (n = 495) physical functioning (PF) and physical component summary (PCS) scores from Short Form-36 questionnaire were significantly lower in individuals with anemia compared to those without. In conclusion, anemia associated with COPD was an important contributor to poor quality of life. (Krishnan et al, 2006)

### 4.2 Health resources

COPD generates a large consumption of resources that involves a significant economic burden worldwide due to its high prevalence and morbidity. Moreover, presences of comorbidities in COPD appear to be a cost multiplier. (Shorr et al, 2008)

The ANTADIR study founded that a reduced hematocrit level was associated with more frequent hospitalizations and a longer mean hospital stay (Chambellan et al, 2005).Two studies mentioned above have been measured the economic impact of anemia in COPD based on large sample of patients. Both documented that anemia significantly and independently contributes to the cost of care for COPD. (Halpern et al, 2006; Shorr et al, 2008).

### 4.3 Mortality

There is some evidence available to suggest that anemia is associated with a reduced survival in COPD. In cohort of stable COPD used to described the BODE index (body mass index, airflow obstruction, dyspnea and exercise capacity) Celli and colleagues showed that patients who died were found to have significantly lower hematocrit levels than those who survived (Celli et al, 2004).

In survival data derived from the ANTADIR study, multivariate analysis proved that hematocrit was important independent predictor of survival in COPD patients receiving LTOT and showed that the survival rate at three years was 24% in patients with hematocrit <35%, and 70% in patients with hematocrit > 55%(Chambellan et al, 2005).These findings are consistent with a recent report also conducted on patients under LTOT in which 67% had a diagnosis of COPD. Hemoglobin and hematocrit were significantly lower in the nonsurvivor group. Multiple regression analysis demonstrated that the main risk factors for mortality after three years of follow-up were male gender, lower values of hemoglobin, hematocrit and carbon dioxide pressure more intense hypoxemia and dyspnea sensation. The cut-off point associated with higher mortality in this study was hemoglobin ≤ 11 g/dl (sensitivity 95% specificity 85%) or hematocrit ≤33%(sensitivity 97% specificity 89%)(Lima et al, 2010).

In the National Emphysema Treatment Trial, in which randomized patients to be treated medically or surgically, also found that the decrease in hemoglobin acted as an independent predictor of mortality (Martinez et al, 2006).

Lastly, Rasmussen and co-workers analyzed the effects of anemia in critically ill patients with COPD admitted to the intensive care unit (ICU) requiring invasive mechanical ventilation. With a cutoff point of hemoglobin to define anemia of 12g/dL, it found that low hemoglobin levels were associated with substantially increased mortality within the first 90 days following admission (Rasmussen et al, 2011).

## 5. Should anemia be treated in COPD?

Throughout this review we have discussed some clinical and pathophysiological aspects that would justify therapeutics efforts to correct anemia in COPD. However, the degree of uncertainty in fundamental aspects, as well limited available evidence do not establish whether the treatment of this condition will result in improvement in COPD outcomes.

Schonhofer et al., published the only two studies in the literature on this subject. After treating anemia by blood transfusion in 20 patients with severe COPD in an ICU, it documented a statistically significant reduction in minute-ventilation and work of breathing, with unloading of the respiratory muscles (Schonhofer et al, 1999) The earlier study involved 5 COPD patients in whom weaning from invasive mechanical ventilation had proved difficult. By increasing hemoglobin levels to over 12 g/dL by blood transfusion, the physicians were able to extubate satisfactorily ( Schonhofer et al, 1998)

Another treatment options to correct anemia as used in other chronic disease such congestive heart failure, cancer or chronic kidney disease have not been explored in COPD (i.e. erythropoietic agents, iron supplements or combined therapy). Is not known whether treating the underlying inflammation could improve the hematological values. Future prospective trials are needed to establish the appropriate threshold for initiation treatment and effect of improvement of hemoglobin on clinical outcomes in COPD population.

## 6. Conclusions

Anemia seems to be a common feature in COPD, although its real prevalence remains to be determined. While the mechanisms involved in the genesis of anemia in COPD are poorly studied and the evidence is scarce, we can talk about an imbalance in hemoglobin levels because there are factors that stimulate erythropoiesis as well as others that blunt this process.

Recent data support that low hemoglobin and hematocrit concentrations can have a detrimental impact on certain respiratory variables in COPD, including mortality. Whether the treatment of anemia will result in improvement in functional outcome measures remains uncertain. However, before a treatment strategy can be devised, the influence of anemia on the natural history of COPD should be properly evaluated in further prospective studies.

## 7. References

Andreas S, Anker SD, Scanlon PD, Somers VK. Neurohumoral activation as a link to systemic manifestations of chronic lung disease. *Chest.* 2005; 128:3618-25.

Barnes PJ, Celli BR. Systemic manifestations and comorbidities of COPD. *Eur Respir J.* 2009; 33:1165-85.

Boutou AK, Stanopoulos I, Pitsiou GG, Kontakiotis T, Kyriazis G, Sichletidis L, Argyropoulou P. Anemia of Chronic Disease in Chronic Obstructive Pulmonary Disease: A Case-Control Study of Cardiopulmonary Exercise Responses. *Respiration*. 2011 [Epub ahead of print]

Casaburi R, Bhasin S, Cosentino L, Porszasz J, Somfay A, Lewis MI, et al. Effects of testosterone and resistance training in men with chronic obstructive pulmonary disease. *Am J Respir Crit Care Med*. 2004;170:870-8.

Celli BR, Cote CG, Marin JM, Casanova C, Montes de Oca M, Méndez RA, et al. The body-mass index, airflow obstruction, dyspnea, and exercise capacity index in chronic obstructive pulmonary disease. *N Engl J Med*. 2004; 350: 1005–1012.

Chambellan A, Chailleux E, Similowski T, ANTADIR Observatory Group. Prognostic value of hematocrit in patients with severe COPD receiving long-term oxygen therapy. *Chest*. 2005; 128: 1201–1208.

Cote C, Zilberberg MD, Mody SH, Dordelly LJ, Celli B. Haemoglobin level and its clinical impact in a cohort of patients with COPD. *Eur Respir J*. 2007;29: 923-9.

Ferrucci L, Maggio M, Bandinelli S, Basaria S, Lauretani F, Ble A, et al. Low testosterone levels and the risk of anemia in older men and women. *Arch Intern Med*. 2006; 166:1380-8.

Gan WQ, Man SF, Senthilselvan A, Sin DD. Association between chronic obstructive pulmonary disease and systemic infl ammation: a systematic review and a meta-analysis. *Thorax*. 2004;59:574-80.

García-Pachón E, Padilla-Navas I. Red cell macrocytosis in COPD patients without respiratory insufficiency: a brief report. *Respir Med*. 2007;101:349-52.

Halpern MT, Zilberberg MD, Schmier JK, Lau EC, Shorr AF. Anemia, costs and mortality in chronic obstructive pulmonary disease. *Cost Eff Resour Alloc*. 2006 16;4:17.

John M, Hoernig S, Doehner W, Okonko DD, Witt C, Anker SD. Anemia and inflammation in COPD. *Chest*. 2005; 127: 825–829.

John M, Lange A, Hoernig S, Witt C, Anker SD. Prevalence of anemia in chronic obstructive pulmonary disease: comparison to other chronic diseases. *Int J Cardiol*. 2006;111:365-70.

Krishnan G, Grant BJ, Muti PC, et al. Association between anemia and quality of life in a population sample of individuals with chronic obstructive pulmonary disease. *BMC Pulm Med*. 2006; 6: 23.

Lima DF, Dela Coleta K, Tanni SE, Silveira LV, Godoy I, Godoy I. Potentially modifiable predictors of mortality in patients treated with long-term oxygen therapy. *Respir Med*. 2011;105:470-6.

MacNee W. Pulmonary and systemic oxidant/antioxidant imbalance in chronic obstructive pulmonary disease. *Proc Am Thorac Soc*. 2005;2:50-60.

Markoulaki D, Kostikas K, Papatheodorou G, Koutsokera A, Alchanatis M, Bakakos P, et al. Eur J Hemoglobin, erythropoietin and systemic inflammation in exacerbations of chronic obstructive pulmonary disease. *Intern Med*. 2011 ;22:103-7.

Martínez FJ, Foster G, Curtis JL, Criner G, Weinmann G, Fishman A, et al; NETT Research Group. Predictors of mortality in patients with emphysema and severe airflow obstruction. *Am J Respir Crit Care Med.* 2006;173:1326-34.

Pham I, Andrivet P, Sediame S, Defouilloy C, Moutereau S, et al. Increased erythropoietin synthesis in patients with COLD or left heart failure is related to alterations in renal haemodynamics. *Eur J Clin Invest.* 2001;31:103-9.

Portillo K, Belda J, Antón P, Casan P. High frequency of anemia in COPD patients admitted in a tertiary hospital. *Rev Clin Esp.* 2007; 207:383-7.

Portillo K. Anemia in COPD: should it be taken into consideration?.Arch Bronconeumol. 2007;43:392-8.

Rasmussen L, Christensen S, Lenler-Petersen P, Johnsen SP. Anemia and 90-day mortality in COPD patients requiring invasive mechanical ventilation. *Clin Epidemiol.* 2011;3:1-5.

Roy CN. Anemia of inflammation. *Hematology Am Soc Hematol Educ Program.* 2010;2010: 276-80.

Sala E, Balaguer C, Villena C, Ríos A, Noguera A, Núñez B,et al. Low erythropoietin plasma levels during exacerbations of COPD. *Respiration.* 2010;80:190-7.

Schonhofer B, Bohrer H, Kohler D. Importance of blood transfusion in anemic patients with COPD and unsuccessful weaning from respirator. *Med Klin.* 1999;Suppl 1:108-10.

Schonhofer B, Wenzel M, Geibel M, Kohler D. Blood transfusion and lung function in chronically anemic patients with severe chronic obstructive pulmonary disease. *Crit Care Med.* 1998;26:1824-8.

Shorr AF, Doyle J, Stern L, Dolgitser M, Zilberberg MD. Anemia in chronic obstructive pulmonary disease: epidemiology and economic implications. *Curr Med Res Opin.* 2008;24:1123-30.923

Similowski T, Agusti A, MacNee W, Schonhofer B. The potential impact of anaemia of chronic disease in COPD. *Eur Respir J.* 2006; 27:390–6.

Soler-Cataluña JJ,Martínez-García MA, Catalán Serra P. Impacto multidimensional de las exacerbaciones de la EPOC. *Arch Bronconeumol.*2010; 46(Supl.11) :12-9.

Tassiopoulos S, Kontos A, Konstantopoulos K, Hadzistavrou C, Vaiopoulos G, Aessopos A, et al. Erythropoietic response to hypoxaemia in diffuse idiopathic pulmonary fibrosis, as opposed to chronic obstructive pulmonary disease. *Respir Med.* 2001;95: 471-5.

Tsantes AE, Papadhimitriou SI, Tassiopoulos ST, Bonovas S, Paterakis G, Meletis I, et al. Red cell macrocytosis in hypoxemic patients with chronic obstructive pulmonary disease. *Respir Med.* 2004;98:1117-23.

Tsantes AE, Tassiopoulos ST, Papadhimitriou SI, Bonovas S, Poulakis N, Vlachou A, et al. Theophylline treatment may adversely affect the anoxia-induced erythropoietic response without suppressing erythropoietin production. *Eur J Clin Pharmacol.* 2003;59:379-83.

Vlahakos D, Kosmas E, Dimopoulou I, Ikonomou E, Jullien G, Vassilakos P, et al. Association between activation of the reninangiotensin system and secondary erythrocytosis in patients with chronic obstructive pulmonary disease. *Am J Med.* 1999;106:158- 64.

Weiss G, Goodnough LT. Anemia of chronic disease. *N Engl J Med.* 2005;352:1011 23.

World Health Organization. Nutritional anemias: report of a WHO scientific group. WHO Technical Report Series 405. Geneva, World Health Organization, 1968; pp. 1–37

# 24

# An Emerging Face of Fanconi Anemia: Cancer

Sevgi Gözdaşoğlu
*Ankara University*
*Turkey*

## 1. Introduction

Fanconi anemia (FA) is a chromosomal instability syndrome characterized by various congenital malformations, progressive pancytopenia, chromosome breakage and predisposition to malignancy (Alter, 2003a). Autosomal recessive, FA is also inherited with X-linked inheritance reported in FA complementation group B (Meetei et al., 2004). FA pathway controls genomic stabilisation in mammalian cells and is referred to as FA pathway of antioncogenesis. Children with FA have a very high risk of developing acute myeloid leukemia (AML) and myelodysplastic syndrome (MDS). The incidence of AML in children with FA is 15.000 times that of children in the general population (Auerbach & Allen, 1991). Acute leukemia is the terminal event in about 5-20% of these cases (Ebell et al., 1989), MDS in about 5-10%, and solid tumors was held responsible in about 5-10% of the remaining cases. Patients with FA are at a high risk of developing solid tumors of the head, neck, esophagus, liver and female genitalia (Alter, 2003c, Rosenberg, Greene & Alter, 2003). In order to clarify the relationship between FA and cancer, the description of FA was recently updated as "an inherited genomic instability disorder, caused by mutations in genes regulating replication-dependent removal of interstrand DNA crosslinks" (Moldovan & D'Andrea, 2009). The research on the complex roles of FA proteins in repairing DNA improved our understanding of cancer biology. In this chapter, my main objective is twofold: to analyze clinical findings, diagnosis and hematological characteristics of FA, and to evaluate the relationship between FA pathway and cancer from the perspective of a pediatrician.

## 2. Fanconi anemia

FA is a familial pancytopenia associated with bone marrow hypoplasia and congenital malformations, originally discovered in three brothers by Fanconi in 1927 (Gözdaşoğlu et al., 1980). 2000 cases were reported in the literature between the years of 1927 and 2009 (Alter, 2011). FA should be considered a syndrome, not a disease due to its heterogeneity. The physical phenotype ranges from normal appearance to manifest congenital malformations, the hematological spectrum ranges from nominal values to those associated with severe aplastic anemia (Alter, 1993b). Clinical heterogeneity in FA follows from genetic heterogeneity. The heterozygote prevalence for FA is estimated to be 1 in 300 in the United States (Alter, 1993a). Homozygote frequency is estimated at 1-3 per million (Joenje et al., 1995). The male-female ratio of occurrence is 1.2:1 (Alter, 2003a). The age of diagnosis ranges from birth to 48 years with an average of 8 years. About 10-20% of families have consanguineous marriage (Alter, 1992).

### 2.1 Congenital abnormalities

Several congenital abnormalities may accompany this disorder such as skeletal abnormalities, hyperpigmentation, renal malformation, microcephaly, hypogonadism and mental and growth retardations (Gözdaşoğlu et al., 1980; Akar & Gözdaşoğlu, 1984). Among skeletal system anomalies, radial ray defects such as hypoplasia of the thumb and the radius are observed most (Figures 1, 2, 3). In addition to congenital hip dislocations, scoliosis, vertebral anomalies, cafe-au-lait spots, diffuse hyperpigmentation and hypopigmentation are frequent. A short stature is prominent in more than half of the cases in utero and following birth. The median height is about 50 percentile in the patients, which can be related to growth hormone deficiency or hypothyroidism. Mycrophtalmia, microcephaly and deafness may be observed, renal anomalies such as unilateral and renal aplasia, renal hypoplasia, horse-shoe kidney and double ureter may be encountered in about a third of the cases. Boys have genital anomalies as hypogenitalia, undescended testis and hypospadias. Girls have uterus anomalies. There have been reports of gastrointestinal defects such as esophageal, duodenal atresia, imperforated anus, tracheo-esophageal fistula, cardiac defects such as patent ductus arteriosus, ventricular septal defect, pulmonary stenosis, aortic stenosis, aortic coarctation, central nervous system anomalies such as hydrocephalus and absence of septum pellucidum (Alter, 2003b; Kwee & Kuyt, 1989; Smith et al., 1989). The FA phenotype can vary within family members; a report of four FA cases within two related consanguineous families who all had the same FANCA mutation demonstrated a wide variation in birth weight, skin pigmentation and the severity of skeletal, renal and genital abnormalities (Koç et al., 1999). Approximately 25-40% of the FA patients in the International Fanconi Anemia Registry (IFAR) do not exhibit any major malformation (Alter, 2003a).

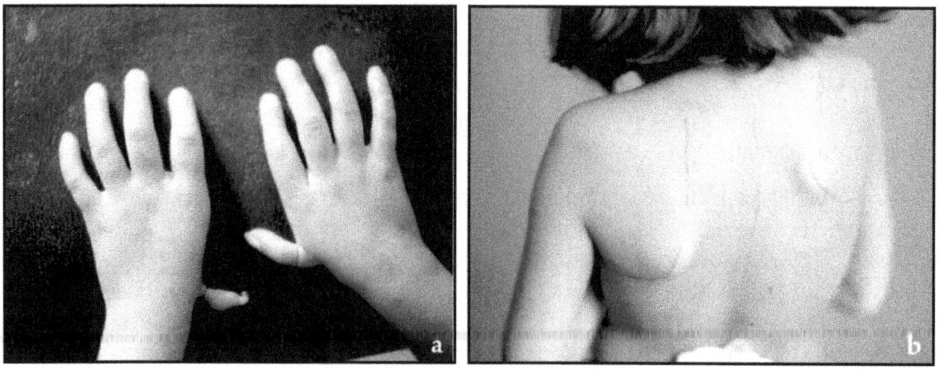


Fig. 1. a) The picture of a 6-year-old girl with Fanconi anemia showing hypoplastic and proximally placed rudimentary thumbs, clinodactyly. b) Sprengel deformity and scoliosis.

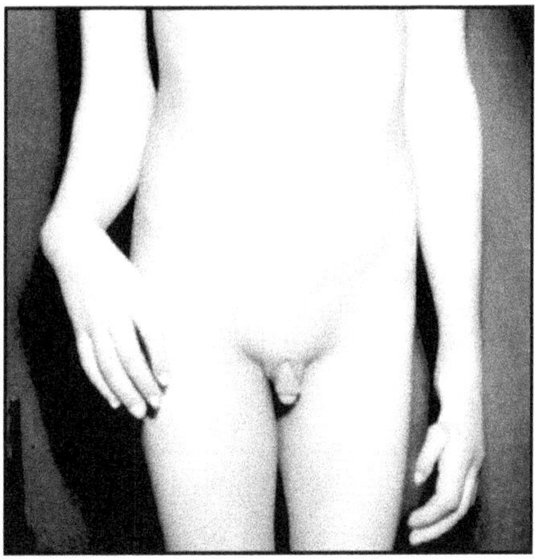

Fig. 2. The picture of a 10-year-old boy with aplastic anemia showing the absence of radius and thumb on the right hand, hypoplastic thumb on the left hand and hypogenitalismus.

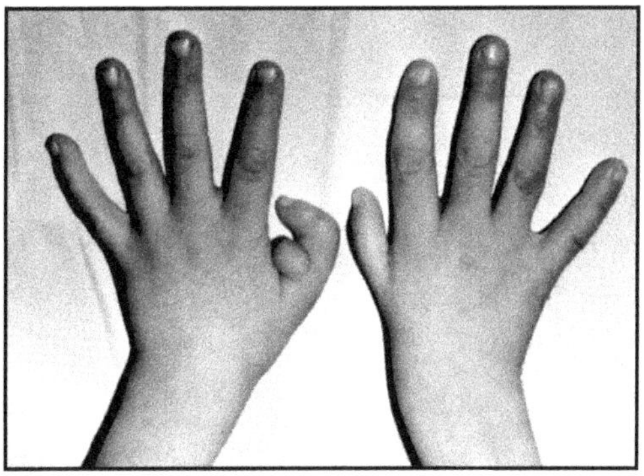

Fig. 3. Bifid left thumb and proximally placed right thumb.

### 2.2 Hematologic abnormalities

In homozygote FA, the most prominent finding is hematologic disorders. The blood count at birth is mostly normal and macrocytosis is generally the first sign of FA. This is followed by thrombocytopenia and anemia. Pancytopenia develops typically at 5-10 years of age, median at seven years (birth to 31 years) (Butturini et al., 1994). IFAR defined hematologic abnormality as hemoglobin level below 10 g/dL, absolute neutrophil count below $1x10^9$/L or platelet count below 100 x $10^9$/L (Alter et al., 2003a). On retrospective analysis of 145 FA patients, some congenital anomalies were seen to carry a potential risk of the development of bone marrow failure. The risk of bone marrow failure in those with radius anomaly is 5.5 times more than those without. The presence of abnormal head, deafness, developmental delay, cardiopulmonary abnormality and abnormal kidney, also kown as 5-item congenital abnormality, increase the risk of bone marrow failure (Rosenberg et al., 2004).

Hematologic disorders are the first sign of FA in young adults not exhibiting any congenital anomalies. Stress erythropoesis exists in FA with characteristics of macrocytosis, increased HbF and the antigen *i* (Table 1). These characteristics may also be found in the anemia free siblings of FA patients (Alter, 2003a). Aspiration from bone marrow reveals marked depression or absence of hematopoietic cells and replacement by fatty tissue containing reticulum cells, lymphocytes, plasma cells and usually tissue mast cells. Nucleated red cells are also decreased in number and they may display megaloblastic features (Fig. 4). Bone marrow biopsy is essential for diagnosis (Lanzkowsky, 1999). In a study based on data from 388 cases with FA, actuarial risk of developing hematopoietic abnormalities was 98% by the age of 40 (Butturini et al., 1994).

Stress erythropoesis
- macrocytosis
- Hb F ↑
- Antigen i

Trombocytopenia, anemia
Pancytopenia median age: 7 years (5-10 years)
Bone marrow failure in radius aplasia; 5.5 ↑

Table 1. Hematological findings in FA.

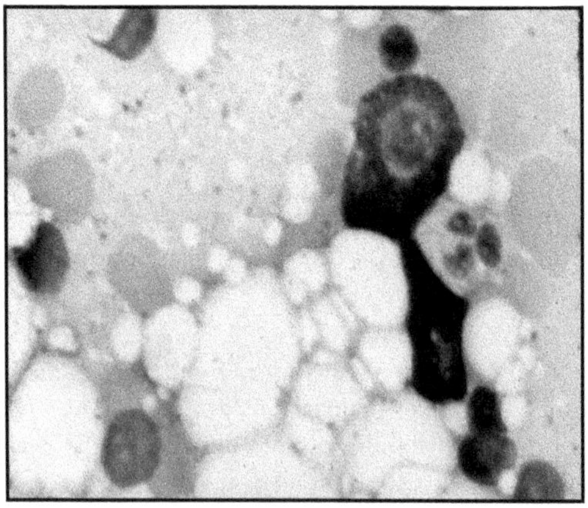

Fig. 4. Fatty tissue and mast cells in the bone marrow.

The most striking feature of FA cells is an increased spontaneous chromosomal instability. Diepoxybutane (DEB) test remains a classical test for diagnosis, involving the detection of chromosomal breaks, gaps, rearrangements, radials, exchange and endoreduplications in peripheral lymphocytes following culturing with clastogenic agents (such as DEB or mitomycin-C) (Fig. 5a, b) (Auerbach et al., 1981). FA homozygotes have a mean of 8.96 breaks per cell in the DEB test according to the IFAR (Alter, 2003a).

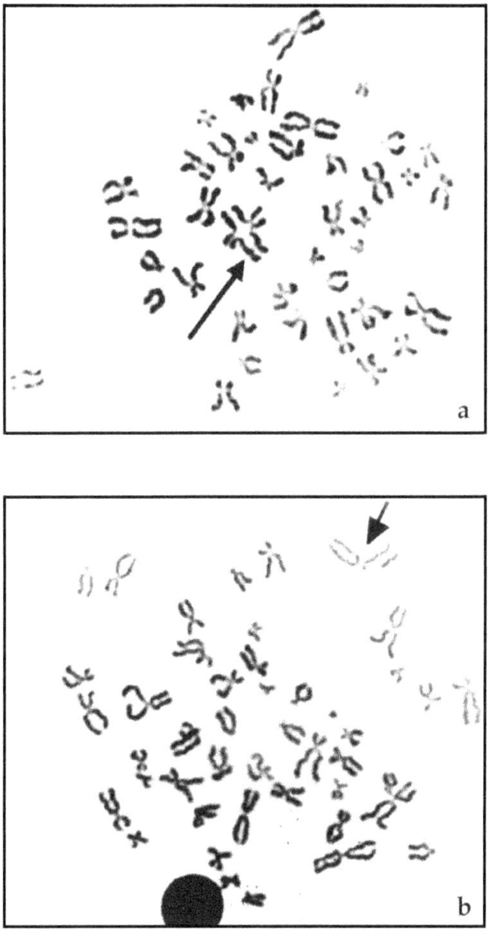

Fig. 5. a) Chromosomal structure abnormalities in the patient with FA. Arrow indicates typical quadriradial chromosome. b) Cytogenetic abnormalities in the metaphase plaque. Arrow indicates chromatid breaks and fragmentation.

Interpretation of the results of DEB test may be complicated by mosaicism. Approximately 25% of patients with FA have evidence of spontaneously occurring mosaicism as manifest by the presence of two subpopulations of lymphocytes, one of which is hypersensitive to cross-linking agents while the other behaves normally in response to these agents. Mosaicism might be associated with a relatively mild hematological course (Lo Ten Foe et al., 1997). DEB test gives a false negative for these patients. DEB testing to establish the diagnosis could be performed on an alternative cell type, such as skin fibroblasts (Alter & Kupfer, 2011). Although DEB test is of crucial importance in the diagnosis of FA, it should be also noted that molecular genetic diagnostic methods have also started to be used in the identification of this disorder.

### 2.3 Cellular disorders and hematopoiesis

Patients with FA generally develop some degree of bone marrow dysfunction ranging from mild asymptomatic cytopenias in any lineage to severe aplastic anemia, MDS or AML. The absence of marrow failure does not rule out FA (Shimamura, 2003). A number of cytokines are critical in the control and regulation of cellular homeostasis in bone marrow. Several cellular disorders associated with FA were reported in a large number of studies. FA cells have important phenotypic abnormalities related to hematopoiesis as shown in Table 2.

| Cellular disorders |
|---|
| Sensitivity to cross- linking agents |
| Prolongation of G2 phases of cell cycles |
| Sensitivity to oxygen |
| Sensitivity to ionized radiation |
| Overproduction of tumor necrosis factor-α |
| Direct defects in DNA repair: |
| - Accumulation of DNA adducts |
| - Defect in repair DNA cross links |
| Genomic instability |
| - Spontaneous chromosome breakage |
| - Hypermutability |
| Increased apoptosis |
| Defective p53 induction |
| Intrinsic stem cell defect |
| Decreased colony growth |

Table 2. Cellular disorders in FA (From Lanzkowsky, P. Manual of Pediatric Hematology and Oncology 1999).

Defective hematopoiesis in FA was shown by the investigation of in vitro bone marrow cell cultures. Interleukin (IL)-6 and granulocyte macrophage-colony stimulating factor expression reduced in many patients with FA (Stark et al., 1993). In another research, the overproduction of tumor necrosis factor-α in FA was also reported (Schultz & Shahidi, 1993). On the other hand, these patients have increased loss of telomere signals compared with controls (Hanson et al., 2001). Abnormal telomere metabolism might play a role in the evoluation of bone marrow failure and malignant transformation in FA (Li et al., 2003). The cytokine changes, increased apoptosis and telomere shortening play a significant role in the microenvironment of bone marrow and the regulation of cellular homeostasis (Fig. 6). Bone marrow failure occurs at a median age of 7 years. Hematopoietic tissue is particularly sensitive to DNA damage caused by radiation or cytotoxic drugs. Genome instability and telomere shortening alter the signals and form mutant clones resistant to apoptosis and consequently AML develops (Lensch et al., 1999; Tischkowitz & Dokal, 2004).

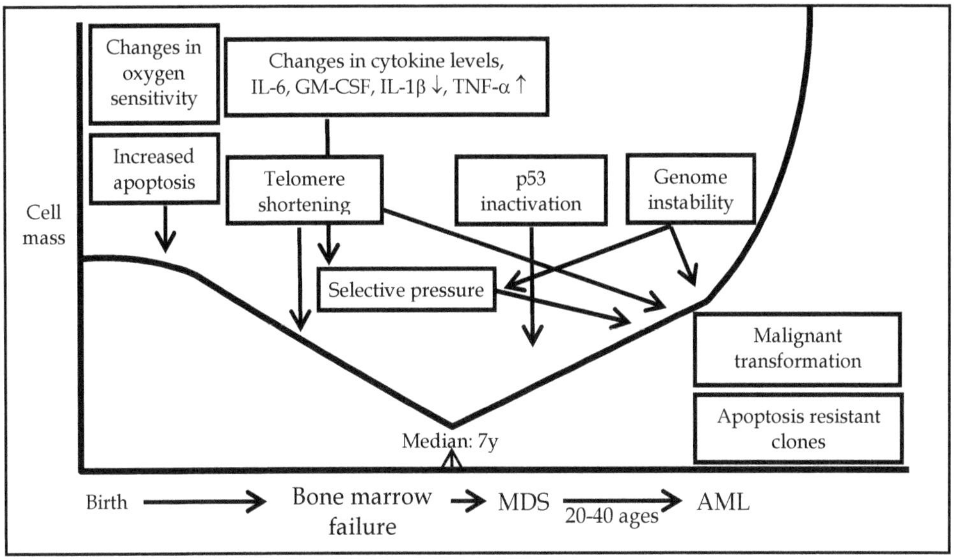


Fig. 6. Defective Hematopoiesis in FA (Adapted from Lensch et al., 1999 and Tischkowitz & Dokal, 2004).

The role of p53 in preventing DNA damage in FA cells was shown in a theoretical model (Kennedy & D'Andrea 2005). As revealed in Fig. 7, when severe DNA damage occurs in FA cells, p53 activates apoptosis and tumor progression is inhibited. If this process occurs in embryonic stem cells, it may cause anomalies. Stem cell loss in bone marrow leads to progressive anemia associated with FA.

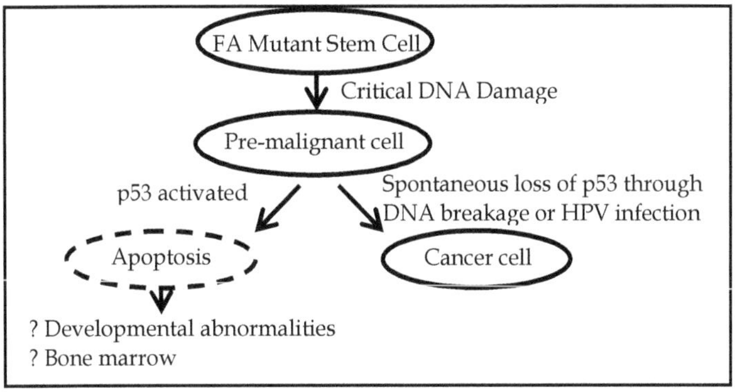


Fig. 7. p53-mediated apoptosis (From Kennedy, R.D. & D'Andrea, A.D., The Fanconi Anemia/BRCA Pathway: New Faces in the Crowd. Genes and Development, 2005; 19:2925-2940).

Loss of p53 or other genes related to apoptosis due to DNA breakage by viral infection or cross-link agents, might inhibit the cell apoptosis. Cells with severe DNA damage continue dividing and this, in turn, may result in malignant transformation. Also a tumor may develop with human papilloma virus (HPV) infections. Since HPV E6 protein decreases the p53 protein level, the apoptotic pathway activation is inhibited. Loss of p53 function may lead to cancer by allowing premalignant cells to survive (Kennedy & D'Andrea 2005).

### 2.4 Complementation groups, genes and DNA repair

Fifteen complementation groups have been identified in patients with FA (Table 3) and new complementation groups may be identified in the future.

| Complementation group | gene | frequency* % | chromosome |
|---|---|---|---|
| FA - A | FANCA | 60 | 16q 24.3 |
| FA - B | FANCB | <1 | Xp 22.3 |
| FA - C | FANCC | 15 | 9q 22.3 |
| FA - DI | BRCA2 | <5 | 13q 12.3 |
| FA - D2 | FANCD2 | <5 | 3p 25.3 |
| FA - E | FANCE | <1 | 6p 21.3 |
| FA - F | FANCF | <1 | 11p 15 |
| FA - G | FANCG | 10 | 9p 13 |
| FA - I | FANCI | <1 | 15q 25 - q 26 |
| FA - J | BRIP1 | <1 | 17q 22 |
| FA - L | FANCL | <1 | 2p 16.1 |
| FA - M | FANC M | <1 | 14q 21.3 |
| FA - N | PALB2 | <1 | 16p 12 |
| FA - O | RAD51C | <1 | 17q 22 |
| FA - P | SLX4 | <1 | 16p 13.3 |

Table 3. FA complementation groups and genes (Adapted from Alter & Kupfer, 2011; Kennedy & D'Andrea, 2005).

FA-A mutations are the most frequent ones observed in about 60% of the cases; FA-C and FA-G mutations are recognized in 15% and 10% of the cases, respectively. While the frequencies of FA-D1 (BRCA2) and FA-D2 are 5% each, the prevalence of other complementation groups is rare (Kennedy & D'Andrea, 2005). The first gene cloned is the FA-C complementation group gene composed of 1674 nucleotides and 14 exons (Fig. 8). Six mutations are recognized in the gene. More than 90% of FA-C mutations are in exon 1 and in exon 4. There is a mild form of FA in mutation related with "dG 322" deletion in exon 1. IV S4 + 4A > T mutations are distinguished for the majority of FA in Ashkenazi Jewish patients having severe phenotype of multiple congenital malformations and early onset of hematological disease (Joenje et al., 1995a, 1995b).

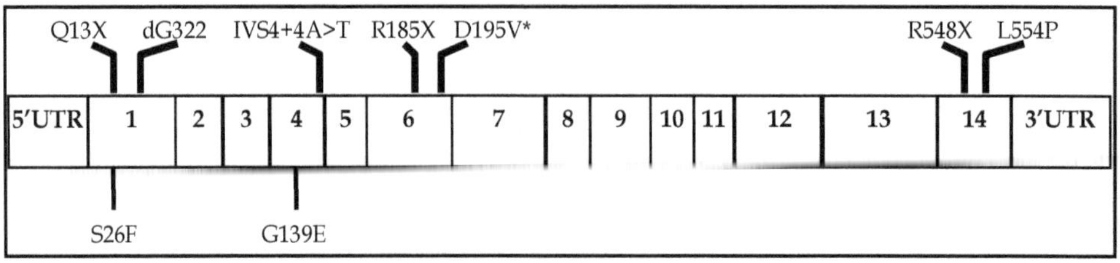


Fig. 8. Mutations in FA-C gene (From Joenje, H. et al., Fanconi Anemia Research: Current Status and Prospects, European Journal of Cancer 1995; 31:268-272).

Several types of, sometimes overlapping, DNA repair processes are identified based on the targeted types of damage. Three types of excision repair processes have been described: base excision repair (BER), nucleotide excision repair (NER) and mismatch repair (MMR). Two additional types of DNA repair, homologous recombination (HR) and nonhomologous end-joining (NHEJ) are employed in response to a double strand break, the most serious type of DNA damage. HR is considered to be an error-free pathway since it uses a copy of the damaged segment. NHEJ is accepted as an error-prone pathway since free ends are joined in the absence of a template which might cause an associated loss of nucleotides or translocation (Risinger & Groden, 2004). FA pathway has an important role in three classic DNA repair processes, namely homologous recombination, nucleotide excision repair andtranslesion synthesis which is DNA polymerization on damaged templates (Moldovan & D'Andrea, 2009).

FA proteins have a significant role in regulating DNA repair by homologous recombination. FA proteins cooperate in a common pathway known as the FA/BRCA pathway. Eight of the FA proteins (A, B, C, E, F, G, L, M and possibly I subunits) form a nuclear core complex required for the monoubiquitination of FANCD2 protein. In response to DNA damage, the FA complex (complex 1) is activated and initiates the monoubiquitination of FANCD2. Then FANCD2 - Ub interacts with BRCA2 in complex 2, leading to repair of the cross-link possibly through homologous recombination and translesion synthesis. The FANCD1 gene is identical to the breast and ovarian cancer susceptibility gene, BRCA2. FANCD2 is deubiquitinated by USP1, thereby inactivating the pathway (Fig. 9). The FA proteins are also important in the arrangement of an intra-S-phase checkpoint (D'Andrea, 2003; Kennedy & D'Andrea, 2005; Wang & D'Andrea, 2004). In the absence of BRCA2, DNA repair cannot be performed by homologous recombination. DNA damage is repaired by nonhomologous end-joining (Fig. 10).

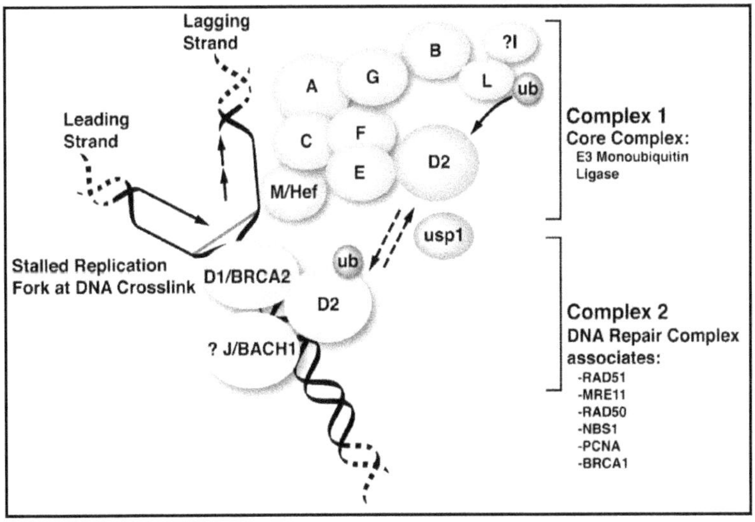


Fig. 9. The FA pathway (From Kennedy, R.D. & D'Andrea, A.D., The Fanconi Anemia/BRCA Pathway: New Faces in the Crowd. Genes and Development 2005; 19: 2925-2940).

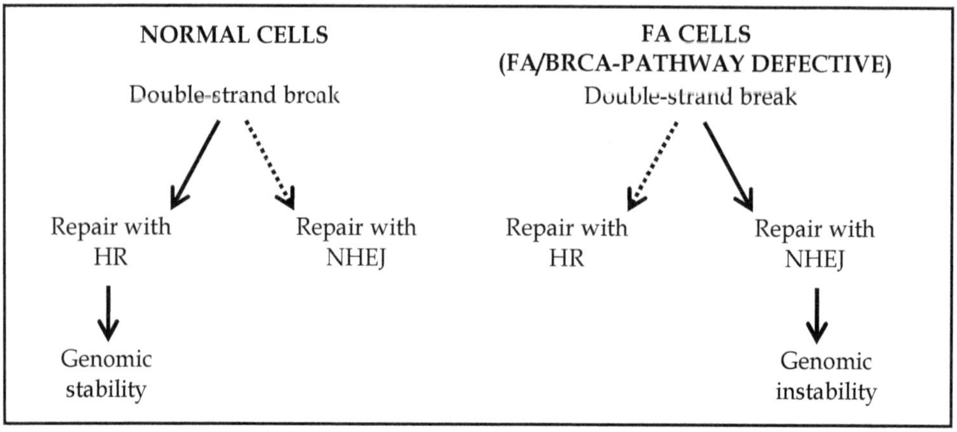


Fig. 10. Repair of double-strand break in normal and FA cells (Adapted from Venkitaraman, 2004). HR: Homologous recombination; NHEJ: Nonhomologous end-joining.

In the cytoplasm, only FANCA, FANCC, FANCF and FANCG proteins are present. Cytoplasmic functions and interactions of FANCC and FANCG are decoded. The FANCC protein binds to NADPH cytochrome P-450 reductase and regulates the major detoxification pathway. FANCC also interacts with glutathion-S-transpherase PI-I, and protects the cell from oxidative stress. FANCC interacts with HSP70 to prevent the apoptosis in hematopoietic cells exposed to IFN-γ and TNF-α. FANCC is required for optimal activation of STAT1 in the JAK/STAT pathway. FANCG protein directly interacts with CYP2E1 and prevents oxidative DNA damage (Thompson et al., 2005).

### 2.5 Fanconi anemia and cancer

Mutations in FA genes cause a disorder characterized by bone marrow failure, developmental defects and cancer proneness (Moldovan & D'Andrea, 2009). The FANCD2 knockout mice exhibit micropthalmia, perinatal lethality, and severe hypogonadism. Fancd2knockout mice also has increased incidences of epithelial cancers such as breast, ovarian and liver cancers (D'Andrea, 2003). FA is a rare cancer susceptibility syndrome that increases the predisposition of the patient to leukemia, squamous cell carcinomas of the head and neck or female genitelia as well as liver tumors. Predisposition to cancer in heterozygotes was also reported by Swift (Alter, 2003a). One thousand three hundred cases of FA were evaluated during the years between 1927 and 2001. Nine percent of these cases had leukemia, 7% had myelodysplastic syndrome, 5% had solid tumors and 3% liver tumors. In approximately 25% of patients with cancer, the malignancy preceded the diagnosis of FA. It is unclear which patients are prone to develop such tumors (Alter, 2003c). In another study, the cumulative incidence of malignancies among 145 patients with FA was 9 leukemias and 18 solid tumors in 14 patients. The ratio of observed to expected neoplasm (O/E) was 50 for all cancers, 48 for all solid tumors and 785 for leukemia. These increased risks were calculated to be statistically significant. The highest solid tumor O/E ratios were 4317 for vulvar cancer, 2362 for esophageal cancer, and 706 for head and neck cancer. The median age of onset of leukemia was 11.3 years, which is significantly lower compared to the median 28.9 years of onset for solid tumors (Rosenberg et al., 2003). Actuarial risk of developing MDS or AML by 40 years of age was 52% (Butturini et al., 1994).

The types of leukemia occurring in FA are primarily non-lymphocytic leukemia although a few lymphoblastic types have also been reported (Alter, 1993a; Yetgin et al., 1994). The incidence of AML in FA patients is 15.000 times more compared to children in the population (Auerbach & Allen, 1991). In these patients, all FAB sub-types occur; the myelomonocytic ($M_4$) and acute monocytic ($M_5$) types (Fig.11, Fig.12) are the most common (Alter, 2003c, Tischkowitz & Dokal, 2004).
Certain cytogenetic abnormalities are commonly seen in these patients with MDS/AML. In one study of the cytogenetic findings of 23 MDS and AML cases in FA homozygotes in high incidence of monosomy 7, 7q-, rearrangement of 1p36, 1q24-34 and 11q22-25, abnormalities was reported (Butturini et al., 1994). The most frequently observed chromosomal abnormalities in FA-associated leukemia are monosomy 7, duplication of 1 q and chromosome 3q abnormalities. Gain of 3q is associated with poor prognosis (Taniguchi & D'Andrea, 2006). As suggested, all FA patients may be considered as preleukemic state and this disorder represents a model for study of the etiology of AML (Auerbach & Allen, 1991). Leukemia may be the first hematologic manifestation of FA (Auerbach et al., 1982). Five out of the 52 patients with FA developing 3 AML, 1 squamous cell carcinoma of the gingiva, 1 hepatocellular carcinoma were mentioned in another clinical research (Altay et al., 1997).

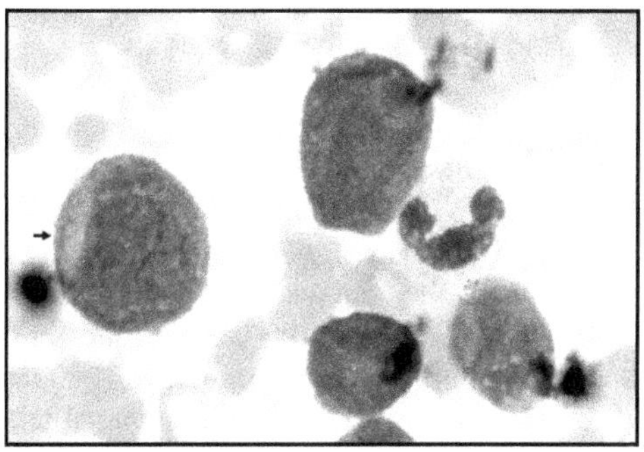

Fig. 11. Auer rods positivity in myeloblast.

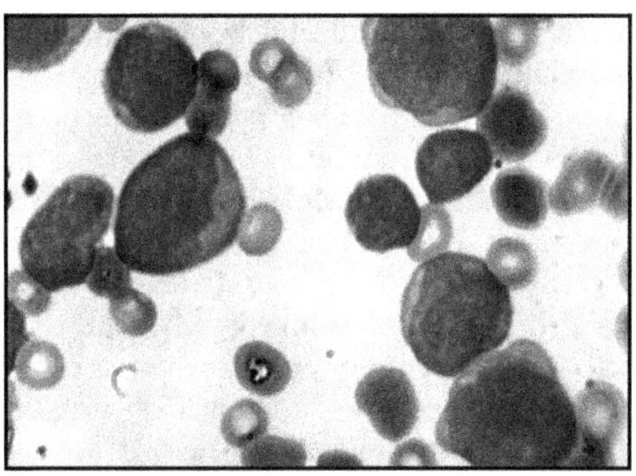

Fig. 12. Monoblasts in the bone marrow.

In our series, four out of 39 cases developed AML and one had two malignancies.There were no other cancers among family members in these four patients whereas the sister of a boy with FA developed acute leukemia in another hospital. (Gözdaşoğlu et al., 1980, Gözdaşoğlu et al., 2009). The majority of solid tumors occurs after the first or second decade of life (Alter, 2011).

FA-D1 complementation group is different from other complementation groups in its severity. In this group, leukemia and solid tumors develop as early as before 5 years of age. A cell line (termed FA-AML1) was obtained from blast cells after a second relapse following the bone marrow transplantation in a 2 years old boy with FA and AML. FA-AML1 is the first AML cell line obtained from a FA patient. FA-AML1 cells have failed to reveal FA phenotype such as hypersensitivity to growth inhibition and chromosomal breakage by the cross-linking agent mitomycin C. Genomic DNA showed biallelic mutations in FANCD1/BRCA2. Genetic reversion has been observed resulting in the loss of the FA cellular phenotype (Ikeda et al., 2003). In another report, a cross-linker-sensitive AML cell line also was derived from a 2 years old boy who had biallelic FANCD1/BRCA2 (Meyer et al., 2005). FA-D1 subgroup, however, can be associated with a high incidence of leukemia and specific solid tumors such as Wilms tumor and medulloblastoma in very early childhood (Hirsch et al., 2004). BRCA2 mutations predisposes to cancers like the familial breast, ovary, prostate and pancreas (Shivji & Venkitaraman, 2004). From several studies on the issue, it is possible to conclude that the diagnosis of leukemia and solid tumors at early age and worse prognosis are the most important features of FA-D1 complementation group.

FA is found as the most common form of inherited bone marrow failure syndrome associated with worst prognosis. A high percentage of patients developed severe bone marrow failure and cancer in a study based on 127 patients whose 66 cases (52%) are with FA. One of the striking findings of this study is the high rate of consanguinity, 68 % of patients with FA. Leukemia in 7 patients (11%), MDS in 11 patients (16%) and solid tumors in 6 patients (9%) out of these 66 cases were diagnosed (Tamary et al., 2010). In another study of 181 patients, however, bone marrow failure in 66 patients, acute myeloid leukemia in 14 patients and solid tumors in 10 patients were determined. The ratio of O/E was 44 for all cancers, 26 for all solid tumors and 868 for acute myeloid leukemia. These increased risks were statistically significant. In this study, absent or abnormal radii and a five-item congenital abnormality score were significant risk factors for bone marrow failure. In three of the 48 patients who received a transplant, the three malignancies, namely tongue, liver and esophagus, occurred after 2, 16 and 17 years following the transplants. The age-specific risk of solid tumors was 3.8-fold higher in cases with transplants compared to the cases without (Rosenberg, Alter & Ebell, 2008). Hematopoietic stem cell transplant (HSCT) is presently the only therapy that can restore normal hematopoiesis in patients with FA. The risk of squamous cell cancers increased for FA patients irrespective of receiving and not receiving the transplants. HSCT conditioning regimes may also increase the occurrence of squamous cell cancers in cases with transplants. Rosenberg et al., compared two groups of patients; 117 receiving transplants and 145 not receiving. It was found that the age-specific risk of squamous cell cancer was 4.4 fold higher in patients who received transplants than who did not. Squamous cell cancers developed at significantly younger ages in the transplanted group. Acute and chronic graft-versus-host diseases were significant squamous cell cancer risk factors, and this cancer was also an adverse risk factor for death in both groups. Survival rate following squamous cell cancer was not significantly different between the two groups (Rosenberg et al., 2005). Liver tumors associated with androgens were reported in the patients with FA (Velazquez& Alter, 2004) and the cumulative probability of liver tumors has been estimated to be 46 % by age 50 (Alter, 2003c).

The patients with FA should be followed in the form of hematologic monitoring and cancer surveillance. Complete blood counts should be taken every 4 months. Annual bone marrow aspirates and biopsies should be performed on all patients. Dental and oropharyngeal(

including naso-laryngoscopy) exams should start at age 10 or within the first year after transplant. Gynecologic examination and Pap semears beginning at age 16, and if necessary, annual esophageal endoscopy should be done as part of cancer surveillance. The patients are advised to avoid toxic agents, smoking and alcohol. Radiographic studies should be minimally utilised. Vaccination of female patients with the human papillomavirus vaccine should be considered starting at nine years of age (Alter,2011).

## 3. Conclusion

FA is a rare autosomal recessive or x-linked inherited chromosomal instability syndrome. Affected individuals have a highly increased risk of developing bone marrow failure, hematologic malignancies and solid tumors. FA-pathway has an important role in repairing DNA damage namely homologous recombination, nucleotide excision repair and translesion synthesis. Fifteen complementation groups and genes that cause FA have been identified. FA-D1 subgroup can be associated with high incidence of leukemia and solid tumors such as Wilms tumor, medulloblastoma, neuroblastoma at early ages. BRCA2 mutations predispose to cancers such as familial breast, ovary, prostate and pancreas. Leukemia in FA is generally very difficult to treat and survival is rare. The deficiency in DNA repair leads to increased sensitivity to the side effects of chemotherapy and the patients are either vulnerable to treatment toxicity or may receive inadequate treatment. The effective treatment modalities have to be further developed. Patients with FA should be followed with regard to AML and solid tumors which should be considered as first manifestations of FA. It is also important to note that the family members of the patients with FA must be scanned for cancer as well. Genetic counseling and psychosocial support should be employed as soon as possible.

## 4. Acknowledgements

This work is dedicated to the loving memory of my late husband Prof. Dr. Rıfat Gözdaşoğlu for his unwavering support throughout my career and his unrelenting dedication to the ethical and respectful treatment of his patients.

## 5. References

Akar, N. & Gözdaşoğlu, S. (1984). Spectrum of Anomalies in Fanconi Anemia, *Human Genetics,* Vol.21, No.1, pp. 75-76, ISSN 0340-6717

Altay, C.; Alikaşifoğlu, M.; Kara, A.; Tunçbilek, E.; Özbek, N.; Schroeder-Kurth, T.M. (1997). Analysis of 65 Turkish Patients with Congenital Aplastic Anemia (Fanconi Anemia and Non-Fanconi Anemia): Hacettepe Experience, *Clinical Genetics,* Vol.51, No.5, pp. 296-302, ISSN 0009-9163

Alter, B.P. & Kupfer, G. (2011). Fanconi Anemia, In: *Gene Reviews-(internet) NCBI Bookshelf, ID: NBK 1401, PMID: 20301575,* R.A. Pagon, T.D. Bird, C.R. Dolan, et al., (Eds.), pp. 1-42

Alter, B.P. (1992). Fanconi's Anemia. Current Concepts, *American Journal of Pediatric Hematology/Oncology,* Vol.14, No.2, pp. 170-176, ISSN 0192-8562

Alter, B.P. (1993a). Annotation. Fanconi's Anemia and its Variability, *British Journal of Haematology,* Vol.85, No.1, pp. 9-14, ISSN 0007-1048

Alter, B.P. (2003b). Cancer in Fanconi Anemia 1927-2001, *Cancer*, Vol.97, No.2, pp. 425-440, ISSN 0008-543X

Alter, B.P. (2003c). Inherited bone marrow failure syndrome, In: *Nathan and Oski's Hematology of Infancy and Childhood*, D.G. Nathan, S.H. Orkin, D. Ginsburg, A.T. Look, (Eds.), pp. 280-299, W.B. Saunders Company, ISBN 0-7216-9317-1, Philadelphia

Alter, B.P. (2005). Fanconi's Anemia, Transplantation and Cancer, *Pediatric Transplantation*, Vol.9, (Suppl.7), pp. 81-86, ISSN 1397-3142

Auerbach, A.D. & Allen, R.G. (1991). Leukemia and Preleukemia in Fanconi Anemia Patients. *Cancer Genetics and Cytogenetics*, Vol.51, No.1, pp. 1-12, ISSN 0165-4608

Auerbach, A.D.; Adler, B. & Chaganti, S.K. (1981). Prenatal and Postnatal Diagnosis and Carrier Detection of Fanconi Anemia by a Cytogenetic Method, *Pediatrics*, Vol.67, No.1, pp. 128-135, ISSN 0031-4005

Auerbach, A.D.; Weiner, M.A.; Warburton, D.; Yeboa, K.; Lu, L. & Broxmeyer, H.E. (1982). Acute Myeloid Leukemia as the First Hematologic Manifestation of Fanconi Anemia, *American Journal of Hematology*, Vol.12, No.3, pp. 289-300, ISSN 0361-8609

Butturini, A.; Gale, R.P.; Verlander, P.C.; Adler-Brecher, B.; Gillio, P. & Auerbach, A.D. (1994). Hematologic Abnormalities in Fanconi Anemia Registry Study, *Blood*, Vol.84, No.5, pp. 1650-1655, ISSN 0006-4971

D'Andrea, A.D. (2003). The Fanconi Road to Cancer, *Genes & Development*, Vol.17, No.16, pp. 1933-1936, ISSN 0890-9369

Ebell, W.; Friedrich, W. & Kohne, E. (1989). Therapeutic Aspects of Fanconi Anemia, In: *Fanconi Anemia Clinical, Cytogenetic and Experimental Aspects*, T.M. Schroeder-Kurth, A.D. Auerbach, G. Obe, (Eds.), pp. 47-60, Springer-Verlog, ISBN 3-540-50401-X, New York, Berlin, Heidelberg

Gözdaşoğlu, S.; Çavdar, A.O.; Arcasoy, A.; Babacan, E.; Sanal, Ö. (1980). Fanconi's Aplastic Anemia, Analysis of 18 Cases, *Acta Haematologica*, Vol.64, No.3, pp. 131-135, ISSN 0001-5792

Gözdaşoğlu, S.; Ertem, M.; Uysal, Z.; Babacan, E.; Yüksel, M.; Bökesoy, I.; Sunguroğlu, A.; Arcasoy, A. & Çavdar, A.O. (2009). Acute Myeloid Leukemia in Turkish Children with Fanconi Anemia. One Center Experience in the Period Between 1964-1995, *Turkish Journal of Hematology*, Vol.26, No.3, pp. 118-122, ISSN 1300-7777

Hanson, H.; Mathew, C.G.; Docherty, Z.; Ogilvie, M. & Mackie, M. (2001). Telomere Shortening in Fanconi Anaemia Demonstrated by a Direct FISH Approach, *Cytogenetic and Genome Research*, Special issue, Vol.93, No.3-4, p.203-206, ISSN 1424-8581

Hirsch, B.; Shimamura, A.; Moreau, L.; Baldinger, S.; Hag-alshiek, M.; Bostrom, B.; Sencer, S.; D'Andrea, A.D. (2004) Association of Biallelic BRCA2/FANCD1 Mutations with Spontaneous Chromosomal Instability and Solid Tumors of Childhood, *Blood*, Vol. 103, No. 7, p. 2554-2559 ISSN 0006-4971

Ikeda, H.; Matsushita, M.; Waisfisz, W.; Kinoshita, A.; Oostra, A.B.; Nieuwint, A.W., deWinder, J.P., Hoatlin, M.E., Kawai, Y., Sasaki, M.S., D'Andrea, A.D., Kawakami, Y., Joenjo, H., (2003). Genetic Reversion in an Acute Myelogenous Leukemia Cell Line from a Fanconi Anemia Patient with Biallelic Mutations in BRCA2, *Cancer Research*, Vol.63, No.10, pp. 2688-2694, ISSN 0008-5472

Joenje, H.; Lo Ten Foe, J.R.; Oostra, A.B. & et al. (1995a). Classification of Fanconi Anemia Patients by Complementation Analysis: Evidence for a Fifth Genetic Subtype, *Blood*, Vol.86, No.6, pp. 2156-2160, ISSN 0006-4971

Joenje, H.; Mathew, C. & Gluckman, E. (1995b). Fanconi Anemia Research: Current Status and Prospects, *European Journal of Cancer,* Vol.31, No.2, pp. 268-272, ISSN 0959-8049

Kennedy, R.D. & D'Andrea, A.D. (2005). The Fanconi Anemia/BRCA Pathway: New Faces in the Crowd, *Genes & Development,* Vol.19, No.24, pp. 2925-2940, ISSN 0890-9369

Koç, A.; Pronk, J.C.; Alikaşifoğlu, M.; Joenje, H. & Altay, Ç. (1999). Variable Pathogenicity of Exon 43del (FAA) in Four Fanconi Anaemia Patients within a Consanguineous Family, *British Jornal of Haematology,* Vol.104, No.1, pp. 127-130, ISSN 007-1048

Kwee, M.L. & Kuyt, L.P. (1989). Fanconi Anemia in the Netherlands, In: *Fanconi Anemia Clinical, Cytogenetic and Experimental Aspects,* T.M. Schroeder-Kurth, A.D. Auerbach, G. Obe, (Eds.), pp. 18-33, Springer-Verlog, ISBN 3-540-50401-X, New York, Berlin, Heidelberg

Lanzkowsky, P. (1999). *Manual of Pediatric Hematology and Oncology,* (third ed.), Academic Pres, ISBN 0-12-436635-x, San Diego, San Francisco, New York, Boston, London, Sydney, Tokyo

Lensch, MW., Rathbun, PK., Olson, SB., Jones, GR &Bagby Jr, GC. (1999). Selective Pressure as an Essential Force in Molecular Evolution of Myeloid Leukemic Clones: A View from the Window of Fanconi Anemia, *Leukemia,* Vol.13, No.11, pp. 1784-1789, ISSN 0887-6924

Li, X.; Leteurtre, F.; Rocha, V.; Guardiola, P.; Berger, R.; Daniel, M.T.; Noguera, M.H.; Maarek, O.; Roux, G.L.; de la Salmoniere, P.; Richard, P. & Glueckman, E. (2003). Abnormal Telomere Metabolism in Fanconi's Anemia Correlates with Genomic Instability and the Probability of Developing Severe Aplastic Anemia, *British Journal of Hematology,* Vol.120, No.5, pp. 836-845, ISSN 0007-1048

Lo Ten Foe, J.R.; Kwee, M.L.; Rooimans, M.A.; Oostra, A.B.; Veerman, A.J.P.; van Well, M.; Pauli, R.M.; Shahidi, N.T.; Dokal, I.; Roberts, I.; Altay, Ç.; Gluckman, E.; Gibson, R.A.; Mathew, C.G.; Arwert, F. & Joenje, H. (1997). Somatic Mosaicism in Fanconi Anemia: Molecular Basis and Clinical Significance, *European Journal of Human Genetics,* Vol.5, No.3, pp. 137-148, ISSN 1018-4813

Meetei, A.R.; Levitus, M.; Xue, Y.; Medhurst, A.L.; Zwann, M.; Ling, C.; Rooimans, M.A.; Bier, P.; Hoatlin, M.; Pals, G.; de Winter, J.P.; Wang, W. & Joenje, H. (2004). X-Linked Inheritance of Fanconi Anemia Complementation Group B, *National Genetics,* Vol.36, No.11, pp. 1219-1224, ISSN 1061-4036

Meyer, S.; Fergusson, W.D; Oostra, A.B. & et al. (2005). A Cross-linker. Sensitive Myeloid Leukemia Cell Line from a 2-year-old Boy with Severe Fanconi Anemia and Biallelic FANCDI/BRCA2 Mutations, *Genes Chromosomes Cancer,* Vol.42, No.4, pp. 404-415, ISSN 1045-2257

Moldovan, G.L. & D'Andrea, A.D. (2009). How the Fanconi Anemia Pathway Guards the Genome, *Annual Review Genetics,* Vol.43, pp. 223-249, ISSN 0066-4197

Risinger, M.A. & Groden, J. (2004). Crosslinks and Crosstalk: Human Cancer Syndromes and DNA Repair Defects, *Cancer Cell,* Vol.6, No.6, pp. 539-545, ISSN 1535-6108

Rosenberg, P.S.; Alter, B.P. & Ebell, W. (2008). Cancer Risks in Fanconi Anemia: Finding from the German Fanconi Anemi Registry, *Haematologica,* Vol.93, No.4, pp. 511-517, ISSN 0390-6078

Rosenberg, P.S.; Greene, M.H. & Alter, B.P. (2003). Cancer Incidence in Person with Fanconi Anemia, *Blood,* Vol.101, No.3, pp. 822-826, ISSN 0006-4971

Rosenberg, P.S.; Huang, Y. & Alter, B.P. (2004). Individualized Risks of First Adverse Events in Patients with Fanconi Anemia, *Blood,* Vol.104, No.2, pp. 350-355, ISSN 0006-4971

Rosenberg, P.S.; Socié, G.; Alter, B.P. & Gluckman, E. (2005). Risk of Head and Neck Squamous Cell Cancer and Death in Patients with Fanconi Anemia Who Did and Did Not Receive Transplants, *Blood,* Vol.105, No.1, pp. 67-73, ISSN 0006-4971

Schultz, J.C. & Shahidi, N.T. (1993). Tumor Necrosis Factor-alpha Overproduction in Fanconi's Anemia, *American Journal of Hematology,* Vol.42, No.2, pp. 196-201, ISSN 0361-8609

Shimamure, A. (2003). Treatment of Hematologic Abnormalities in FA, In: *Fanconi Anemia, Standards for Clinical Care,* pp. 17-37, Fanconi Anemia Research Fund, Inc., Second Edition, Eugene, Oregon

Shivji, M.K.K. & Venkitaraman, A.R. (2004). DNA Recombination, Chromosomal Stability and Carcinogenesis: Insights into the Role of BRCA2, *DNA Repair,* Vol.3, No.8-9, pp. 835-843, ISSN 1568-7864

Smith, S.; Marx, M.P.; Jordaan, C.J. & van Niekerk, C.H. (1989). Clinical Aspects of a Cluster of 42 Patients in South Africa with Fanconi Anemia, In: Fanconi Anemia Clinical Cytogenetic and Experimental Aspects, T.M. Schroeder-Kurth, A.D. Auerbach, G. Obe, (Eds.), pp. 18-33, Springer-Verlag, ISBN 3-540-50401-X, Newyork, Berlin, Heidelberg

Stark, R.; Andre, C.; Thierry, D.; Cherel, M.; Galibert, F. & Gluckman, E. (1993). The Expression of Cytokine and Cytokine Receptor Genes in Long-term Bone Marrow Culture in Congenital and Acquired Bone Marrow Hypoplasias, *British Journal of Haematology,* Vol.83, No.4, pp. 560-566, ISSN 0007-1048

Tamary, H.; Nishri, D.; Yacobovich, J.; Zilber, R.; Dgany, D.; Krasnow, T.; Aviner, S.; Stepensky, P.; Ravel-Vilk, S.; Bitan, M.; Kaplinsky, C.; Barak, A.B.; Elhasid, R.; Kapelusnik, J.; Koren, A.; Levin, C.; Attias, D.; Laor, R.; Yaniv, I.; Rosenberg, P.S. & Alter, B.P. (2010). Frequency and Natural History of Inherited Bone Marrow Failure Syndromes: The Israeli Inherited Bone Marrow Failure Registry, *Haematologica,* Vol.95, No.8, pp. 1300-1307, ISSN 0390-6078

Taniguchi, T. & D'Andrea, A.D. (2006). The Molecular Pathogenesis of Fanconi Anemia: Recent Progress, *Blood,* Vol.107, No.11, pp. 4223-4233, ISSN 0006-4971

Thompson, L.H.; Hinz, J.M.; Yamada, N.A. & Jones, N.J. (2005). How Fanconi Anemia Proteins Promote the Four Rs: Replication, Recombination, Repair, and Recovery, *Environmental and Molecular Mutagenesis,* Vol.45, No.2-3, pp. 128-142, ISSN 0893-6692

Tischkowitz, M. & Dokal, I. (2004). Fanconi Anaemia and Leukemia - Clinical and Molecular Aspects, *British Journal of Haematology,* Vol.126, No.2, pp. 176-191, ISSN 0007-1048

Velazquez, I. & Alter, B.P. (2004). Androgens and Liver Tumors: Fanconi's Anemia and Non-Fanconi's Conditions, *American Journal of Hematology,* Vol.77, No.3, pp. 257-267, ISSN 0361-8609

Venkitaraman, A.R. (2004). Tracing the Network Connecting BRCA and Fanconi Anaemia Proteins. *Nature Reviews Cancer,* Vol.4, No.4, pp. 266-276, ISSN 1474-175X

Wang, X.Z. & D'Andrea, A.D. (2004). The Interplay of Fanconi Anemia Proteins in the DNA Damage Response, *DNA Repair,* Vol.3, No.8-9, pp. 1063-1069, ISSN 1568-7864

Yetgin, S.; Tuncer, M.; Güler, E.; Duru, F. & Kaşifoğlu, M.A. (1994). Acute Lymphoblastic Leukemia in Fanconi's Anemia, *American Journal of Hematology,* Vol.45, No.1, p. 101, ISSN 0361-8609

# 25

# The Molecular Connection Between Aluminum Toxicity, Anemia, Inflammation and Obesity: Therapeutic Cues

Adam Bignucolo, Joseph Lemire, Christopher Auger, Zachary Castonguay, Varun Appanna and Vasu D. Appanna
*Laurentian University*
*Canada*

## 1. Introduction

Anemia is reported to be the most common blood disorder. A variety of anemic conditions affecting various groups of people exist and each of the types of anemia has different underlying causes. Iron (Fe) deficiency, a potent instigator of anemia, is the most common mineral deficiency and its effects have been linked to slow physical development and impaired cognitive function along with behavioral and learning disturbances (De Giudice *et al*, 2009). Exacerbating the iron deficiency epidemic is obesity, a disease defined by an excess accumulation of body fat leading to adverse health effects. It has been demonstrated that there is an association between poor iron status and obesity. The relationship between the two conditions has been shown in children, adolescents and adults including post-menopausal women.
Obesity is now considered an independent factor contributing to iron deficiency (McClung *et al*, 2009). Gaining incredible importance as a global health issue, obesity rates are increasing worldwide. The World Health Organization estimated that in 2005, 1.6 billion adults were overweight (body mass index (BMI) =25), and over 400 million adults were obese (BMI =30). Notably, there is an increase in the incidence of childhood and adolescent obesity in industrialized countries where the number of affected population has more than doubled over the past few decades. A similar trend has been observed in developing countries such as Egypt, Brazil and Mexico. What used to be considered a "rich" country issue has now become a worldwide epidemic and the situation is continuously worsening (Hintze *et al*, 2010).

## 2. Hepcidin: Function and regulation

A significant proportion of the world's population is iron-deficient, obese, or both. This makes an understanding of the mechanisms underlying obesity-induced iron deficiency and anemia crucial. Recently, the discovery of the peptide hormone hepcidin, a regulator of organismal iron metabolism has shed light on the relationship between anemia and obesity. Hepcidin is a 25 amino acid long peptide secreted by the liver and adipose tissue that was initially studied for its modulation of iron-homeostasis during infection. Increases in hepcidin levels cause the depletion of serum iron levels and prevent the efflux of iron through the cellular iron exporter ferroportin from hepatocytes, enterocytes and macrophages (**Figure 1**). Therefore, hepcidin is the iron/inflammation/oxygen sensor that can act as a signal for numerous physiological responses including i) the decreased dietary iron uptake during an overload situation, ii) the anemia seen during infection to prevent free iron from promoting pathogen proliferation and iii) an increase of iron uptake during hypoxia (Atkinson *et* al, 2011; Choi *et al,* 2007; Vecchi *et al*, 2009).

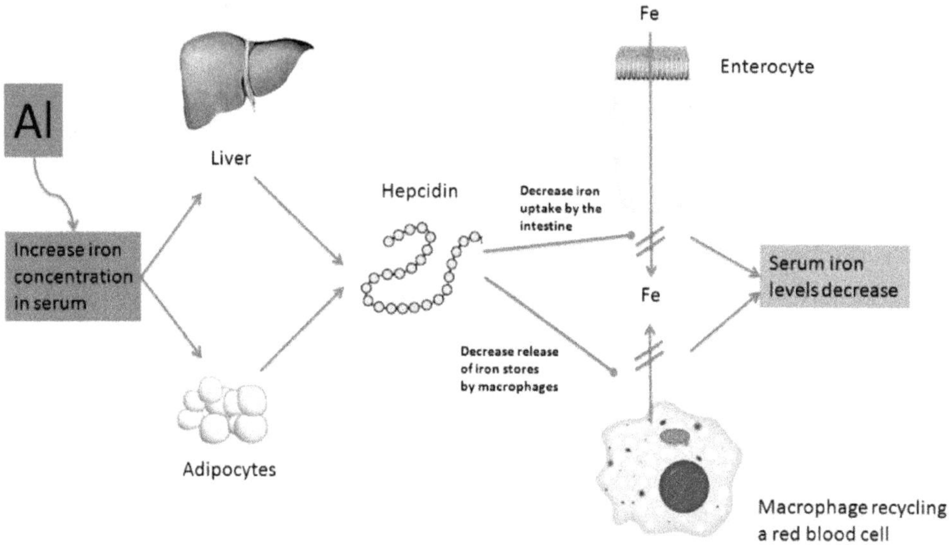


Fig. 1. Al toxicity leads to an increased Fe concentration in the serum of the body. High blood Fe levels cause the liver and adipose tissue to secrete hepcidin, a Fe homeostasis regulator, which signals the decrease in Fe absorption by enterocytes as well as a decrease in Fe release from cellular stores such as red blood cells.

Interestingly, chronic inflammation is one of the hallmarks of obesity (Ausk *et al,* 2008, Yanoff *et al,* 2007). Adipose tissue in obese mice has been shown to be considerably more hypoxic than adipose tissue from lean mice. As a result of the difference in $O_2$ tension there is an important shift in gene expression, not only for expected genes induced by hypoxia but also the increased levels of inflammatory cytokines including interleukin-6 (IL-6) (Lee *et al,* 2005). The latter appears to be the mediator of the induction of hepatic hepcidin secretion during inflammation. IL-6 and other hepcidin-inducing factors such as the adipokine leptin may explain the increased hepcidin levels in obese individuals compared to healthy patients (Barisani *et al,* 2008; Choi *et al,* 2007; Hintze *et al,* 2010).

## 3. The link between Fe-deficiency, anemia, inflammation and obesity

When studied separately, the development of anemia, inflammation and obesity have all been associated with aluminum (Al) toxicity. It is well established that Al disrupts iron homeostasis leading to the dysfunction of essential biochemical processes dependent on this redox-active ion. Al negatively influences the absorption of iron via the intestine, hinders its transport in the serum, and displaces iron by binding to transferrin (**Figure 2**) (Turgut *et al*, 2007).

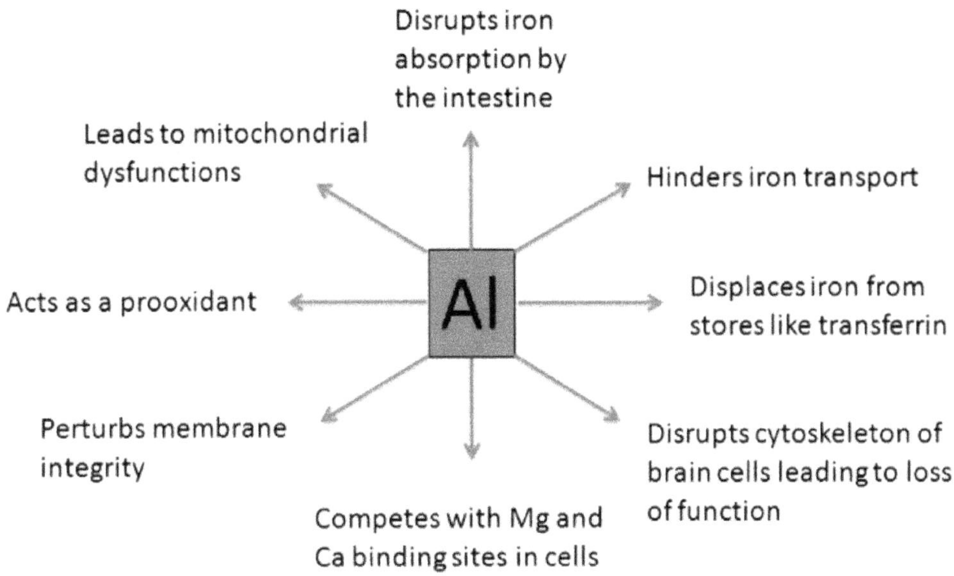


Fig. 2. Al has various toxic effects on cellular processes, notably on Fe homeostasis.

Al plays an important role in the immune response by being a trigger of the inflammatory cascade. For this reason, Al salts are administered with vaccines and act as adjuvants. Al stimulates an inflammatory response which promotes the effectiveness of the immune system to respond to the vaccine and acquire immunity. The effect of Al toxicity on fatty acid metabolism is just starting to emerge. The modulation of energy metabolism at the mitochondrial level caused by this metal leads to an accumulation of triglycerides and an increase in fat deposits. In addition, there is a marked increase in very low density lipoprotein (VLDL) secretion caused by Al toxicity. This phenomenon is directly related to the accumulation of fatty tissue observed during obesity. The information presented in this chapter delineates the molecular mechanism of Al toxicity and thus affords insights into the implication of this metal in dysfunctional Fe homeostasis, inflammation, obesity and anemia.

## 4. Aluminum and the environment

Aluminum is an environmentally abundant element that has a wide variety of uses and industrial applications. Industrialization and anthropogenic activities have led to a further increase in bioavailable Al. Exposure to this non-redox active metal occurs in daily life where the major sources of exposure for the average individual are diet and drinking water. Additional aluminum exposure can be brought upon by certain medications such as antacids, while individuals can also be subjected to high Al levels due to occupational exposure from breathing in contaminated air. Although drinking water was first thought to be the main delivery method of Al to the body, it was shown that 95% of the exposure to the element occurs through diet whereas the soluble water form of Al only accounts for 1-2%. The average human Al intake ranges between a total of 4 to 9 mg/day. Although small, these values are easily influenced by factors such as the type of food consumed in one's diet, the country/place of residence, one's age and sex. Alternate sources contribute to the amount of Al an individual is subjected to (**Table 1**), with antacids representing a significant dose, as they are generally composed of aluminum hydroxide salts (Lopez *et al,* 2002; *et al,* 2006; Yokel *et al,* 2008b).

| Source | Al exposure contribution |
|---|---|
| Antacids | 5000000 µg/day |
| Environmental air inhalation | 4-20 µg/day |
| Industrial air inhalation | 25000 µg/day |
| Antiperspirants | 70000 µg/day |
| Cigarettes | 500-2000 µg/cigarette |
| Vaccines | 1-8 µg/day |
| Allergy immunotherapy | 7-40 µg/day |

Table 1. Various sources of Al and their average Al exposure contribution (Yokel *et al,* 2008b).

The use of aluminum salts is not restricted to stomach acidity neutralizing agents, but are rather quite frequently used in the food industry. Sodium aluminum phosphates (SALPs) are generally recognized as safe (GRAS) FDA-approved food additives that contribute the most important source of Al to the diet. Basic SALP ($Na_8Al_2(OH_2)((PO)_4)_4$) is one of the many emulsifying salts added to processed cheese, cheese food and cheese spread. This salt is added to cheese since it reacts with proteins resulting in modifications that produce a smooth, uniform film around each fat droplet, preventing separation and bleeding of fat from cheese. Ultimately this allows for a soft texture, easy melting characteristics and desirable slicing properties. The FDA approves up to 3% concentrations of basic SALP. Unprocessed cheese has been shown to have an Al concentration of < 10 mg Al/kg. In contrast the aluminum levels in processed cheese can range from 320-1440 mg Al/kg. Cheese is not the only processed food containing higher levels of aluminum. Both fruit juices and soft drinks contain aluminum levels ranging from 49.3 to 1144.6 µg/l in fruit juices and from 44.6 to 1053.3 µg/l in soft drinks respectively (Lopez *et al,* 2002). The benefits of processed foods include a longer shelf life, change in taste and texture, minimal meal preparation and lower cost. The increased consumption of processed food has been shown to be related to the rise in obesity rates in industrialized nations for many reasons including the high simple sugar levels. Perhaps the high levels of Al found in processed food are amplifying the risk of obesity that is associated with food processing (**Figure 3**) (Yokel *et al,* 2008a; 2008b; 2006).

The food processing industry is responsible for an increase in bioavailable Al, however it is not working alone. Industrialization has led to a higher frequency of acid rain which in turn lowers the pH in soil. Consequently, Al is leaching into groundwater thus causing the bioaccumulation of this toxic metal in various non-processed food such as vegetation and livestock. Once consumed, these sources increase the accumulation of aluminum in the body. Various fresh food sources contain relatively high levels of Al, as shown in **Table 2.**

| Food Group | Mean Al concentration (mg/kg of fresh weight) | Food Group | Mean Al concentration (mg/kg of fresh weight) |
|---|---|---|---|
| Bread | 6.6 | Potatoes | 0.9 |
| Poultry | 0.3 | Canned vegetables | 0.97 |
| Fish | 6.1 | Fresh fruit | 0.29 |
| Oils & fats | 1.1 | Fruit products | 0.82 |
| Eggs | 0.14 | Milk | 0.07 |
| Green vegetables | 3.1 | Nuts | 4.0 |

Table 2. Occurrence of Al in food according to the Food Standards Agency, United Kingdom.

Aluminum toxicity has been extensively studied for its implication in neurodegenerative diseases such as Alzheimer's disease (AD) and multiple sclerosis (MS). The brain is an important Al accumulating organ, yet Al can also concentrate more severely in other tissues of the human body (**Figure 4**) (Gomez *et al,* 2008; Rondeau *et al, 2008*). Nonetheless, aluminum salts such as aluminum hydroxides and aluminum phosphates are routinely used in medical practices as the only licensed adjuvants in vaccines. Aluminum adjuvants, referred to as "alum", are proven effective in stimulating an immune response towards the vaccine being administered. However, the mode of action remains unclear. It is generally accepted that the alum particles adhere to the surface of the antigen (Ag), forming an Ag deposit at the injection site. This process maximizes the interaction time between the Ag and the immune system's antigen presenting cells (APCs) which initiate a response cascade (**Figure 4**). Alum have also been shown to act on the immune system's compliment system of the immune machinery, along with causing the formation of granulomas containing antibody (Ab)-producing cells and other immune response mediators. Recent studies have illustrated the ability of alum to stimulate the release of pro-inflammatory cytokines such as IL-1β and IL-18 that have pleiotropic functions, including adjuvant capacity. Although several mechanisms are proposed (**Figure 5**), the exact way by which aluminum promotes inflammation has yet to be solved (Aimanianda *et al,* 2009; HogenEsch, 2002; Li *et al,* 2008). Nonetheless, Al is an active instigator of inflammation (Campbell *et al,* 2002). Regardless of the source of Al the reality remains that the element is bioavailable and at significant concentrations. For this reason, the toxic effects of Al are of interest to the human population and the study of these effects could help explain Al-associated dysfunctions such as neurodegenerative diseases, obesity and chronic inflammation. More importantly, the link between these disease states, aluminum toxicity and anemia is beginning to be understood.

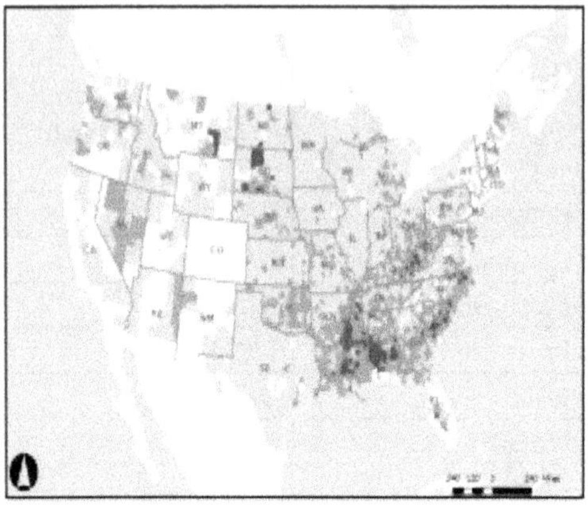

A)

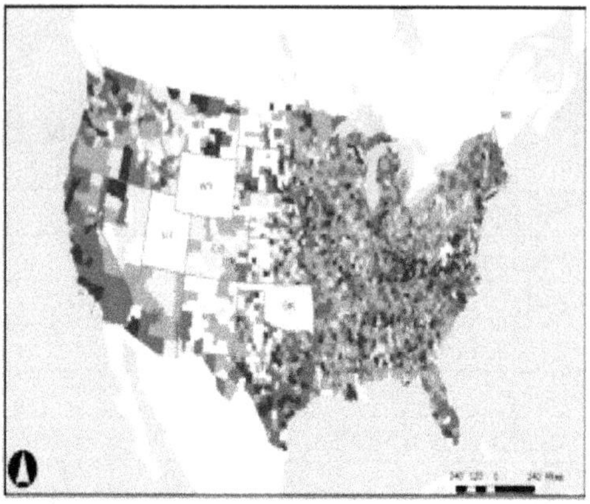

B)

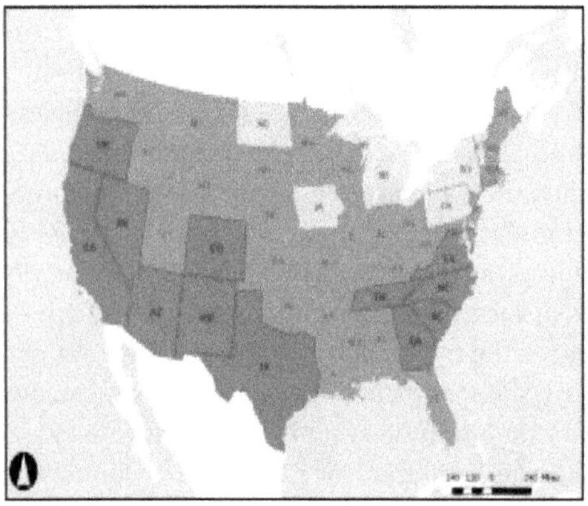

C)

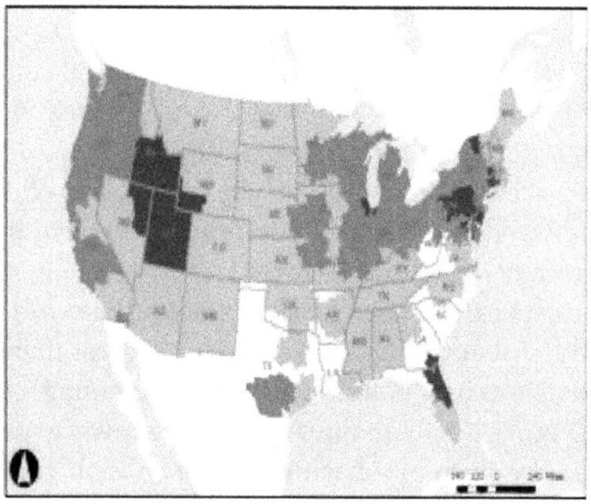

D)

Fig. 3. These maps illustrate the link between processed food (commonly served in the fast food industry or found in prepared meals) and the obesity epidemic in the United-States. **A) Adult obesity rate in 2007**. Grey (12.5% - 25%). Light blue (25.1% - 30%). Blue (30.1% - 35%). Dark blue (35.1% - 43.5%); **B) Low-income preschool obesity rate in 2008**. Light pink (2.1% - 10%). Pink (10.1% - 14%). Red (14.1% - 18%). Dark red (18.1% - 39.7%); **C) Fast food expenditure per capita in 2007**. Light pink ($402.10 - $500.00). Pink ($500.01 - $700.00). Red ($700.01 - $1,043.86). **D) Prepared food (lbs) per capita in 2006**. Grey (229 - 280lbs). Light green (281 - 300lbs). Green (301 - 320lbs). Dark green (321-374lbs). (Centers for Disease Control and Prevention).

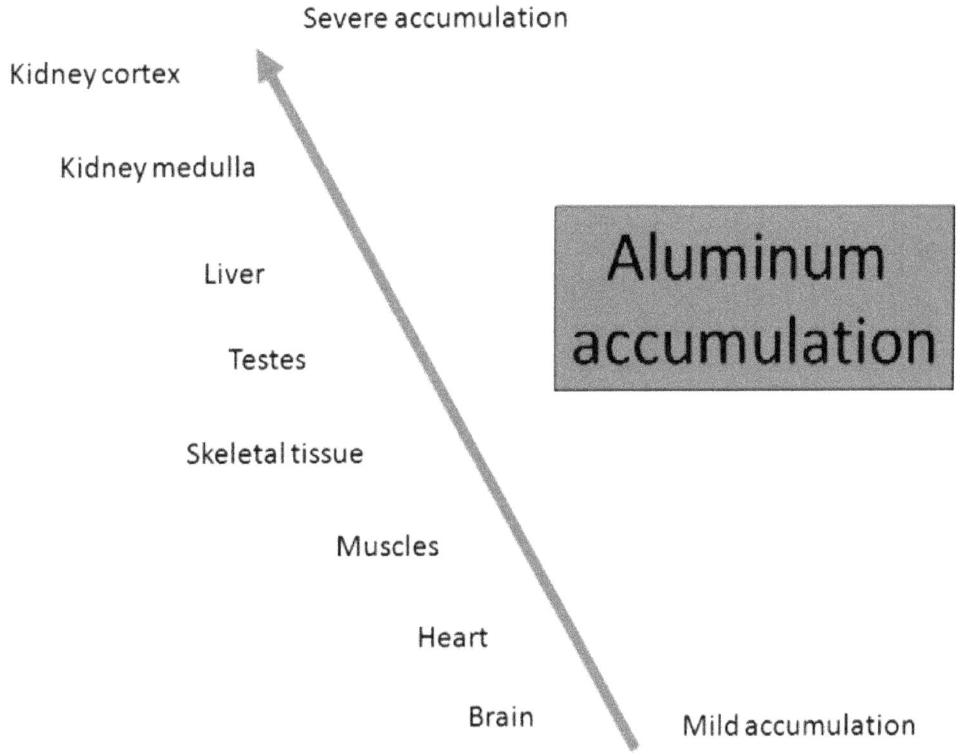


Fig. 4. The hierarchy of Al accumulation in the various tissues of the human body. Although the brain is an important location for Al accumulation, there are many other organs that accumulate much greater concentrations of Al (Ward *et al,* 2001).

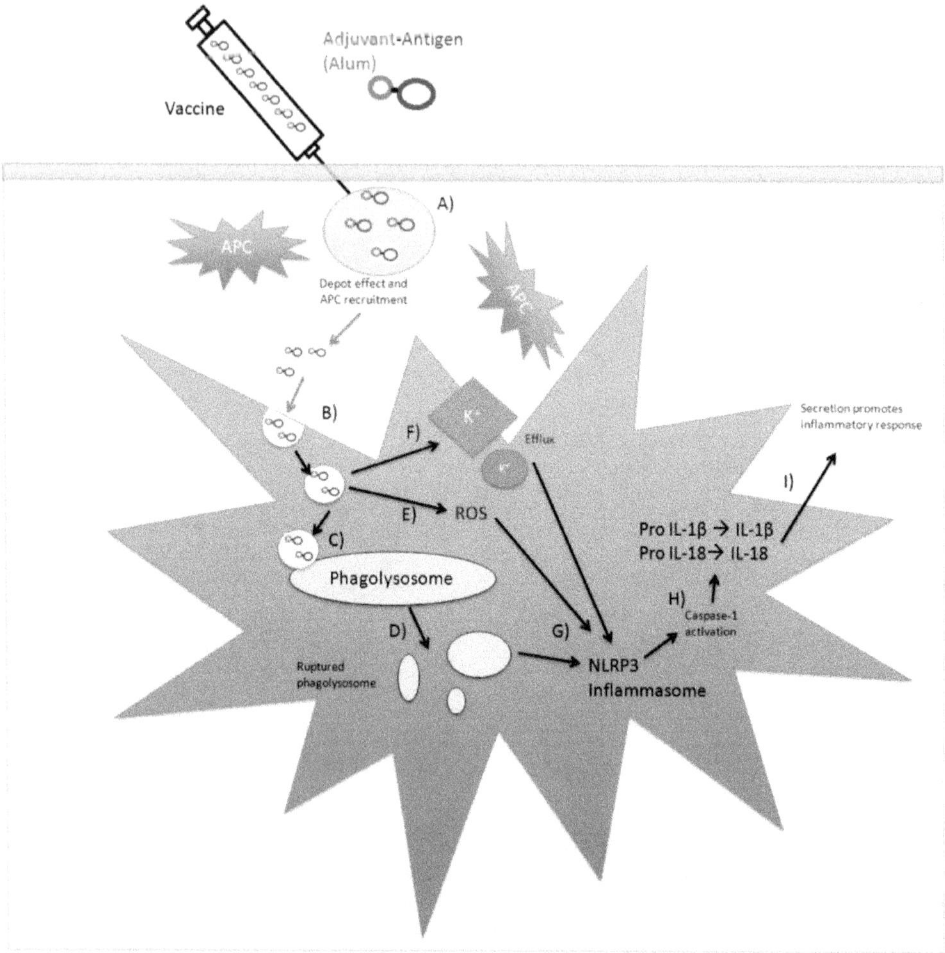


Fig. 5. Proposed mechanism of action for Al being used as an adjuvant A) As a vaccine is injected into the skin, the alum adjuvant bound to the Ag form a deposit at the injection site. This promotes APC recruitment and maximizes the interaction between the Ag and the immune system's cells. B) The innate immune system cells intake the Alum salts. C) The engulfed adjuvants interact with the phagolysosome of the APCs. D) Intereaction with the Alum salts leads to rupture of the phagolysosomes and the release of activators of NLRP3 inflammasome (not shown in image). E) Al within the cell promotes the formation of ROS which also activates the NLRP3 inflammasome. F) The Alum salts also lead to potassium ($K^+$) efflux, thus further activating the NLRP3 inflammasome. G) The NLRP3 inflammasome, an intracellular innate immune response system, senses the K+ efflux, the ROS formation and the lysosomal damage and activates caspase-1. H) Caspase-1 processes pro-IL-1β and pro-IL-18 into IL-1β and IL-18, respectively, resulting in the release of these mature cytokines (Modified from Aimanianda *et al,* 2009; HogenEsch, 2002; Li, 2008).

## 5. Aluminum and dyslipidemia: A metabolic perspective

Metal toxicity has been linked to cancers, neurological disorders, nephrological complications and pulmonary diseases. Environmental pollution is a growing concern in today's society causing the increased bioavailability of metals that pose a serious threat to living organisms. Toxic elements like mercury (Hg) and lead (Pb) have been extensively studied. While Hg has been shown to react with critical thiol moieties and impede normal immunological responses and mental cognition, Pb dislocates the essential zinc (Zn) found in enzymes responsible for heme production. Ultimately these toxic metals lead to various diseases (Mailloux *et al*, 2007b). The molecular aspects of Al toxicity have begun to emerge. It has been reported that a variety of ion channels are inactivated by micromolar quantities of Al, subsequently disrupting biological membranes. In addition, Al has an ionic radius that resembles that of magnesium (Mg), which leads to its interaction with naturally-occurring Mg-dependent enzymes. Al has also been shown to perturb cytoskeletal structure of astrocytoma cells causing a disruption of their shape and hence their biological function. Exposure to Al, however, is primarily characterized by the disruption of Fe homeostasis which in turn interferes with essential biochemical processes that are dependent on this metal (Lemire *et al*, 2009; Mailloux *et al*, 2011).

Fe is an important cofactor of many enzymes and a structural component of proteins. It is redox-active and therefore can act as an electron acceptor and donor, a critical attribute for its involvement in metabolic processes. Notably, Fe is required for protein components such as iron-sulfur clusters (Fe-S clusters) and hemes. When Al interacts with these constituents, it mimics the Fe atoms forcing the liberation of the transition metal and its subsequent intracellular accumulation. Free Fe poses a threat to cells as it leads to the formation of reactive oxygen species (ROS) through Fenton chemistry (figure 6). The Al-triggered oxidative environment enhances the toxic effect of the trivalent metal. Together, Al and its concomitant ROS greatly affect cellular metabolism. Metabolism is the foundation of any biological system and metabolic processes allow organisms to react and adapt to intracellular and extracellular fluctuations. It enables the maintenance of an environment suitable for the production and storage of energy and for cellular growth (Kim *et al*, 2007; Mailloux *et al*, 2011; Vergara *et al*, 2008).

The importance of Fe as a cofactor in metabolic processes is made evident in energy metabolism. The redox active metal is essential for the ATP-producing machinery in the mitochondria of eukaryotes. The central metabolic pathway known as the tricarboxylic acid cycle (TCA cycle), along with the electron transport chain (ETC) which is responsible for oxidative phosphorylation, are composed of enzymes that depend on Fe for proper functioning. For example, the Fe-containing enzyme aconitase (ACN) is considered the "gatekeeper" to the TCA cycle. ACN are Fe-S cluster proteins that catalyze the reversible isomerization of citrate to isocitrate. The enzymatically active form of the ACN Fe-S clusters are predominantly [4Fe-4S]. In mammalian systems, ACN with [3Fe-4S] clusters play an alternate role, acting as an oxygen sensor therefore aiding in energy homeostasis. This form of the enzyme serves as a regulatory protein that controls the stability and translation of messenger RNAs (mRNAs) encoding proteins involved in iron and energy homeostasis. The regulatory ACN is referred to as iron-responsive protein, which binds to iron-responsible elements localized in the RNA-stem loop (figure 7). This action leads to the modulation of gene expression (Middaugh *et al*, 2005).

It has been demonstrated that cells exposed to Al have severely impeded mitochondrial functions. Most importantly, these cells appear to have limited ATP production due to diminished TCA cycle and oxidative phosphorylation activity. As the trivalent metal Al displaces Fe in key enzymes of the TCA cycle such as ACN, fumarase (FUM) along with the Fe found in enzymes of the ETC (notably succinate dehydrogenase (SDH) and cytochrome C oxidase (Cyt c ox)), an evident shift in metabolism occurs as these enzymes become inactive. Impairment of ACN by Al triggers a decrease in NADH production by the TCA cycle. NADH is a reducing equivalent essential for oxidative phosphorylation, thus as the levels of NADH diminish and Al displaces Fe from ETC enzymes, mitochondrial production of ATP is hindered (figure 8). This perturbation in oxidative phosphorylation is advantageous during Al exposure since the ETC is a known endogenous ROS generator. Inefficient electron transport through the chain leads to the univalent reduction of oxygen, a process that creates free radical species that exacerbates the toxic effect of Al. It is in a cell's favor to maintain redox homeostasis by limiting its own production of oxidative species during Al-stressed conditions. In order to meet its energy demands, Al-stressed cells evoke the anaerobic respiratory machinery to produce ATP, notably substrate level phosphorylation (SLP) (Mailloux *et al*, 2011; 2007a; 2007b; Middaugh *et al*, 2005; Lemire *et al*, 2011a).

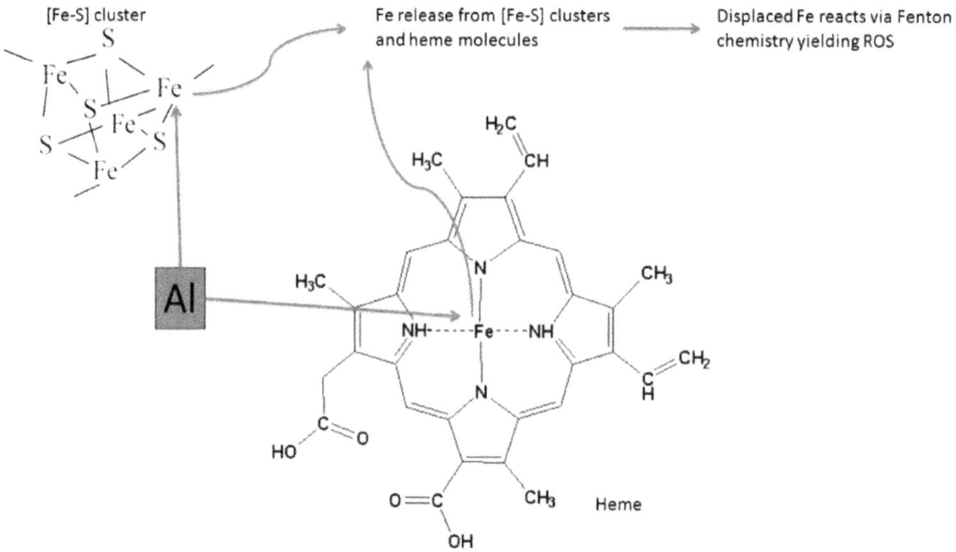


Fig. 6. Al displaces the Fe in biological molecules such as heme and [Fe-S] clusters. The presence of free Fe leads to the formation of ROS.

Al can severely impede mitochondrial function, however the consequences of its effects are not limited to a decrease in energy production. The disruption of oxidative phosphorylation by the trivalent metal evokes not only a limited supply of ATP but also an increased lipid production. This phenomenon is common in obese individuals who tend to experience diminished levels of ATP and an accumulation of fatty tissue. In human liver cells, it has been demonstrated that dyslipidemia is due to the ability of Al to perturb iron metabolism and promote oxidative stress. By displacing Fe in metabolically active enzymes, Al favors a hypoxic environment and stimulates lipogenesis. Lipogenesis is the series of chemical reactions leading to the carboxylation and subsequent polymerization of acetyl CoA through the use of the anabolic nucleotide NADPH. Under Al toxicity, pivotal enzymes in the lipid production pathway of hepatocytes show an increase in activity. First, acetyl-CoA carboxylase (ACC) is up-regulated under ROS and Al-stress conditions. This enzyme is responsible for the production of malonyl-CoA, an inhibitor of the transport of lipids into the mitochondria and an activator of lipogenesis. Second, glycerol-3-phosphate dehydrogenase (G3PDH) diverts trioses from glycolysis into the lipid generating machinery by producing glycerol, the backbone of triglycerides. Finally, the much-needed supply of NADPH for lipogenesis during Al toxicity is ensured by an ensemble of enzymes including glucose-6-phosphate dehydrogenase (G6PDH), 6-phosphogluconate dehydrogenase (6PGDH), malic enzyme (ME), $NADP^+$-dependent glutamate dehydrogenase (GDH), NAD kinase (NADK) and $NADP^+$-dependent isocitrate dehydrogenase (IDH) (**Figure 9**). Since Al disrupts Fe homeostasis, rendering the TCA cycle and oxidative phosphorylation inactive, carbon sources coming from upstream metabolism are funneled towards the production of fatty acids. Al toxicity instigates the metabolic shift from NADH production to the synthesis of the anabolic reducing agent and antioxidant, NADPH (**Figure 10**) (Mailloux *et al*, 2011; 2007b; Lemire *et al*, 2008).

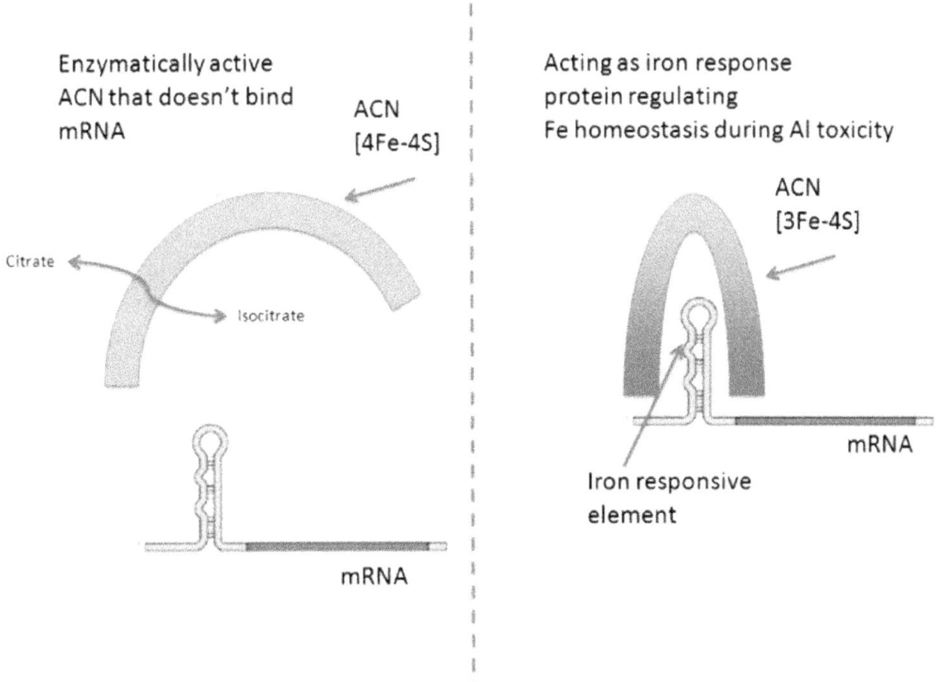


Fig. 7. ACN is recognized as the "gatekeeper" to the TCA cycle. When the [4Fe-4S] cluster is intact, the protein is enzymatically active. However under conditions that favor the [3Fe-4S] form of the enzyme, such as Fe starvation, Al toxicity and oxidative stress, the protein is no longer metabolically active. ACN [3Fe-4S] acts as the Fe response protein which regulates Fe homeostasis at the gene expression level by binding to the Fe responsive element in mRNA coding for various genes involved in Fe metabolism.

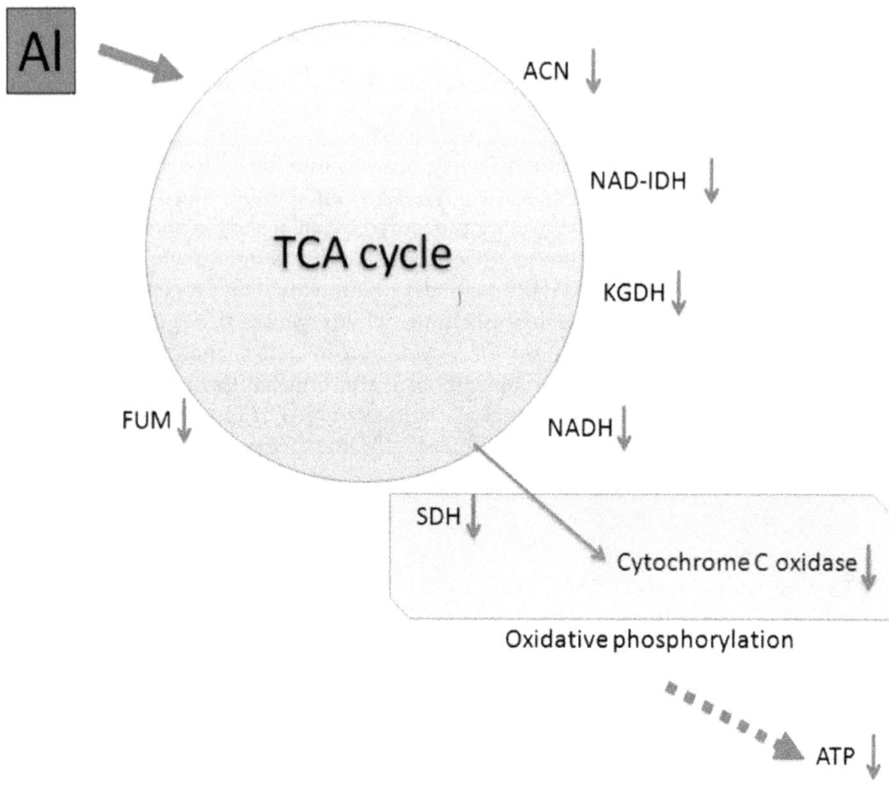


Fig. 8. Al toxicity leads to a disruption of the central metabolic pathways known as the TCA cycle. ACN, IDH (NAD-dependent), KGDH and FUM are all hindered under Al stress. This limits the production of NADH and therefore oxidative phosphorylation lacks the substrate for ATP production. Furthermore, the activity of the ETC enzymes SDH and Cyt C oxidase is perturbed under Al toxicity.

The Al-triggered increase in lipogenesis in liver cells has been recently demonstrated. When cultured hepatocytes are stressed with Al, there is a marked increase in lipoproteins and cholesterol levels in comparison to non-stressed cultures. ApoB-100 is a glycoprotein that plays a critical role in the formation of very low density lipoproteins (VLDL) and low density lipoproteins (LDL). As apoB-100 accumulates, insoluble intracellular aggregates form leading to their co-translational or post-translational degradation. However, nascent apoB-100 is stabilized by the presence of lipids, a process mediated by the microsomal triglyceride transfer protein (MTP), ultimately leading to the formation of VLDL and LDL. Al leads to the increased lipid production needed to stabilize apoB-100, allowing the maturation of VLDL molecules which are subsequently excreted out of the cell. Once out of the cells VLDL molecules can be transported to different organs via a receptor-mediated process. The concentration of the apoB-100 glycoprotein in the spent media of cultured liver cells is directly proportional to the concentration of Al utilized, thus showing direct evidence of the link between Al toxicity, lipogenesis and fatty acid accumulation. What is of further interest is the fact that the carbon source used to grow the cultured cells has an effect on the concentration of lipids accumulated and the monosaccharide D-fructose, a common product in processed food and a compound chemically linked to cancer development and obesity, lead to enhanced VLDL secretion in the Al-stressed hepatocytes (figure 9) (Mailloux *et al, 2007b).*

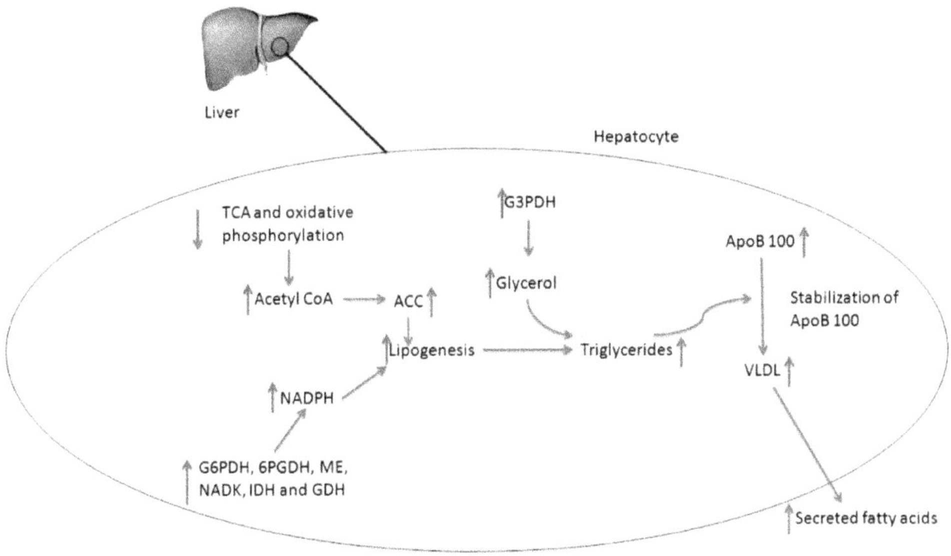


Fig. 9. Al toxicity leads to an increase in lipogenesis which can be observed by the increased levels of VLDL excreted by Al-stressed hepatocytes. As Al disables the TCA cycle and oxidative phosphorylation, there is an accumulation of acetyl-CoA, an important cofactor for lipogensis. Al also induces an increase in NADPH production through IDH and G6PDH along with an increase in glycerol synthesis, two essential substrates for triglyceride synthesis. The elevated levels of lipids in the cell stabilized the glycoprotein ApoB-100, leading to the formation and secretion of VLDL (Mailloux *et al,* 2007b).

The accumulation of lipids during Al exposure is partially due to the increased lipogenesis brought upon by a hindered mitochondrial TCA cycle and ETC. However, the Al stressed cells are also unable to degrade lipids, a phenomenon which also contributes to the accumulation of fatty acids. L-Carnitine is a non-essential amino acid involved in the transport of fatty acid-derived acyl groups into the mitochondria, a key step in the lipid degradation process known as β-oxidation. During Al-stressed conditions, L-carnitine levels have been shown to decrease in both liver and brain cells. The synthesis of L-carnitine is a multistep enzymatic process that requires the participation of lysine, methionine and α-ketoglutarate (KG). The decrease in L-carnitine levels appear to be triggered by the diminished activity and expression of two key enzymes involved in its synthesis, namely γ-butyrobetainealdehyde dehydrogenase (BADH) and butyrobetaine dioxygenase (BBDOX) (Lemire *et al,* 2011b). Along with the downregulated enzymes, the impeded TCA cycle blocks the steady supply of KG needed for L-carnitine synthesis. Al-toxicity is associated with the formation of ROS and under oxidative stress cells undergo metabolic reconfigurations. As previously mentioned the TCA cycle is modulated during Al exposure and therefore also during oxidative stress. An important aspect of this metabolic adaptation is the downregulation of KG dehydrogenase (KGDH). This enzyme is particularly sensitive to ROS due to the reactivity of its covalently bound lipoic acid cofactor with oxidizing species. It has been shown that oxidation products in the lipid membranes can go on to react with membrane bound proteins. For example the aldehydic product of lipid peroxidation, 4-hydroxy-2-nonenal (HNE), reacts with the lipoic acid of KGDH, leading to the disruption of enzyme activity. The advantage of KGDH downregulation is the accumulation of the potent antioxidant KG. Like other ketoacids such as pyruvate and oxaloacetate, KG reacts with and nullifies ROS releasing succinate (KG's respective product) and $CO_2$, by a process referred to as non-enzymatic decarboxylation. As KG is being syphoned towards ROS sequestration, L-carnitine synthesis decreases due to a lack of this pivotal cofactor (**Figure 11**) (Lemire *et al*, 2011b).

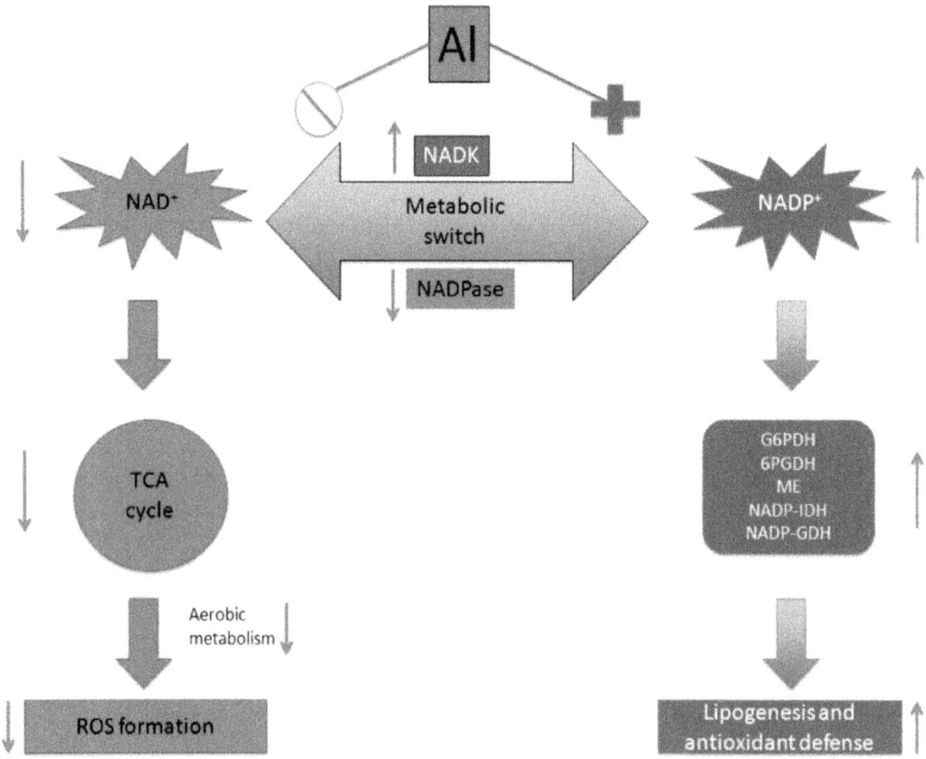


Fig. 10. Al leads to decreased levels of $NAD^+$ through the inhibition of the TCA cycle. Under Al toxicity, aerobic metabolism comes to a halt in order to prevent further ROS formation by endogenous sources such as the electron transport chain in the mitochondria. Al triggers the metabolic shift gated by NADK towards $NADP^+$ production. This substrate is subsequently reduced by various enzymes to produce NADPH. This last compound is essential in antioxidant defense and just as importantly, for lipogenesis (Mailloux *et al, 2007b).*

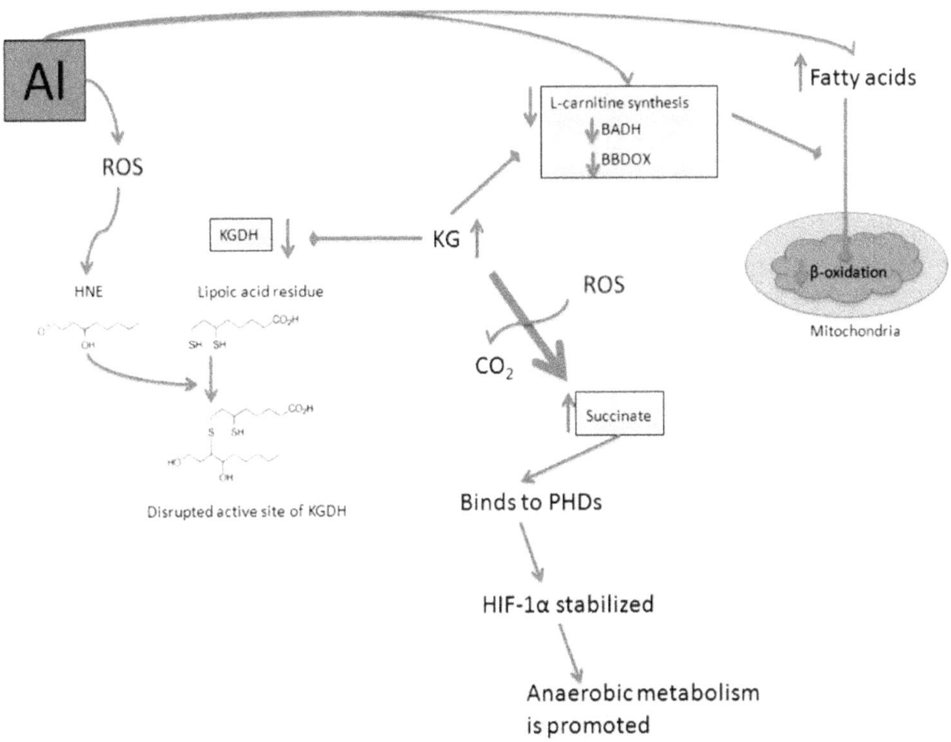


Fig. 11. Al leads to the formation of ROS, which ultimately disrupts KGDH activity (through interactions with the lipoic acid residue in the enzyme's active site). The resulting KG is accumulated in the cell and funneled towards ROS scavenging yielding an accumulation of succinate. Elevated levels of succinate leads to the stabilization of the transcription factor HIF-1α leading to the promotion of anaerobic metabolism. The supply of KG is utilized for sequestration of ROS and L-carnitine synthesis is hindered. Hence, there is decreased expression of key enzymes in the synthesis pathway. This amino acid is responsible for fatty acid transport into the mitochondria for degradation (β-oxidation) and so accumulation of lipids caused by Al is further enabled by a decrease in fatty acid catabolism (Lemire *et al*, 2011b).

The concomitant production of succinate during ROS scavenging by KG is a key contributor to the switch to anaerobic respiration. This adaptive response is initiated by the heterodimeric transcription factor HIF-1. HIF-1 consists of HIF-1α, HIF-2α and HIF-1β subunits. HIF-1α is extremely sensitive to oxygen tension and, under normoxic conditions (when the ETC can function properly), HIF-1α is quickly degraded by prolyl hydroxylases (PHDs) and the ubiquitin-proteosomal degradation pathway. When the proline residues undergo hydroxylation (via PHD), HIF-1α is targeted for degradation by the proteosome. Succinate is known to perturb substrate binding sites in PHD thus interfering with the degradation of HIF-1α. As Al and ROS lead to an accumulation of succinate due to an altered TCA cycle, HIF-1α is stabilized and anaerobic metabolism is promoted (Mailloux *et al*, 2009; 2007a; 2006; Peyssonnaux *et al*, 2007).

## 6. Aluminum: The missing link between obesity, chronic inflammation and anemia

It is well established that Al disrupts Fe homeostasis. As exposure to this toxin leads to decreased absorption of Fe in the intestine, hinders its transport in the serum, and displaces Fe by binding to transferrin, the involvement of Al in anemia is evident. In a similar fashion to insulin resistance in diabetic individuals, which leads to high levels of glucose in the serum and low intracellular glucose concentrations, Al toxicity causes a disproportionate ratio of serum and cellular Fe levels. When the body experiences Al toxicity, Fe is displaced and released into the bloodstream. This increase in serum Fe tricks the body into thinking there is an excess of Fe, which would lead to limited Fe uptake and release (regulated by hepcidin), when in fact the Al exposed cells are in an anemic state (Del Giudice *et al*, 2009). However, the effects of Al-altered Fe metabolism extend beyond these aforementioned phenomena. As described in the previous section, Al displaces Fe from important enzymatically active proteins leading to a disruption of metabolic processes. This event results in a dysfunctional mitochondria geared towards lipogenesis rather than energy production. An excess fat accumulation and an increase in adipose tissue evoked by Al toxicity can lead to obesity (Mailloux *et al*, 2011). Obese individuals are faced with many obstacles including being at greater risk for cardiovascular diseases, diabetes, obstructive sleep apnea, certain cancers and osteoarthritis (Ausk *et al*, 2008). One of the hallmarks of obesity is chronic inflammation. Inflammation associated with obesity may be linked to Al exposure, a well known and readily used adjuvant. There exists a correlation between unhealthy eating habits and obesity and so an increased intake of processed and "fast" foods by an individual would suggest an increased exposure to Al. This Al could be responsible for the chronic inflammatory response observed in obese patients.

Fe release from various proteins including the [Fe-S] clusters and hemes of enzymes is facilitated by Al. This would cause an increase in free Fe in the body, an event which is hazardous to an organism due to potential ROS formation and promotion of pathogen infection. The body's response to increase Fe levels is the secretion of the hormonal peptide hepcidin. Secreted by the liver and adipose tissues, this peptide limits absorption of Fe by the intestine and release from stores. When gene deletions for hepcidin were performed in mice, unregulated hyperabsorption of Fe in the intestine and unregulated discharge of Fe from spleen macrophages was observed. Overexpression of the hepcidin gene in the mice led to Fe deficiencies and death. It is therefore obvious that this peptide is the regulator of Fe homeostasis.

As an organism is exposed to Al, multiple effects can be observed. The dysfunctional mitochondria leads to increased intracellular lipid accumulation. Obesity sets in and chronic inflammation occurs. Fe homeostasis is disrupted. Together, these events may favor an increase in hepcidin levels in the serum which would limit further absorption of Fe, ultimately causing Al-induced anemia (figure 12) (Ganz, 2003). As Al is associated with ROS toxicity and metabolic shifts leading to the accumulation of the ketoacid antioxidants, such as KG and pyruvate, perhaps dietary supplementation with these potent scavengers might offset the effects of the metal toxin.

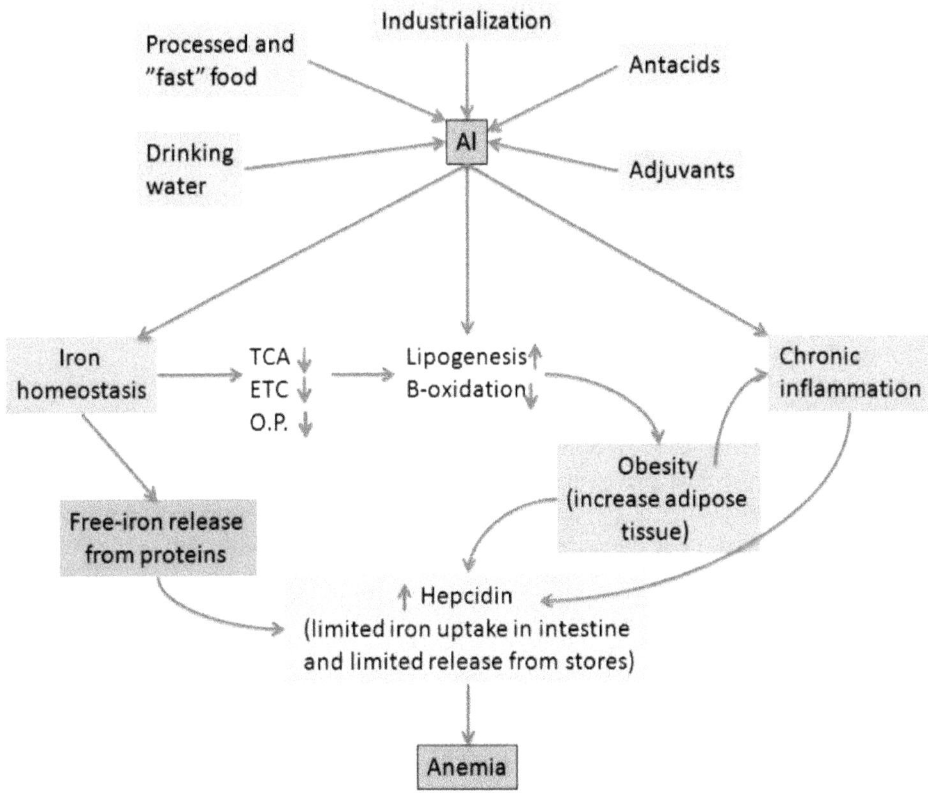


Fig. 12. A global outlook on the implications of Al toxicity leading to disruption of Fe homeostasis, increased lipogenesis and induction of chronic inflammation. Ultimately Al causes the release of Fe into the bloodstream which can signal the secretion of hepcidin by the liver and adipose tissue leading to the limited Fe uptake in the intestine and limited release from cellular stores. Al, by mimicking Fe, tricks the body into thinking it has an overload of the redox active metal and the body response leads to an Al induced anemic state.

## 7. The therapeutic potential of α-ketoacids

An important factor contributing to Al toxicity is its ability to generate an oxidative environment within the cell. As Al displaces Fe, this redox-active element can participate in ROS-generating reactions leading to the formation of toxic moieties such as hydrogen peroxide ($H_2O_2$), superoxide ($O_2\cdot^-$) and the hydroxyl radical ($\cdot OH$). Due to the nature of our oxygen-rich environment, cells are constantly challenged with the burden of oxidative stress. Situations such as Al toxicity worsen the oxidative load that aerobic organisms are exposed to. Hence, organisms possess a battery of antioxidant systems that maintain the redox balance of their cells. With the classical antioxidants molecules such as glutathione

(GSH), ascorbic acid (AA) and vitamin E being extensively studied, the importance of α-ketoacids as ROS scavengers has begun to emerge.

α-Ketoacids are organic compounds that contain a carboxylic acid group adjacent to a ketone group. They play an essential role in cellular metabolism as intermediates in many pathways including the TCA cycle and glycolysis. Examples of biologically relevant α-ketoacids include pyruvate, α-ketoglutarate, oxaloacetate and glyoxylate. The antioxidant potential of these substrates has been demonstrated in a variety of ways. For example, in the soil microbe *Pseudomonas fluorescens* the α-ketoacids KG and pyruvate are readily accumulated for ROS scavenging in conditions of oxidative stress induced by exogenous $H_2O_2$, menadione (a $O_2^{\cdot-}$ generator), and Al (Mailloux *et al,* 2008). Similarly, metabolic adaptations occur in cultured human hepatocytes and astrocytes leading to the accumulation of these α-ketoacids when the cells are exposed to Al and other oxidizing agents (Lemire *et al,* 2011, Mailloux *et al,* 2011).

In a clinical setting, numerous studies have shown the benefits of α-ketoacid supplementation in an effort to prevent or rectify oxidative damage. An area of this research includes the prevention of cataract formation by pyruvate. Cataracts cause the clouding that develops in the crystalline lens of the eye, which can vary from a slight or complete degree of opacity and obstruction of the passage of light. Cataract formation has been linked to diabetes, hypertension and the over-exposure to UV-radiation. Although treatment with surgery and replacement with synthetic implants are options, there is a push for the development of pharmacological means of cataract prevention, which would reduce invasiveness and cause less secondary effects. The UV-radiation hypothesis of cataract formation states that photons penetrate through to the cornea and subsequently cause the generation of photochemically derived ROS in the aqueous humour and lens of the eye. Fittingly, cataract formation is accompanied by many signs of oxidative stress such as excessive protein glycation and lipid peroxidation, depletion of GSH and a decrease in ATP levels. *In vitro* incubation of mice and rat eye lens with pyruvate demonstrated the beneficial effect of this α-ketoacid in preventing cataract formation by scavenging ROS. These studies demonstrate the therapeutic potential of pyruvate in offsetting the cataractogenesis effects of solar radiation and other factors that act via ROS toxicity (Hegde, 2007, Hegde, 2005).

The use of α-ketoacids in the detoxification of ROS has been shown in many other cases. In numerous brain pathologies such as neurodegenerative diseases or in acute injuries such as ischemia or trauma, $H_2O_2$ is a suspected culprit in the development of neuropathogenesis. A study by Desagher *et al.* examined the ability of pyruvate to improve the survival of cultured striatal neurons exposed to oxidative agents. Pyruvate protected neurons against both $H_2O_2$ added to the external medium and $O_2^{\cdot-}$ endogenously produced through the redox cycling agent menadione. The neuroprotective effect of pyruvate appeared to result from the ability of the α-ketoacid to undergo non-enzymatic decarboxylation in the presence of ROS. In addition, several other α-ketoacids including α-ketobutyrate, which is not an energy substrate, also provided the neuroprotective effect of pyruvate. This study also showed that optimal neuroprotection was achieved with relatively low concentrations of pyruvate (>1mM) and that due to its low toxicity and its capacity to cross the blood-brain barrier, this α-ketoacid opens a new therapeutic perspective in ROS associated-brain pathologies (Desagher, 1997).

The advantages of α-ketoacid supplementation for the cardiovascular system have been demonstrated in numerous settings including cardiopulmonary bypass surgery, cardiopulmonary resuscitation, myocardial stunning, and cardiac failure. An important factor in these situations includes the trauma brought upon by myocardial ischemia. As the muscles of the heart are re-oxygenated after a prolonged anaerobic period, the tissue is faced with a depleted energy supply and a massive burst of ROS formation. Therapy with pyruvate has been shown to decrease the damage caused to the ischemic myocardium after reperfusion (Mallet *et al.*, 2005).

The clinical use of α-ketoacids along with their natural occurrence as an antioxidant shows promise of a new line of therapeutic drugs against a wide variety of diseases and dysfunctions. Since Al toxicity is linked to disease states such as obesity, chronic inflammation and anemia, α-ketoacids supplementation may perhaps offer a treatment for the effects of this ROS-forming metal toxin.

## 8. Acknowledgments

Research in our laboratory is funded by Laurentian University, Industry Canada and NATO. Adam Bignucolo is a recipient of the OGSST TEMBEC Scholarship. Joseph Lemire is a recipient of the Alexander Graham Bell Doctoral Canada Graduate Scholarship. Christopher Auger is a recipient of the Ontario Graduate Scholarship.

## 9. References

Aimanianda, V., Haensler, J., Lacroix-Desmazes, S., Kaveri, S.V., & Baryr, J. (2009) Novel cellular and molecular mechanisms of induction of immune responses by aluminum adjuvants. *Trends in Pharmacological Sciences.* Vol. 30(6): 287-295

Atkinson, M.A., & White, C.T. (2011) Hepcidin in anemia of chronic kidney disease: review for the pediatric nephrologist. *Pediatric Nephrology.* (in press)

Ausk, K.J., & Ioannou, G.N. (2008) Is obesity associated with anemia of chronic disease? A population-based study. *Obesity.* Vol. 16: 2356-2361

Barisani, D., Pelucchi, S., Mariani, R., Galimberti, S., Trombini, P., Fumagalli, D., Meneveri, R., Nemeth, E., Ganz, T., & Piperno, A. (2008) Hepcidin and iron-related gene expression in subjects with dysmetabolic hepatic iron overload. *Journal of Hepatology.* Vol. 49: 123-133

Campbell, A., Yang, E., Tsai-turton, M., & Bondy, S. (2002) Pro-inflammatory effects of aluminum in human glioblastoma cells. *Brain Research.* Vol. 933: 60-65

Choi, S-O., Cho, Y-S., Kim, H-L., & Park, J-W. (2007) ROS mediate the hypoxic repression of the *hepcidin* gene by inhibition C/EBPα and STAT-3. *Biochemical and Biophysical Research Communications.* Vol. 356: 312-317

Del Giudice, E.M., Santoro, N., Amato, A., Brienza, C., Calabro, P., Wiegerinck, E.T., Cirillo, G., Tartaglione, N., Grandone, A., Swinkels, D.W., & Perrone, L. (2009) Hepcidin in obese children as a potential mediator of the association between obesity and iron deficiency. *Journal of Clinical Endocrinology and Metabolism.* Vol. 94: 5102-5107

Desagher, S., Glowinski, J., & Prémont, J. (1997) Pyruvate protects neurons against hydrogen peroxide- induced toxicity. *Journal of Neuroscience.* Vol. 17(23): 9060–9067

Ganz, T. (2003) Hepcidin, a key regulator of iron metabolism and mediator of anemia of inflammation. *Blood.* Vol. 102(3): 783-788

Gomez, M., Esparza, J.L., Cabre, M., Garcia, M., & Domingo, J.L. (2008) Aluminum exposure through diet: metal levels in AβPP transgenis mice, a model for Alzheimer's disease. *Toxicology.* Vol. 249: 214-219

Hegde, K.R., Kovtun, S., & Varma, S.D. (2007) Induction of ultraviolet cataracts in vitro: prevention by pyruvate. *Journal of Ocular Pharmacology and Therapeutics.* Vol 23(5): 492-502

Hegde, K.R. & Varma, S.D. (2005) Prevention of cataract by pyruvate in experimentally diabetic mice. *Molecular and Cellular Biochemistry.* Vol. 269: 115–120

Hintze, K.J., Snow, D., Nabor, D., & Timbimboo, H. (2010) Adipocyte hypoxia increases hepatocyte hepcidin expression. *Biological Trace Element Research.* (in press)

HogenEsch, H. (2002) Mechanisms of stimulation of the immune response by aluminum adjuvants. *Vaccine.* Vol. 20: 534-539

Kim, Y., Olivi, L., Cheong, J.H., Maertens, A., & Bressler, J.P. (2007) Aluminum stimulate uptake of non- transferrin bound iron and transferrin bound iron in human glial cells. *Toxicology and Applied Pharmacology.* Vol 220: 349-356

Lee, P., Peng, H., Gelbart, T., Wang, L., & Beutler, E. (2005) Regulation of hepcidin transcription by interleukin-1 and interleukin-6. *PNAS.* Vol. 102(6): 1906-1910

Lemire, J., & Appanna, V. (2011a) Aluminum toxicity and astrocyte dysfunction: a metabolic link to neurological disorders. *Journal of Inorganic Biochemistry.* (in press)

Lemire, J., Mailloux, R.J., Darwich, R., Auger, C., & Appanna, V. (2011b) The disruption of L-carnitine metabolism by aluminum toxicity and oxidative stress promotes dyslipidemia in human astrocytic and hepatic cells. *Toxicology letters.* Vol. 203: 219-226

Lemire, J., Mailloux, R.J., Puiseux-Dao, S., & Appanna, V. (2009) Aluminum-induced defective mitochondrial metabolism perturbs cytoskeletal dynamics in human astrocytoma cells. *Journal of Neuroscience research.* Vol. 87: 1474-1483

Lemire, J., Kumar, P., Mailloux, R.J., Cossar, K., & Appanna, V. (2008) Metabolic adaptation and oxaloacetate homeostasis in *P.fluorescens* exposed to aluminum toxicity.

Li, H., Willingham, S.B., Ting, J., & Re, F. (2008) Cutting edge: inflammasome activation by alum and alum's adjuvant effect are mediated by NLRP3. *The Journal of Immunology.* Vol. 181: 17-21

Lopez, F.F., Cabrera, C., Lorenzo, M.L., & Lopez, M.C. (2002) Aluminum content of drinking waters, fruit juices and soft drinks: contribution on dietary intake. *The Science of the Total Environment.* Vol. 292: 205-213

Mailloux, R.J., Lemire, J., & Appanna, V. (2011) Hepatic response to aluminum toxicity: dyslipidemia and liver diseases. *Experimental Cell Research.* (in press)

Mailloux, R.J., Puiseux-Dao, S., & Appanna, V. (2009) α-ketoglutarate abrogates the nuclear localization of HIF-1α in aluminum-exposed hepatocytes. *Biochimie.* Vol. 91: 408-415

Mailloux, R.J., Lemire, J., Kalyuzhnyi, S., & Appanna, V. (2008) A novel metabolic network leads to enhanced citrate biogenesis in *Pseudomonas fluorescens* exposed to aluminum toxicity. *Extremophiles.* Vol. 12: 451-459

Mailloux, R.J. & Appanna, V. (2007a) Aluminum toxicity triggers the nuclear translocation of HIF-1α and promotes anaerobiosis in hepatocytes. *Toxicology in Vitro.* Vol. 21: 16-24

Mailloux, R.J., Lemire, J., & Appanna, V. (2007b) Aluminum-induced mitochondrial dysfunction leads to lipid accumulation in human hepatocytes: a link to obesity. *Cellular Physiology and Biochemistry.* Vol. 20: 627-638

Mailloux, R.J., Hamel, R., & Appanna, V. (2006) Aluminum toxicity elicits a dysfunctional TCA cycle and succinate accumulation in hepatocytes. *Journal of Biochemical and Molecular Toxicology.* Vol. 20(4): 198-208

Mallet, R.T., Sun, J., Knott., E.M., Sharma, A.B., & Olivencia-Yurvati, A.H. (2005) Metabolic cardioprotection by pyruvate: recent progress. *Experimental and Biological Medicine.* Vol. 230(7): 435-443

McClung, J.P., & Karl, J.P. (2009) Iron deficiency and obesity: the contribution of inflammation and diminished iron absorption. *Nutrition Reviews.* Vol. 67(2): 100-104

Middaugh, J., Hamel, R., Hean-Baptiste, G., Beriault, R., Chenier, D., & Appanna, V. (2005) Aluminum triggers decreased aconitase activity via Fe-S cluster disruption and the overexpression of isocitrate dehydrogenase and isocitrate lyase: a metabolic network mediating cellular survival. *The Journal of Biological Chemistry.* Vol. 280(5): 3159-3165

Peyssonnaux, C., Zinkermagel, A., Schuepbach, R., Rankin, E., Vaulont, S., Haase, V., Nizet, V., & Johnson, R. (2007) Regulation of iron homeostasis by the hypoxi-inducible transcription factors (HIFs). *The Journal of Clinical Investigation.* Vol. 117(7): 1926-1932

Rondeau, V., Jacqumin-Gadda, H., Commenges, D., Helmer, C., & Dartigues, J-F. (2008) Aluminum and silica in drinking water and the risk of Alzeihmer's disease or cognitive decline: findings from 15- year follow-up of the PAQUID cohort. *American Journal of Epidemiology.* Vol. 169(4): 489-496

Turgut, S., Bor-Kucukaty, M., Emmungil, G., Atsak, P., & Turgut, G. (2007) The effect of low dose aluminum on hemorheological and hematological parameters in rats. *Archives of Toxicology.* Vol. 81: 11-17

Vecchi, C., Montosi, G., Zhang, K., Lamberti, I., Duncan, S., Kaufman, R., & Pietrangelo, A. (2009) ER stress controls iron metabolism through induction of hepcidin. *Science.* Vol 325: 877-880

Vergara, S.V., & Thiele, D.J. (2008) Post-transcriptional regulation of gene expression in response to iron deficiency: coordinated metabolic reprogramming by yeast mRNA-binding proteins. *Biochemical Society Transactions.* Vol. 36(5): 1088-1090

Ward, R.J., Zhang, Y, & Critchon, R.R. (2001) Aluminum toxicity and iron homeostasis. *Journal of Inorganic Biochemistry.* Vol. 87: 9-14

Yanoff, I.B., Menzie, C.M., Denkinger, B., Sebring., N.G., McHugh, T., Remaley, A.T., & Yanovski, J.A. (2007) Inflammation and iron deficiency in the hypoferremia of obesity. *International Journal of Obesity.* Vol. 31: 1412-1419

Yokel, R.A., & Florence, R.L. (2008a) Aluminum bioavailability from tea infusion. *Food and Chemical Toxicology.* Vol. 46: 3659-3663

Yokel, R.A., Hicks, C.L., & Florence, R.L. (2008b) Aluminum bioavailability from basic sodium aluminum phosphate, an approved food additive emulsifying agent, incorporated in cheese. *Food and Chemical Toxicology*. Vol. 46: 2261-2266

Yokel, R.A., & Florence, R.L. (2006) Aluminum bioavailability from the approved food additive leavening agent acidic sodium aluminum phosphate, incorportated into a baked is lower than from water. *Toxicology*. Vol. 227: 86-93

26

# Hemolysis and Anemia Induced by Dapsone Hydroxylamine

Gabriella Donà[1], Eugenio Ragazzi[2], Giulio Clari[1] and Luciana Bordin[1,*]
[1]*Department of Biological Chemistry, University of Padova,*
[2]*Department of Pharmacology and Anesthesiology, University of Padova*
*Italy*

## 1. Introduction

Dapsone (4,4'-diaminodiphenylsulfone, DDS) has been used for over half a century in the treatment of leprosy, for anti-inflammatory conditions and, in the chlorproguanil-dapsone and artesunate–dapsone–proguanil combinations, for treating malaria. It is also a second-line treatment for AIDS-related Pneumocystis pneumonia (Sangiolo et al., 2005), and is increasingly applied to a variety of immuno-related conditions (Bahadir et al., 2004; Ujiie et al., 2006), despite its well-documented toxicity, which is closely related to its routes of biotransformation.

Dapsone is mono and diacetylated and the monoacetylated derivative and the parent drug can be oxidised by cytochrome P (CYP) family to hydroxylamines, both of which are methaemoglobin formers. However, both dapsone and mono-N-acetyl dapsone are 97% to 100% bound to plasma proteins. Both hydroxylamines are auto-oxidisable to nitroso arenes, which can covalently bind proteins. In erythrocytes, hydroxylamines react with hemoglobin to form methemoglobin and nitrosoarenes and produce reactive oxygen species (ROS). In turn, ROS reacts with glutathione (GSH) and with hemoglobin thiols to generate thiyl radicals (RS· where R is residue from glutathione or hemoglobin cysteine residue). The thiyl free radicals are responsible for glutathione-protein mixed disulfide and skeletal protein-hemoglobin disulfide formation, which causes alterations in cell morphology (McMillan et al., 2005; Bradshaw et al., 1997) (Fig. 1).

Mono- and diacetylated metabolites of dapsone (MADDS and DADDS) are not associated with toxicity (Coleman et al., 1991), although N-hydroxylation of the parent drug and MADDS lead to the formation of the toxic hydroxylamines DDS-NHOH and MADDS-NHOH (Israili et al., 1973; Coleman et al., 1989) (Fig. 1). These species, formed either by CYP2C9 (Winter et al., 2000), one isoform of the cytochrome P450 (CYP) family, or other oxidative enzyme systems, are linked with several immune-mediated hypersensitivity reactions (Vyas et al., 2006). The hydroxylamines are also responsible for the clinical methaemoglobinaemia associated with dapsone therapy (DT) (Israili et al., 1973; Schiff et al., 2006).

DDS-NHOH cannot be directly detected in human plasma as it is rapidly taken up by erythrocytes prior to its redox cycling with haemoglobin, forming methaemoglobin (Coleman & Jacobus, 1993). In any case, the metabolic elimination of dapsone is N-hydroxylation, which accounts for between 30% and 40% of an oral dapsone dose, and the efficiency of N-hydroxylation is related to dapsone clearance (May et al., 1990; May et al., 1992; Bluhm et al., 1999). Dapsone therapy includes a daily administration of 50-100 mg for leprosy and 100-300 mg for dermatitis herpetiformis (Leonard and Fry, 1991), leading to serum concentrations of 0.5-5 mg/L (equivalent to 2-20 microM); therapeutical doses up to 400 mg have been reported in literature (Elonen et al., 1979; Zuidema et al., 1986), as well as some cases of intoxication with DDS, such as after an overdose with 10 g of DDS, leading to serum concentrations of 120 mg/L (about 0.5 mM, comparable to those used in our in vitro experiments). Another case of intoxication produced methaemoglobinemia at serum concentrations of 18.8 mg/L (76 μM) (Woodhouse et al., 1983). The acetylation ratio (MADDS:DDS) shows a genetically determined bimodal distribution, allowing the definition of 'slow' and 'rapid' acetylators (Zuidema et al., 1986).

## 2. DDS-NHOH toxicity

Adverse effects of dapsone therapy are the cause of an idiosyncratic reaction, called dapsone hypersensitivity syndrome (DHS) (Orion et al., 2005; Sener et al., 2006), and, more frequently, dose-related methaemoglobinaemia and haemolytic anemia (Cream, 1970).

DHS includes a number of adverse effects including fever, rash, and internal organ involvement, all related to the bioactivation of DDS into DDS-NHOH (Prussick R & Shear NH, 1996). Bioactivated drug represent the first step in the formation of toxic intermediates, which bind covalently to or modify various molecules through the process defined haptenation, where a small molecule can elicit an immune response by attaching to a large carrier, such as a protein. Once the body has generated antibodies to a hapten-carrier adduct, it will usually initiate an immune response.

It has been recently demonstrated that skin (Roychowdhury et al., 2007) and human keratinocytes are able to convert DDS to hydroxylamine by the action of myeloperoxidase (MPO). Once formed, these highly reactive metabolites can bind to cellular proteins and act as haptens, promoting autoimmunity in susceptible individuals (Vyas et al., 2006).

DDS mediated haemolytic anemia is closely related to erythrocyte membrane alterations leading to premature cell removal, which can occur both extravascularly, by spleen-mediated subtraction of damaged erythrocytes, or intravascularly, by DDS induced cell fragility. All haematological side effects reported for DDS therapy are due to the N-hydroxy metabolites of the drug, dapsone hydroxylamine (DDS-NHOH).

## 3. Erythrocytes and DDS-NHOH toxicity

### 3.1 In vitro alterations of normal erythrocyte membranes

DDS-NHOH undergoes a coupled oxidation-reduction reaction with haemoglobin and molecular oxygen yielding methaemoglobin and ROS formation (ferryl haem and hydroxyl radicals) (Fig. 1), respectively (Bradshaw et al., 1997).

To date, no direct evidence of the mechanism whereby DDS-NHOH shortens the erythrocyte lifespan has ever been reported. Only the fact that DDS-NHOH affects the integrity of the erythrocyte lipid bilayer has been excluded, since neither lipid peroxidation nor phosphatidylserine (PS) externalisation have ever been detected (McMillan et al., 1998; McMillan et al., 2005).

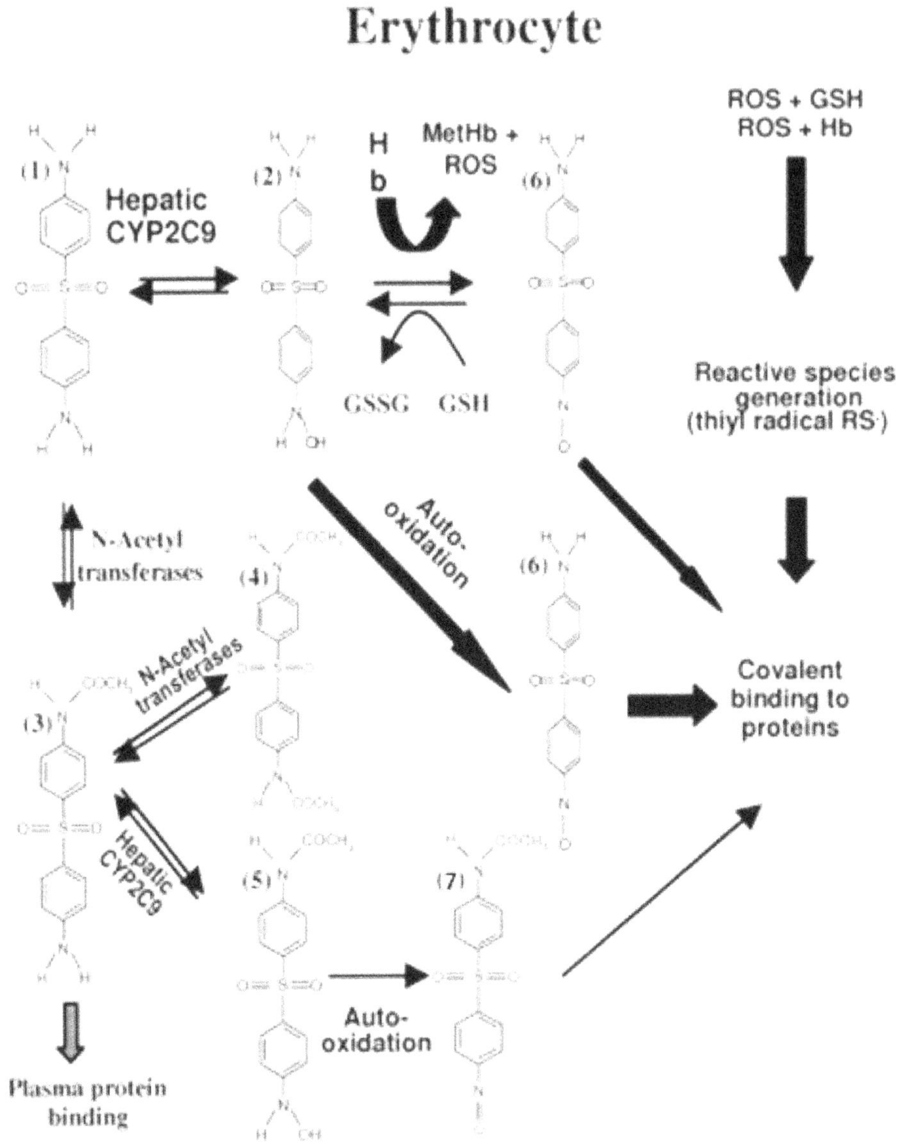


Fig. 1. Scheme showing main features of metabolic fate of dapsone in man. (1) Dapsone; (2) dapsone hydroxylamine; (3) monoacetyl dapsone (MADDS), (4) diacetyl dapsone (DADDS); (5) monoacetyl dapsone hydroxylamine; (6) dapsone nitrosoarene derivatives (7) . monoacetyl dapsone nitrosoarene derivative.

In a recent report (Bordin et al., 2010a) we proposed tyrosine phosphorylation (Tyr-P) level of erythrocyte membrane as diagnostic method to evaluate erythrocyte membrane status.
In human erythrocytes, Tyr-P of membrane proteins is the result of the antithetic actions of protein tyrosine kinases (TPKs) and protein tyrosine phosphatases (PTPs) and involves mainly

band 3 protein. This is the most abundant membrane protein of red blood cells and is divided into three regions: an external domain, enriched in glycosyl chains that probably allow band 3 protein to be recognised as a specific antigens (Bratosin et al., 1998); a transmembrane domain, representing the anionic exchanger of cells; and a cytosol portion (Wang, 1994), containing all phosphorylatable residues. Although serine/threonine (Ser/Thr)-phosphorylation of the band 3 cytosol domain has been demonstrated to regulate the anion flux rate (Baggio et al., 1993a,; Baggio et al., 1993b), Tyr-P is involved in multiple functions, including regulation of glycolysis (Low et al., 1993), alteration of erythrocyte morphology (Bordin et al., 1995) and volume (Musch et al., 1999), and senescence (Bordin et al., 2009; Pantaleo et al., 2009).

When triggered by oxidative (diamide) or hyperosmotic stress, the band 3 Tyr-P level can predict both pathological and particular physiological conditions. In glucose-6-phosphate dehydrogenase (G6PD) deficiency, the higher band 3 Tyr-P level, compared with normal control cells, correlates well with chronic impairment of cell anti-oxidative defences (Bordin et al., 2005b); conversely, the lower band 3 Tyr-P level observed in pregnancy is synonymous of characteristically increased anti-oxidative defences (Bordin et al., 2006).

Methemoglobinemia occurs to some extent in all patients receiving DDS and becomes less pronounced as treatment is continued because of an adaptative increase in the activity of NADH-dependent reductase in erythrocytes (Orion et al., 2005). Methemoglobin (MetHb) production is due to oxidation of hemoglobin by nitroso species which react with NADPH (Kiese et al., 1966) or glutathione (GSH) (Coleman et al., 1994) to regenerate hydroxylamines. Reilly and co-workers (Reilly et al., 1999) showed that GSH, rather than NADPH, is the key reducing specie responsible for regenerating hydroxylamine metabolites and that any GSH consumed must be rapidly regenerated.

We observed that DDS-NHOH, when added to intact erythrocytes in in vitro experiments, triggered the formation of both MetHb and Tyr-P level of band 3 (Bordin et al., 2010b). This last process was time and dose-dependent by DDS-NHOH but only for the early 30 minutes of incubation and to 0.3 mM concentration. Increasing incubation time (50 min) and effector dose (0.6 mM), band 3 Tyr-P decreased to negligible level.

We compared these effects with those induced by diamide (Bordin et al., 2005a), which increased protein phosphorylation level by inhibiting tyrosine phosphatase activities by directly oxidising cysteine located in the catalytic domain of the enzyme (Hecht & Zick, 1992), and by inducing immediate band 3 clustering (Bordin et al., 2006; Fiore et al., 2008).

Our findings showed that both Tyr-kinase and phosphatase activities were promptly inhibited by DDS-NHOH in both dose- and time-dependent manners, and total inactivation was reached in both after 60 min incubation with 0.15 and 0.3 mM. At 0.6 mM, DDS-NHOH treatment was almost completely inhibitory after only 15 minutes of incubation. This suggests that the triggering of band 3 Tyr-P is not due to an imbalance between enzymatic activities but, more probably, by a favoured substrate-kinase interaction, at least up to 0.3 mM within 30 min. Longer incubation times or higher compound concentrations resulted in the total disappearance of band 3 Tyr-P, as well as total enzyme inhibition. This time-dependent increasing effect of DDS-NHOH indicated that there is progression in the action mechanism of the compound.

In addition, it has been previously demonstrated that band 3 structural alterations can be useful to further reveal the status of membranes (Bordin et al., 2006). DDS-NHOH treatment induced band 3 aggregation in high molecular weight aggregates (HMWA) mainly located in the Triton-soluble part of the membrane. This effector differentiated greatly from diamide: its time-dependent effect increased in a sort of amplifying system, leading to further increases in band 3 HMWA, but, more interestingly, also to their total relocation within the membrane, accompanied by reorganization of both PTKs (Brunati et al., 2000) and PTPs (Bordin et al., 2002), independently from band 3 Tyr-P level. This new membrane set up was easily recognized and marked by autologous IgG, representative of damaged cells (Bordin et al., 2010b).

This raises the hypothesis that the gradual band 3 Tyr-P tailing off within the first 45 min may represent the time threshold between the formation of two differently located band 3 aggregates - Triton-soluble, and, successively, cytoskeleton bound. Accordingly, the Tyr-phosphorylative process may be considered a cellular defence against the incoming oxidative modifications induced by DDS-NHOH. In this process, introduction of negative charges, represented by phosphate groups, to band 3 protein would slow down its aggregation, at least up to the total arrest of the phosphorylative process. Subsequently, modifications would continue more profoundly, inducing not only more marked clustering of band 3 but also totally redistributing HMWA from soluble to insoluble (cytoskeleton) membrane fractions. This is further suggested by total rearrangement of band 3 HMWA at 0.6 mM DDS-NHOH: in these conditions, band 3 Tyr-P is very slight, and band 3 HMWA were located in the cytoskeleton even after 30 min incubation (Bordin et al., 2010b).

This may fit the hypothesis that reactive radicals also generate a second species of radicals, probably a thiyl radical (McMillan et al., 2005), more reactive and efficacious in generating so many and drastic alterations in membrane structure and composition.

Taken together, the direct evidence of the mechanism whereby DDS-NHOH shortens the erythrocyte lifespan is consistent with progressive oxidative alteration starting from cytosol, where it induces methaemoglobin formation (Israili et al., 1973; Schiff et al., 2006), glutathione oxidation, and initial impairment of Tyr-protein kinase and phosphatase activities. Later, the effect of DDS-NHOH advances, with progressive reorganisation of membrane/proteins, as evidenced by enzyme recruitment and the formation of band 3 aggregates (HMWA) (Bordin et al., 2010b). Lastly, general membrane reorganisation is achieved, with protein relocation from the Triton-soluble compartment to the cytoskeleton and with autologous antibody recognition (Bordin et al., 2010b). The fact that DDS-NHOH affects the integrity of the erythrocyte lipid bilayer has been excluded, since neither lipid peroxidation nor phosphatidylserine externalisation have ever been detected (McMillan et al., 1998; McMillan et al., 2005).

### 3.2 Erythrocyte membrane alterations in Glucose-6-Phosphate Dehydrogenase (G6PD) deficient patients in dapsone therapy

In order to verify whether the above mechanism of DDS-NHOH-induced membrane reorganisation was the mechanism effectively leading to erythrocyte denaturation/removal in vivo, we analysed membranes from two patients in dapsone treatment (DT) for dermatitis herpetiformis (Bordin et al., 2010b). The two patients were diagnosed as suffering from dermatitis herpetiformis (DH) according to skin biopsies and cell surface deposition of IgA, and were given oral dapsone. At admission, both had normal blood and urine samples. Their treatment started with 100 mg/day DT, as usual dose (Leonard & Fry 1991).

Patient 1 remained successfully in treatment for the length of the study; blood was withdrawn before and during dapsone administration (after 14 days' treatment).

Patient 2, was hospitalised for a haemolytic episode following 3 days of 100 mg/day DT ($P2_{100}$). His laboratory tests revealed that he had Glucose-6-Phosphate Dehydrogenase (G6PD) deficiency, class II, according to the WHO directive (Betke et al., 1967). G6PD residual activity in red cells was < 10%, measured spectrophotometrically at 340 nm on a

Sigma diagnostic kit (Sigma-Aldrich, Italy). Dapsone was discontinued for a month, after which laboratory test results had returned to normal range. Dapsone treatment (DT) was later re-administered, starting with two days with 30 mg/day, and then 50 mg/day, with partial relief but not total remission of symptoms.

Blood samples from both patients were taken before and during treatments. Samples from patient 1 were called P1 and $P1_{100}$ to indicate samples before administration and during 100 mg/day DT; erythrocytes from patient 2 were called P2, $P2_{30}$, and $P2_{50}$ to indicate samples withdrawn before and after 2 days at 30 mg/day, or after 3 days at 50 mg/day DT, respectively. Erythrocytes were analysed for their band 3 HMWA and IgG bound contents. DT in patient 1 (P1) induced a slight increase in band 3 HMWA, which was correlated with an increase in bound IgG (Fig. 2, panel A). Erythrocyte membranes from patient 2 showed a higher level of basal band 3 HMWA (P2), which increased (+18%) during the 30 mg/day DT, but reached a dramatic level at 50 mg/day (+215%). The effect was correlated with a 30% increase in bound IgG in $P2_{30}$ and with more than 120% in $P2_{50}$.

$P1_{100}$ was chosen as arbitrary unit to indicate erythrocyte membrane alterations (band 3 HMWA and IgG binding) induced by DT (A) or band 3 Tyr-P induced by diamide (B) in normal patients.

In addition, when analysed for Tyr-P level extent, membranes from erythrocytes of both patients showed that the basal level of band 3 Tyr-P was negligible. Successive analysis of glutathione content evidenced that DT induced a decrease in total GSH content in both patients (Bordin et al., 2010b). However, $P1_{100}$ maintained about 85% of total glutathione in reduced form (GSH), but P2 showed progressive depletion of glutathione, with an alarming rise in oxidised glutathione (GS-SG) which, at $P2_{50}$, reached almost 60% of total glutathione. To induce weak oxidative stress, addition of 0.3 mM diamide to isolated erythrocytes from both patients was performed. $P1_{100}$ showed a reduction in total glutathione content and a rise of GS-SG. P2 and $P2_{30}$ highlighted a net reduction in the amount of total glutathione which, at $P2_{50}$, was only 50%, compared with the glutathione content of P2. Diamide induced net increase in the GS-SG form, which reached almost 100% glutathione at $P2_{50}$.

When analysed also for their Tyr-P content after 0.3 mM diamide treatment (inconsistent with Tyr-P triggering in normal subjects), patients presented clear differences (Bordin et al., 2006) (Fig. 2, panel B). The first patient showed a slight trace of band 3 Tyr-P only after DT ($P1_{100}$). Instead, P2 evidenced net band 3 Tyr-P (as expected, due to his G6PDdeficiency), which dramatically escalated on increasing DT (Fig. 2 panel B). Syk and SHP-2 content in membranes from P2 also rose after DT, in both the absence and presence of diamide incubation (Bordin et al., 2010b).

This is in line with what evidenced in vitro from normal erythrocytes: in normal subjects, therapy leads to weakening of anti-oxidant defences (as indicated by decreased GSH content) and triggers membrane reorganisation, as indicated by increased band 3 HMWA formation (Fig. 2, panel A) and higher sensitivity towards diamide-induced oxidative stress. When dapsone was administered to G6PDd patient (P2), drops in both haemoglobin content and haematocrit were observed at $P2_{50}$, suggesting the onset of the haemolytic process. This cannot be explained by the simple fall in GSH content since, even at 50 mg/day dapsone ($P2_{50}$), almost one-third of total glutathione is in reduced form, but incapable of preventing DT-induced erythrocyte modification. In other words, glutathione is not sufficient to counteract membrane oxidisation induced by dapsone, because its metabolite, DDS-NHOH, acts on different substrates in a time-dependent progressive ROS formation. That hydroxylamine is the responsible of the alterations is confirmed by the fact that DT induces the same membrane alterations than those previously shown in *in vitro* experiments with DDS-NHOH, such as band 3 HMWA formation and IgG binding increase. Instead, band 3 Tyr-P was not detected, even in $P2_{50}$ erythrocytes, although Tyr-protein kinases and/or phosphatases were not inhibited in these conditions, as indicated by the following diamide-induced band 3 Tyr-P of patients' erythrocytes (especially in P2). This was probably because the concentration of this effector is insufficient to have immediate effects on the enzymes, like those evidenced in in vitro experiments, which would be representative of high toxicity. Band 3 Tyr-P level, therefore, is to be dependent on the net alteration of erythrocyte membrane following DT.

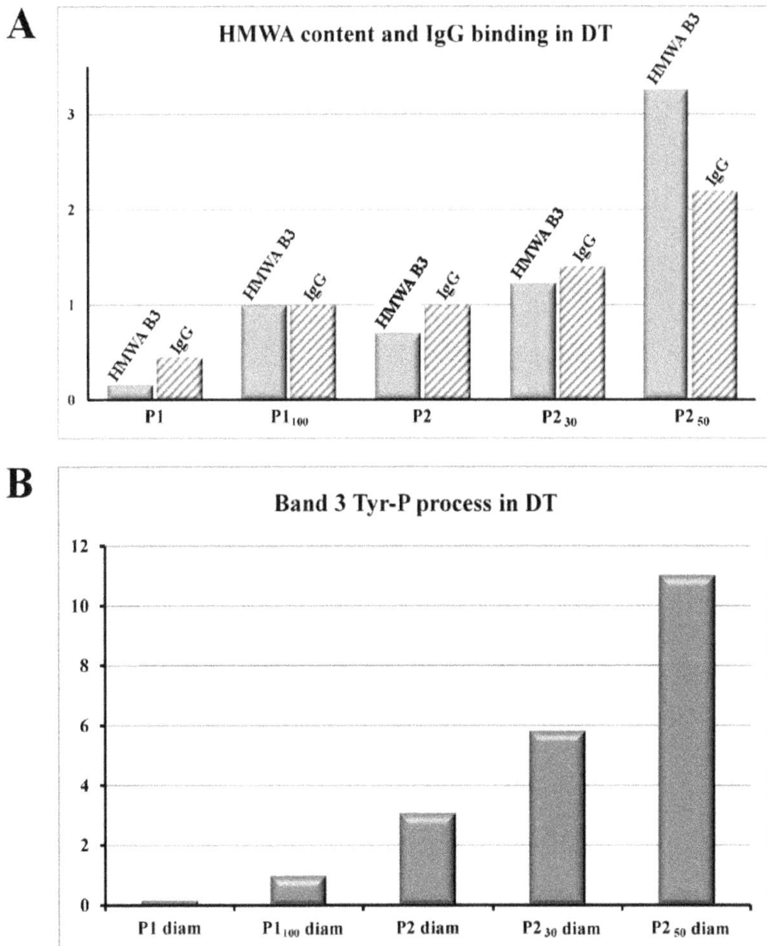


Fig. 2. Effect of dapsone treatment (DT) on erythrocyte membrane rearrangement. Erythrocytes from patients 1 and 2 before (P1 and P2) and after DT ($P1_{100}$ and $P2_{30}$ and $P2_{50}$) were directly analysed for high molecular weight aggregate (HMWA) of band 3 and IgG binding (panel A), or incubated with 0.3 mM diamide to trigger band 3 Tyr-P level (panel B).

### 3.3 DDS-NHOH-induced alterations in erythrocyte from endometriotic patients: Potential toxicity in inflammatory disease

In the above paragraph, it has been reported that band 3 Tyr-P levels were negligible in erythrocytes from patients during DT, and diamide addition was useful to investigate membrane status, mainly cell capacity of counteracting additional oxidative stress.

To evidence the direct effect of pre-existing inflammatory status on DDS-NHOH treatment, we compared band 3 Tyr-P levels induced by increasing concentrations of DDS-NHOH on erythrocytes from endometriotic patients with that obtained in normal erythrocytes (Figures 3 and 4).

Figure 3 shows band 3 Tyr-P obtained with 0.15, 0.3 and 0.6 mM DDS-NHOH in erythrocytes from endometriotic patients (panel A, lanes b-d), which result much higher than that obtained in the control (lane a) with 0.3 mM (concentration able to induce maximum Tyr-P level in normal erythrocytes (Bordin et al., 2010b).

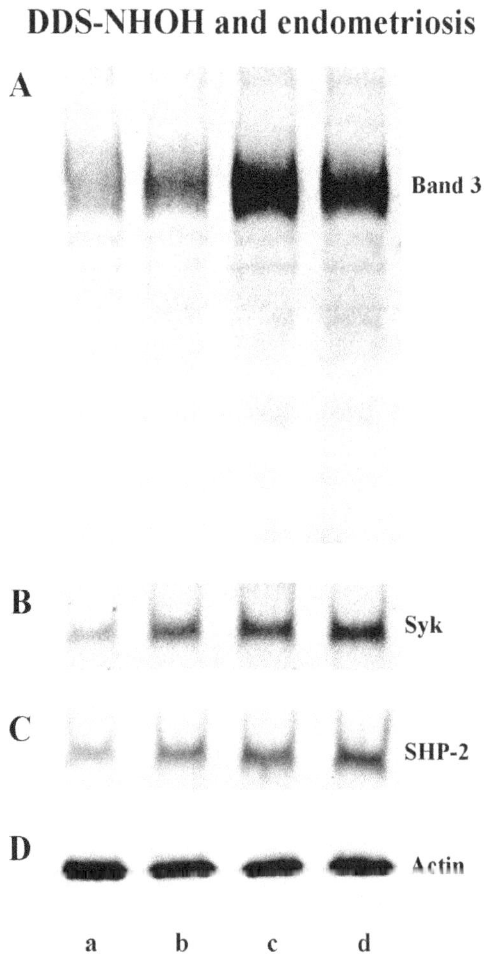


Fig. 3. DDS-NHOH effect on band 3 Tyr-P level (panel A), Syk (panel B) and SHP-2 (panel C) recruitments.

This higher sensitivity of endometriotic erythrocytes towards hydroxylamine was further confirmed by the increased amounts of enzymes, Syk PTK (panel B) and SHP-2 PTP (panel C) bound to membranes following DDS-NHOH treatment. In addition, band 3 HMWA, synonymous of a predisposition of the cell to be recognized by IgG and removed from circulation (Bordin et al., 2010b, Arese et al., 2005; Ciccoli et al., 2004; Kay, 2005; Lutz et al., 1987), were markedly higher in endometriotic cells (Fig. 4) following DDS-NHOH treatment (lanes b-d, compared with lane a, control erythrocytes incubated with 0.3 mM DDS-NHOH).

In order to verify if the patterns of figures 3 and 4 obtained in vitro would mirror potential toxicity for endometriotic patients in DT, we compared them with those obtained by incubating erythrocytes from G6PDd patients in the same above conditions (Fig. 5). Diamide-induced band 3 Tyr-P level and Syk and SHP-2 recruitments were very similar between G6PDd and endometriotic patients, the former reaching the highest values for all parameters, especially when compared with healthy controls.

The high similarity present in in vitro DDS-NHOH treatment between G6PDd and endometriosis erythrocytes strengthens the idea that inflammation status-related alteration would predispose cell to be highly sensitive to the presence of arylamine derivatives, which would lead to potential toxicity to DT.

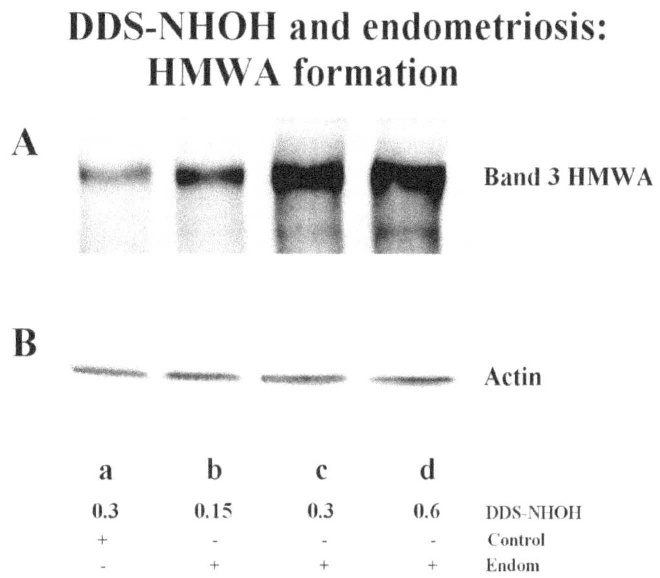


Fig. 4. Effect of increasing DDS-NHOH on band 3 HMWA formation in normal (lane a) and endometriotic patients (lanes b-d).

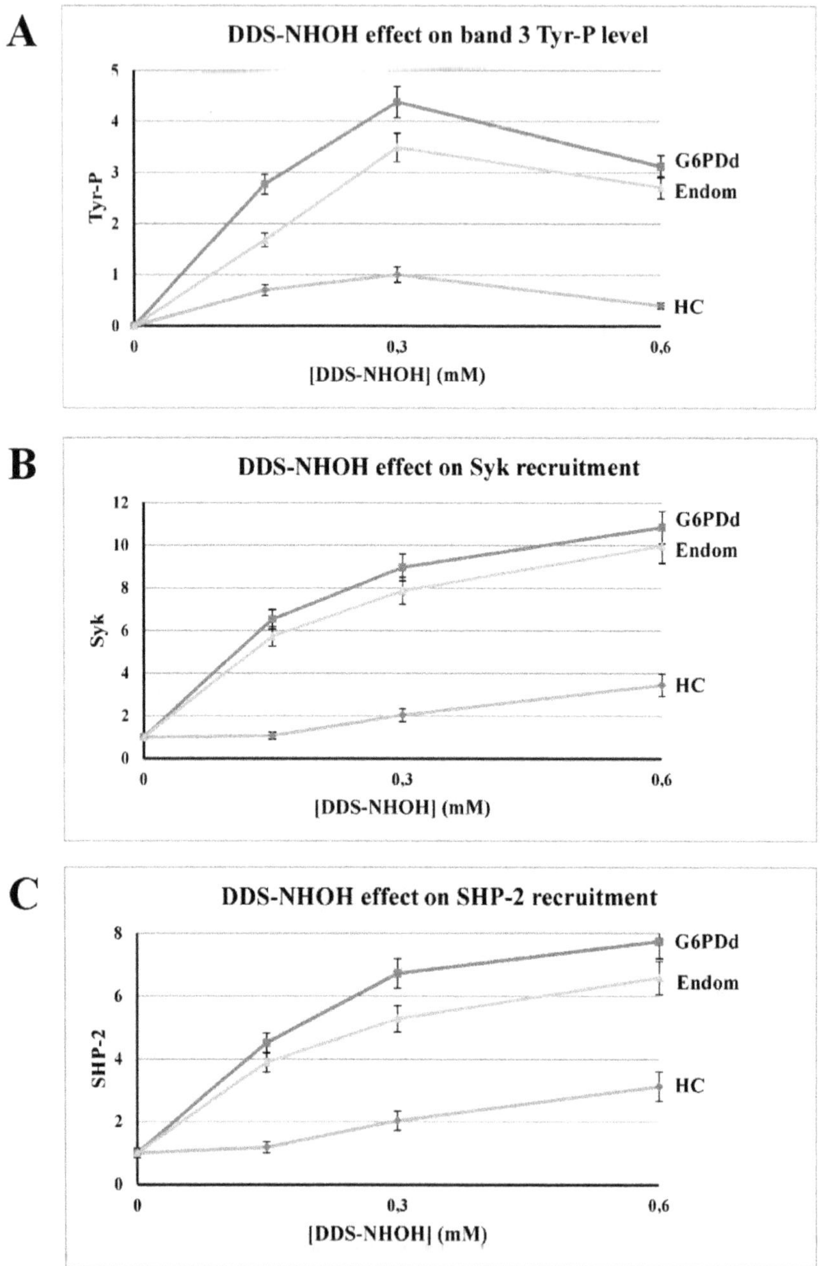


Fig. 5. DDS-NHOH effect on erythrocytes: membrane band 3 Tyr-P level (Panel A), Syk (Panel B) and SHP-2 (Panel C) recruitments, in in vitro experiments: comparison among Healthy Controls (HC), G6PDd and Endometriotic (Endom) patients.

## 4. Conclusions

G6PD in the hexose (HMP) shunt regulates the production of NADPH, an obligatory substrate for several redox systems, in particular for glutathione, which protects the cell from oxidative stress. It has been previously shown that conditions of oxidative stress lowering NADPH content immediately raise the HMP shunt rate up to 30-fold. Red blood cells with G6PD deficiency cannot increase their shunt sufficiently during an oxidative load, and thus show a weakened cellular redox defence (Jacobasch & Rapoport 1996). In several antimalarial, antipyretics or analgesic drugs' treatments, G6PD deficient patients can not provide an adequate antioxidant defence and their erythrocytes present degenerative parameters, revealing the formation of anomalies in cell morphology and deformability (Jacobasch & Rapoport 1996). Oxidative stress induces haemoglobin (Hb) denaturation and membrane binding of hemichromes, Heinz body precursors, and provokes aggregation of band 3 and deposition of antibodies and complement C3c fragments. In fact, it has been described that membrane clustering of band 3 can allow immune recognition by naturally occurring antibodies, inducing antibody-dependent phagocytosis of senescent/alterate erythrocytes (Arese et al., 2005; Kay, 1984; Low et al. 1985; Schluter & Drenekhanh 1986; Lutz et al. 1988; Arese & De Flora 1990; Hebbel, 1990). Also, band 3 Tyr-P level induced by pathological conditions, could make structural alterations, which probably lead cell into apoptosis, by exposing new band 3 epitopes and favouring cell removal from circulation. Both can induce membrane alterations as well as binding of multivalent ligands, leading to hemolysis (Bottini et al., 1997).

All these facts, together with the G6PDd cell inability to response powerfully to oxidants, indicates that the physiological status of band 3 is essential for erythrocytes survival/apoptosis.

In G6PDd anti-oxidative defences are much lower than those present in endometriosis, which has been demonstrated to correlate with chronic oxidative assault induced by inflammation, rather than impairment in glutathione (GSH) restoring. In addition, pre-existing membrane alterations have been postulated even for endometriotic erythrocytes, as indicated by their higher sensitivity to diamide (Bordin et al., 2010a). In fact, diamide-triggered band 3 Tyr-P level was two or three times higher than those of controls, owed to an altered redox system, predisposing membrane proteins to be more markedly oxidized. This was confirmed by the observation that total cell glutathione does not differ from that of healthy controls (data not shown) but, once the erythrocytes are incubated with diamide, patients' GSH contents are far lower, probably due to membrane oxidative status alterations which retained glutathione under the form of protein glutathionylation (Bordin et al., 2010a).

Our study confirms previous reports, stressing that sensitiveness to the compound is clearly idiosyncratic and dependent on the patho/physiological patients' status (May et al., 1990; May et al., 1992; Wertheim et al., 2006).

From these considerations, the assessment of the pre-existent oxidative status of erythrocytes should be carefully evaluated prior to the choice of the appropriate therapy.

## 5. References

Arese, P. & De Flora, A. (1990). Pathophysiology of hemolysis in glucose-6-phosphate dehydrogenase deficiency. *Seminars in Hematolology*, Vol.27, No.1, pp. 1-40.

Arese, P.; Turrini, F. & Schwarzer, E. (2005). Band 3/complement-mediated recognition and removal of normally senescent and pathological human erythrocytes. *Cellular Physiology and Biochemistry*, Vol.16, No.4-6, pp. 133-146.

Baggio, B., Bordin, L.; Clari, G.; Gambero, G. & Moret, V. (1993a). Functional correlation between the Ser/Thr-phosphorylation of band 3 and band 3-mediated transmembrane anion transport in human erythrocytes. *Biochimica and Biophysica Acta*, Vol.1148, No.1, pp. 157-160.

Baggio, B.; Bordin, L.; Gambaro, G.; Piccoli, A.; Marzaro, G. & Clari, G. (1993b). Evidence of a link between band 3 phosphorylation and anion transport in patients with "idiopathic" calcium oxalate nephrolithiasis. *Mineral and Electrolyte Metabolism*, Vol.19, No.1, pp. 17-20.

Bahadir, S.; Cobanoglu, U.; Cimsit, G.; Yayli, S. & Alpay, K. (2004). Erythema dyschromicum perstans: response to dapsone therapy. *International Journal of Dermatolology*, Vol.43, No.3, pp. 220-222.

Betke, K.; Beutler, E.; Brewer, G.J.; Kirkman. H.N.; Luzzato, L.; Motulsky, A.G.; Ramot, B. & Siniscalco, M. (1967). Standardization of procedures for the study of glucose-6-phosphate dehydrogenase. *Report of a WHO scientific group-WHO*, Technical Report-Serial 366.

Bluhm, R.E.; Adedoyin, A.; McCarver, D.G. & Branch R.A. (1999). Development of dapsone toxicity in patients with inflammatory dermatoses: activity of acetylation and hydroxylation of dapsone as risk factors. *Clinical Pharmacology & Therapeutics*, Vol.65, No.6, pp. 598-605.

Bordin, L.; Brunati, A.M.; Donella-Deana, A.; Baggio, B.; Toninello, A. & Clari, G. (2002). Band 3 is a anchor protein and a target for SHP-2 tyrosine phosphatases in human erythrocytes. *Blood*, Vol.100, No.1, pp. 276-282.

Bordin, L.; Clari, G.; Moro, I.; Dalla Vecchia, F. & Moret, V. (1995). Functional link between phosphorylation state of membrane proteins and morphological changes of human erythrocytes. *Biochemical and Biophysical Research Communications*, Vol.213, No.1, pp. 249-257.

Bordin, L.; Fiore, C.; Bragadin, M.; Brunati, A.M. & Clari, G. (2009). Regulation of membrane band 3 Tyr-phosphorylation by proteolysis of p72(Syk) and possible involvement in senescence process. *Acta Biochimica et Biophysica Sinica*, Vol.41, No.10, pp. 846-851.

Bordin, L.; Fiore, C.; Donà, G.; Andrisani, A.; Ambrosini, G.; Faggian, D.; Plebani, M.; Clari, G. & Armanini, D. (2010a). Evaluation of erythrocyte band 3 phosphotyrosine level, glutathione content, CA-125, and human epididymal secretory protein E4 as combined parameters in endometriosis. *Fertility and Sterility*, Vol.94, No.5, pp. 1616-1621.

Bordin, L.; Fiore, C.; Zen, F.; Coleman, M.D.; Ragazzi, E. & Clari, G. (2010b) Dapsone hydroxylamine induces premature removal of human erythrocytes by membrane reorganization and antibody binding. *British Journal of Pharmacology*, Vol.161, No.5, pp. 1186-1199.

Bordin, L.; Ion-Popa, F.; Brunati, A.M.; Clari, G. & Low, P.S. (2005a). Effector-induced Syk-mediated phosphorylation in human erythrocytes. *Biochimica et Biophysica Acta*, Vol.1745, No.1, pp. 20-28.

Bordin, L.; Quartesan, S.; Zen, F.; Vianello, F. & Clari, G. (2006). Band 3 Tyr-phosphorylation in human erythrocytes from non-pregnant and pregnant women. *Biochimica et Biophysica Acta,* Vol.1758, No.5, pp. 611-619.

Bordin, L.; Zen, F.; Ion-Popa, F.; Barbetta, M.; Baggio, B. & Clari, G. (2005b). Band 3 Tyr-phosphorylation in normal and glucose-6-phospate dehydrogenase-deficient human erythrocytes. *Molecular Membrane Biology,* Vol.22, No.5, pp. 411-420.

Bottini, E.; Bottini, F.G.; Borgiani, P. & Businco, L. (1997). Association between ACP1 and favism: a possible biochemical mechanism. *Blood,* Vol.89, No.7, pp. 2613-2615.

Bradshaw, T.P.; McMillan, D.C.; Crouch, R.K, & Jollow, D.J. (1997). Formation of free radicals and protein mixed disulfides in rat red cells exposed to dapsone hydroxylamine. *Free Radical Biology and Medicine,* Vol.22, No.7, pp. 1183-1193.

Bratosin, D.; Mazurier, J.; Tissier, J.P.; Estaquier, J.; Huart, J.J.; Ameisen J.C.; Aminoff, D. & Montreuil, J. (1998). Cellular and molecular mechanisms of senescent erythrocyte phagocytosis by macrophages. A review. *Biochimie,* Vol.80, No.2, pp. 173-195.

Brunati, A.M.; Bordin, L.; Clari, G.; James, P.; Quadroni, M.; Baritono, E.; Pinna, L.A. & Donella-Deana, A. (2000). Sequential phosphorylation of protein band 3 by Syk and Lyn tyrosine kinases in intact human erythrocytes: identification of primary and secondary phosphorylation sites. *Blood,* Vol.96, No.4, pp. 1550-1557.

Ciccoli, L.; Rossi, V.; Leoncini, S.; Signorini, C.; Blanco-Garcia, J.; Aldinucci, C.; Buonocore, G. & Comporti, M. (2004). Iron release, superoxide production and binding of autologous IgG to band 3 dimers in newborn and adult erythrocytes exposed to hypoxia and hypoxia-reoxygenation. *Biochimica et Biophysica Acta,* Vol.1672, No.3, pp. 203-213.

Coleman, M.D.; Breckenridge, A.M. & Park, B.K. (1989). Bioactivation of dapsone to a cytotoxic metabolite by human hepatic microsomal enzymes. *British Journal of Clinical Pharmacology,* Vol.28, No.4, pp. 389-395.

Coleman, M.D. & Jacobus, D.P. (1993). Reduction of dapsone hydroxylamine to dapsone during methaemoglobin formation in human erythrocytes in vitro. *Biochemical Pharmacology,* Vol.45, No.5, pp. 1027-1033.

Coleman, M.D.; Simpson, J. & Jacobus, D.P. (1994). Reduction of dapsone hydroxylamine to dapsone during methaemoglobin formation in human erythrocytes in vitro. IV: Implications for the development of agranulocytosis. *Biochemical Pharmacology,* Vol.48, No.7, pp. 1349-1354.

Coleman, M.D.; Tingle, M.D.; Hussain, F.; Storr, R.C. & Park, B.K. (1991). An investigation into the haematological toxicity of structural analogues of dapsone in vivo and in vitro. *The Journal of Pharmacy and Pharmacology,* Vol.43, No.11, pp. 779-784.

Cream, J.J. & Scott, G.L. (1970). Anaemia in dermatitis herpetiformis. The role of dapsone-induced haemolysis and malabsorption. *The British Journal of Dermatology,* Vol.82, No.4, pp. 333-338.

Elonen, E.; Neuvonen, P.J.; Halmekoski, J. & Mattila, M.J. (1979). Acute dapsone intoxication: a case with prolonged symptoms. *Clinical Toxicology,* Vol.14, No.1, pp. 79-85.

Fiore, C.; Bordin, L.; Pellati, D.; Armanini, D. & Clari, G. (2008). Effect of glycyrrhetinic acid on membrane band 3 in human erythrocytes. *Archives of Biochemistry and Biophysics,* Vol.479, No.1, pp. 46-51.

Hebbel, R.P. (1990). The sickle erythrocyte in double jeopardy: autoxidation and iron decompartmentalization. *Seminars in Hematology,* Vol.27, No.1, pp. 51-69.

Hecht, D. & Zick, Y. (1992). Selective inhibition of protein tyrosine phosphatase activities by H2O2 and vanadate in vitro. *Biochemistry and Biophysic Research Communication,* Vol.188, No.2, pp. 773-779.

Israili, Z.H.; Cucinell, S.A.; Vaught, J.; Davis, E.; Lesser, J.M. & Dayton, P.G. (1973). Studies of the metabolism of dapsone in man and experimental animals: formation of N-hydroxy metabolites. *The Journal of Pharmacology and Experimental Therapeutics,* Vol.187, No.1, pp. 138-151.

Jacobasch, G. & Rapoport, S.M. (1996). Hemolytic anemias due to erythrocyte enzyme deficiencies. *Molecular Aspects of Medicine,* Vol.17, No.2, pp. 143-170.

Kay, M.M. (1984). Localization of senescent cell antigen on band 3. *Proceedings of the National Academy of Sciences of the United States of America,* Vol.81, No.18, pp. 5753-5757.

Kay, M. (2005). Immunoregulation of cellular life span. *Annals of the New York Academy of Sciences,* Vol.1057, pp. 85-111.

Kiese, M., Rauscher, E. & Weger, N. (1966). The role of N,N-dimethylaniline-N-oxide in the formation of hemiglobin following the absorption of N,N-dimethylaniline. *Naunyn -chmiedebergs Archive fur Pharmakologie und Experimentelle Pathologie,* Vol.254, No.3, pp. 253-260.

Leonard, J.N. & Fry, L. (1991). Treatment and management of dermatitis herpetiformis. *Clinics in Dermatology,* Vol. 9, No.3, pp. 403-408.

Low, P.S.; Rathinavelu, P. & Harrison, M.L. (1993). Regulation of glycolysis via reversible enzyme binding to the membrane protein band 3. *The Journal of Biological Chemistry,* Vol.268, No.20, pp. 14627-14631.

Low, P.S.; Waugh, S.M.; Zinke, K. & Drenckhahn, D. (1985). The role of hemoglobin denaturation and band 3 clustering in red blood cell aging. *Science,* Vol.227, No.4686, pp. 531-533.

Lutz, H.U.; Bussolino, F.; Flepp, R.; Fasler, S.; Stammler, P.; Kazatchkine, M.D. & Arese, P. (1987). Naturally occurring anti-band-3 antibodies and complement together mediate phagocytosis of oxidatively stressed human erythrocytes. *Proceedings of the National Academy of Sciences of the United States of America,* Vol. 84, No. 21, pp. 7368-7376.

Lutz, H.U.; Fasler, S.; Stammler, P.; Bussolino, F. & Arese, P. (1988). Naturally occurring anti-band 3 antibodies and complement in phagocytosis of oxidatively-stressed and in clearance of senescent red cells. *Blood Cells,* Vol. 14, No.1, pp. 175-195.

May, D.G.; Arns, P.A.; Richards, W.O.; Porter, J.; Ryder, D.; Fleming, C.M.; Wilkinson, G.R. & Branch, R.A. (1992). The disposition of dapsone in cirrhosis. *Clinical Pharmacology and Therapeutics,* Vol.51, No.6, pp. 689-700.

May, D.G.; Porter, J.A.; Uetrecht, J.P.; Wilkinson, G.R. & Branch, R.A. (1990). The contribution of N-hydroxylation and acetylation to dapsone pharmacokinetics in normal subjects. *Clinical Pharmacology and Therapeutics,* Vol. 48, No. 6, pp. 619-627.

McMillan, D.C.; Jensen, C.R. & Jollow, D.J. (1998). Role of lipid peroxidation in dapsone-induced hemolytic anemia. *The Journal of Pharmacology and Experimental Pharmaceutics,* Vol.287, No.3, pp. 868-876.

McMillan, D.C.; Powell, C.L.; Bowman, Z.S.; Morrow, J.D. & Jollow, D.J. (2005). Lipid versus proteins as major targets of pro-oxidant, direct-acting hemolytic agents. *Toxicological Sciences*, Vol. 88, No.1, pp. 274-283.

Musch, M.W.; Hubert, E.M. & Goldstein, L. (1999). Volume expansion stimulates p72(syk) and p56(lyn) in skate erythrocytes. *The Journal of Biological Chemistry*, Vol.274, No.2, pp. 7923-7928.

Orion, E.; Matz, H. & Wolf, R. (2005). The life-threatening complications of dermatologic therapies. *Clinics in Dermatology*, Vol.23, No.2, pp. 182-192.

Pantaleo, A.; Ferru E.; Giribaldi, G.; Mannu, F.; Carta, F.; Matte, A.; De Franceschi, L. & Turrini, F. (2009). Oxidized and poorly glycosylated band 3 is selectively phosphorylated by Syk kinase to form large membrane clusters in normal and G6PD-deficient red blood cells. *The Biochemical Journal*, Vol.418, No.2, pp. 359-367.

Prussick, R. & Shear, N.H. (1996) Dapsone hypersensitivity syndrome. *Journal of the American Academy of Dermatology*, Vol.35, No.2, pp. 346-349.

Reilly, T.P.; Woster, P.M. & Svensson, C.K. (1999). Methemoglobin formation by hydroxylamine metabolites of sulfamethoxazole and dapsone: implications for differences in adverse drug reactions. *The Journal of Pharmacology and Experimental Therapeutics*, Vol.288, No.3, pp. 951-959.

Roychowdhury, S.; Cram, A.E.; Aly, A. & Svensson, C.K. (2007). Detection of haptenated proteins in organotypic human skin explant cultures exposed to dapsone. *Drug Metabolism and Disposition,* Vol.35, No.9, pp. 1463-1465.

Sangiolo, D.; Storer, B.; Nash, R.; Corey, L.; Davis, C.; Flowers, M.; Hackman, R.C. & Boeckh, M. (2005). Toxicity and efficacy of daily dapsone as Pneumocystis jiroveci prophylaxis after hematopoietic stem cell transplantation: a case-control study. *Biology and Blood Marrow Transplantation*, Vol.11, No.7, pp. 521-529.

Schiff, D.E.; Roberts, W.D. & Sue YJ (2006). Methaemoglobinemia associated with dapsone therapy in a child with pneumonia and chronic immune thrombocytopenic purpura. *Journal of Pediatric Hematology/ Oncology*, Vol.28, No.6, pp. 395-398.

Schluter, K. & Drenekhanh, D. (1986). Co-clustering of denaturated hemoglobin with band 3: its role in binding of autoantibodies against band 3 to abnormal and aged erythrocytes, *Proceedings of the National Academy of Sciences of the United States of America*, Vol.83, No.16, pp. 6137-6141.

Sener, O.; Doganci, L.; Safali, M.; Besirbellioglu, B.; Bulucu, F. & Pahsa, A. (2006) Severe dapsone hypersensitivity syndrome. *Journal of Investigational Allergology and Clinical Immunology*, Vol.16, No.4, pp. 268-270.

Ujiie, H.; Shimizu, T.; Ito, M.; Arita, K. & Shimizu H (2006). Lupus erythematosus profundus successfully treated with dapsone: review of the literature. *Archives of Dermatology*, Vol.142, No.3, pp. 399-401.

Vyas, P.M.; Roychowdhury, S.; Koukouritaki, S.B.; Hines, R.N.; Krueger, S.K.; Williams, D.E.; Nauseef, W.M. & Svensson, C.K. (2006). Enzyme-mediated protein haptenation of dapsone and sulfamethoxazole in human keratinocytes: II. Expression and role of flavin-containing monooxygenases and peroxydases. *The Journal of Pharmacology and Experimental Therapeutics*, Vol.319, No.1, pp. 497-505.

Wang, D.N. (1994). Band 3 protein: structure, flexibility and function. *FEBS Letters*, Vol.346, No.1, pp. 26-31.

Wertheim, M.S.; Males, J.J.; Cook, S.D. & Tole, M.D. (2006). Dapsone induced haemolytic anaemia in patients treated for ocular cicatricial pemphigoid. *The British Journal of Ophthalmology*, Vol. 90, No.4, pp. 516.

Winter, H.R.; Wang, Y. & Unadkat, J.D. (2000). CYP2C8/9 mediate dapsone N-hydroxylation at clinical concentrations of dapsone. *Drug Metabolicm and Disposition*, Vol.28, No.8, pp. 865-868.

Woodhouse, K.W.; Henderson, D.B.; Charlton, B.; Peaston, R.T. & Rawlins, M.D. (1983). Acute dapsone poisoning: clinical features and pharmacokinetic studies. *Human Toxicology*, Vol.2, No.3, pp. 507-510.

Zuidema, J.; Hilbers-Modderman, E.S. & Merkus, F.W. (1986). Clinical pharmacokinetics of dapsone. *Clinical Pharmacokinetics*, Vol.11, No.4, pp. 299-315.